P9-DTX-355

Psychotropic Drug Information Handbook

3rd Edition

Psychotropic Drug Information Handbook

3rd Edition

Matthew A. Fuller, PharmD, BCPS, BCPP, FASHP
Clinical Pharmacy Specialist, Psychiatry
Cleveland Department of Veterans Affairs Medical Center
Brecksville, Ohio
Associate Clinical Professor of Psychiatry
Clinical Instructor of Psychology
Case Western Reserve University
Cleveland, Ohio
Adjunct Associate Professor of Clinical Pharmacy
University of Toledo
Toledo, Ohio

Martha Sajatovic, MD
Associate Professor of Psychiatry
Case Western Reserve University
Cleveland, Ohio

LEXI-COMP, INC
Hudson (Cleveland), OH

AMERICAN
PHARMACEUTICAL
ASSOCIATION APhA

NOTICE

This handbook is intended to serve the user as a handy quick reference and not as a complete drug information resource. It does not include information on every therapeutic agent available. The publication covers commonly used drugs and is specifically designed to present certain important aspects of drug data in a more concise format than is generally found in medical literature or product material supplied by manufacturers.

The nature of drug information is that it is constantly evolving because of ongoing research and clinical experience and is often subject to interpretation. While great care has been taken to ensure the accuracy of the information presented, the reader is advised that the authors, editors, reviewers, contributors, and publishers cannot be responsible for the continued currency of the information or for any errors, omissions, or the application of this information, or for any consequences arising therefrom. Therefore, the author(s) and/or the publisher shall have no liability to any person or entity with regard to claims, loss, or damage caused, or alleged to be caused, directly or indirectly, by the use of information contained herein. Because of the dynamic nature of drug information, readers are advised that decisions regarding drug therapy must be based on the independent judgment of the clinician, changing information about a drug (eg, as reflected in the literature and manufacturer's most current product (information), and changing medical practices. The editors are not responsible for any inaccuracy of quotation or for any false or misleading implication that may arise due to the text or formulas as used or due to the quotation of revisions no longer official.

The editors, authors, and contributors have written this book in their private capacities. No official support or endorsement by any federal agency or pharmaceutical company is intended or inferred.

The publishers have made every effort to trace the copyright holders for borrowed material. If they have inadvertently overlooked any, they will be pleased to make the necessary arrangements at the first opportunity.

If you have any suggestions or questions regarding any information presented in this handbook, please contact our drug information pharmacist at

1-877-837-LEXI (5394)

This manual was produced using the FormuLex™ Program —
a complete publishing service of Lexi-Comp Inc.

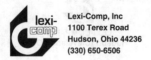

Lexi-Comp, Inc
1100 Terex Road
Hudson, Ohio 44236
(330) 650-6506

ISBN 1-930598-79-3

TABLE OF CONTENTS

ABOUT THE AUTHORS

MATTHEW A. FULLER, PharmD

Dr Fuller received his Bachelor of Science in Pharmacy from Ohio Northern University and then earned a Doctor of Pharmacy degree from the University of Cincinnati. A residency in hospital pharmacy was completed at Bethesda hospital in Zanesville, Ohio. After completion of his training, Dr Fuller accepted a position at the Veterans Affairs Medical Center in Cleveland, Ohio

Dr Fuller has over 15 years of experience in psychiatric psychopharmacology in a variety of clinical settings including acute care and ambulatory care. Dr Fuller is currently a Clinical Pharmacy Specialist in Psychiatry at the Veterans Affairs Medical Center in Cleveland, Ohio. He is also an Associate Clinical Professor of Psychiatry and Clinical Instructor of Psychology at Case Western Reserve University in Cleveland, Ohio and Adjunct Associate Professor of Clinical Pharmacy at the University of Toledo in Toledo, Ohio. In this position, Dr Fuller is responsible for providing service, education and research. He is also the Director of the ASHP accredited Psychopharmacy Residency Program.

Dr Fuller has received several awards including the Upjohn Excellence in Research Award and the OSHP Hospital Pharmacist of the Year Award in 1994. In 1996 he received the CSHP Evelyn Gray Scott Award (Pharmacist of the Year). In 2001 he received the OSHP Pharmacy Practice Research Award.

Dr Fuller is Board Certified by the Board of Pharmaceutical Specialties in both Pharmacotherapy and Psychopharmacy. He speaks regularly on the topic of psychotropic use and has published articles and abstracts on various issues in psychiatric psychopharmacology. His research interests include the psychopharmacologic treatment of schizophrenia and bipolar disorder.

Dr Fuller is a member of numerous professional organizations, including the American Society of Health-System Pharmacists (ASHP), where he was recently designated as a fellow. He completed his term as a member of the Commission on Therapeutics and is a member of the Clinical Specialist Section; Ohio Society of Health-System Pharmacists (OSHP) where he has served as an Educational Affairs Division member and a House of Delegates member; American College of Clinical Pharmacy (ACCP), Ohio College of Clinical Pharmacy where he served as secretary/treasurer, Cleveland Society of Health-System Pharmacist (CSHP) where he has served as the education chair and treasurer. He is a member of the National Alliance for the Mentally Ill (NAMI) and also serves as a reviewer for pharmacy and psychiatric journals.

MARTHA SAJATOVIC, MD

Dr Sajatovic is Associate Professor of Psychiatry at Case Western Reserve University School of Medicine in Cleveland, Ohio. She is a clinician and researcher with particular interest in health outcomes for individuals with serious mental illness. She also has a strong interest in assessment instruments in psychiatry, and frequently serves as a consultant to pharmaceutical companies for rating scales training, as well as publishing in this area.

Dr Sajatovic received her BS in biology at Ohio State University and completed medical school at the Medical College of Ohio at Toledo. She completed her residency training in psychiatry at University Hospitals of Cleveland where she was Chief Resident in Research. Following completion of her residency, Dr Sajatovic was a Clinical Director of Inpatient Schizophrenia Research at University Hospitals of Cleveland, and later, was the Associate Chief of Psychiatry and Chief of the

Mood Disorders Program at the Cleveland Veterans Affairs Medical Center in Cleveland, Ohio. Dr Sajatovic has extensive experience with the management of serious mental illness through her work as a state hospital Chief Clinical Officer (Cleveland Campus Northcoast Behavioral Healthcare), in her own private practice, and in consulting with agencies providing community services to the seriously mentally ill.

Dr Sajatovic has published a number of original papers on treatment of serious mental illness and treatment outcomes including work with special populations such as the elderly, women with psychosis, and individuals with developmental disorder. She has been a guest lecturer at numerous academic and community settings including speaking to consumer and family advocacy groups for individuals with psychiatric illness. Dr Sajatovic has a long-standing commitment to education including supervision of medical students and residents in psychiatry, lecturing at Case Western Reserve University School of Medicine, psychiatric resident supervision, and seminar teaching for residents in psychiatry.

EDITORIAL ADVISORY PANEL

Bernard L. Kasten, Jr, MD, FCAP
Vice-President/Chief Medical Officer
Quest Diagnostics Inc
Teteroboro, New Jersey

Polly E. Kintzel, PharmD, BCPS, BCOP
Clinical Pharmacy Specialist
Bone Marrow Transplantation,
Detroit Medical Center
Harper Hospital
Detroit, Michigan

Donna M. Kraus, PharmD, FAPhA
Associate Professor of Pharmacy Practice
Departments of Pharmacy Practice
and Pediatrics
Pediatric Clinical Pharmacist
University of Illinois at Chicago
Chicago, Illinois

Charles Lacy, RPh, PharmD, FCSHP
Coordinator of Clinical Services
Director, Drug Information Services
Cedars-Sinai Health System
Los Angeles, California

Brenda R. Lance, RN, MSN
Nurse Coordinator
Ritzman Infusion Services
Akron, Ohio

Leonard L. Lance, RPh, BSPharm
Clinical Pharmacist
Lexi-Comp Inc
Hudson, Ohio

Jerrold B. Leikin, MD, FACP, FACEP, FACMT, FAACT
Director, Medical Toxicology
Evanston Northwestern Healthcare-OMEGA
Glenbrook Hospital
Glenview, Illinois
Associate Director
Toxikon Consortium at Cook County Hospital
Chicago, Illinois

Timothy F. Meiller, DDS, PhD
Professor
Diagnostic Sciences and Pathology
Baltimore College of Dental Surgery
Professor of Oncology
Greenebaum Cancer Center
University of Maryland at Baltimore
Baltimore, Maryland

Franklin A. Michota, Jr, MD
*Head, Section of Hospital and
Preoperative Medicine*
Department of General Internal Medicine
Cleveland Clinic Foundation
Cleveland, Ohio

Eugene S. Olsowka, MD, PhD
Pathologist
Institute of Pathology PC
Saginaw, Michigan

Dwight K. Oxley, MD
Medical Director
Wesley Medical Center
Wichita, Kansas

Thomas E. Page, MA
Drug Recognition Expert and Instructor
Pasadena, CA

Frank P. Paloucek, PharmD, ABAT
Clinical Associate Professor
University of Illinois
Chicago, Illinois

Christopher J. Papasian, PhD
*Director of Diagnostic Microbiology
and Immunology Laboratories*
Truman Medical Center
Kansas City, Missouri

Bradley G. Phillips, PharmD, BCPS
Associate Professor
University of Iowa College of Pharmacy
Clinical Pharmacist
Veterans Affairs Medical Center
Iowa City, Iowa

Luis F. Ramirez, MD
Adjunct Associate Professor of Psychiatry
Case Western Reserve University
Cleveland, Ohio

Todd P. Semla, PharmD
*Associate Director of the Psychopharmacology
Clinical and Research Center*
Department of Psychiatry and
Behavioral Sciences
Evanston Northwestern Healthcare
Evanston, Illinois
*Clinical Assistant Professor of Pharmacy
Practice in Medicine,
Section of Geriatric Medicine*
University of Illinois at Chicago
Chicago, Illinois

Dominic A. Solimando, Jr, MA
Oncology Pharmacist
President, Oncology Pharmacy Services, Inc
Arlington, VA

Virend K. Somers, MD, DPhil
*Consultant in Hypertension and in
Cardiovascular Disease*
Mayo Medical School
Rochester, MN

Carol K. Taketomo, PharmD
Pharmacy Manager
Children's Hospital of Los Angeles
Los Angeles, California

Beatrice B. Turkoski, RN, PhD
*Professor, Advanced Pharmacology and
Applied Therapeutics*
Kent State University School of Nursing
Kent, Ohio

Richard L. Wynn, PhD
Professor and Chairman of Pharmacology
Baltimore College of Dental Surgery
Dental School
University of Maryland at Baltimore
Baltimore, Maryland

PREFACE

Our third edition of the *Psychotropic Drug Information Handbook* continues our efforts to provide an up-to-date, easy-to-use, portable source of drug information for mental healthcare professionals. To this aim, we have added new psychotropic monographs and have updated our existing monographs with new indications, contraindications, warning/precautions, adverse effects, drug interactions, dosing information, and dosage forms that may have changed over the past year. Further, to ease finding drug information, we have added a dictionary style index system on the top of the pages in the alphabetical listing of drugs.

The main feedback we received from the marketplace this year was the desire for information regarding child/adolescent dosing for the psychotropic drugs. We took this to heart and have added this information where it exists. This work could not have been done without the help of a consultant whom we would like to recognize. Barbara L. Gracious MD, Assistant Professor of Psychiatry and Pediatrics at Case Western Reserve University and Director of Child Psychiatry Training and Education at University Hospitals of Cleveland.

We continue to offer a complete drug information source designed for the mental healthcare practitioner titled *Drug Information for Mental Health*.

We hope that we have met our goal in that this handbook proves a useful tool for the mental healthcare professional. We greatly appreciate your feedback and continue to encourage this so that we can continue to meet our goals and your reference needs. Your comments and suggestions are taken seriously when future editions are written. As always, we look forward to hearing from you.

— Matthew A. Fuller and Martha Sajatovic

ACKNOWLEDGMENTS

Psychotropic Drug Information Handbook exists in its present form as the result of the concerted efforts of the following individuals: Robert D. Kerscher, publisher and president of Lexi-Comp Inc; Lynn D. Coppinger, managing editor; Barbara F. Kerscher, production manager; David C. Marcus, director of information systems; Ginger S. Stein, project manager; Paul A. Rhine, product manager; Tracey J. Reinecke, graphic designer; and Julian I. Graubart, American Pharmaceutical Association (APhA), Director of Books and Electronic Products.

Special acknowledgment to all Lexi-Comp staff for their contributions to this book.

Much of the material contained in this book was a result of pharmacy contributors throughout the United States and Canada. Lexi-Comp has assisted many medical institutions to develop hospital-specific formulary manuals that contains clinical drug information as well as dosing. Working with these clinical pharmacists, hospital pharmacy and therapeutics committees, and hospital drug information centers, Lexi-Comp has developed an evolutionary drug database that reflects the practice of pharmacy in these major institutions.

Special thanks from Dr Fuller to his parents, Raymond and Mary Fuller, who afforded him the opportunity to write this book; and to his wife and son, Jeanette and Samuel, who generously gave of their time and support.

A special thanks from Dr Sajatovic goes to her parents, Nick and Martha Sajatovic, to her husband, Douglas N. Flagg, MD, and to her sons, Alexander and Andrew for their continuous patience and support.

DESCRIPTION OF FIELDS AND SECTIONS IN THIS HANDBOOK

The *Psychotropic Drug Information Handbook* is divided into five sections.

The first section is a compilation of introductory text pertinent to the use of this book.

The drug information section of the handbook, in which all drugs are listed alphabetically, details information appropriate to each drug. Extensive cross-referencing is provided by brand names and synonyms.

The third section is comprised of several text chapters dealing with various subjects and issues relevant to the management of the psychiatric patient.

The fourth section is an invaluable appendix with charts, tables, nomograms, algorithms, management guidelines, and conversion information which can be helpful for patient care.

The last section of this handbook incorporates two indices, a pharmacologic category index and an alphabetical index which includes generic names, brand names (U.S. and Canadian), synonyms, text chapter headings, and appendix listings.

The **Alphabetical Listing of Drugs** is presented in a consistent format and provides the following fields of information:

Generic Name	U.S. adopted name
Pronunciation	Phonetic pronunciation guide
Related Information	Cross-reference to other pertinent drug information found elsewhere in this handbook
U.S. Brand Names	U.S. trade names (manufacturer-specific)
Canadian Brand Names	Trade names found in Canada
Synonyms	Other names or accepted abbreviations of the generic drug
Pharmacologic Category	Unique systematic classification of medications
Generic Available	Indicates if a generic form is available for psychotropic medications
Use	Information pertaining to appropriate FDA-approved indications of the drug.
Unlabeled/ Investigational Use	Information pertaining to non-FDA approved and investigational indications of the drug
Restrictions	The controlled substance classification from the Drug Enforcement Agency (DEA). U.S. schedules are I-V. Schedules vary by country and sometimes state (ie, Massachusetts uses I-VI).
Pregnancy Risk Factor	Five categories established by the FDA to indicate the potential of a systemically absorbed drug for causing birth defects
Pregnancy/Breast-Feeding Implications	Information pertinent to or associated with the use of the psychotropic drug as it relates to clinical effects on the fetus, breast-feeding/lactation, and clinical effects on the infant
Contraindications	Information pertaining to inappropriate use of the drug
Warnings/Precautions	Precautionary considerations, hazardous conditions related to use of the drug, and disease states or patient populations in which the drug should be cautiously used
Adverse Reactions	Side effects are grouped by percentage of incidence (if known) and/or body system

DESCRIPTION OF FIELDS AND SECTIONS IN THIS HANDBOOK *(Continued)*

Overdosage/Toxicology	Comments and/or considerations are offered when appropriate and include signs/symptoms of excess drug and suggested management of the patient
Drug Interactions	Description of the interaction between the drug listed in the monograph and other drugs or drug classes. May include possible mechanisms and effect of combined therapy. May also include a strategy to manage the patient on combined therapy (ie, quinidine).
Ethanol/Nutrition/Herb Interactions	Information regarding potential interactions with food, nutritionals (including herbal products or vitamins), or ethanol.
Stability	Information regarding reconstitution, storage, and compatibility
Mechanism of Action	How the drug works in the body to elicit a response
Pharmacodynamics/ Kinetics	The magnitude of a drug's effect depends on the drug concentration at the site of action. The pharmacodynamics are expressed in terms of onset of action and duration of action. Pharmacokinetics are expressed in terms of absorption, distribution (including appearance in breast milk and crossing of the placenta), protein binding, metabolism, bioavailability, half-life, time to peak serum concentration, and elimination.
Usual Dosage	The amount of the drug to be typically given or taken during therapy for children and adults; also includes any dosing adjustment/comments for renal impairment or hepatic failure
Child/Adolescent Considerations	Information from clinical trials for children and adolescent patients
Dietary Considerations	Includes information on how the medication should be taken relative to meals or food
Administration	Information regarding recommended final concentrations, rates of administration for parenteral drugs, or other guidelines when giving psychotropic medications
Monitoring Parameters	Laboratory tests and patient physical parameters that should be monitored for safety and efficacy
Reference Range	Therapeutic and toxic serum concentrations including peak and trough levels
Test Interactions	Listing of assay interferences when relevant; (B) = Blood; (S) = Serum; (U) = Urine
Patient Information	Specific information pertinent for the patient
Nursing Implications	Includes additional instructions for the administration of the drug and monitoring tips from the nursing perspective
Additional Information	Information about sodium content and/or pertinent information about specific brands
Dosage Forms	Information with regard to form, strength, and availability of the drug

FDA PREGNANCY CATEGORIES

Throughout this book there is a field labeled Pregnancy Risk Factor (PRF) and the letter A, B, C, D, or X immediately following which signifies a category. The FDA has established these five categories to indicate the potential of a systemically absorbed drug for causing birth defects. The key differentiation among the categories rests upon the reliability of documentation and the risk:benefit ratio. Pregnancy Category X is particularly notable in that if any data exists that may implicate a drug as a teratogen and the risk:benefit ratio is clearly negative, the drug is contraindicated during pregnancy.

These categories are summarized as follows:

A	Controlled studies in pregnant women fail to demonstrate a risk to the fetus in the first trimester with no evidence of risk in later trimesters. The possibility of fetal harm appears remote.
B	Either animal-reproduction studies have not demonstrated a fetal risk but there are no controlled studies in pregnant women, or animal-reproduction studies have shown an adverse effect (other than a decrease in fertility) that was not confirmed in controlled studies in women in the first trimester and there is no evidence of a risk in later trimesters.
C	Either studies in animals have revealed adverse effects on the fetus (teratogenic or embryocidal effects or other) and there are no controlled studies in women, or studies in women and animals are not available. Drugs should be given only if the potential benefits justify the potential risk to the fetus.
D	There is positive evidence of human fetal risk, but the benefits from use in pregnant women may be acceptable despite the risk (eg, if the drug is needed in a life-threatening situation or for a serious disease for which safer drugs cannot be used or are ineffective).
X	Studies in animals or human beings have demonstrated fetal abnormalities or there is evidence of fetal risk based on human experience, or both, and the risk of the use of the drug in pregnant women clearly outweighs any possible benefit. The drug is contraindicated in women who are or may become pregnant.

DRUGS IN PREGNANCY

Analgesics
Acceptable: Acetaminophen, meperidine, methadone
Controversial: Codeine, propoxyphene
Unacceptable: Nonsteroidal anti-inflammatory agents, salicylates, phenazo-pyridine

Antimicrobials
Acceptable: Penicillins, 1st and 2nd generation cephalosporins, erythromycin (base and EES), clotrimazole, miconazole, nystatin, isoniazid*, lindane, acyclovir, metronidazole
Controversial: 3rd generation cephalosporins, aminoglycosides, nitrofuran-toin†
Unacceptable: Erythromycin estolate, chloramphenicol, sulfa, tetracyclines

ENT
Acceptable: Diphenhydramine*, dextromethorphan
Controversial: Pseudoephedrine
Unacceptable: Brompheniramine, cyproheptadine, dimenhydrinate

FDA PREGNANCY CATEGORIES *(Continued)*

GI
>**Acceptable:** Trimethobenzamide, antacids*, simethicone, other H₂-blockers, psyllium, bisacodyl, docusate
>**Controversial:** Metoclopramide, prochlorperazine

Neurologic
>**Controversial:** Phenytoin, phenobarbital
>**Unacceptable:** Carbamazepine, valproic acid, ergotamine

Pulmonary
>**Acceptable:** Theophylline, metaproterenol, terbutaline, inhaled steroids
>**Unacceptable:** Epinephrine, oral steroids

Psychiatric
>**Controversial:** Hydroxyzine*, lithium*, tricyclics, SSRIs, antipsychotics, stimulants
>**Unacceptable:** Anticonvulsants

Other
>**Acceptable:** Heparin, insulin
>**Unacceptable:** Warfarin, sulfonylureas

*Do not use in first trimester
†Do not use in third trimester

SAFE WRITING

Health professionals and their support personnel frequently produce handwritten copies of information they see in print; therefore, such information is subjected to even greater possibilities for error or misinterpretation on the part of others. Thus, particular care must be given to how drug names and strengths are expressed when creating written healthcare documents.

The following are a few examples of safe writing rules suggested by the Institute for Safe Medication Practices, Inc.*

1. There should be a space between a number and its units as it is easier to read. There should be no periods after the abbreviations mg or mL.

Correct	Incorrect
10 mg	10mg
100 mg	100mg

2. Never place a decimal and a zero after a whole number (2 mg is correct and 2.0 mg is **incorrect**). If the decimal point is not seen because it falls on a line or because individuals are working from copies where the decimal point is not seen, this causes a tenfold overdose.

3. Just the opposite is true for numbers less than one. Always place a zero before a naked decimal (0.5 mL is correct, .5 mL is **incorrect**).

4. Never abbreviate the word unit. The handwritten U or u, looks like a 0 (zero), and may cause a tenfold overdose error to be made.

5. IU is not a safe abbreviation for international units. The handwritten IU looks like IV. Write out international units or use int. units.

6. Q.D. is not a safe abbreviation for once daily, as when the Q is followed by a sloppy dot, it looks like QID which means four times daily.

7. O.D. is not a safe abbreviation for once daily, as it is properly interpreted as meaning "right eye" and has caused liquid medications such as saturated solution of potassium iodide and Lugol's solution to be administered incorrectly. There is no safe abbreviation for once daily. It must be written out in full.

8. Do not use chemical names such as 6-mercaptopurine or 6-thioguanine, as sixfold overdoses have been given when these were not recognized as chemical names. The proper names of these drugs are mercaptopurine or thioguanine.

9. Do not abbreviate drug names (5FC, 6MP, 5-ASA, MTX, HCTZ, CPZ, PBZ, etc) as they are misinterpreted and cause error.

10. Do not use the apothecary system or symbols.

11. Do not abbreviate microgram as μg; instead use mcg as there is less likelihood of misinterpretation.

SAFE WRITING *(Continued)*

12. When writing an outpatient prescription, write a complete prescription. A complete prescription can prevent the prescriber, the pharmacist, and/or the patient from making a mistake and can eliminate the need for further clarification. The legible prescriptions should contain:

    a. patient's full name

    b. for pediatric or geriatric patients: their age (or weight where applicable)

    c. drug name, dosage form and strength; if a drug is new or rarely prescribed, print this information

    d. number or amount to be dispensed

    e. complete instructions for the patient, including the purpose of the medication

    f. when there are recognized contraindications for a prescribed drug, indicate to the pharmacist that you are aware of this fact (ie, when prescribing a potassium salt for a patient receiving an ACE inhibitor, write "K serum level being monitored")

*From "Safe Writing" by Davis NM, PharmD and Cohen MR, MS, Lecturers and Consultants for Safe Medication Practices, 1143 Wright Drive, Huntington Valley, PA 19006. Phone: (215) 947-7566.

ALPHABETICAL LISTING OF DRUGS

- ◆ **Absinthe** *see* Wormwood *on page 435*
- ◆ **Acetaminophen, Dichloralphenazone, and Isometheptene** *see* Acetaminophen, Isometheptene, and Dichloralphenazone *on page 14*

Acetaminophen, Isometheptene, and Dichloralphenazone

(a seet a MIN oh fen, eye soe me THEP teen, & dye KLOR al FEN a zone)

U.S. Brand Names Isocom®; Isopap®; Midchlor®; Midrin®; Migratine®

Synonyms Acetaminophen, Dichloralphenazone, and Isometheptene; Dichloralphenazone, Acetaminophen, and Isometheptene; Dichloralphenazone, Isometheptene, and Acetaminophen; Isometheptene, Acetaminophen, and Dichloralphenazone; Isometheptene, Dichloralphenazone, and Acetaminophen

Pharmacologic Category Analgesic, Miscellaneous

Use Relief of migraine and tension headache

Restrictions C-IV

Usual Dosage Adults: Oral:

Migraine headache: 2 capsules to start, followed by 1 capsule every hour until relief is obtained (maximum: 5 capsules/12 hours)

Tension headache: 1-2 capsules every 4 hours (maximum: 8 capsules/24 hours)

Dosage Forms Capsule: Acetaminophen 325 mg, isometheptene mucate 65 mg, dichloralphenazone 100 mg

- ◆ **Adamantanamine Hydrochloride** *see* Amantadine *on page 19*
- ◆ **Adderall®** *see* Dextroamphetamine and Amphetamine *on page 107*
- ◆ **Addiction Treatments** *see page 550*
- ◆ **Adipex-P®** *see* Phentermine *on page 307*
- ◆ **Akineton®** *see* Biperiden *on page 47*
- ◆ **Alertec® (Can)** *see* Modafinil *on page 247*
- ◆ **Allerdryl® (Can)** *see* Diphenhydramine *on page 116*
- ◆ **AllerMax® [OTC]** *see* Diphenhydramine *on page 116*
- ◆ **Allernix® (Can)** *see* Diphenhydramine *on page 116*
- ◆ *Allium savitum* *see* Garlic *on page 166*

Almotriptan (al moh TRIP tan)

Related Information

Patient Information - Miscellaneous Medications - Antimigraine Medications *on page 521*

U.S. Brand Names Axert™

Synonyms Almotriptan Malate

Pharmacologic Category Serotonin 5-HT$_{1D}$ Receptor Agonist

Generic Available No

Use Acute treatment of migraine with or without aura

Pregnancy Risk Factor C

Pregnancy/Breast-Feeding Implications There are no adequate, well-controlled studies in pregnant women. Use in pregnancy should be limited to situations where benefit outweighs risk to fetus. Excretion in breast milk unknown; use caution.

Contraindications Hypersensitivity to almotriptan or any component of the formulation; use as prophylactic therapy for migraine; hemiplegic or basilar migraine; cluster headache; known or suspected ischemic heart disease (angina pectoris, MI, documented silent ischemia, coronary artery vasospasm, Prinzmetal's variant angina); peripheral vascular syndromes (including ischemic bowel disease); uncontrolled hypertension; use within 24 hours of another 5-HT$_1$ agonist; use within 24 hours of ergotamine derivative; concurrent administration or within 2 weeks of discontinuing an MAO inhibitor (specifically MAO type A inhibitors)

Warnings/Precautions Almotriptan is indicated only in patients ≥18 years of age with a clear diagnosis of migraine headache. If a patient does not respond to the first dose, the diagnosis of migraine should be reconsidered. Do not give to patients with risk factors for CAD until a cardiovascular evaluation has been performed; if evaluation is satisfactory, the healthcare provider should administer the first dose and cardiovascular status should be periodically evaluated. Cardiac events (coronary artery vasospasm, transient ischemia, myocardial infarction, ventricular tachycardia/fibrillation, cardiac arrest, and death), cerebral/subarachnoid hemorrhage, stroke, peripheral vascular ischemia and colonic ischemia have been reported with 5-HT₁ agonist administration. Significant elevation in blood pressure, including hypertensive crisis, has also been reported on rare occasions in patients with and without a history of hypertension. Use with caution in liver or renal dysfunction. Safety and efficacy in pediatric patients have not been established.

Adverse Reactions

1% to 10%:

Central nervous system: Headache (>1%), dizziness (>1%), somnolence (>1%)

Gastrointestinal: Nausea (1% to 2%), xerostomia (1%)

Neuromuscular & skeletal: Paresthesia (1%)

<1%: Abdominal cramps, abdominal pain, abnormal coordination, anxiety, arthralgia, arthritis, back pain, bronchitis, chest pain, chills, colitis, conjunctivitis, coronary artery vasospasm, creatine phosphokinase increased, depressive symptoms, dermatitis, diaphoresis, diarrhea, diplopia, dream changes, dry eyes, dysmenorrhea, dyspepsia, dyspnea, ear pain, epistaxis, erythema, esophageal reflux, euphoria, eye irritation, eye pain, fatigue, fever, gastritis, gastroenteritis, GGTP increased, hyperacusis, hypercholesterolemia, hypesthesia, hyperglycemia, hyper-reflexia, hypertension, hypertonia, hyperventilation, impaired concentration, insomnia, laryngismus, laryngitis, muscular weakness, myalgia, myocardial ischemia, myocardial infarction, myopathy, neck pain, nervousness, neuropathy, nightmares, nystagmus, otitis media, palpitations, parosmia, pharyngitis, photosensitivity reaction, pruritus, rash, restlessness, rhinitis, rigid neck, salivation increased, scotoma, shakiness, sinusitis, sneezing, stimulation, syncope, tachycardia, taste alterations, thirst, tinnitus, tremor, vasodilation, ventricular fibrillation, ventricular tachycardia, vertigo, vomiting, weakness

Overdosage/Toxicology Hypertension or more serious cardiovascular symptoms may occur. Clinical and electrocardiographic monitoring needed for at least 20 hours even if patient asymptomatic. Treatment is symptoms-directed and supportive.

Drug Interactions CYP2D6 and 3A4 enzyme substrate

CYP3A4 inhibitors: Likely to increase almotriptan serum concentration. Effect seen with ketoconazole. Inhibitors include amiodarone, cimetidine, clarithromycin, erythromycin, delavirdine, diltiazem, dirithromycin, itraconazole, ketoconazole, nefazodone, nevirapine, propoxyphene, quinupristin-dalfopristin, ritonavir, saquinavir, verapamil, zafirlukast, zileuton. Monitor for increased almotriptan response.

Ergot-containing drugs: Prolong vasospastic reactions; do not use almotriptan or ergot-containing drugs within 24 hours of each other.

Ketoconazole: Increases almotriptan serum concentration. Monitor for increased almotriptan response.

MAO inhibitors (moclobemide [MAO type A inhibitor]): Almotriptan clearance decreased by 27%; C_{max} increased by 6%. Avoid concurrent administration of MAO inhibitors or within 2 weeks of discontinuing an MAO inhibitor, specifically MAO type A inhibitors.

Selegiline: Selegiline is a selective MAO type B inhibitor; while not specifically contraindicated, combination has not been studied.

Verapamil: Increased almotriptan serum concentration by 24%. Dose adjustment not necessary.

SSRIs: Concurrent use may lead to symptoms of hyper-reflexia, weakness, and lack of coordination; monitor.

Stability Store at 15°C to 30°C (59°F to 86°F).

(Continued)

Almotriptan *(Continued)*

Mechanism of Action Selective agonist for serotonin (5-HT$_{1B}$, 5-HT$_{1D}$, 5-HT$_{1F}$ receptors) in cranial arteries; causes vasoconstriction and reduce sterile inflammation associated with antidromic neuronal transmission correlating with relief of migraine

Pharmacodynamics/Kinetics
Absorption: Well absorbed
Distribution: V$_d$: 180-200 L
Protein binding: ~35%
Metabolism: MAO type A oxidative deamination (~27% of dose); via CYP3A4 and 2D6 oxidation (~12% of the dose); metabolized to inactive metabolites
Bioavailability: 70%
Half life: 3-4 hours
Time to peak: 1-3 hours after administration
Excretion: In urine (40% unchanged); in feces (13% unchanged and metabolized)

Usual Dosage Oral: Adults: Migraine: Initial: 6.25-12.5 mg in a single dose; if the headache returns, repeat the dose after 2 hours; no more than 2 doses in 24-hour period
Note: If the first dose is ineffective, diagnosis needs to be re-evaluated. Safety of treating more than 4 migraines/month has not been established.
Dosage adjustment in renal impairment: Initial: 6.25 mg in a single dose; maximum daily dose: ≤12.5 mg
Dosage adjustment in hepatic impairment: Initial: 6.25 mg in a single dose; maximum daily dose: ≤12.5 mg

Dietary Considerations Food: May be taken without regard to meals

Patient Information This drug is to be used to reduce your migraine not to prevent or reduce the number of attacks. Take exactly as directed. If headache returns or is not fully resolved, the dose may be repeated after 2 hours. Do not use more than two doses in 24 hours. Do not take within 24 hours of other migraine medication without consulting prescriber. You may experience dizziness, fatigue, or drowsiness (use caution when driving or engaging in tasks that require alertness until response to drug is known). Report immediately chest pain, palpitations, feeling of tightness or pressure in chest, jaw, or throat; acute headache or dizziness; muscle cramping, pain, or tremors; skin rash; hallucinations, anxiety, panic; or other adverse reactions.

Dosage Forms Tablet, as malate: 6.25 mg, 12.5 mg

♦ **Almotriptan Malate** *see Almotriptan on page 14*

Alprazolam *(al PRAY zoe lam)*

Related Information
Anxiolytic/Hypnotic Use in Long-Term Care Facilities *on page 562*
Benzodiazepines Comparison Chart *on page 566*
Federal OBRA Regulations Recommended Maximum Doses *on page 583*
Patient Information - Anxiolytics & Sedative Hypnotics (Benzodiazepines) *on page 483*

U.S. Brand Names Xanax®

Canadian Brand Names Apo®-Alpraz; Novo-Alprazol; Nu-Alprax

Pharmacologic Category Benzodiazepine

Generic Available Yes

Use Treatment of anxiety disorder (GAD); panic disorder, with or without agoraphobia; anxiety associated with depression

Unlabeled/Investigational Use Anxiety in children

Restrictions C-IV

Pregnancy Risk Factor D

Contraindications Hypersensitivity to alprazolam or any component of the formulation (cross-sensitivity with other benzodiazepines may exist); narrow-angle glaucoma; concurrent use of ketoconazole and itraconazole; pregnancy

Warnings/Precautions Rebound or withdrawal symptoms, including seizures may occur 18 hours to 3 days following abrupt discontinuation or large decreases in dose (more common in patients receiving >4 mg/day or prolonged treatment). Dose reductions or tapering must be approached with extreme caution. Between dose, anxiety may also occur. Use with caution in patients receiving concurrent CYP3A4 inhibitors, particularly when these agents are added to therapy. Has weak uricosuric properties, use with caution in renal impairment or predisposition to urate nephropathy. Use with caution in elderly or debilitated patients, patients with hepatic disease (including alcoholics), renal impairment, or obese patients.

Causes CNS depression (dose-related) resulting in sedation, dizziness, confusion, or ataxia which may impair physical and mental capabilities. Patients must be cautioned about performing tasks which require mental alertness (ie, operating machinery or driving). Use with caution in patients receiving other CNS depressants or psychoactive agents. Effects with other sedative drugs or ethanol may be potentiated. Benzodiazepines have been associated with falls and traumatic injury and should be used with extreme caution in patients who are at risk of these events (especially the elderly). Use with caution in patients with respiratory disease or impaired gag reflex.

Use caution in patients with depression, particularly if suicidal risk may be present. Episodes of mania or hypomania have occurred in depressed patients treated with alprazolam. May cause physical or psychological dependence - use with caution in patients with a history of drug dependence. Acute withdrawal, including seizures, may be precipitated in patients after administration of flumazenil to patients receiving long-term benzodiazepine therapy.

Benzodiazepines have been associated with anterograde amnesia. Paradoxical reactions, including hyperactive or aggressive behavior, have been reported with benzodiazepines, particularly in adolescent/pediatric or psychiatric patients. Does not have analgesic, antidepressant, or antipsychotic properties.

Adverse Reactions
>10%:
  Central nervous system: Drowsiness, fatigue, ataxia, lightheadedness, memory impairment, dysarthria, irritability
  Endocrine & metabolic: Decreased libido, menstrual disorders
  Gastrointestinal: Xerostomia, decreased salivation, increased or decreased appetite, weight gain/loss
  Genitourinary: Micturition difficulties
1% to 10%:
  Cardiovascular: Hypotension
  Central nervous system: Confusion, dizziness, disinhibition, akathisia, increased libido
  Dermatologic: Dermatitis, rash
  Gastrointestinal: Increased salivation
  Genitourinary: Sexual dysfunction, incontinence
  Neuromuscular & skeletal: Rigidity, tremor, muscle cramps
  Otic: Tinnitus
  Respiratory: Nasal congestion

Overdosage/Toxicology
  Signs and symptoms: Somnolence, confusion, coma, and diminished reflexes; treatment for benzodiazepine overdose is supportive
  Treatment: Rarely is mechanical ventilation required; flumazenil has been shown to selectively block the binding of benzodiazepines to CNS receptors, resulting in a reversal of benzodiazepine-induced sedation; however, its use may not alter the course of overdose

Drug Interactions CYP3A3/4 enzyme substrate
  CNS depressants: Sedative effects and/or respiratory depression may be additive with CNS depressants. Includes ethanol, barbiturates, narcotic analgesics, and other sedative agents; monitor for increased effect
  (Continued)

Alprazolam *(Continued)*

Enzyme inducers: Metabolism of some benzodiazepines may be increased, decreasing their therapeutic effect; consider using an alternative sedative/hypnotic agent. Potential inducers include phenobarbital, phenytoin, carbamazepine, rifampin, and rifabutin.

CYP3A3/4 inhibitors: Serum level and/or toxicity of some benzodiazepines may be increased. Inhibitors include amiodarone, cimetidine, clarithromycin, erythromycin, delavirdine, diltiazem, dirithromycin, disulfiram, fluoxetine, fluvoxamine, grapefruit juice, indinavir, itraconazole, ketoconazole, nefazodone, nevirapine, propoxyphene, quinupristin-dalfopristin, ritonavir, saquinavir, verapamil, zafirlukast, zileuton; monitor for altered benzodiazepine response

Levodopa: Therapeutic effects may be diminished in some patients following the addition of a benzodiazepine; limited/inconsistent data

Oral contraceptives: May decrease the clearance of some benzodiazepines (those which undergo oxidative metabolism); monitor for increased benzodiazepine effect

Theophylline: May partially antagonize some of the effects of benzodiazepines; monitor for decreased response; may require higher doses for sedation

Ethanol/Nutrition/Herb Interactions

Ethanol: Avoid ethanol (may increase CNS depression).

Food: Alprazolam serum concentration is unlikely to be increased by grapefruit juice because of alprazolam's high oral bioavailability.

Herb/Nutraceutical: St John's wort may decrease alprazolam levels. Avoid valerian, St John's wort, kava kava, gotu kola (may increase CNS depression).

Mechanism of Action Binds to stereospecific benzodiazepine receptors on the postsynaptic GABA neuron at several sites within the central nervous system, including the limbic system, reticular formation. Enhancement of the inhibitory effect of GABA on neuronal excitability results by increased neuronal membrane permeability to chloride ions. This shift in chloride ions results in hyperpolarization (a less excitable state) and stabilization.

Pharmacodynamics/Kinetics

Distribution: V_d: 0.9-1.2 L/kg; distributes into breast milk

Protein binding: 80%

Metabolism: Extensive in the liver; major metabolite is inactive

Half-life: 12-15 hours

Time to peak serum concentration: Within 1-2 hours

Elimination: Excretion of metabolites and parent compound in urine

Usual Dosage Oral:

Children: Anxiety (unlabeled use): Initial: 0.005 mg/kg or 0.125 mg/dose 3 times/day; increase in increments of 0.125-0.25 mg, up to a maximum of 0.02 mg/kg/dose or 0.06 mg/kg/day (0.375-3 mg/day)

Adults:
Anxiety: Effective doses are 0.5-4 mg/day in divided doses; the manufacturer recommends starting at 0.25-0.5 mg 3 times/day; titrate dose upward; maximum: 4 mg/day

Depression: Average dose required: 2.5-3 mg/day in divided doses

Alcohol withdrawal: Usual dose: 2-2.5 mg/day in divided doses

Panic disorder: Many patients obtain relief at 2 mg/day, as much as 10 mg/day may be required

Elderly: Elderly patients may be more sensitive to the effects of alprazolam including ataxia and oversedation. The elderly may also have impaired renal function leading to decreased clearance. The smallest effective dose should be used.

Dosing adjustment in hepatic impairment: Reduce dose by 50% to 60% or avoid in cirrhosis

Note: Treatment >4 months should be re-evaluated to determine the patient's need for the drug

Child/Adolescent Considerations Children <18 years: Anxiety: Dose not established; investigationally, in children 7-16 years of age (n=13), initial doses of 0.005

mg/kg or 0.125 mg/dose were given 3 times/day for situational anxiety; increments of 0.125-0.25 mg were used to increase doses to maximum of 0.02 mg/kg/dose or 0.06 mg/kg/day; a range of 0.375-3 mg/day was needed.

Note: A more recent study in 17 children (8-17 years of age) with overanxious disorder or avoidant disorders used initial daily doses of 0.25 mg for children <40 kg and 0.5 mg for those >40 kg. The dose was titrated at 2-day intervals to a maximum of 0.04 mg/kg/day. Required doses ranged from 0.5-3.5 mg/day (mean: 1.6 mg/day). Based on clinical global ratings, alprazolam appeared to be better than placebo, however, this difference was **not** statistically significant; further studies are needed (Simeon, 1992).

Administration Can be administered sublingually with comparable onset and completeness of absorption.

Monitoring Parameters Respiratory and cardiovascular status

Test Interactions ↑ alkaline phosphatase

Patient Information Avoid alcohol and other CNS depressants; avoid activities needing good psychomotor coordination until CNS effects are known; drug may cause physical or psychological dependence; avoid abrupt discontinuation after prolonged use

Nursing Implications Assist with ambulation during beginning therapy, raise bed rails and keep room partially illuminated at night; monitor for CNS respiratory depression

Additional Information Not intended for management of anxieties and minor distresses associated with everyday life. Treatment longer than 4 months should be re-evaluated to determine the patient's need for the drug. Patients who become physically dependent on alprazolam tend to have a difficult time discontinuing it; withdrawal symptoms may be severe. To minimize withdrawal symptoms, taper dosage slowly; do not discontinue abruptly. Abrupt discontinuation after sustained use (generally >10 days) may cause withdrawal symptoms.

Dosage Forms
Solution, oral: 1 mg/mL (30 mL)
Tablet: 0.25 mg, 0.5 mg, 1 mg, 2 mg

♦ **Altamisa** *see Feverfew on page 143*
♦ **Alti-Bromocriptine (Can)** *see Bromocriptine on page 49*

Amantadine *(a MAN ta deen)*

Related Information
Antiparkinsonian Agents Comparison Chart *on page 556*
Discontinuation of Psychotropic Drugs - Withdrawal Symptoms and Recommendations *on page 582*
Patient Information - Agents for Treatment of Extrapyramidal Symptoms *on page 493*

U.S. Brand Names Symadine®; Symmetrel®

Canadian Brand Names Endantadine®; PMS-Amantadine

Synonyms Adamantanamine Hydrochloride; Amantadine Hydrochloride

Pharmacologic Category Anti-Parkinson's Agent (Dopamine Agonist); Antiviral Agent

Generic Available Yes

Use Prophylaxis and treatment of influenza A viral infection; treatment of parkinsonism; treatment of drug-induced extrapyramidal reactions

Unlabeled/Investigational Use Creutzfeldt-Jakob disease

Pregnancy Risk Factor C

Contraindications Hypersensitivity to amantadine or any component of the formulation

Warnings/Precautions Use with caution in patients with liver disease, history of recurrent and eczematoid dermatitis, uncontrolled psychosis or severe psychoneurosis, seizures, and in those receiving CNS stimulant drugs; reduce dose in renal disease. When treating Parkinson's disease, do not discontinue abruptly. In many patients, the therapeutic benefits of amantadine are limited to a few months. *(Continued)*

Amantadine *(Continued)*

Elderly patients may be more susceptible to CNS effects (using 2 divided daily doses may minimize this effect). Has been associated with neuroleptic malignant syndrome (associated with dose reduction or abrupt discontinuation). Has not been shown to prevent bacterial infection or complications when used as prophylaxis or treatment of influenza A. Use with caution in patients with CHF, peripheral edema, or orthostatic hypotension. Avoid in angle closure glaucoma.

Adverse Reactions

1% to 10%:

Cardiovascular: Orthostatic hypotension, peripheral edema

Central nervous system: Insomnia, depression, anxiety, irritability, dizziness, hallucinations, ataxia, headache, somnolence, nervousness, dream abnormality, agitation, fatigue, confusion

Dermatologic: Livedo reticularis

Gastrointestinal: Nausea, anorexia, constipation, diarrhea, xerostomia

Respiratory: Dry nose

<1%: Amnesia, congestive heart failure, decreased libido, dyspnea, eczematoid dermatitis, euphoria, hyperkinesis, hypertension, instances of convulsions, leukopenia, neutropenia, oculogyric episodes, psychosis, rash, slurred speech, urinary retention, visual disturbances, vomiting, weakness

Overdosage/Toxicology

Signs and symptoms: Nausea, vomiting, slurred speech, blurred vision, lethargy, hallucinations, seizures, myoclonic jerking

Treatment: Should be directed at reducing the CNS stimulation and at maintaining cardiovascular function; minimize or discontinue use of other psychotropics that may contribute to adverse effects. Seizures can be treated with diazepam 5-10 mg I.V. every 15 minutes as needed; up to a total of 30 mg in adults (0.25-0.4 mg/kg/dose I.V. every 15 minutes as needed up to a total of 10 mg for children) while a lidocaine infusion may be required for the cardiac dysrhythmias

Drug Interactions

Anticholinergics may potentiate CNS side effects of amantadine; monitor for altered response. Includes benztropine and trihexyphenidyl, as well as agents with anticholinergic activity such as quinidine, tricyclics, and antihistamines.

Thiazide diuretics: Hydrochlorothiazide has been reported to increase the potential for toxicity with amantadine (limited documentation); monitor response

Triamterene: Has been reported to increase the potential for toxicity with amantadine (limited documentation); monitor response

Trimethoprim: Has been reported to increase the potential for toxicity with amantadine (limited documentation); monitor for acute confusion

Ethanol/Nutrition/Herb Interactions Ethanol: Avoid ethanol (may increase CNS adverse effects).

Stability Protect from freezing

Mechanism of Action As an antiviral, blocks the uncoating of influenza A virus preventing penetration of virus into host; antiparkinsonian activity may be due to its blocking the reuptake of dopamine into presynaptic neurons or by increasing dopamine release from presynaptic fibers

Pharmacodynamics/Kinetics

Onset of antidyskinetic action: Within 48 hours

Absorption: Well absorbed from GI tract

Distribution: To saliva, tear film, and nasal secretions; in animals, tissue (especially lung) concentrations higher than serum concentrations, crosses blood-brain barrier

V_d:

Normal: 1.5-6.1 L/kg

Renal failure: 5.1±0.2 L/kg

Protein binding:

Normal renal function: ~67%

Hemodialysis patients: ~59%

Metabolism: Not appreciable, small amounts of an acetyl metabolite identified

Bioavailability: 86% to 90%

Half-life:

Normal renal function: 16 ± 6 hours (9-31 hours)

End-stage renal disease: 7-10 days

Time to peak: 1-4 hours

Elimination: 80% to 90% excreted unchanged in urine by glomerular filtration and tubular secretion

Total clearance: 2.5-10.5 L/hour

Usual Dosage

Children: Influenza:

1-9 years (<45 kg): 5-9 mg/kg/day in 1-2 divided doses to a maximum of 150 mg/day

10-12 years: 100-200 mg/day in 1-2 divided doses

Influenza prophylaxis: Administer for 10-21 days following exposure if the vaccine is concurrently given or for 90 days following exposure if the vaccine is unavailable or contraindicated and re-exposure is possible

Adults:

Drug-induced extrapyramidal reactions: 100 mg twice daily; may increase to 300-400 mg/day, if needed

Parkinson's disease or Creutzfeldt-Jakob disease (unlabeled use): 100 mg twice daily as sole therapy; may increase to 400 mg/day if needed with close monitoring; initial dose: 100 mg/day if with other serious illness or with high doses of other anti-Parkinson drugs

Influenza A viral infection: 200 mg/day in 1-2 divided doses; initiate within 24-48 hours after onset of symptoms; discontinue as soon as possible based on clinical response (generally within 3-5 days or within 24-48 hours after symptoms disappear)

Influenza prophylaxis: 200 mg/day in 1-2 doses; minimum 10-day course of therapy following exposure if the vaccine is concurrently given or for 90 days following exposure if the vaccine is unavailable or contraindicated and re-exposure is possible

Elderly patients should take the drug in 2 daily doses rather than a single dose to avoid adverse neurologic reactions

Dosing interval in renal impairment:

Cl_{cr} 50-60 mL/minute: Administer 200 mg alternating with 100 mg/day

Cl_{cr} 30-50 mL/minute: Administer 100 mg/day

Cl_{cr} 20-30 mL/minute: Administer 200 mg twice weekly

Cl_{cr} 10-20 mL/minute: Administer 100 mg 3 times/week

Cl_{cr} <10 mL/minute: Administer 200 mg alternating with 100 mg every 7 days

Hemodialysis: Slightly hemodialyzable (5% to 20%); no supplemental dose is needed

Peritoneal dialysis: No supplemental dose is needed

Continuous arterio-venous or venous-venous hemofiltration: No supplemental dose is needed

Monitoring Parameters Renal function, Parkinson's symptoms, mental status, influenza symptoms, blood pressure

Patient Information Do not abruptly discontinue therapy, it may precipitate a parkinsonian crisis; may impair ability to perform activities requiring mental alertness or coordination. Must take throughout flu season or for 2 weeks following vaccination for effective prophylaxis.

Nursing Implications If insomnia occurs, the last daily dose should be given several hours before retiring; assess parkinsonian symptoms prior to and throughout course of therapy

Additional Information Patients with intolerable CNS side effects often do better with rimantadine.

Dosage Forms

Capsule, as hydrochloride: 100 mg

Syrup, as hydrochloride: 50 mg/5 mL (120 mL, 480 mL)

Tablet, as hydrochloride: 100 mg

- ♦ **Amantadine Hydrochloride** *see* Amantadine *on page 19*
- ♦ **Amaphen**® *see* Butalbital Compound *on page 59*
- ♦ **Amber Touch-and-Feel** *see* St John's Wort *on page 382*
- ♦ **Ambien**™ *see* Zolpidem *on page 445*
- ♦ **Amerge**® *see* Naratriptan *on page 257*
- ♦ **Amfepramone** *see* Diethylpropion *on page 114*
- ♦ **Amino-Opti-E**® **[OTC]** *see* Vitamin E *on page 433*

Amitriptyline (a mee TRIP ti leen)

Related Information

Antidepressant Agents Comparison Chart *on page 553*

Discontinuation of Psychotropic Drugs - Withdrawal Symptoms and Recommendations *on page 582*

Federal OBRA Regulations Recommended Maximum Doses *on page 583*

Patient Information - Antidepressants (TCAs) *on page 454*

Teratogenic Risks of Psychotropic Medications *on page 594*

U.S. Brand Names Elavil®; Vanatrip®

Canadian Brand Names Apo®-Amitriptyline; Levate®; Novo-Tryptin

Synonyms Amitriptyline Hydrochloride

Pharmacologic Category Antidepressant, Tricyclic (Tertiary Amine)

Generic Available Yes

Use Relief of symptoms of depression

Unlabeled/Investigational Use Analgesic for certain chronic and neuropathic pain; prophylaxis against migraine headaches; treatment of depressive disorders in children

Pregnancy Risk Factor D

Contraindications Hypersensitivity to amitriptyline or any component of the formulation (cross-sensitivity with other tricyclics may occur); use of MAO inhibitors within past 14 days; recovery from acute myocardial infarction; concurrent use of cisapride; pregnancy

Warnings/Precautions Often causes drowsiness/sedation, resulting in impaired performance of tasks requiring alertness (ie, operating machinery or driving). Sedative effects may be additive with other CNS depressants and/or ethanol. The degree of sedation is very high relative to other antidepressants. May worsen psychosis in some patients or precipitate a shift to mania or hypomania in patients with bipolar disease. May cause hyponatremia/SIADH. May increase the risks associated with electroconvulsive therapy. This agent should be discontinued, when possible, prior to elective surgery. Therapy should not be abruptly discontinued in patients receiving high doses for prolonged periods.

May cause orthostatic hypotension; the risk of this problem is very high relative to other antidepressants. Use with caution in patients at risk of hypotension or in patients where transient hypotensive episodes would be poorly tolerated (cardiovascular disease or cerebrovascular disease). The degree of anticholinergic blockade produced by this agent is very high relative to other cyclic antidepressants; use with caution in patients with urinary retention, benign prostatic hypertrophy, narrow-angle glaucoma, xerostomia, visual problems, constipation, or a history of bowel obstruction. May alter glucose control - use with caution in patients with diabetes.

Use caution in patients with depression, particularly if suicidal risk may be present. Use with caution in patients with a history of cardiovascular disease (including previous MI, stroke, tachycardia, or conduction abnormalities). The risk of conduction abnormalities with this agent is high relative to other antidepressants. May lower seizure threshold - use caution in patients with a previous seizure disorder or condition predisposing to seizures such as brain damage, alcoholism, or concurrent therapy with other drugs which lower the seizure threshold. Use with caution in hyperthyroid patients or those receiving thyroid supplementation. Use with caution in patients with hepatic or renal dysfunction and in elderly patients. Not recommended for use in patients <12 years of age.

Adverse Reactions Anticholinergic effects may be pronounced; moderate to marked sedation can occur (tolerance to these effects usually occurs).

Cardiovascular: Orthostatic hypotension, tachycardia, nonspecific EKG changes, changes in AV conduction

Central nervous system: Restlessness, dizziness, insomnia, sedation, fatigue, anxiety, impaired cognitive function, seizures, extrapyramidal symptoms

Dermatologic: Allergic rash, urticaria, photosensitivity

Gastrointestinal: Weight gain, xerostomia, constipation

Genitourinary: Urinary retention

Ocular: Blurred vision, mydriasis

Miscellaneous: Diaphoresis

Overdosage/Toxicology

Signs and symptoms: Agitation, confusion, hallucinations, urinary retention, hypothermia, hypotension, ventricular tachycardia, seizures

Treatment: Following initiation of essential overdose management, toxic symptoms should be treated. Ventricular arrhythmias often respond to phenytoin 15-20 mg/kg (adults) with concurrent systemic alkalinization (sodium bicarbonate 0.5-2 mEq/kg I.V.). Arrhythmias unresponsive to this therapy may respond to lidocaine 1mg/kg I.V. followed by a titrated infusion. Physostigmine (1-2 mg I.V. slowly for adults or 0.5 mg I.V. slowly for children) may be indicated in reversing cardiac arrhythmias that are due to vagal blockade or for anticholinergic effects, but should only be used as a last measure in life-threatening situations. Seizures usually respond to diazepam I.V. boluses (5-10 mg for adults up to 30 mg or 0.25-0.4 mg/kg/dose for children up to 10 mg/dose). If seizures are unresponsive or recur, phenytoin or phenobarbital may be required.

Drug Interactions CYP1A2, 2C9, 2C19, 2D6, and 3A3/4 enzyme substrate

Altretamine: Concurrent use may cause orthostatic hypertension

Amphetamines: TCAs may enhance the effect of amphetamines; monitor for adverse CV effects

Anticholinergics: Combined use with TCAs may produce additive anticholinergic effects

Antihypertensives: Amitriptyline inhibits the antihypertensive response to bethanidine, clonidine, debrisoquin, guanadrel, guanethidine, guanabenz, guanfacine; monitor BP; consider alternate antihypertensive agent

Beta-agonists: When combined with TCAs may predispose patients to cardiac arrhythmias

Bupropion: May increase the levels of tricyclic antidepressants. Based on limited information; monitor response

Carbamazepine: Tricyclic antidepressants may increase carbamazepine levels; monitor

Cholestyramine and colestipol: May bind TCAs and reduce their absorption; monitor for altered response

Cisapride: May increase the risk of QT_c prolongation and/or arrhythmia; concurrent use is contraindicated.

Clonidine: Abrupt discontinuation of clonidine may cause hypertensive crisis, amitriptyline may enhance the response (also see note on antihypertensives)

CNS depressants: Sedative effects may be additive with TCAs; monitor for increased effect; includes benzodiazepines, barbiturates, antipsychotics, ethanol, and other sedative medications.

CYP1A2 inhibitors: Metabolism of amitriptyline may be decreased; increasing clinical effect or toxicity; inhibitors include cimetidine, ciprofloxacin, fluvoxamine, isoniazid, ritonavir, and zileuton

CYP2C8/9 inhibitors: Serum levels and/or toxicity of some tricyclic antidepressants may be increased; inhibitors include amiodarone, cimetidine, fluvoxamine, some NSAIDs, metronidazole, ritonavir, sulfonamides, troglitazone, valproic acid, and zafirlukast; monitor for increased effect/toxicity

CYP2C19 inhibitors: Serum levels of amitriptyline may be increased; inhibitors include cimetidine, felbamate, fluconazole, fluoxetine, fluvoxamine, omeprazole, teniposide, tolbutamide, and troglitazone

(Continued)

Amitriptyline *(Continued)*

CYP2D6 inhibitors: Serum levels and/or toxicity of some tricyclic antidepressants may be increased; inhibitors include amiodarone, cimetidine, delavirdine, fluoxetine, paroxetine, propafenone, quinidine, and ritonavir; monitor for increased effect/toxicity

CYP3A3/4 inhibitors: Serum level and/or toxicity of some tricyclic antidepressants may be increased. Inhibitors include amiodarone, cimetidine, clarithromycin, erythromycin, delavirdine, diltiazem, dirithromycin, disulfiram, fluoxetine, fluvoxamine, grapefruit juice, indinavir, itraconazole, ketoconazole, nefazodone, nevirapine, propoxyphene, quinupristin-dalfopristin, ritonavir, saquinavir, verapamil, zafirlukast, zileuton. Monitor for altered effects; a decrease in TCA dosage may be required

Enzyme inducers: May increase the metabolism of amitriptyline resulting in decreased effect; includes carbamazepine, phenobarbital, phenytoin, and rifampin; monitor for decreased response

Epinephrine (and other direct alpha-agonists): Pressor response to I.V. epinephrine, norepinephrine, and phenylephrine may be enhanced in patients receiving TCAs (**Note:** Effect is unlikely with epinephrine or levonordefrin dosages typically administered as infiltration in combination with local anesthetics)

Fenfluramine: May increase tricyclic antidepressant levels/effects

Hypoglycemic agents (including insulin): TCAs may enhance the hypoglycemic effects of tolazamide, chlorpropamide, or insulin; monitor for changes in blood glucose levels; reported with chlorpropamide, tolazamide, and insulin

Levodopa: Tricyclic antidepressants may decrease the absorption (bioavailability) of levodopa; rare hypertensive episodes have also been attributed to this combination

Linezolid: Hyperpyrexia, hypertension, tachycardia, confusion, seizures, and **deaths have been reported** with agents which inhibit MAO (serotonin syndrome); this combination should be avoided

Lithium: Concurrent use with a TCA may increase the risk for neurotoxicity

MAO inhibitors: Hyperpyrexia, hypertension, tachycardia, confusion, seizures, and **deaths have been reported** (serotonin syndrome); this combination should be avoided

Methylphenidate: Metabolism of amitriptyline may be decreased

Phenothiazines: Serum concentrations of some TCAs may be increased; in addition, TCAs may increase concentration of phenothiazines; monitor for altered clinical response

QT_c prolonging agents: Concurrent use of tricyclic agents with other drugs which may prolong QT_c interval may increase the risk of potentially fatal arrhythmias; includes type Ia and type III antiarrhythmics agents, selected quinolones (sparfloxacin, gatifloxacin, moxifloxacin, grepafloxacin), cisapride, and other agents

Sucralfate: Absorption of tricyclic antidepressants may be reduced with coadministration

Sympathomimetics, indirect-acting: Tricyclic antidepressants may result in a decreased sensitivity to indirect-acting sympathomimetics; includes dopamine and ephedrine; also see interaction with epinephrine (and direct-acting sympathomimetics)

Tramadol: Tramadol's risk of seizures may be increased with TCAs

Valproic acid: May increase serum concentrations/adverse effects of some tricyclic antidepressants

Warfarin (and other oral anticoagulants): Amitriptyline may increase the anticoagulant effect in patients stabilized on warfarin; monitor INR

Ethanol/Nutrition/Herb Interactions

Ethanol: Avoid ethanol (may increase CNS depression).

Food: Grapefruit juice may inhibit the metabolism of some TCAs and clinical toxicity may result.

Herb/Nutraceutical: St John's wort may decrease amitriptyline levels. Avoid valerian, St John's wort, kava kava, gotu kola (may increase CNS depression).

Stability Protect injection and Elavil® 10 mg tablets from light

Mechanism of Action Increases the synaptic concentration of serotonin and/or norepinephrine in the central nervous system by inhibition of their reuptake by the presynaptic neuronal membrane

Pharmacodynamics/Kinetics

Onset of therapeutic effect: 7-21 days

Desired therapeutic effect (for depression) may take as long as 4-6 weeks

When used for migraine headache prophylaxis, therapeutic effect may take as long as 6 weeks; a higher dosage may be required in a heavy smoker because of increased metabolism

Distribution: Crosses placenta; enters breast milk

Metabolism: In the liver to nortriptyline (active), hydroxy derivatives, and conjugated derivatives; metabolism may be impaired in the elderly

Half-life: Adults: 9-25 hours (15-hour average)

Time to peak serum concentration: Within 4 hours

Elimination: Renal excretion of 18% as unchanged drug; small amounts eliminated in feces by bile

Usual Dosage

Children:

Chronic pain management (unlabeled use): Oral: Initial: 0.1 mg/kg at bedtime, may advance as tolerated over 2-3 weeks to 0.5-2 mg/kg at bedtime

Depressive disorders (unlabeled use): Oral: Initial doses of 1 mg/kg/day given in 3 divided doses with increases to 1.5 mg/kg/day have been reported in a small number of children (n=9) 9-12 years of age; clinically, doses up to 3 mg/kg/day (5 mg/kg/day if monitored closely) have been proposed

Adolescents: Depressive disorders: Oral: Initial: 25-50 mg/day; may administer in divided doses; increase gradually to 100 mg/day in divided doses

Adults:

Depression:

Oral: 50-150 mg/day single dose at bedtime or in divided doses; dose may be gradually increased up to 300 mg/day

I.M.: 20-30 mg 4 times/day

Pain management (unlabeled use): Oral: Initial: 25 mg at bedtime; may increase as tolerated to 100 mg/day

Dosing interval in hepatic impairment: Use with caution and monitor plasma levels and patient response

Hemodialysis: Nondialyzable

Administration Not recommended for I.V.

Monitoring Parameters Monitor blood pressure and pulse rate prior to and during initial therapy; evaluate mental status; monitor weight; EKG in older adults and patients with cardiac disease

Reference Range Therapeutic: Amitriptyline and nortriptyline 100-250 ng/mL (SI: 360-900 nmol/L); nortriptyline 50-150 ng/mL (SI: 190-570 nmol/L); Toxic: >0.5 µg/mL; plasma levels do not always correlate with clinical effectiveness

Test Interactions ↑ glucose

Patient Information Avoid alcohol ingestion; do not discontinue medication abruptly; may cause urine to turn blue-green; may cause drowsiness; full effect may not occur for 3-6 weeks; dry mouth may be helped by sips of water, sugarless gum, or hard candy

Nursing Implications May increase appetite and possibly a craving for sweets

Dosage Forms

Injection, as hydrochloride: 10 mg/mL (10 mL)

Tablet, as hydrochloride: 10 mg, 25 mg, 50 mg, 75 mg, 100 mg, 150 mg

Amitriptyline and Chlordiazepoxide

(a mee TRIP ti leen & klor dye az e POKS ide)

Related Information

Patient Information - Antidepressants (TCAs) *on page 454*

Patient Information - Anxiolytics & Sedative Hypnotics (Benzodiazepines) *on page 483*

(Continued)

Amitriptyline and Chlordiazepoxide *(Continued)*

U.S. Brand Names Limbitrol®; Limbitrol® DS

Synonyms Chlordiazepoxide and Amitriptyline

Pharmacologic Category Antidepressant, Tricyclic (Tertiary Amine)

Generic Available Yes

Use Treatment of moderate to severe anxiety and/or agitation and depression

Restrictions C-IV

Pregnancy Risk Factor D

Contraindications Hypersensitivity to benzodiazepines, tricyclic antidepressants, or any component of the formulation; depression of CNS; MAO inhibitors; acute recovery phase following myocardial infarction; angle-closure glaucoma; pregnancy

Warnings/Precautions See individual agents

Adverse Reactions See individual agents

Drug Interactions

Based on **amitriptyline** component: CYP1A2, 2C9, 2C19, 2D6, and 3A3/4 enzyme substrate

Altretamine: Concurrent use may cause orthostatic hypertension

Amphetamines: TCAs may enhance the effect of amphetamines; monitor for adverse CV effects

Anticholinergics: Combined use with TCAs may produce additive anticholinergic effects

Antihypertensives: Amitriptyline inhibits the antihypertensive response to bethanidine, clonidine, debrisoquin, guanadrel, guanethidine, guanabenz, guanfacine; monitor BP; consider alternate antihypertensive agent

Beta-agonists: When combined with TCAs may predispose patients to cardiac arrhythmias

Bupropion: May increase the levels of tricyclic antidepressants. Based on limited information; monitor response

Carbamazepine: Tricyclic antidepressants may increase carbamazepine levels; monitor

Cholestyramine and colestipol: May bind TCAs and reduce their absorption; monitor for altered response

Clonidine: Abrupt discontinuation of clonidine may cause hypertensive crisis, amitriptyline may enhance the response (also see note on antihypertensives)

CNS depressants: Sedative effects may be additive with TCAs; monitor for increased effect; includes benzodiazepines, barbiturates, antipsychotics, ethanol, and other sedative medications.

CYP1A2 inhibitors: Metabolism of amitriptyline may be decreased; increasing clinical effect or toxicity; inhibitors include cimetidine, ciprofloxacin, fluvoxamine, isoniazid, ritonavir, and zileuton.

CYP2C8/9 inhibitors: Serum levels and/or toxicity of some tricyclic antidepressants may be increased; inhibitors include amiodarone, cimetidine, fluvoxamine, some NSAIDs, metronidazole, ritonavir, sulfonamides, troglitazone, valproic acid, and zafirlukast; monitor for increased effect/toxicity

CYP2C19 inhibitors: Serum levels of amitriptyline may be increased; inhibitors include cimetidine, felbamate, fluconazole, fluoxetine, fluvoxamine, omeprazole, teniposide, tolbutamide, and troglitazone

CYP2D6 inhibitors: Serum levels and/or toxicity of some tricyclic antidepressants may be increased; inhibitors include amiodarone, cimetidine, delavirdine, fluoxetine, paroxetine, propafenone, quinidine, and ritonavir; monitor for increased effect/toxicity

CYP3A3/4 inhibitors: Serum level and/or toxicity of some tricyclic antidepressants may be increased. Inhibitors include amiodarone, cimetidine, clarithromycin, erythromycin, delavirdine, diltiazem, dirithromycin, disulfiram, fluoxetine, fluvoxamine, grapefruit juice, indinavir, itraconazole, ketoconazole, nefazodone, nevirapine, propoxyphene, quinupristin-dalfopristin, ritonavir, saquinavir, verapamil, zafirlukast, zileuton. Monitor for altered effects; a decrease in TCA dosage may be required

Enzyme inducers: May increase the metabolism of amitriptyline resulting in decreased effect; includes carbamazepine, phenobarbital, phenytoin, and rifampin; monitor for decreased response

Epinephrine (and other direct alpha-agonists): Pressor response to I.V. epinephrine, norepinephrine, and phenylephrine may be enhanced in patients receiving TCAs (**Note:** Effect is unlikely with epinephrine or levonordefrin dosages typically administered as infiltration in combination with local anesthetics)

Fenfluramine: May increase tricyclic antidepressant levels/effects

Hypoglycemic agents (including insulin): TCAs may enhance the hypoglycemic effects of tolazamide, chlorpropamide, or insulin; monitor for changes in blood glucose levels; reported with chlorpropamide, tolazamide, and insulin

Levodopa: Tricyclic antidepressants may decrease the absorption (bioavailability) of levodopa; rare hypertensive episodes have also been attributed to this combination

Linezolid: Hyperpyrexia, hypertension, tachycardia, confusion, seizures, and **deaths have been reported** with agents which inhibit MAO (serotonin syndrome); this combination should be avoided

Lithium: Concurrent use with a TCA may increase the risk for neurotoxicity

MAO inhibitors: Hyperpyrexia, hypertension, tachycardia, confusion, seizures, and **deaths have been reported** (serotonin syndrome); this combination should be avoided

Methylphenidate: Metabolism of amitriptyline may be decreased

Phenothiazines: Serum concentrations of some TCAs may be increased; in addition, TCAs may increase concentration of phenothiazines; monitor for altered clinical response

QT_c-prolonging agents: Concurrent use of tricyclic agents with other drugs which may prolong QT_c interval may increase the risk of potentially fatal arrhythmias; includes type Ia and type III antiarrhythmics agents, selected quinolones (sparfloxacin, gatifloxacin, moxifloxacin, grepafloxacin), cisapride, and other agents

Sucralfate: Absorption of tricyclic antidepressants may be reduced with coadministration

Sympathomimetics, indirect-acting: Tricyclic antidepressants may result in a decreased sensitivity to indirect-acting sympathomimetics; includes dopamine and ephedrine; also see interaction with epinephrine (and direct-acting sympathomimetics)

Tramadol: Tramadol's risk of seizures may be increased with TCAs

Valproic acid: May increase serum concentrations/adverse effects of some tricyclic antidepressants

Warfarin (and other oral anticoagulants): Amitriptyline may increase the anticoagulant effect in patients stabilized on warfarin; monitor INR

Based on **chlordiazepoxide** component: CYP3A3/4 enzyme substrate

CNS depressants: Sedative effects and/or respiratory depression may be additive with CNS depressants; includes ethanol, barbiturates, narcotic analgesics, and other sedative agents; monitor for increased effect

CYP enzyme inducers: Metabolism of some benzodiazepines may be increased, decreasing their therapeutic effect; consider using an alternative sedative/hypnotic agent; potential inducers include phenobarbital, phenytoin, carbamazepine, rifampin, and rifabutin

CYP3A3/4 inhibitors: Serum level and/or toxicity of some benzodiazepines may be increased; inhibitors include amiodarone, cimetidine, clarithromycin, erythromycin, delavirdine, diltiazem, dirithromycin, disulfiram, fluoxetine, fluvoxamine, grapefruit juice, indinavir, itraconazole, ketoconazole, nevirapine, propoxyphene, quinupristin-dalfopristin, ritonavir, saquinavir, verapamil, zafirlukast, zileuton; monitor for altered benzodiazepine response

Levodopa: Therapeutic effects may be diminished in some patients following the addition of a benzodiazepine; limited/inconsistent data

Oral contraceptives: May decrease the clearance of some benzodiazepines (those which undergo oxidative metabolism); monitor for increased benzodiazepine effect

(Continued)

Amitriptyline and Chlordiazepoxide *(Continued)*

Theophylline: May partially antagonize some of the effects of benzodiazepines; monitor for decreased response; may require higher doses for sedation

Usual Dosage Initial: 3-4 tablets in divided doses; this may be increased to 6 tablets/day as required; some patients respond to smaller doses and can be maintained on 2 tablets

Dosage Forms

Tablet:

5-12.5: Amitriptyline hydrochloride 12.5 mg and chlordiazepoxide 5 mg

10-25: Amitriptyline hydrochloride 25 mg and chlordiazepoxide 10 mg

Amitriptyline and Perphenazine

(a mee TRIP ti leen & per FEN a zeen)

Related Information

Patient Information - Antidepressants (TCAs) *on page 454*

U.S. Brand Names Etrafon®; Triavil®

Canadian Brand Names Elavil Plus®

Synonyms Perphenazine and Amitriptyline

Pharmacologic Category Antidepressant, Tricyclic (Tertiary Amine); Antipsychotic Agent, Phenothiazine, Piperazine

Generic Available Yes

Use Treatment of patients with moderate to severe anxiety and depression

Unlabeled/Investigational Use Depression with psychotic features

Pregnancy Risk Factor D

Contraindications Hypersensitivity to amitriptyline, perphenazine, or any component of the formulation (cross-sensitivity with other phenothiazines may exist); pregnancy; angle-closure glaucoma; bone marrow depression; severe liver or cardiac disease

Warnings/Precautions Safe use of tricyclic antidepressants in children <12 years of age has not been established; amitriptyline should not be abruptly discontinued in patients receiving high doses for prolonged periods; do not drink alcoholic beverages

Adverse Reactions

Based on **amitriptyline** component: Anticholinergic effects may be pronounced; moderate to marked sedation can occur (tolerance to these effects usually occurs).

Cardiovascular: Orthostatic hypotension, tachycardia, nonspecific EKG changes, changes in AV conduction

Central nervous system: Restlessness, dizziness, insomnia, sedation, fatigue, anxiety, impaired cognitive function, seizures, extrapyramidal symptoms

Dermatologic: Allergic rash, urticaria, photosensitivity

Gastrointestinal: Weight gain, xerostomia, constipation

Genitourinary: Urinary retention

Ocular: Blurred vision, mydriasis

Miscellaneous: Diaphoresis

Based on **perphenazine** component:

Cardiovascular: Hypotension, orthostatic hypotension, hypertension, tachycardia, bradycardia, dizziness, cardiac arrest

Central nervous system: Extrapyramidal symptoms (pseudoparkinsonism, akathisia, dystonias, tardive dyskinesia), dizziness, cerebral edema, seizures, headache, drowsiness, paradoxical excitement, restlessness, hyperactivity, insomnia, neuroleptic malignant syndrome (NMS), impairment of temperature regulation

Dermatologic: Increased sensitivity to sun, rash, discoloration of skin (blue-gray)

Endocrine & metabolic: Hypoglycemia, hyperglycemia, galactorrhea, lactation, breast enlargement, gynecomastia, menstrual irregularity, amenorrhea, SIADH, changes in libido

Gastrointestinal: Constipation, weight gain, vomiting, stomach pain, nausea, xerostomia, salivation, diarrhea, anorexia, ileus

Genitourinary: Difficulty in urination, ejaculatory disturbances, incontinence, polyuria, ejaculating dysfunction, priapism

Hematologic: Agranulocytosis, leukopenia, eosinophilia, hemolytic anemia, thrombocytopenic purpura, pancytopenia

Hepatic: Cholestatic jaundice, hepatotoxicity

Neuromuscular & skeletal: Tremor

Ocular: Pigmentary retinopathy, blurred vision, cornea and lens changes

Respiratory: Nasal congestion

Miscellaneous: Diaphoresis

Drug Interactions

Based on **amitriptyline** component: CYP1A2, 2C9, 2C19, 2D6, and 3A3/4 enzyme substrate

Altretamine: Concurrent use may cause orthostatic hypertension

Amphetamines: TCAs may enhance the effect of amphetamines; monitor for adverse CV effects

Anticholinergics: Combined use with TCAs may produce additive anticholinergic effects

Antihypertensives: Amitriptyline inhibits the antihypertensive response to bethanidine, clonidine, debrisoquin, guanadrel, guanethidine, guanabenz, guanfacine; monitor BP; consider alternate antihypertensive agent

Beta-agonists: When combined with TCAs may predispose patients to cardiac arrhythmias

Bupropion: May increase the levels of tricyclic antidepressants. Based on limited information; monitor response

Carbamazepine: Tricyclic antidepressants may increase carbamazepine levels; monitor

Cholestyramine and colestipol: May bind TCAs and reduce their absorption; monitor for altered response

Clonidine: Abrupt discontinuation of clonidine may cause hypertensive crisis, amitriptyline may enhance the response (also see note on antihypertensives)

CNS depressants: Sedative effects may be additive with TCAs; monitor for increased effect; includes benzodiazepines, barbiturates, antipsychotics, ethanol, and other sedative medications

CYP1A2 inhibitors: Metabolism of amitriptyline may be decreased; increasing clinical effect or toxicity; inhibitors include cimetidine, ciprofloxacin, fluvoxamine, isoniazid, ritonavir, and zileuton

CYP2C8/9 inhibitors: Serum levels and/or toxicity of some tricyclic antidepressants may be increased; inhibitors include amiodarone, cimetidine, fluvoxamine, some NSAIDs, metronidazole, ritonavir, sulfonamides, troglitazone, valproic acid, and zafirlukast; monitor for increased effect/toxicity

CYP2C19 inhibitors: Serum levels of amitriptyline may be increased; inhibitors include cimetidine, felbamate, fluconazole, fluoxetine, fluvoxamine, omeprazole, teniposide, tolbutamide, and troglitazone

CYP2D6 inhibitors: Serum levels and/or toxicity of some tricyclic antidepressants may be increased; inhibitors include amiodarone, cimetidine, delavirdine, fluoxetine, paroxetine, propafenone, quinidine, and ritonavir; monitor for increased effect/toxicity

CYP3A4 inhibitors: Serum level and/or toxicity of some tricyclic antidepressants may be increased. Inhibitors include amiodarone, cimetidine, clarithromycin, erythromycin, delavirdine, diltiazem, dirithromycin, disulfiram, fluoxetine, fluvoxamine, grapefruit juice, indinavir, itraconazole, ketoconazole, nefazodone, nevirapine, propoxyphene, quinupristin-dalfopristin, ritonavir, saquinavir, verapamil, zafirlukast, zileuton. Monitor for altered effects; a decrease in TCA dosage may be required

Enzyme inducers: May increase the metabolism of amitriptyline resulting in decreased effect; includes carbamazepine, phenobarbital, phenytoin, and rifampin; monitor for decreased response

(Continued)

Amitriptyline and Perphenazine *(Continued)*

Epinephrine (and other direct alpha-agonists): Pressor response to I.V. epinephrine, norepinephrine, and phenylephrine may be enhanced in patients receiving TCAs (**Note:** Effect is unlikely with epinephrine or levonordefrin dosages typically administered as infiltration in combination with local anesthetics)

Fenfluramine: May increase tricyclic antidepressant levels/effects

Hypoglycemic agents (including insulin): TCAs may enhance the hypoglycemic effects of tolazamide, chlorpropamide, or insulin; monitor for changes in blood glucose levels; reported with chlorpropamide, tolazamide, and insulin

Levodopa: Tricyclic antidepressants may decrease the absorption (bioavailability) of levodopa; rare hypertensive episodes have also been attributed to this combination

Linezolid: Hyperpyrexia, hypertension, tachycardia, confusion, seizures, and **deaths have been reported** with agents which inhibit MAO (serotonin syndrome); this combination should be avoided

Lithium: Concurrent use with a TCA may increase the risk for neurotoxicity

MAO inhibitors: Hyperpyrexia, hypertension, tachycardia, confusion, seizures, and **deaths have been reported** (serotonin syndrome); this combination should be avoided

Methylphenidate: Metabolism of amitriptyline may be decreased

Phenothiazines: Serum concentrations of some TCAs may be increased; in addition, TCAs may increase concentration of phenothiazines; monitor for altered clinical response

QT$_c$-prolonging agents: Concurrent use of tricyclic agents with other drugs which may prolong QT$_c$ interval may increase the risk of potentially fatal arrhythmias; includes type Ia and type III antiarrhythmics agents, selected quinolones (sparfloxacin, gatifloxacin, moxifloxacin, grepafloxacin), cisapride, and other agents

Sucralfate: Absorption of tricyclic antidepressants may be reduced with coadministration

Sympathomimetics, indirect-acting: Tricyclic antidepressants may result in a decreased sensitivity to indirect-acting sympathomimetics; includes dopamine and ephedrine; also see interaction with epinephrine (and direct-acting sympathomimetics)

Tramadol: Tramadol's risk of seizures may be increased with TCAs

Valproic acid: May increase serum concentrations/adverse effects of some tricyclic antidepressants

Warfarin (and other oral anticoagulants): Amitriptyline may increase the anticoagulant effect in patients stabilized on warfarin; monitor INR

Based on **perphenazine** component: CYP2D6 enzyme substrate; CYP2D6 enzyme inhibitor

Aluminum salts: May decrease the absorption of phenothiazines; monitor

Amphetamines: Efficacy may be diminished by antipsychotics; in addition, amphetamines may increase psychotic symptoms; avoid concurrent use

Anticholinergics: May inhibit the therapeutic response to phenothiazines and excess anticholinergic effects may occur; includes benztropine, trihexyphenidyl, biperiden, and drugs with significant anticholinergic activity (TCAs, antihistamines, disopyramide)

Antihypertensives: Concurrent use of phenothiazines with an antihypertensive may produce additive hypotensive effects (particularly orthostasis)

Bromocriptine: Phenothiazines inhibit the ability of bromocriptine to lower serum prolactin concentrations

CNS depressants: Sedative effects may be additive with phenothiazines; monitor for increased effect; includes barbiturates, benzodiazepines, narcotic analgesics, ethanol, and other sedative agents

CYP2D6 inhibitors: Metabolism of phenothiazines may be decreased; increasing clinical effect or toxicity; inhibitors include amiodarone, cimetidine, delavirdine, fluoxetine, paroxetine, propafenone, quinidine, and ritonavir; monitor for increased effect/toxicity

Enzyme inducers: May enhance the hepatic metabolism of phenothiazines; larger doses may be required; includes rifampin, rifabutin, barbiturates, phenytoin, and cigarette smoking

Epinephrine: Chlorpromazine (and possibly other low potency antipsychotics) may diminish the pressor effects of epinephrine

Guanethidine and guanadrel: Antihypertensive effects may be inhibited by phenothiazines

Levodopa: Phenothiazines may inhibit the antiparkinsonian effect of levodopa; avoid this combination

Lithium: Phenothiazines may produce neurotoxicity with lithium; this is a rare effect

Phenytoin: May reduce serum levels of phenothiazines; phenothiazines may increase phenytoin serum levels

Propranolol: Serum concentrations of phenothiazines may be increased; propranolol also increases phenothiazine concentrations

Polypeptide antibiotics: Rare cases of respiratory paralysis have been reported with concurrent use of phenothiazines

QT_c prolonging agents: Effects on QT_c interval may be additive with phenothiazines, increasing the risk of malignant arrhythmias; includes type Ia antiarrhythmics, TCAs, and some quinolone antibiotics (sparfloxacin, moxifloxacin, and gatifloxacin)

Sulfadoxine-pyrimethamine: May increase phenothiazine concentrations

Tricyclic antidepressants: Concurrent use may produce increased toxicity or altered therapeutic response

Trazodone: Phenothiazines and trazodone may produce additive hypotensive effects

Valproic acid: Serum levels may be increased by phenothiazines

Ethanol/Nutrition/Herb Interactions Ethanol: Avoid ethanol (due to increased sedation)

Usual Dosage Oral: 1 tablet 2-4 times/day

Monitoring Parameters Blood pressure and pulse rate prior to and during initial therapy; evaluate mental status; monitor weight; extrapyramidal symptoms

Patient Information Do not drink alcoholic beverages

Nursing Implications Monitor blood pressure and pulse rate prior to and during initial therapy; evaluate mental status; monitor weight; may increase appetite and possibly a craving for sweets; offer patient sugarless hard candy for dry mouth

Dosage Forms
Tablet:
2-10: Amitriptyline hydrochloride 10 mg and perphenazine 2 mg
4-10: Amitriptyline hydrochloride 10 mg and perphenazine 4 mg
2-25: Amitriptyline hydrochloride 25 mg and perphenazine 2 mg
4-25: Amitriptyline hydrochloride 25 mg and perphenazine 4 mg
4-50: Amitriptyline hydrochloride 50 mg and perphenazine 4 mg

♦ **Amitriptyline Hydrochloride** see Amitriptyline on page 22

Amobarbital (am oh BAR bi tal)
Related Information
Anxiolytic/Hypnotic Use in Long-Term Care Facilities on page 562
Federal OBRA Regulations Recommended Maximum Doses on page 583
Patient Information - Anxiolytics & Sedative Hypnotics (Barbiturates) on page 485
U.S. Brand Names Amytal®
Canadian Brand Names Amobarbital®
Synonyms Amylobarbitone
Pharmacologic Category Barbiturate
Generic Available Yes: Capsule
Use
Oral: Hypnotic in short-term treatment of insomnia; reduce anxiety and provide sedation preoperatively
(Continued)

Amobarbital *(Continued)*

I.M., I.V.: Control status epilepticus or acute seizure episodes; control acute episodes of agitated behavior in psychosis and in "Amytal® Interviewing" for narcoanalysis

Restrictions C-II

Pregnancy Risk Factor D

Contraindications Hypersensitivity to barbiturates or any component of the formulation; marked hepatic impairment; dyspnea or airway obstruction; porphyria

Warnings/Precautions Safety has not been established in children <6 years of age. Use with caution in patients with CHF, hepatic or renal impairment, hypovolemic shock; when administered I.V., respiratory depression and hypotension are possible, have equipment and personnel available; this I.V. medication should be given only to hospitalized patients. Do not administer to patients in acute pain. Use caution in elderly, debilitated, renally impaired, hepatic impairment, or pediatric patients. May cause paradoxical responses, including agitation and hyperactivity, particularly in acute pain and pediatric patients. Use with caution in patients with depression or suicidal tendencies, or in patients with a history of drug abuse. Tolerance, psychological and physical dependence may occur with prolonged use. May cause CNS depression, which may impair physical or mental abilities. Patients must be cautioned about performing tasks which require mental alertness (ie, operating machinery or driving). Effects with other sedative drugs or ethanol may be potentiated. Use with caution in patients with hypoadrenalism.

Adverse Reactions

>10%:

Central nervous system: Dizziness, lightheadedness, "hangover" effect, drowsiness, CNS depression, fever

Local: Pain at injection site

1% to 10%:

Central nervous system: Confusion, mental depression, unusual excitement, nervousness, faint feeling, headache, insomnia, nightmares

Gastrointestinal: Nausea, vomiting, constipation

<1%: Agranulocytosis, apnea, exfoliative dermatitis, hallucinations, hypotension, laryngospasm, megaloblastic anemia, rash, respiratory depression, Stevens-Johnson syndrome, thrombocytopenia, thrombophlebitis, urticaria

Overdosage/Toxicology

Signs and symptoms: Unsteady gait, slurred speech, confusion, jaundice, hypothermia, fever, hypotension

Treatment: If hypotension occurs, administer I.V. fluids and place the patient in the Trendelenburg position. If unresponsive, an I.V. vasopressor (eg, dopamine, epinephrine) may be required. Forced alkaline diuresis is of no value in the treatment of intoxications with short-acting barbiturates. Charcoal hemoperfusion or hemodialysis may be useful in the harder to treat intoxications, especially in the presence of very high serum barbiturate levels.

Drug Interactions CYP1A2, 2B6, 2C, 2C8, 2C9, 2C18, 2C19, 3A3/4, and 3A5-7 enzyme inducer. **Note:** Barbiturates are cytochrome P450 enzyme inducers. Patients should be monitored when these drugs are started or stopped for a decreased or increased therapeutic effect respectively.

Acetaminophen: Barbiturates may enhance the hepatotoxic potential of acetaminophen overdoses

Antiarrhythmics: Barbiturates may increase the metabolism of antiarrhythmics, decreasing their clinical effect; includes disopyramide, propafenone, and quinidine

Anticonvulsants: Barbiturates may increase the metabolism of anticonvulsants; includes ethosuximide, felbamate (possibly), lamotrigine, phenytoin, tiagabine, topiramate, and zonisamide; does not appear to affect gabapentin or levetiracetam

Antineoplastics: Limited evidence suggests that enzyme-inducing anticonvulsant therapy may reduce the effectiveness of some chemotherapy regimens (specifically in ALL); teniposide and methotrexate may be cleared more rapidly in these patients

Antipsychotics: Barbiturates may enhance the metabolism (decrease the efficacy) of antipsychotics; monitor for altered response; dose adjustment may be needed

Beta-blockers: Metabolism of beta-blockers may be increased and clinical effect decreased; atenolol and nadolol are unlikely to interact given their renal elimination

Calcium channel blockers: Barbiturates may enhance the metabolism of calcium channel blockers, decreasing their clinical effect

Chloramphenicol: Barbiturates may increase the metabolism of chloramphenicol and chloramphenicol may inhibit barbiturate metabolism; monitor for altered response

Cimetidine: Barbiturates may enhance the metabolism of cimetidine, decreasing its clinical effect

CNS depressants: Sedative effects and/or respiratory depression with barbiturates may be additive with other CNS depressants; monitor for increased effect; includes ethanol, sedatives, antidepressants, narcotic analgesics, and benzodiazepines

Corticosteroids: Barbiturates may enhance the metabolism of corticosteroids, decreasing their clinical effect

Cyclosporine: Levels may be decreased by barbiturates; monitor

Doxycycline: Barbiturates may enhance the metabolism of doxycycline, decreasing its clinical effect; higher dosages may be required

Estrogens: Barbiturates may increase the metabolism of estrogens and reduce their efficacy

Felbamate may inhibit the metabolism of barbiturates and barbiturates may increase the metabolism of felbamate

Griseofulvin: Barbiturates may impair the absorption of griseofulvin, and griseofulvin metabolism may be increased by barbiturates, decreasing clinical effect

Guanfacine: Effect may be decreased by barbiturates

Immunosuppressants: Barbiturates may enhance the metabolism of immunosuppressants, decreasing its clinical effect; includes both cyclosporine and tacrolimus

Loop diuretics: Metabolism may be increased and clinical effects decreased; established for furosemide, effect with other loop diuretics not established

MAO inhibitors: Metabolism of barbiturates may be inhibited, increasing clinical effect or toxicity of the barbiturates

Methadone: Barbiturates may enhance the metabolism of methadone resulting in methadone withdrawal

Methoxyflurane: Barbiturates may enhance the nephrotoxic effects of methoxyflurane

Oral contraceptives: Barbiturates may enhance the metabolism of oral contraceptives, decreasing their clinical effect; an alternative method of contraception should be considered

Theophylline: Barbiturates may increase metabolism of theophylline derivatives and decrease their clinical effect

Tricyclic antidepressants: Barbiturates may increase metabolism of tricyclic antidepressants and decrease their clinical effect; sedative effects may be additive

Valproic acid: Metabolism of barbiturates may be inhibited by valproic acid; monitor for excessive sedation; a dose reduction may be needed

Warfarin: Barbiturates inhibit the hypoprothrombinemic effects of oral anticoagulants via increased metabolism; this combination should generally be avoided

Ethanol/Nutrition/Herb Interactions Ethanol: Avoid ethanol (may increase CNS depression).

Stability Hydrolyzes when exposed to air; use contents of vial within 30 minutes after constitution; use only clear solution

(Continued)

Amobarbital *(Continued)*

Mechanism of Action Interferes with transmission of impulses from the thalamus to the cortex of the brain resulting in an imbalance in central inhibitory and facilitatory mechanisms

Pharmacodynamics/Kinetics

Onset of action:

Oral: Within 1 hour

I.V.: Within 5 minutes

Distribution: Readily crosses the placenta; small amounts appear in breast milk

Metabolism: Chiefly in the liver by microsomal enzymes

Half-life, biphasic:

Initial: 40 minutes

Terminal: 20 hours

Usual Dosage

Children: Oral:

Sedation: 6 mg/kg/day divided every 6-8 hours

Insomnia: 2 mg/kg or 70 mg/m^2/day in 4 equally divided doses

Hypnotic: 2-3 mg/kg

Adults:

Insomnia: Oral: 65-200 mg at bedtime

Sedation: Oral: 30-50 mg 2-3 times/day

Preanesthetic: Oral: 200 mg 1-2 hours before surgery

Hypnotic:

Oral: 65-200 mg at bedtime

I.M., I.V.: 65-500 mg, should not exceed 500 mg I.M. or 1000 mg I.V.

Acute episode of agitated behavior:

Oral: 30-50 mg 2-3 times/day

I.M., I.V.: 65-500 mg, should not exceed 500 mg I.M. or 1000 mg I.V.

Status epilepticus/acute seizure episode: I.M., I.V.: 65-500 mg, should not exceed 500 mg I.M. or 1000 mg I.V.

Amobarbital (Amytal®) interview: I.V.: 50 mg/minute for total dose up to 300 mg

Administration I.M. injection should be deep to prevent against pain, sterile abscess, and sloughing

Monitoring Parameters Vital signs should be monitored during injection and for several hours after administration

Reference Range

Therapeutic: 1-5 µg/mL (SI: 4-22 µmol/L)

Toxic: >10 µg/mL (SI: >44 µmol/L)

Lethal: >50 µg/mL

Test Interactions ↑ ammonia (B); ↓ bilirubin (S)

Patient Information Avoid alcohol ingestion; physical dependency may result when used for an extended period of time (1-3 months); do not try to get out of bed without assistance, will cause drowsiness

Nursing Implications Raise bed rails at night

Dosage Forms

Capsule, as sodium: 65 mg, 200 mg

Injection, as sodium: 250 mg, 500 mg

Tablet: 30 mg, 50 mg, 100 mg

Amobarbital and Secobarbital

(am oh BAR bi tal & see koe BAR bi tal)

Related Information

Patient Information - Anxiolytics & Sedative Hypnotics (Barbiturates) *on page 485*

U.S. Brand Names Tuinal®

Canadian Brand Names Tuinal

Synonyms Secobarbital and Amobarbital

Pharmacologic Category Barbiturate

Generic Available No

Use Short-term treatment of insomnia

Restrictions C-II

Pregnancy Risk Factor D

Contraindications Hypersensitivity to secobarbital, amobarbital, or any component of the formulation; CNS depression; marked liver impairment; latent porphyria

Warnings/Precautions Safety has not been established in children <6 years of age; potential for drug dependency exists; avoid alcoholic beverages; use with caution in patients with CHF, hepatic or renal impairment; hypovolemic shock

Adverse Reactions

>10%:

Central nervous system: Dizziness, lightheadedness, drowsiness, "hangover" effect

Local: Pain at injection site

1% to 10%:

Central nervous system: Confusion, mental depression, unusual excitement, nervousness, faint feeling, headache, insomnia, nightmares

Gastrointestinal: Constipation, nausea, vomiting

<1%: Agranulocytosis, dermatitis, exfoliative, hallucinations, hypotension, megaloblastic anemia, respiratory depression, skin rash, Stevens-Johnson syndrome, thrombocytopenia, thrombophlebitis

Drug Interactions Amobarbital: CYP1A2, 2B6, 2C, 2C8, 2C9, 2C18, 2C19, 3A3/4, and 3A5-7 enzyme inducer. **Note:** Barbiturates are cytochrome P450 enzyme inducers. Patients should be monitored when these drugs are started or stopped for a decreased or increased therapeutic effect respectively.

Acetaminophen: Barbiturates may enhance the hepatotoxic potential of acetaminophen overdoses

Antiarrhythmics: Barbiturates may increase the metabolism of antiarrhythmics, decreasing their clinical effect; includes disopyramide, propafenone, and quinidine

Anticonvulsants: Barbiturates may increase the metabolism of anticonvulsants; includes ethosuximide, felbamate (possibly), lamotrigine, phenytoin, tiagabine, topiramate, and zonisamide; does not appear to affect gabapentin or levetiracetam

Antineoplastics: Limited evidence suggests that enzyme-inducing anticonvulsant therapy may reduce the effectiveness of some chemotherapy regimens (specifically in ALL); teniposide and methotrexate may be cleared more rapidly in these patients

Antipsychotics: Barbiturates may enhance the metabolism (decrease the efficacy) of antipsychotics; monitor for altered response; dose adjustment may be needed

Beta-blockers: Metabolism of beta-blockers may be increased and clinical effect decreased. Atenolol and nadolol are unlikely to interact given their renal elimination.

Calcium channel blockers: Barbiturates may enhance the metabolism of calcium channel blockers, decreasing their clinical effect

Chloramphenicol: Barbiturates may increase the metabolism of chloramphenicol and chloramphenicol may inhibit barbiturate metabolism; monitor for altered response

Cimetidine: Barbiturates may enhance the metabolism of cimetidine, decreasing its clinical effect

CNS depressants: Sedative effects and/or respiratory depression with barbiturates may be additive with other CNS depressants; monitor for increased effect; includes ethanol, sedatives, antidepressants, narcotic analgesics, and benzodiazepines

Corticosteroids: Barbiturates may enhance the metabolism of corticosteroids, decreasing their clinical effect

Cyclosporine: Levels may be decreased by barbiturates; monitor

Doxycycline: Barbiturates may enhance the metabolism of doxycycline, decreasing its clinical effect; higher dosages may be required

(Continued)

Amobarbital and Secobarbital *(Continued)*

Estrogens: Barbiturates may increase the metabolism of estrogens and reduce their efficacy

Felbamate may inhibit the metabolism of barbiturates and barbiturates may increase the metabolism of felbamate

Griseofulvin: Barbiturates may impair the absorption of griseofulvin, and griseofulvin metabolism may be increased by barbiturates, decreasing clinical effect

Guanfacine: Effect may be decreased by barbiturates

Immunosuppressants: Barbiturates may enhance the metabolism of immunosuppressants, decreasing its clinical effect; includes both cyclosporine and tacrolimus

Loop diuretics: Metabolism may be increased and clinical effects decreased; established for furosemide, effect with other loop diuretics not established

MAO inhibitors: Metabolism of barbiturates may be inhibited, increasing clinical effect or toxicity of the barbiturates

Methadone: Barbiturates may enhance the metabolism of methadone resulting in methadone withdrawal

Methoxyflurane: Barbiturates may enhance the nephrotoxic effects of methoxyflurane

Oral contraceptives: Barbiturates may enhance the metabolism of oral contraceptives, decreasing their clinical effect; an alternative method of contraception should be considered

Theophylline: Barbiturates may increase metabolism of theophylline derivatives and decrease their clinical effect

Tricyclic antidepressants: Barbiturates may increase metabolism of tricyclic antidepressants and decrease their clinical effect; sedative effects may be additive

Valproic acid: Metabolism of barbiturates may be inhibited by valproic acid; monitor for excessive sedation; a dose reduction may be needed

Warfarin: Barbiturates inhibit the hypoprothrombinemic effects of oral anticoagulants via increased metabolism; this combination should generally be avoided

Usual Dosage Adults: Oral: 1-2 capsules at bedtime

Dosage Forms

Capsule:

100: Amobarbital 50 mg and secobarbital 50 mg

200: Amobarbital 100 mg and secobarbital 100 mg

Amoxapine *(a MOKS a peen)*

Related Information

Antidepressant Agents Comparison Chart *on page 553*

Discontinuation of Psychotropic Drugs - Withdrawal Symptoms and Recommendations *on page 582*

Federal OBRA Regulations Recommended Maximum Doses *on page 583*

Patient Information - Antidepressants (TCAs) *on page 454*

Teratogenic Risks of Psychotropic Medications *on page 594*

U.S. Brand Names Asendin®

Canadian Brand Names Asendin

Pharmacologic Category Antidepressant, Tricyclic (Secondary Amine)

Generic Available Yes

Use Treatment of depression, psychotic depression, depression accompanied by anxiety or agitation

Pregnancy Risk Factor C

Contraindications Hypersensitivity to amoxapine or any component of the formulation; use of MAO inhibitors within past 14 days; recovery from acute myocardial infarction

Warnings/Precautions May cause sedation, resulting in impaired performance of tasks requiring alertness (ie, operating machinery or driving). Sedative effects may be additive with other CNS depressants and/or ethanol. The degree of sedation is moderate relative to other antidepressants. May worsen psychosis in some patients or precipitate a shift to mania or hypomania in patients with bipolar disease. May increase the risks associated with electroconvulsive therapy. This agent should be discontinued, when possible, prior to elective surgery. Therapy should not be abruptly discontinued in patients receiving high doses for prolonged periods.

May cause extrapyramidal reactions, including pseudoparkinsonism, acute dystonic reactions, akathisia, and tardive dyskinesia (risk of these reactions is low). May be associated with neuroleptic malignant syndrome.

May cause orthostatic hypotension (risk is moderate relative to other antidepressants) - use with caution in patients at risk of hypotension or in patients where transient hypotensive episodes would be poorly tolerated (cardiovascular disease or cerebrovascular disease). The degree of anticholinergic blockade produced by this agent is moderate relative to other cyclic antidepressants - use caution in patients with urinary retention, benign prostatic hypertrophy, narrow-angle glaucoma, xerostomia, visual problems, constipation, or history of bowel obstruction.

Use caution in patients with depression, particularly if suicidal risk may be present. Use with caution in patients with a history of cardiovascular disease (including previous MI, stroke, tachycardia, or conduction abnormalities). The risk conduction abnormalities with this agent is moderate relative to other antidepressants. May lower seizure threshold - use caution in patients with a previous seizure disorder or condition predisposing to seizures such as brain damage, alcoholism, or concurrent therapy with other drugs which lower the seizure threshold. Use with caution in hyperthyroid patients or those receiving thyroid supplementation. Use with caution in patients with hepatic or renal dysfunction and in elderly patients.

Adverse Reactions

>10%:
    Central nervous system: Drowsiness
    Gastrointestinal: Xerostomia, constipation
1% to 10%:
    Central nervous system: Dizziness, headache, confusion, nervousness, restlessness, insomnia, ataxia, excitement, anxiety
    Dermatologic: Edema, skin rash
    Endocrine: Elevated prolactin levels
    Gastrointestinal: Nausea
    Neuromuscular & skeletal: Tremor, weakness
    Ocular: Blurred vision
    Miscellaneous: Diaphoresis
<1%: Abdominal pain, abnormal taste, agranulocytosis, allergic reactions, breast enlargement, delayed micturition, diarrhea, elevated liver enzymes, epigastric distress, extrapyramidal symptoms, flatulence, galactorrhea, hypertension, hypotension, impotence, incoordination, increased intraocular pressure, increased or decreased libido, lacrimation, leukopenia, menstrual irregularity, mydriasis, nasal stuffiness, neuroleptic malignant syndrome, numbness, painful ejaculation, paresthesia, photosensitivity, seizures, SIADH, syncope, tachycardia, tardive dyskinesia, testicular edema, tinnitus, urinary retention, vomiting

Overdosage/Toxicology

Signs and symptoms: Grand mal convulsions, acidosis, coma, renal failure

Treatment: Following initiation of essential overdose management, toxic symptoms should be treated. Ventricular arrhythmias often respond to phenytoin 15-20 mg/kg (adults) with concurrent systemic alkalinization (sodium bicarbonate 0.5-2 mEq/kg I.V.). Arrhythmias unresponsive to this therapy may respond to lidocaine 1mg/kg I.V. followed by a titrated infusion. Physostigmine (1-2 mg I.V. slowly for adults or 0.5 mg I.V. slowly for children) may be indicated in reversing cardiac arrhythmias that are due to vagal blockade or for anticholinergic effects, but should only be used as a last measure in life-threatening situations. Seizures usually respond to diazepam I.V. boluses (5-10 mg for adults up to 30 mg or 0.25-0.4 mg/kg/dose for children up to 10 mg/dose). If seizures are unresponsive or recur, phenytoin or phenobarbital may be required.

Drug Interactions CYP1A2, 2C9, 2C19, 2D6, and 3A3/4 enzyme substrate

(Continued)

Amoxapine *(Continued)*

Anticholinergics: Combined use with TCAs may produce additive anticholinergic effects

Altretamine: Concurrent use may cause orthostatic hypertension

Amphetamines: TCAs may enhance the effect of amphetamines; monitor for adverse CV effects

Antihypertensives: Amitriptyline inhibits the antihypertensive response to bethanidine, clonidine, debrisoquin, guanadrel, guanethidine, guanabenz, guanfacine; monitor BP; consider alternate antihypertensive agent

Beta-agonists: When combined with TCAs may predispose patients to cardiac arrhythmias

Bupropion: May increase the levels of tricyclic antidepressants; based on limited information; monitor response

Carbamazepine: Tricyclic antidepressants may increase carbamazepine levels; monitor

Cholestyramine and colestipol: May bind TCAs and reduce their absorption; monitor for altered response

Clonidine: Abrupt discontinuation of clonidine may cause hypertensive crisis, amitriptyline may enhance the response

CNS depressants: Sedative effects may be additive with TCAs; monitor for increased effect; includes benzodiazepines, barbiturates, antipsychotics, ethanol and other sedative medications

CYP1A2 inhibitors: Metabolism of amoxapine may be decreased, increasing clinical effect or toxicity; inhibitors include cimetidine, ciprofloxacin, fluvoxamine, isoniazid, ritonavir, and zileuton

CYP2C8/9 inhibitors: Serum levels and/or toxicity of some tricyclic antidepressants may be increased; inhibitors include amiodarone, cimetidine, fluvoxamine, some NSAIDs, metronidazole, ritonavir, sulfonamides, troglitazone, valproic acid, and zafirlukast; monitor for increased effect/toxicity

CYP2C19 inhibitors: Serum levels of some cyclic antidepressants may be increased; inhibitors include cimetidine, felbamate, fluconazole, fluoxetine, fluvoxamine, omeprazole, teniposide, tolbutamide, and troglitazone

CYP2D6 inhibitors: Serum levels and/or toxicity of some tricyclic antidepressants may be increased; inhibitors include amiodarone, cimetidine, delavirdine, fluoxetine, paroxetine, propafenone, quinidine, and ritonavir. Monitor for increased effect/toxicity

CYP3A3/4 inhibitors: Serum level and/or toxicity of some tricyclic antidepressants may be increased; inhibitors include amiodarone, cimetidine, clarithromycin, erythromycin, delavirdine, diltiazem, dirithromycin, disulfiram, fluoxetine, fluvoxamine, grapefruit juice, indinavir, itraconazole, ketoconazole, nevirapine, propoxyphene, quinupristin-dalfopristin, ritonavir, saquinavir, verapamil, zafirlukast, zileuton; monitor for altered effects; a decrease in TCA dosage may be required

Enzyme inducers: May increase the metabolism of amitriptyline resulting in decreased effect; includes carbamazepine, phenobarbital, phenytoin, and rifampin; monitor for decreased response

Epinephrine (and other direct alpha-agonists): Pressor response to I.V. epinephrine, norepinephrine, and phenylephrine may be enhanced in patients receiving TCAs (**Note:** Effect is unlikely with epinephrine or levonordefrin dosages typically administered as infiltration in combination with local anesthetics)

Fenfluramine: May increase tricyclic antidepressant levels/effects

Hypoglycemic agents (including insulin): TCAs may enhance the hypoglycemic effects of tolazamide, chlorpropamide, or insulin; monitor for changes in blood glucose levels; reported with chlorpropamide, tolazamide, and insulin

Levodopa: Tricyclic antidepressants may decrease the absorption (bioavailability) of levodopa; rare hypertensive episodes have also been attributed to this combination

Linezolid: Hyperpyrexia, hypertension, tachycardia, confusion, seizures, and **deaths have been reported** with agents which inhibit MAO (serotonin syndrome); this combination should be avoided

Lithium: Concurrent use with a TCA may increase the risk for neurotoxicity

MAO inhibitors: Hyperpyrexia, hypertension, tachycardia, confusion, seizures, and **deaths have been reported** (serotonin syndrome); this combination should be avoided

Methylphenidate: Metabolism of amitriptyline may be decreased

Phenothiazines: Serum concentrations of some TCAs may be increased; in addition, TCAs may increase concentration of phenothiazines; monitor for altered clinical response

QT_c-prolonging agents: Concurrent use of tricyclic agents with other drugs which may prolong QT_c interval may increase the risk of potentially fatal arrhythmias; includes type Ia and type III antiarrhythmics agents, selected quinolones (sparfloxacin, gatifloxacin, moxifloxacin, grepafloxacin), cisapride, and other agents

Sucralfate: Absorption of tricyclic antidepressants may be reduced with coadministration.

Sympathomimetics, indirect-acting: Tricyclic antidepressants may result in a decreased sensitivity to indirect-acting sympathomimetics; includes dopamine and ephedrine; also see interaction with epinephrine (and direct-acting sympathomimetics)

Tramadol: Tramadol's risk of seizures may be increased with TCAs

Valproic acid: May increase serum concentrations/adverse effects of some tricyclic antidepressants

Warfarin (and other oral anticoagulants): Amitriptyline may increase the anticoagulant effect in patients stabilized on warfarin; monitor INR

Ethanol/Nutrition/Herb Interactions

Ethanol: Avoid ethanol (may increase CNS depression).

Food: Grapefruit juice may inhibit the metabolism of some TCAs and clinical toxicity may result.

Herb/Nutraceutical: Avoid valerian, St John's wort, SAMe, kava kava.

Mechanism of Action Reduces the reuptake of serotonin and norepinephrine. The metabolite, 7-OH-amoxapine has significant dopamine receptor blocking activity similar to haloperidol.

Pharmacodynamics/Kinetics

Onset of antidepressant effect: Usually occurs after 1-2 weeks, but may require 4-6 weeks

Absorption: Oral: Rapidly and well absorbed

Distribution: V_d: 0.9-1.2 L/kg; distributes into breast milk

Protein binding: 80%

Metabolism: Extensive in the liver

Half-life:

Parent drug: 11-16 hours

Active metabolite (8-hydroxy): Adults: 30 hours

Time to peak serum concentration: Within 1-2 hours

Elimination: Excretion of metabolites and parent compound in urine

Usual Dosage Oral:

Children: Not established in children <16 years of age.

Adolescents: Initial: 25-50 mg/day; increase gradually to 100 mg/day; may administer as divided doses or as a single dose at bedtime

Adults: Initial: 25 mg 2-3 times/day, if tolerated, dosage may be increased to 100 mg 2-3 times/day; may be given in a single bedtime dose when dosage <300 mg/day

Elderly: Initial: 25 mg at bedtime increased by 25 mg weekly for outpatients and every 3 days for inpatients if tolerated; usual dose: 50-150 mg/day, but doses up to 300 mg may be necessary

Maximum daily dose:

Inpatient: 600 mg

Outpatient: 400 mg

Monitoring Parameters Monitor blood pressure and pulse rate prior to and during initial therapy evaluate mental status; monitor weight; EKG in older adults

(Continued)

Amoxapine *(Continued)*

Reference Range Therapeutic: Amoxapine: 20-100 ng/mL (SI: 64-319 nmol/L); 8-OH amoxapine: 150-400 ng/mL (SI: 478-1275 nmol/L); both: 200-500 ng/mL (SI: 637-1594 nmol/L)

Test Interactions ↑ glucose

Patient Information Dry mouth may be helped by sips of water, sugarless gum, or hard candy; avoid alcohol; very important to maintain established dosage regimen; photosensitivity to sunlight can occur, do not discontinue abruptly; full effect may not occur for 4-6 weeks; full dosage may be taken at bedtime to avoid daytime sedation

Nursing Implications May increase appetite and possibly a craving for sweets; recognize signs of neuroleptic malignant syndrome and tardive dyskinesia

Additional Information Extrapyramidal reactions and tardive dyskinesia may occur.

Dosage Forms Tablet: 25 mg, 50 mg, 100 mg, 150 mg

Amphetamine *(am FET a meen)*

Related Information

Hallucinogenic Drugs *on page 585*
Patient Information - Stimulants *on page 481*
Stimulant Agents Used for ADHD *on page 593*

Synonyms Amphetamine Sulfate; Racemic Amphetamine Sulfate

Pharmacologic Category Stimulant

Generic Available Yes

Use Treatment of narcolepsy; attention-deficit/hyperactivity disorder (ADHD); exogenous obesity

Unlabeled/Investigational Use Potential augmenting agent for antidepressants; abnormal behavioral syndrome in children (minimal brain dysfunction)

Restrictions C-II

Pregnancy Risk Factor C

Contraindications Hypersensitivity or idiosyncrasy to amphetamine or other sympathomimetic amines. Patients with advanced arteriosclerosis, symptomatic cardiovascular disease, moderate to severe hypertension (stage II or III), hyperthyroidism, glaucoma, diabetes mellitus, agitated states, patients with a history of drug abuse, and during or within 14 days following MAO inhibitor therapy. Stimulant medications are contraindicated for use in children with attention-deficit/hyperactivity disorders and concomitant Tourette's syndrome or tics.

Warnings/Precautions Use with caution in patients with bipolar disorder, cardiovascular disease, seizure disorders, insomnia, porphyria, or mild hypertension (stage I). May exacerbate symptoms of behavior and thought disorder in psychotic patients. Potential for drug dependency exists - avoid abrupt discontinuation in patients who have received for prolonged periods. Stimulant use in children has been associated with growth suppression. Stimulants may unmask tics in individuals with coexisting Tourette's syndrome.

Adverse Reactions

Cardiovascular: Arrhythmia (high dose), palpitations, elevation in blood pressure, tachycardia, chest pain

Central nervous system: Overstimulation, restlessness, insomnia, dizziness, euphoria, dyskinesia, dysphoria, headache, exacerbation of motor incoordination, tics, Tourette's syndrome; may rarely see psychosis

Dermatologic: Urticaria

Endocrine & metabolic: Changes in libido

Gastrointestinal: Xerostomia, unpleasant taste, diarrhea, constipation; anorexia and weight loss may occur as undesirable effects when amphetamines aroused for other than anorectic effect

Genitourinary: Impotence

Neuromuscular & skeletal: Tremor

Miscellaneous: Delayed bone growth

Overdosage/Toxicology Treatment: There is no specific antidote for amphetamine intoxication and the bulk of the treatment is supportive. Hyperactivity and agitation usually respond to reduced sensory input; however, with extreme agitation, haloperidol (2-5 mg I.M. for adults) may be required. Hyperthermia is best treated with external cooling measures, or when severe or unresponsive, muscle paralysis with pancuronium may be needed. Hypertension is usually transient and generally does not require treatment unless severe. For diastolic blood pressures >110 mm Hg, a nitroprusside infusion should be initiated. Seizures usually respond to diazepam IVP and/or phenytoin maintenance regimens.

Drug Interactions CYP2D6 enzyme substrate

Acidifiers: Very large doses of potassium acid phosphate or ammonium chloride may increase the renal elimination of amphetamines due to urinary acidification

Alkalinizers: Large doses of sodium bicarbonate or other alkalinizers may increase renal tubular reabsorption (decreased elimination) and diminish the effect of amphetamine; includes potassium or sodium citrate and acetate

Antipsychotics: Efficacy of amphetamines may be decreased by antipsychotics; in addition, amphetamines may induce an increase in psychotic symptoms in some patients

CYP2D6 inhibitors: Metabolism of amphetamine may be decreased, increasing clinical effect or toxicity; inhibitors include amiodarone, cimetidine, delavirdine, fluoxetine, paroxetine, propafenone, quinidine, and ritonavir; monitor for increased effect/toxicity

Enzyme inducers: Metabolism of amphetamine may be increased, decreasing clinical effect; inducers include barbiturates, carbamazepine, phenytoin, and rifampin

Furazolidone: Amphetamines may induce hypertensive episodes in patients receiving furazolidone

Guanethidine: Amphetamines inhibit the antihypertensive response to guanethidine; probably also may occur with guanadrel

MAO inhibitors: Severe hypertensive episodes have occurred with amphetamine when used in patients receiving MAO inhibitors; concurrent use or use within 14 days is contraindicated

Norepinephrine: Amphetamines may enhance the pressor response to norepinephrine

Sibutramine: Concurrent use of sibutramine and amphetamines may cause severe hypertension and tachycardia; use is contraindicated in product

SSRIs: Amphetamines may increase the potential for serotonin syndrome when used concurrently with selective serotonin reuptake inhibitors (including fluoxetine, fluvoxamine, paroxetine, and sertraline)

Tricyclic antidepressants: Concurrent use of amphetamines with TCAs may result in hypertension and CNS stimulation; avoid this combination

Mechanism of Action The amphetamines are noncatecholamine sympathomimetic amines with CNS stimulant activity. They require breakdown by monoamine oxidase for inactivation; produce central nervous system and respiratory stimulation, a pressor response, mydriasis, bronchodilation, and contraction of the urinary sphincter; thought to have a direct effect on both alpha- and beta-receptor sites in the peripheral system, as well as release stores of norepinephrine in adrenergic nerve terminals. The central nervous system action is thought to occur in the cerebral cortex and reticular activating system. The anorexigenic effect is probably secondary to the CNS-stimulating effect; the site of action is probably the hypothalamic feeding center.

Pharmacodynamics/Kinetics

Onset of action: 1 hour

Duration: 4-24 hours

Usual Dosage Oral:

Narcolepsy:

Children:

6-12 years: 5 mg/day in divided doses; increase by 5 mg at weekly intervals

>12 years: 10 mg/day in divided doses; increase by 10 mg at weekly intervals

Adults: 5-60 mg/day in 2-3 divided doses

(Continued)

Amphetamine *(Continued)*

ADHD: Children:

3-5 years: 2.5 mg/day; increase by 2.5 mg at weekly intervals up to maximum dose of 40 mg/day in divided doses

>6 years: 5 mg/day, increase by 5 mg at weekly intervals up to maximum dose of 40 mg/day in divided doses

Short-term adjunct to exogenous obesity: Children >12 years and Adults: 5-30 mg/day in divided doses

Monitoring Parameters CNS

Reference Range Therapeutic: 20-30 ng/mL; Toxic: >200 ng/mL

Patient Information Take during day to avoid insomnia; do not discontinue abruptly, may cause physical and psychological dependence with prolonged use; sometimes used only during school year to minimize potential long-term effects

Nursing Implications Monitor CNS, dose should not be given in evening or at bedtime

Dosage Forms Tablet, as sulfate: 5 mg, 10 mg

- ♦ **Amphetamine and Dextroamphetamine** *see* Dextroamphetamine and Amphetamine *on page 107*
- ♦ **Amphetamine Sulfate** *see* Amphetamine *on page 40*
- ♦ **Amylobarbitone** *see* Amobarbital *on page 31*
- ♦ **Amytal**® *see* Amobarbital *on page 31*
- ♦ **Anafranil**® *see* Clomipramine *on page 82*
- ♦ **Anergan**® *see* Promethazine *on page 337*
- ♦ **Anexate**® **(Can)** *see* Flumazenil *on page 143*
- ♦ **Anoquan**® *see* Butalbital Compound *on page 59*
- ♦ **Antabuse**® *see* Disulfiram *on page 119*
- ♦ **Anticholinergic Effects of Common Psychotropic Agents** *see page 551*
- ♦ **Antidepressant Agents Comparison Chart** *see page 553*
- ♦ **Antiparkinsonian Agents Comparison Chart** *see page 556*
- ♦ **Antipsychotic Agents Comparison Chart** *see page 557*
- ♦ **Antipsychotic Medication Guidelines** *see page 559*
- ♦ **ANX**® *see* Hydroxyzine *on page 178*
- ♦ **Anxiolytic/Hypnotic Use in Long-Term Care Facilities** *see page 562*
- ♦ **Aphrodyne**™ *see* Yohimbine *on page 436*
- ♦ **Apo**®**-Alpraz (Can)** *see* Alprazolam *on page 16*
- ♦ **Apo**®**-Amitriptyline (Can)** *see* Amitriptyline *on page 22*
- ♦ **Apo**® **Bro ocriptine (Can)** *see* Bromocriptine *on page 49*
- ♦ **Apo**®**-Carbamazepine (Can)** *see* Carbamazepine *on page 61*
- ♦ **Apo**®**-Chlordiazepoxide (Can)** *see* Chlordiazepoxide *on page 71*
- ♦ **Apo**®**-Chlorpromazine (Can)** *see* Chlorpromazine *on page 74*
- ♦ **Apo**®**-Clomipramine (Can)** *see* Clomipramine *on page 82*
- ♦ **Apo**®**-Clonidine (Can)** *see* Clonidine *on page 88*
- ♦ **Apo**®**-Clorazepate (Can)** *see* Clorazepate *on page 92*
- ♦ **Apo**®**-Diazepam (Can)** *see* Diazepam *on page 110*
- ♦ **Apo**®**-Doxepin (Can)** *see* Doxepin *on page 123*
- ♦ **Apo**®**-Fluphenazine [Hydrochloride] (Can)** *see* Fluphenazine *on page 151*
- ♦ **Apo**®**-Flurazepam (Can)** *see* Flurazepam *on page 155*
- ♦ **Apo**®**-Fluvoxamine (Can)** *see* Fluvoxamine *on page 157*
- ♦ **Apo**®**-Hydroxyzine (Can)** *see* Hydroxyzine *on page 178*
- ♦ **Apo**®**-Imipramine (Can)** *see* Imipramine *on page 180*
- ♦ **Apo**®**-Lorazepam (Can)** *see* Lorazepam *on page 209*
- ♦ **Apo**®**-Meprobamate (Can)** *see* Meprobamate *on page 223*
- ♦ **Apo**®**-Nortriptyline (Can)** *see* Nortriptyline *on page 267*
- ♦ **Apo**®**-Oxazepam (Can)** *see* Oxazepam *on page 276*

♦ **Apo®-Perphenazine (Can)** *see* Perphenazine *on page 295*
♦ **Apo®-Pindol (Can)** *see* Pindolol *on page 319*
♦ **Apo®-Primidone (Can)** *see* Primidone *on page 325*
♦ **Apo®-Propranolol (Can)** *see* Propranolol *on page 340*
♦ **Apo®-Temazepam (Can)** *see* Temazepam *on page 388*
♦ **Apo®-Thioridazine (Can)** *see* Thioridazine *on page 393*
♦ **Apo®-Triazo (Can)** *see* Triazolam *on page 410*
♦ **Apo®-Trihex (Can)** *see* Trihexyphenidyl *on page 418*
♦ **Apo®-Trimip (Can)** *see* Trimipramine *on page 421*
♦ **Aquachloral® Supprettes®** *see* Chloral Hydrate *on page 69*
♦ **Aquasol E® [OTC]** *see* Vitamin E *on page 433*
♦ **Aricept®** *see* Donepezil *on page 121*
♦ **Artane®** *see* Trihexyphenidyl *on page 418*
♦ **Artemisia absinthium** *see* Wormwood *on page 435*
♦ **Asendin®** *see* Amoxapine *on page 36*
♦ **Atapryl®** *see* Selegiline *on page 370*
♦ **Atarax®** *see* Hydroxyzine *on page 178*
♦ **Ativan®** *see* Lorazepam *on page 209*
♦ **Atypical Antipsychotics** *see page 565*
♦ **Aventyl®** *see* Nortriptyline *on page 267*
♦ **Awa** *see* Kava *on page 186*
♦ **Axert™** *see* Almotriptan *on page 14*
♦ **Axotal®** *see* Butalbital Compound *on page 59*

Ayahuasca
Pharmacologic Category Herb
Use Religious purposes in South America (as a sacrament)
Adverse Reactions Central nervous system: Hallucinations
Overdosage/Toxicology
Decontamination: Do **not** induce emesis; lavage within 60 minutes/activated charcoal with cathartic
Treatment: Supportive therapy; benzodiazepines may be useful for sedation
Drug Interactions Although this interaction has not been described, use of this tea with specific serotonin reuptake inhibitors may precipitate the serotonin syndrome
Usual Dosage 2 mL/kg of the tea
Additional Information Average levels of DMT and tetrahydroharmine following a dose of 2 mL/kg: ~15.8 ng/mL and 90.8 ng/mL respectively

♦ **B-A-C®** *see* Butalbital Compound *on page 59*
♦ **Bachelor's Buttons** *see* Feverfew *on page 143*
♦ **Bancap®** *see* Butalbital Compound *on page 59*
♦ **Banophen® [OTC]** *see* Diphenhydramine *on page 116*
♦ **Barbilixir® (Can)** *see* Phenobarbital *on page 302*
♦ **Benadryl® [OTC]** *see* Diphenhydramine *on page 116*
♦ **Benzhexol Hydrochloride** *see* Trihexyphenidyl *on page 418*
♦ **Benzodiazepines Comparison Chart** *see page 566*

Benzphetamine (benz FET a meen)
U.S. Brand Names Didrex®
Synonyms Benzphetamine Hydrochloride
Pharmacologic Category Anorexiant
Generic Available No
Use Short-term adjunct in exogenous obesity
Restrictions C-III
Pregnancy Risk Factor X
(Continued)

Benzphetamine *(Continued)*

Contraindications Hypersensitivity or idiosyncrasy to sympathomimetic amines. Patients with advanced arteriosclerosis, symptomatic cardiovascular disease, moderate to severe hypertension (stage II or III), hyperthyroidism, glaucoma, agitated states, patients with a history of drug abuse, pregnancy, and during or within 14 days following MAO inhibitor therapy. Concurrent use with other anorectic agents; stimulant medications are contraindicated for use in children with attention-deficit/hyperactivity disorders **and concomitant** Tourette's syndrome or tics. Not recommended for children <12 years of age.

Warnings/Precautions Cardiovascular disease, nephritis, angina pectoris, hypertension, glaucoma, patients with a history of drug abuse; stimulants may unmask tics in individuals with coexisting Tourette's syndrome

Adverse Reactions Frequency not defined.

Cardiovascular: Hypertension, palpitations, tachycardia, chest pain, T-wave changes, arrhythmias, pulmonary hypertension, valvulopathy

Central nervous system: Euphoria, nervousness, insomnia, restlessness, dizziness, anxiety, headache, agitation, confusion, mental depression, psychosis, CVA, seizure

Dermatologic: Alopecia, urticaria, skin rash, ecchymosis, erythema

Endocrine & metabolic: Changes in libido, gynecomastia, menstrual irregularities, porphyria

Gastrointestinal: Nausea, vomiting, abdominal cramps, constipation, xerostomia, metallic taste

Genitourinary: Impotence

Hematologic: Bone marrow depression, agranulocytosis, leukopenia

Neuromuscular & skeletal: Tremor

Ocular: Blurred vision, mydriasis

Overdosage/Toxicology Treatment: There is no specific antidote for amphetamine intoxication and the bulk of the treatment is supportive. Hyperactivity and agitation usually respond to reduced sensory input, however, with extreme agitation haloperidol (2-5 mg I.M. for adults) may be required. Hyperthermia is best treated with external cooling measures, or when severe or unresponsive, muscle paralysis with pancuronium may be needed. Hypertension is usually transient and generally does not require treatment unless severe. For diastolic blood pressures >110 mm Hg, a nitroprusside infusion should be initiated. Seizures usually respond to diazepam IVP and/or phenytoin maintenance regimens.

Drug Interactions CYP3A3/4 enzyme substrate

Acidifiers: Very large doses of potassium acid phosphate or ammonium chloride may increase the renal elimination of amphetamines due to urinary acidification

Alkalinizers: Large doses of sodium bicarbonate or other alkalinizers may increase renal tubular reabsorption (decreased elimination) and diminish the effect of amphetamine; includes potassium or sodium citrate and acetate

Antipsychotics: Efficacy of amphetamines may be decreased by antipsychotics; in addition, amphetamines may induce an increase in psychotic symptoms in some patients

CYP3A3/4 inhibitors: Serum level and/or toxicity of benzphetamine may be increased. Inhibitors include amiodarone, cimetidine, clarithromycin, erythromycin, delavirdine, diltiazem, dirithromycin, disulfiram, fluoxetine, fluvoxamine, grapefruit juice, indinavir, itraconazole, ketoconazole, nefazodone, nevirapine, propoxyphene, quinupristin-dalfopristin, ritonavir, saquinavir, verapamil, zafirlukast, zileuton. Monitor for altered effects; a decrease in benzphetamine dosage may be required.

Enzyme inducers: Metabolism of amphetamine may be increased, decreasing clinical effect; inducers include barbiturates, carbamazepine, phenytoin, and rifampin

Furazolidone: Amphetamines may induce hypertensive episodes in patients receiving furazolidone

Guanethidine: Amphetamines inhibit the antihypertensive response to guanethidine; probably also may occur with guanadrel

MAO inhibitors: Severe hypertensive episodes have occurred with amphetamine when used in patients receiving MAO inhibitors; concurrent use or use within 14 days is contraindicated

Norepinephrine: Amphetamines may enhance the pressor response to norepinephrine

Sibutramine: Concurrent use of sibutramine and amphetamines may cause severe hypertension and tachycardia; use is contraindicated in product

SSRIs: Amphetamines may increase the potential for serotonin syndrome when used concurrently with selective serotonin reuptake inhibitors (including fluoxetine, fluvoxamine, paroxetine, and sertraline)

Tricyclic antidepressants: Concurrent of amphetamines with TCAs may result in hypertension and CNS stimulation; avoid this combination

Mechanism of Action Noncatechol sympathomimetic amines with pharmacologic actions similar to ephedrine; require breakdown by monoamine oxidase for inactivation; produce central nervous system and respiratory stimulation, a pressor response, mydriasis, bronchodilation, and contraction of the urinary sphincter; thought to have a direct effect on both alpha- and beta-receptor sites in the peripheral system, as well as release stores of norepinephrine in adrenergic nerve terminals; central nervous system action is thought to occur in the cerebral cortex and reticular activating system; anorexigenic effect is probably secondary to the CNS-stimulating effect; the site of action is probably the hypothalamic feeding center

Usual Dosage Adults: Oral: Dose should be individualized based on patient response: Initial: 25-50 mg once daily; titrate to 25-50 mg 1-3 times/day; once-daily dosing should be administered midmorning or midafternoon; maximum dose: 50 mg 3 times/day

Patient Information Take during the day to avoid insomnia; do not discontinue abruptly, may be addicting with prolonged use

Nursing Implications Monitor CNS

Dosage Forms Tablet, as hydrochloride: 50 mg

♦ **Benzphetamine Hydrochloride** *see* Benzphetamine *on page 43*

Benztropine (BENZ troe peen)

Related Information

Antiparkinsonian Agents Comparison Chart *on page 556*
Clozapine-Induced Side Effects *on page 568*
Discontinuation of Psychotropic Drugs - Withdrawal Symptoms and Recommendations *on page 582*
Patient Information - Agents for Treatment of Extrapyramidal Symptoms *on page 493*

U.S. Brand Names Cogentin®

Canadian Brand Names PMS-Benztropine

Synonyms Benztropine Mesylate

Pharmacologic Category Anticholinergic Agent; Anti-Parkinson's Agent (Anticholinergic)

Generic Available Yes: Tablet

Use Adjunctive treatment of Parkinson's disease; treatment of drug-induced extrapyramidal effects (except tardive dyskinesia)

Pregnancy Risk Factor C

Contraindications Hypersensitivity to benztropine or any component of the formulation; pyloric or duodenal obstruction, stenosing peptic ulcers; bladder neck obstructions; achalasia; myasthenia gravis; children <3 years of age

Warnings/Precautions Use with caution in older children (dose has not been established). Use with caution in hot weather or during exercise. May cause anhidrosis and hyperthermia, which may be severe. The risk is increased in hot environments, particularly in the elderly, alcoholics, patients with CNS disease, and those with prolonged outdoor exposure.
(Continued)

Benztropine *(Continued)*

Elderly patients frequently develop increased sensitivity and require strict dosage regulation - side effects may be more severe in elderly patients with atherosclerotic changes. Use with caution in patients with tachycardia, cardiac arrhythmias, hypertension, hypotension, prostatic hypertrophy (especially in the elderly), any tendency toward urinary retention, liver or kidney disorders, and obstructive disease of the GI or GU tract. When given in large doses or to susceptible patients, may cause weakness and inability to move particular muscle groups.

May be associated with confusion or hallucinations (generally at higher dosages). Intensification of symptoms or toxic psychosis may occur in patients with mental disorders. Benztropine does not relieve symptoms of tardive dyskinesia.

Adverse Reactions

Cardiovascular: Tachycardia

Central nervous system: Confusion, disorientation, memory impairment, toxic psychosis, visual hallucinations

Dermatologic: Rash

Endocrine & metabolic: Heat stroke, hyperthermia

Gastrointestinal: Xerostomia, nausea, vomiting, constipation, ileus

Genitourinary: Urinary retention, dysuria

Ocular: Blurred vision, mydriasis

Miscellaneous: Fever

Overdosage/Toxicology

Signs and symptoms: CNS depression, confusion, nervousness, hallucinations, dizziness, blurred vision, nausea, vomiting, hyperthermia

Treatment: For anticholinergic overdose with severe life-threatening symptoms, physostigmine 1-2 mg (0.5 or 0.02 mg/kg for children) I.V. or S.C., slowly may be given to reverse these effects. Anticholinergic toxicity is caused by strong binding of the drug to cholinergic receptors. Anticholinesterase inhibitors reduce acetylcholinesterase, the enzyme that breaks down acetylcholine and thereby allows acetylcholine to accumulate and compete for receptor binding with the offending anticholinergic.

Drug Interactions

Amantadine, rimantadine: Central and/or peripheral anticholinergic syndrome can occur when administered with amantadine or rimantadine

Anticholinergic agents: Central and/or peripheral anticholinergic syndrome can occur when administered with narcotic analgesics, phenothiazines and other antipsychotics (especially with high anticholinergic activity), tricyclic antidepressants, quinidine and some other antiarrhythmics, and antihistamines

Atenolol: Anticholinergics may increase the bioavailability of atenolol (and possibly other beta-blockers); monitor for increased effect

Cholinergic agents: Anticholinergics may antagonize the therapeutic effect of cholinergic agents; includes tacrine and donepezil

Digoxin: Anticholinergics may decrease gastric degradation and increase the amount of digoxin absorbed by delaying gastric emptying

Levodopa: Anticholinergics may increase gastric degradation and decrease the amount of levodopa absorbed by delaying gastric emptying

Neuroleptics: Anticholinergics may antagonize the therapeutic effects of neuroleptics

Ethanol/Nutrition/Herb Interactions
Ethanol: Avoid ethanol (may increase CNS depression).

Mechanism of Action
Possesses both anticholinergic and antihistaminic effects. *In vitro* anticholinergic activity approximates that of atropine; *in vivo* it is only about half as active as atropine. Animal data suggest its antihistaminic activity and duration of action approach that of pyrilamine maleate. May also inhibit the reuptake and storage of dopamine and thereby, prolong the action of dopamine.

Pharmacodynamics/Kinetics

Onset of action:

Oral: Within 1 hour

I.M./I.V.: Within 15 minutes
Duration of action: 6-48 hours (wide range)

Usual Dosage Use in children ≤3 years of age should be reserved for life-threatening emergencies

Drug-induced extrapyramidal reaction: Oral, I.M., I.V.:
  Children >3 years: 0.02-0.05 mg/kg/dose 1-2 times/day
  Adults: 1-4 mg/dose 1-2 times/day
Acute dystonia: Adults: I.M., I.V.: 1-2 mg
Parkinsonism: Oral:
  Adults: 0.5-6 mg/day in 1-2 divided doses; if one dose is greater, administer at bedtime; titrate dose in 0.5 mg increments at 5- to 6-day intervals
  Elderly: Initial: 0.5 mg once or twice daily; increase by 0.5 mg as needed at 5-6 days; maximum: 4 mg/day

Monitoring Parameters Symptoms of EPS or Parkinson's, pulse, anticholinergic effects

Patient Information Take after meals or with food if GI upset occurs; do not discontinue drug abruptly; notify physician if adverse GI effects, rapid or pounding heartbeat, confusion, eye pain, rash, fever, or heat intolerance occurs. Observe caution when performing hazardous tasks or those that require alertness such as driving, as may cause drowsiness. Avoid alcohol and other CNS depressants. May cause dry mouth - adequate fluid intake or hard sugar-free candy may relieve. Difficult urination or constipation may occur - notify physician if effects persist; may increase susceptibility to heat stroke.

Nursing Implications No significant difference in onset of I.M. or I.V. injection, therefore, there is usually no need to use the I.V. route. Improvement is sometimes noticeable a few minutes after injection.

Dosage Forms
Injection, as mesylate: 1 mg/mL (2 mL)
Tablet, as mesylate: 0.5 mg, 1 mg, 2 mg

♦ **Benztropine Mesylate** see Benztropine on page 45

Biperiden (bye PER i den)

Related Information
Antiparkinsonian Agents Comparison Chart on page 556
Discontinuation of Psychotropic Drugs - Withdrawal Symptoms and Recommendations on page 582
Patient Information - Agents for Treatment of Extrapyramidal Symptoms on page 493

U.S. Brand Names Akineton®

Canadian Brand Names Akineton

Synonyms Biperiden Hydrochloride; Biperiden Lactate

Pharmacologic Category Anticholinergic Agent; Anti-Parkinson's Agent (Anticholinergic)

Generic Available No

Use Adjunct in the therapy of all forms of Parkinsonism; control of extrapyramidal symptoms secondary to antipsychotics

Pregnancy Risk Factor C

Contraindications Hypersensitivity to biperiden or any component of the formulation; narrow-angle glaucoma; bowel obstruction, megacolon

Warnings/Precautions Use with caution in patients with narrow-angle glaucoma, peptic ulcer, urinary tract obstruction, hyperthyroidism; some preparations contain sodium bisulfite

Adverse Reactions
Cardiovascular: Orthostatic hypotension, bradycardia (I.V.)
Central nervous system: Drowsiness, euphoria, disorientation, agitation
Gastrointestinal: Constipation, xerostomia
Genitourinary: Urinary retention
Ocular: Blurred vision
(Continued)

Biperiden (Continued)

Overdosage/Toxicology

Signs and symptoms: CNS stimulation or depression; overdose may result in death in infants and children

Treatment: No specific treatment for overdose, however, most of its clinical toxicity is due to anticholinergic effects; anticholinesterase inhibitors may be useful by reducing acetylcholinesterase. Anticholinesterase inhibitors include physostigmine, neostigmine, pyridostigmine and edrophonium; for anticholinergic overdose with severe life-threatening symptoms, physostigmine 1-2 mg (0.5 or 0.02 mg/kg for children) I.V., slowly may be given to reverse these effects.

Drug Interactions

Amantadine, rimantadine: Central and/or peripheral anticholinergic syndrome can occur when administered with amantadine or rimantadine

Anticholinergic agents: Central and/or peripheral anticholinergic syndrome can occur when administered with narcotic analgesics, phenothiazines and other antipsychotics (especially with high anticholinergic activity), tricyclic antidepressants, quinidine and some other antiarrhythmics, and antihistamines

Atenolol: Anticholinergics may increase the bioavailability of atenolol (and possibly other beta-blockers); monitor for increased effect

Cholinergic agents: Anticholinergics may antagonize the therapeutic effect of cholinergic agents; includes tacrine and donepezil

Digoxin: Anticholinergics may decrease gastric degradation and increase the amount of digoxin absorbed by delaying gastric emptying

Levodopa: Anticholinergics may increase gastric degradation and decrease the amount of levodopa absorbed by delaying gastric emptying

Neuroleptics: Anticholinergics may antagonize the therapeutic effects of neuroleptics

Ethanol/Nutrition/Herb Interactions

Ethanol: Avoid ethanol (may increase sedation).

Mechanism of Action

Biperiden is a weak peripheral anticholinergic agent with nicotinolytic activity. The beneficial effects in Parkinson's disease and neuroleptic-induced extrapyramidal reactions are believed to be due to the inhibition of striatal cholinergic receptors.

Pharmacodynamics/Kinetics

Bioavailability: 29%

Half-life: 18.4-24.3 hours

Time to peak serum concentration: 1-1.5 hours

Usual Dosage

Adults:

Parkinsonism: Oral: 2 mg 3-4 times/day

Extrapyramidal:

Oral: 2 mg 1-3 times/day

I.M., I.V.: 2 mg every 30 minutes up to 4 doses or 8 mg/day

Administration

I.V. must be given slowly

Monitoring Parameters

Symptoms of EPS or Parkinson's, pulse, anticholinergic effects (ie, CNS, bowel, and bladder function)

Patient Information

May cause drowsiness

Nursing Implications

No significant difference in onset of I.M. or I.V. injection, therefore, there is usually no need to use the I.V. route. Improvement is sometimes noticeable a few minutes after injection. Do not discontinue drug abruptly.

Dosage Forms

Injection, as lactate: 5 mg/mL (1 mL)

Tablet, as hydrochloride: 2 mg

- ♦ **Biperiden Hydrochloride** see Biperiden on page 47
- ♦ **Biperiden Lactate** see Biperiden on page 47
- ♦ **Black Draught® [OTC]** see Senna on page 373
- ♦ **Black Susans** see Echinacea on page 129
- ♦ **Body Mass Index (BMI)** see page 569

♦ **Bontril PDM®** *see* Phendimetrazine *on page 298*
♦ **Bontril® Slow-Release** *see* Phendimetrazine *on page 298*
♦ **Brevital® Sodium** *see* Methohexital *on page 233*
♦ **Brietal Sodium® (Can)** *see* Methohexital *on page 233*

Bromocriptine (broe moe KRIP teen)

Related Information
Discontinuation of Psychotropic Drugs - Withdrawal Symptoms and Recommendations *on page 582*

U.S. Brand Names Parlodel®
Canadian Brand Names Alti-Bromocriptine; Apo® Bro ocriptine
Synonyms Bromocriptine Mesylate
Pharmacologic Category Anti-Parkinson's Agent (Dopamine Agonist); Ergot Derivative
Generic Available No
Use
Amenorrhea with or without galactorrhea; infertility or hypogonadism; prolactin-secreting adenomas; acromegaly; Parkinson's disease

A previous indication for prevention of postpartum lactation was withdrawn voluntarily by Sandoz Pharmaceuticals Corporation

Unlabeled/Investigational Use Neuroleptic malignant syndrome
Pregnancy Risk Factor B
Contraindications Hypersensitivity to bromocriptine, ergot alkaloids, or any component of the formulation; uncontrolled hypertension; severe ischemic heart disease or peripheral vascular disorders; pregnancy (risk to benefit evaluation must be performed in women who become pregnant during treatment for acromegaly, prolactinoma, or Parkinson's disease - hypertension during treatment should generally result in efforts to withdraw)

Warnings/Precautions Use with caution in patients with impaired renal or hepatic function, a history of psychosis, or cardiovascular disease (myocardial infarction, arrhythmia). Patients who receive bromocriptine during and immediately following pregnancy as a continuation of previous therapy (ie, acromegaly) should be closely monitored for cardiovascular effects. Discontinuation of bromocriptine in patients with macroadenomas has been associated with rapid regrowth of tumor and increased prolactin serum levels. Use with caution in patients with a history of peptic ulcer disease, dementia, or concurrent antihypertensive therapy. Safety and effectiveness in patients <15 years of age have not been established.

Adverse Reactions
>10%:
  Central nervous system: Headache, dizziness
  Gastrointestinal: Nausea
1% to 10%:
  Cardiovascular: Orthostatic hypotension
  Central nervous system: Fatigue, lightheadedness, drowsiness
  Gastrointestinal: Anorexia, vomiting, abdominal cramps, constipation
  Respiratory: Nasal congestion
<1%: Arrhythmias, hair loss, insomnia, paranoia, visual hallucinations

Overdosage/Toxicology
Signs and symptoms: Nausea, vomiting, hypotension
Treatment: Hypotension, when unresponsive to I.V. fluids or Trendelenburg positioning, often responds to norepinephrine infusions started at 0.1-0.2 mcg/kg/minute followed by a titrated infusion.

Drug Interactions CYP3A3/4 enzyme substrate
Antipsychotics: Antipsychotics may inhibit bromocriptine's therapeutic effects (diminished ability to lower prolactin)
CYP3A3/4 inhibitors: Serum level and/or toxicity of bromocriptine may be increased; inhibitors include amiodarone, cimetidine, clarithromycin, erythromycin, delavirdine, diltiazem, dirithromycin, disulfiram, fluoxetine, fluvoxamine, grapefruit juice, indinavir, itraconazole, ketoconazole, nevirapine, propoxyphene, (Continued)

Bromocriptine *(Continued)*

quinupristin-dalfopristin, ritonavir, saquinavir, verapamil, zafirlukast, zileuton; monitor for altered effects; a decrease in bromocriptine dosage may be required

Entacapone: Fibrotic complications (retroperitoneal or pulmonary fibrosis) have been associated with combinations of entacapone and bromocriptine

Ethanol: May increase the sensitivity of receptors to bromocriptine; monitor for increase effect

Sympathomimetics: May increase risk of hypertension and seizure; isometheptene and phenylpropanolamine (and other sympathomimetics) should be avoided in patients receiving bromocriptine

Ethanol/Nutrition/Herb Interactions

Ethanol: Avoid ethanol (may increase GI side effects or ethanol intolerance).

Herb/Nutraceutical: St John's wort may decrease bromocriptine levels.

Mechanism of Action Semisynthetic ergot alkaloid derivative and a dopamine receptor agonist which activates postsynaptic dopamine receptors in the tuberoin-fundibular and nigrostriatal pathways

Pharmacodynamics/Kinetics

Protein binding: 90% to 96%

Metabolism: Majority of drug metabolized in the liver

Half-life (biphasic):

Initial: 6-8 hours

Terminal: 50 hours

Time to peak serum concentration: Oral: Within 1-2 hours

Elimination: In bile; only 2% to 6% excreted unchanged in urine

Usual Dosage Adults: Oral:

Parkinsonism: 1.25 mg 2 times/day, increased by 2.5 mg/day in 2- to 4-week intervals (usual dose range is 30-90 mg/day in 3 divided doses), though elderly patients can usually be managed on lower doses

Neuroleptic malignant syndrome: 2.5-5 mg 3 times/day

Hyperprolactinemia: 2.5 mg 2-3 times/day

Acromegaly: Initial: 1.25-2.5 mg increasing as necessary every 3-7 days; usual dose: 20-30 mg/day

Prolactin-secreting adenomas: Initial: 1.25-2.5 mg/day; daily range 2.5-10 mg.

Dosing adjustment in hepatic impairment: No guidelines are available, however, may be necessary

Dietary Considerations May be administered with food to decrease GI distress.

Monitoring Parameters Monitor blood pressure closely as well as hepatic, hematopoietic, and cardiovascular function

Patient Information Take with food or milk; drowsiness commonly occurs upon initiation of therapy; limit use of alcohol; avoid exposure to cold; incidence of side effects is high (68%) with nausea the most common; hypotension occurs commonly with initiation of therapy, usually upon rising after prolonged sitting or lying; discontinue immediately if pregnant; may restore fertility; women desiring not to become pregnant should use mechanical contraceptive means

Nursing Implications Raise bed rails and institute safety measures; aid patient with ambulation; may cause postural hypotension and drowsiness

Additional Information Usually used with levodopa or levodopa/carbidopa to treat Parkinson's disease. When adding bromocriptine, the dose of levodopa/carbidopa can usually be decreased.

Dosage Forms

Capsule, as mesylate: 5 mg

Tablet, as mesylate: 2.5 mg

♦ **Bromocriptine Mesylate** *see* Bromocriptine *on page 49*

♦ **Buprenex**® *see* Buprenorphine *on page 50*

Buprenorphine *(byoo pre NOR feen)*

U.S. Brand Names Buprenex®

Synonyms Buprenorphine Hydrochloride

Pharmacologic Category Analgesic, Narcotic

Generic Available Yes

Use Management of moderate to severe pain

Unlabeled/Investigational Use Heroin and opioid withdrawal

Restrictions C-V

Pregnancy Risk Factor C

Contraindications Hypersensitivity to buprenorphine or any component of the formulation

Warnings/Precautions May cause respiratory depression - use caution in patients with respiratory disease or pre-existing respiratory depression. Potential for drug dependency exists, abrupt cessation may precipitate withdrawal. Use caution in elderly, debilitated, or pediatric patients. Use with caution in patients with depression or suicidal tendencies, or in patients with a history of drug abuse. Tolerance, psychological and physical dependence may occur with prolonged use. Use with caution in patients with hepatic, pulmonary, or renal function impairment. May cause CNS depression, which may impair physical or mental abilities. Patients must be cautioned about performing tasks which require mental alertness (ie, operating machinery or driving). Effects with other sedative drugs or ethanol may be potentiated. Elderly may be more sensitive to CNS depressant and constipating effects. Use with caution in patients with head injury or increased ICP, biliary tract dysfunction, pancreatitis, patients with history of ileus or bowel obstruction, glaucoma, hyperthyroidism, adrenal insufficiency, prostatic hypertrophy, urinary stricture, CNS depression, toxic psychosis, alcoholism, delirium tremens, or kyphoscoliosis. Partial antagonist activity may precipitate acute narcotic withdrawal in opioid-dependent individuals.

Adverse Reactions

>10%: Central nervous system: Sedation

1% to 10%:

Cardiovascular: Hypotension

Central nervous system: Respiratory depression, dizziness, headache

Gastrointestinal: Vomiting, nausea

Ocular: Miosis

Miscellaneous: Diaphoresis

<1%: Blurred vision, bradycardia, confusion, constipation, cyanosis, depression, diplopia, dyspnea, euphoria, hypertension, nervousness, paresthesia, pruritus, slurred speech, tachycardia, urinary retention, xerostomia

Overdosage/Toxicology

Signs and symptoms: CNS depression, pinpoint pupils, hypotension, bradycardia

Treatment: Support of the patient's airway, establishment of an I.V. line, and administration of naloxone 2 mg I.V. (0.01 mg/kg for children) with repeat administration as necessary up to a total of 10 mg

Drug Interactions

Cimetidine: May increase sedation from narcotic analgesics; however, histamine blockers may attenuate the cardiovascular response from histamine release associated with narcotic analgesics

CNS depressants: May produce additive respiratory and CNS depression; includes benzodiazepines, barbiturates, ethanol, and other sedatives. Respiratory and CV collapse was reported in a patient who received diazepam and buprenorphine.

Naltrexone: May antagonize the effect of narcotic analgesics; concurrent use or use within 7-10 days is contraindicated

Ethanol/Nutrition/Herb Interactions

Ethanol: Avoid ethanol (may increase CNS depression).

Herb/Nutraceutical: Avoid valerian, St John's wort, kava kava, gotu kola (may increase CNS depression).

Stability Protect from excessive heat (>40°C/104°F) and light

Compatible with 0.9% sodium chloride, lactated Ringer's solution, 5% dextrose in water, scopolamine, haloperidol, glycopyrrolate, droperidol, and hydroxyzine

Incompatible with diazepam, lorazepam

(Continued)

Buprenorphine *(Continued)*

Mechanism of Action Buprenorphine exerts its analgesic effect via high affinity binding to μ opiate receptors in the CNS; displays both agonist and antagonist activity

Pharmacodynamics/Kinetics
Onset of analgesia: Within 10-30 minutes
Duration: 6-8 hours
Absorption: I.M., S.C.: 30% to 40%
Distribution: V_d: 97-187 L/kg
Protein binding: High
Metabolism: Mainly in the liver; undergoes extensive first-pass metabolism
Half-life: 2.2-3 hours
Elimination: 70% excreted in feces via bile and 20% in urine as unchanged drug

Usual Dosage Long-term use is not recommended
I.M., slow I.V.:
Children ≥13 years and Adults:
Moderate to severe pain: 0.3-0.6 mg every 6 hours as needed
Heroin or opiate withdrawal (unlabeled use): Variable; 0.1-0.4 mg every 6 hours
Elderly: Moderate to severe pain: 0.15 mg every 6 hours; elderly patients are more likely to suffer from confusion and drowsiness compared to younger patients

Monitoring Parameters Pain relief, respiratory and mental status, CNS depression, blood pressure

Patient Information May cause drowsiness; avoid alcoholic beverages; may be habit forming

Nursing Implications Gradual withdrawal of drug is necessary to avoid withdrawal symptoms

Additional Information 0.3 mg = 10 mg morphine or 75 mg meperidine, has longer duration of action than either agent

Dosage Forms Injection, as hydrochloride: 0.3 mg/mL (1 mL)

♦ **Buprenorphine Hydrochloride** see Buprenorphine on page 50

Bupropion *(byoo PROE pee on)*

Related Information
Addiction Treatments on page 550
Antidepressant Agents Comparison Chart on page 553
Patient Information - Antidepressants (Bupropion) on page 456

U.S. Brand Names Wellbutrin®; Wellbutrin SR®; Zyban™
Canadian Brand Names Wellbutrin; Zyban
Pharmacologic Category Antidepressant, Dopamine-Reuptake Inhibitor
Generic Available Yes: Wellbutrin® strength only
Use Treatment of depression; adjunct in smoking cessation
Unlabeled/Investigational Use Attention-deficit/hyperactivity disorder (ADHD)
Pregnancy Risk Factor B
Contraindications Hypersensitivity to bupropion or any component of the formulation; seizure disorder; anorexia/bulimia; use of MAO inhibitors within 14 days
Warnings/Precautions Seizure risk is increased at total daily dosage >450 mg, individual dosages >150 mg, or by sudden, large increments in dose. The risk of seizures is increased in patients with a history of seizures, head trauma, CNS tumor, abrupt discontinuation of sedative-hypnotics or alcohol, medications which lower seizure threshold, stimulants, or hypoglycemic agents. May cause CNS stimulation (restlessness, anxiety, insomnia) or anorexia. Use with caution in patients where weight loss is not desirable. The incidence of sexual dysfunction with bupropion is generally lower than with SSRIs.

Use caution in patients with cardiovascular disease, history of hypertension, or coronary artery disease; treatment-emergent hypertension (including some severe cases) has been reported, both with bupropion alone and in combination with nicotine transdermal systems.

Use with caution in patients with hepatic or renal dysfunction and in elderly patients. Elderly patients may be at greater risk of accumulation during chronic dosing. May cause motor or cognitive impairment in some patients, use with caution if tasks requiring alertness such as operating machinery or driving are undertaken. May worsen psychosis in some patients or precipitate a shift to mania or hypomania in patients with bipolar disease. Use caution in patients with depression, particularly if suicidal risk may be present.

Arthralgia, myalgia, and fever with rash and other symptoms suggestive of delayed hypersensitivity resembling serum sickness reported

Adverse Reactions
>10%:
  Cardiovascular: Tachycardia
  Central nervous system: Agitation, insomnia, headache, dizziness, sedation
  Gastrointestinal: Nausea, vomiting, xerostomia, constipation
  Neuromuscular & skeletal: Tremor
  Ocular: Blurred vision
  Respiratory: Rhinitis
  Miscellaneous: Diaphoresis
1% to 10%:
  Cardiovascular: Hypertension (2.5% alone, up to 6.1% in combination with nicotine patch), palpitations
  Central nervous system: Anxiety, nervousness, confusion, hostility, abnormal dreams
  Dermatologic: Rash, acne, dry skin
  Endocrine & metabolic: Hyper- or hypoglycemia
  Gastrointestinal: Anorexia, diarrhea, dyspepsia
  Neuromuscular & skeletal: Arthralgia, myalgia
  Otic: Tinnitus
Postintroduction adverse reactions: Arthralgia, myalgia, and fever with rash and other symptoms suggestive of delayed hypersensitivity resembling serum sickness reported
Hypertension (in some cases severe) requiring acute treatment has been reported in patients receiving bupropion alone and in combination with nicotine replacement therapy, orthostatic hypotension, third degree heart block, extrasystoles, myocardial infarction, phlebitis, pulmonary embolism

Overdosage/Toxicology
Signs and symptoms: Labored breathing, salivation, arched back, ataxia, convulsions
Treatment: Supportive; I.V. diazepam is useful in treating seizures

Drug Interactions CYP2B6 enzyme substrate, CYP3A3/4 enzyme substrate (minor)
  Note: Seizure threshold-lowering agents: Use with caution in individuals receiving other agents that may lower seizure threshold (antipsychotics, antidepressants, fluoroquinolones, theophylline, abrupt discontinuation of benzodiazepines, systemic steroids)
  Cimetidine: May increase effect of bupropion (due to effect on bupropion metabolites)
  Levodopa: Toxicity of bupropion is enhanced by levodopa
  MAO inhibitors: Toxicity of bupropion is enhanced by MAO inhibitors (phenelzine); concurrent use in contraindicated
  Nicotine: Treatment-emergent hypertension may occur; monitor BP in patients treated with bupropion and nicotine patch
  Selegiline: When used in low doses (<10 mg/day), risk of interaction is theoretically lower than with nonselective MAO inhibitors
  Tricyclic antidepressants: Serum levels may be increased by bupropion; in addition, these agents lower seizure threshold (see "Note")
(Continued)

Bupropion *(Continued)*

Ethanol/Nutrition/Herb Interactions
Ethanol: Ethanol (may increase CNS depression).

Herb/Nutraceutical : Avoid valerian, St John's wort, SAMe, gotu kola, kava kava (may increase CNS depression).

Mechanism of Action
Antidepressant structurally different from all other previously marketed antidepressants; like other antidepressants the mechanism of bupropion's activity is not fully understood; weak inhibitor of the neuronal uptake of serotonin, norepinephrine, and dopamine

Pharmacodynamics/Kinetics
Absorption: Rapidly absorbed from GI tract

Distribution: V_d: 19-21 L/kg

Protein binding: 82% to 88%

Metabolism: Extensively in the liver to multiple metabolites

Half-life: 14 hours

Time to peak serum concentration: Oral: Within 3 hours

Usual Dosage Oral:
Children and Adolescents: ADHD (unlabeled use): 1.4-6 mg/kg/day

Adults:

Depression:

Immediate release: 100 mg 3 times/day; begin at 100 mg twice daily; may increase to a maximum dose of 450 mg/day

Sustained release: Initial: 150 mg/day in the morning; may increase to 150 mg twice daily by day 4 if tolerated; target dose: 300 mg/day given as 150 mg twice daily; maximum dose: 400 mg/day given as 200 mg twice daily

Smoking cessation: Initiate with 150 mg once daily for 3 days; increase to 150 mg twice daily; treatment should continue for 7-12 weeks

Elderly: Depression: 50-100 mg/day, increase by 50-100 mg every 3-4 days as tolerated; there is evidence that the elderly respond at 150 mg/day in divided doses, but some may require a higher dose

Dosing adjustment/comments in renal or hepatic impairment: Patients with renal or hepatic failure should receive a reduced dosage initially and be closely monitored

Child/Adolescent Considerations
Attention-deficit/hyperactivity disorder (ADHD): 1.4-5.7 mg/kg/day (mean: 3.3 mg/kg/day) was utilized in 15 ADHD subjects 7-17 years of age (Barrickman, 1995); 72 children with ADHD (6-12 years of age) received 3-6 mg/kg/day (Conners, 1996); adolescents with conduct disorder and substance use disorder were titrated to a maximum fixed daily dose of 300 mg (Riggs, 1998).

Monitoring Parameters
Body weight

Reference Range
Therapeutic levels (trough, 12 hours after last dose): 50-100 ng/mL

Test Interactions
Decreased prolactin levels

Patient Information
Be aware that bupropion is marketed under different names and should not be taken together; Zyban™ is for smoking cessation and Wellbutrin® is for treatment of depression. Take in equally divided doses 3-4 times/day to minimize the risk of seizures; avoid alcohol; do not take more than recommended dose or more than 150 mg in a single dose; do not discontinue abruptly, may take 3-4 weeks for full effect; may impair driving or other motor or cognitive skills and judgment

Nursing Implications
Be aware that drug may cause seizures

Dosage Forms
Tablet (Wellbutrin®): 75 mg, 100 mg

Tablet, sustained release:

Wellbutrin® SR: 100 mg, 150 mg

Zyban™: 150 mg

♦ **BuSpar®** *see* Buspirone *on page 55*

♦ **Buspirex (Can)** *see* Buspirone *on page 55*

Buspirone (byoo SPYE rone)

Related Information

Nonbenzodiazepine Anxiolytics and Hypnotics *on page 589*

Patient Information - Anxiolytics & Sedative Hypnotics (Buspirone) *on page 487*

Teratogenic Risks of Psychotropic Medications *on page 594*

U.S. Brand Names BuSpar®

Canadian Brand Names Buspar; Buspirex; Bustab

Synonyms Buspirone Hydrochloride

Pharmacologic Category Antianxiety Agent, Miscellaneous

Generic Available No

Use Management of generalized anxiety disorder (GAD)

Unlabeled/Investigational Use Management of aggression in mental retardation and secondary mental disorders; major depression; potential augmenting agent for antidepressants; premenstrual syndrome

Pregnancy Risk Factor B

Contraindications Hypersensitivity to buspirone or any component of the formulation

Warnings/Precautions Safety and efficacy not established in children <18 years of age; use in hepatic or renal impairment is not recommended; does not prevent or treat withdrawal from benzodiazepines. Low potential for cognitive or motor impairment. Use with MAO inhibitors may result in hypertensive reactions.

Adverse Reactions

>10%: Central nervous system: Dizziness

1% to 10%:

Central nervous system: Drowsiness, EPS, serotonin syndrome, confusion, nervousness, lightheadedness, excitement, anger, hostility, headache

Dermatologic: Rash

Gastrointestinal: Diarrhea, nausea

Neuromuscular & skeletal: Muscle weakness, numbness, paresthesia, incoordination, tremor

Ocular: Blurred vision, tunnel vision

Miscellaneous: Diaphoresis, allergic reactions

Overdosage/Toxicology

Signs and symptoms: Dizziness, drowsiness, pinpoint pupils, nausea, vomiting

Treatment: There is no known antidote for buspirone and most therapies are supportive and symptomatic in nature

Drug Interactions CYP3A3/4 enzyme substrate

Calcium channel blockers: Diltiazem and verapamil may increase serum concentrations of buspirone; consider a dihydropyridine calcium channel blocker

CYP3A3/4 inhibitors: Serum level and/or toxicity of buspirone may be increased; inhibitors include amiodarone, cimetidine, clarithromycin, erythromycin, delavirdine, diltiazem, dirithromycin, disulfiram, fluoxetine, fluvoxamine, grapefruit juice, indinavir, itraconazole, ketoconazole, nefazodone, nevirapine, propoxyphene, quinupristin-dalfopristin, ritonavir, saquinavir, verapamil, zafirlukast, zileuton; monitor for altered effects; a decrease in buspirone dosage may be required

Enzyme inducers: May reduce serum concentrations of buspirone resulting in loss of efficacy; includes barbiturates, carbamazepine, phenytoin, rifabutin and rifampin

MAO inhibitors: Buspirone should not be used concurrently with an MAO inhibitor due to reports of increased blood pressure; includes classic MAO inhibitors and linezolid (due to ability to inhibit MAO)

Selegiline: Theoretically, risk of interaction with selective MAO type B inhibitor would be less than with nonselective inhibitors; however, this combination is generally best avoided

SSRIs: Concurrent use of buspirone with SSRIs may cause serotonin syndrome. Some SSRIs may increase buspirone serum concentrations (see CYP3A3/4 inhibitors). Buspirone may increase the efficacy of fluoxetine in some patients; (Continued)

Buspirone *(Continued)*

however, the anxiolytic activity of buspirone may be lost when combined with SSRIs (fluoxetine).

Trazodone: Concurrent use of buspirone with trazodone may cause serotonin syndrome

Ethanol/Nutrition/Herb Interactions

Ethanol: Ethanol (may increase CNS depression).

Food: Food may decrease the absorption of buspirone, but it may also decrease the first-pass metabolism, thereby increasing the bioavailability of buspirone. Grapefruit juice may cause increased buspirone concentrations; avoid concurrent use.

Herb/Nutraceutical: St John's wort may decrease buspirone levels or increase CNS depression. Avoid valerian, gotu kola, kava kava (may increase CNS depression).

Mechanism of Action The mechanism of action of buspirone is unknown. Buspirone has a high affinity for serotonin 5-HT_{1A} and 5-HT_2 receptors, without affecting benzodiazepine-GABA receptors; buspirone has moderate affinity for dopamine D_2 receptors

Pharmacodynamics/Kinetics

Protein binding: 95%

Metabolism: In the liver by oxidation and undergoes extensive first-pass metabolism

Half-life: 2-3 hours

Time to peak serum concentration: Oral: Within 0.7-1.5 hours

Usual Dosage Oral:

Generalized anxiety disorder:

Children and Adolescents: Initial: 5 mg daily; increase in increments of 5 mg/day at weekly intervals as needed, to a maximum dose of 60 mg/day divided into 2-3 doses

Adults: Oral: 15 mg/day (7.5 mg twice daily); may increase in increments of 5 mg/day every 2-4 days to a maximum of 60 mg/day; target dose for most people is 30 mg/day (15 mg twice daily)

Dosing adjustment in renal or hepatic impairment: Buspirone is metabolized by the liver and excreted by the kidneys. Patients with impaired hepatic or renal function demonstrated increased plasma levels and a prolonged half-life of buspirone. Therefore, use in patients with severe hepatic or renal impairment cannot be recommended.

Child/Adolescent Considerations Anxiety disorders: One pilot study of 15 children, 6-14 years of age (mean: 10 years), with mixed anxiety disorders, used initial doses of 5 mg/day; doses were individualized with increases in increments of 5 mg/day weekly as needed, to a maximum dose of 20 mg/day divided into 2 doses (mean dose required: 18.6 mg/day). Some authors (Carrey, 1996 and Kutcher, 1992), based on their clinical experience, recommend higher doses. Open-label study in 25 prepubertal inpatients (mean age: 8 years) with anxiety symptoms and moderately-aggressive behavior utilized a mean optimal dose of 28 mg/day (Pfeffer, 1997). Dosages ranging from 15-45 mg/day were utilized in children 6-17 years of age with pervasive developmental disorders (Buitelaar, 1998).

Monitoring Parameters Mental status, symptoms of anxiety

Test Interactions ↑ AST, ALT, growth hormone(s), prolactin (S)

Patient Information Take with food; report any change in senses (ie, smelling, hearing, vision); cautious use with alcohol is recommended; cannot be substituted for benzodiazepines unless directed by a physician; takes 2-3 weeks to see the full effect of this medication; if you miss a dose, do **not** double your next dose

Nursing Implications Monitor mental status

Additional Information Has shown little potential for abuse; needs continuous use. Because of slow onset, not appropriate for "as needed" (prn) use or for brief, situational anxiety. Ineffective for treatment of benzodiazepine or alcohol withdrawal.

Dosage Forms Tablet, as hydrochloride: 5 mg, 10 mg, 15 mg, 30 mg

♦ **Buspirone Hydrochloride** *see* Buspirone *on page 55*

♦ **Bustab (Can)** *see* Buspirone *on page 55*

Butabarbital Sodium (byoo ta BAR bi tal SOW dee um)

Related Information

Anxiolytic/Hypnotic Use in Long-Term Care Facilities *on page 562*
Federal OBRA Regulations Recommended Maximum Doses *on page 583*
Patient Information - Anxiolytics & Sedative Hypnotics (Barbiturates) *on page 485*

U.S. Brand Names Butisol Sodium®

Canadian Brand Names Butisol

Pharmacologic Category Barbiturate

Generic Available Yes

Use Sedative; hypnotic

Restrictions C-III

Pregnancy Risk Factor D

Contraindications Hypersensitivity to barbiturates or any component of the formulation; porphyria; pregnancy

Warnings/Precautions May cause CNS depression, which may impair physical or mental abilities. Patients must be cautioned about performing tasks which require mental alertness (ie, operating machinery or driving). Effects with other sedative drugs or ethanol may be potentiated. May cause respiratory depression or hypotension. Use with caution in hemodynamically unstable patients or patients with respiratory disease. Potential for drug dependency exists; abrupt cessation may precipitate withdrawal, including status epilepticus in epileptic patients. Do not administer to patients in acute pain. Use caution in elderly, debilitated, renally impaired, hepatic impairment, or pediatric patients. May cause paradoxical responses, including agitation and hyperactivity, particularly in acute pain and pediatric patients. Use with caution in patients with depression or suicidal tendencies, or in patients with a history of drug abuse. Tolerance, psychological and physical dependence may occur with prolonged use.

Adverse Reactions

>10%: Central nervous system: Dizziness, lightheadedness, drowsiness, "hangover" effect

1% to 10%:
Central nervous system: Confusion, mental depression, unusual excitement, nervousness, faint feeling, headache, insomnia, nightmares
Gastrointestinal: Constipation, nausea, vomiting

<1%: Agranulocytosis, angioedema, dependence, exfoliative dermatitis, hallucinations, hypotension, megaloblastic anemia, rash, respiratory depression, Stevens-Johnson syndrome, thrombocytopenia, thrombophlebitis

Overdosage/Toxicology

Signs and symptoms: Slurred speech, confusion, nystagmus, tachycardia, hypotension

Treatment: If hypotension occurs, administer I.V. fluids and place the patient in the Trendelenburg position; if unresponsive, an I.V. vasopressor (eg, dopamine, epinephrine) may be required. Forced alkaline diuresis is of no value in the treatment of intoxications with short-acting barbiturates. Charcoal hemoperfusion or hemodialysis may be useful in the harder to treat intoxications, especially in the presence of very high serum barbiturate levels.

Drug Interactions Note: Barbiturates are cytochrome P450 enzyme inducers. Patients should be monitored when these drugs are started or stopped for a decreased or increased therapeutic effect respectively.

Acetaminophen: Barbiturates may enhance the hepatotoxic potential of acetaminophen overdoses

Antiarrhythmics: Barbiturates may increase the metabolism of antiarrhythmics, decreasing their clinical effect; includes disopyramide, propafenone, and quinidine

(Continued)

Butabarbital Sodium *(Continued)*

Anticonvulsants: Barbiturates may increase the metabolism of anticonvulsants; includes ethosuximide, felbamate (possibly), lamotrigine, phenytoin, tiagabine, topiramate, and zonisamide; does not appear to affect gabapentin, or levetiracetam

Antineoplastics: Limited evidence suggests that enzyme-inducing anticonvulsant therapy may reduce the effectiveness of some chemotherapy regimens (specifically in ALL); teniposide and methotrexate may be cleared more rapidly in these patients

Antipsychotics: Barbiturates may enhance the metabolism (decrease the efficacy) of antipsychotics; monitor for altered response; dose adjustment may be needed

Beta-blockers: Metabolism of beta-blockers may be increased and clinical effect decreased; atenolol and nadolol are unlikely to interact given their renal elimination

Calcium channel blockers: Barbiturates may enhance the metabolism of calcium channel blockers, decreasing their clinical effect

Chloramphenicol: Barbiturates may increase the metabolism of chloramphenicol and chloramphenicol may inhibit barbiturate metabolism; monitor for altered response

Cimetidine: Barbiturates may enhance the metabolism of cimetidine, decreasing its clinical effect

CNS depressants: Sedative effects and/or respiratory depression with barbiturates may be additive with other CNS depressants; monitor for increased effect; includes ethanol, sedatives, antidepressants, narcotic analgesics, and benzodiazepines

Corticosteroids: Barbiturates may enhance the metabolism of corticosteroids, decreasing their clinical effect

Cyclosporine: Levels may be decreased by barbiturates; monitor

Immunosuppressants: Barbiturates may enhance the metabolism of immunosuppressants, decreasing its clinical effect; includes both cyclosporine and tacrolimus

Doxycycline: Barbiturates may enhance the metabolism of doxycycline, decreasing its clinical effect; higher dosages may be required

Estrogens: Barbiturates may increase the metabolism of estrogens and reduce their efficacy

Felbamate may inhibit the metabolism of barbiturates and barbiturates may increase the metabolism of felbamate

Griseofulvin: Barbiturates may impair the absorption of griseofulvin, and griseofulvin metabolism may be increased by barbiturates, decreasing clinical effect

Guanfacine: Effect may be decreased by barbiturates

Loop diuretics: Metabolism may be increased and clinical effects decreased; established for furosemide, effect with other loop diuretics not established

MAO inhibitors: Metabolism of barbiturates may be inhibited, increasing clinical effect or toxicity of the barbiturates

Methadone: Barbiturates may enhance the metabolism of methadone resulting in methadone withdrawal

Methoxyflurane: Barbiturates may enhance the nephrotoxic effects of methoxyflurane

Oral contraceptives: Barbiturates may enhance the metabolism of oral contraceptives, decreasing their clinical effect; an alternative method of contraception should be considered

Theophylline: Barbiturates may increase metabolism of theophylline derivatives and decrease their clinical effect

Tricyclic antidepressants: Barbiturates may increase metabolism of tricyclic antidepressants and decrease their clinical effect; sedative effects may be additive

Valproic acid: Metabolism of barbiturates may be inhibited by valproic acid; monitor for excessive sedation; a dose reduction may be needed

Warfarin: Barbiturates inhibit the hypoprothrombinemic effects of oral anticoagulants via increased metabolism; this combination should generally be avoided

Ethanol/Nutrition/Herb Interactions

Ethanol: Avoid ethanol (may increase CNS depression).

Herb/Nutraceutical: Avoid valerian, St John's wort, kava kava, gotu kola (may increase CNS depression).

Mechanism of Action Interferes with transmission of impulses from the thalamus to the cortex of the brain resulting in an imbalance in central inhibitory and facilitatory mechanisms

Pharmacodynamics/Kinetics

Distribution: V_d: 0.8 L/kg

Protein binding: 26%

Metabolism: In the liver

Half-life: 40-140 hours

Time to peak serum concentration: Oral: Within 40-60 minutes

Elimination: In urine as metabolites

Usual Dosage Oral:

Children: Preop sedative: 2-6 mg/kg/dose (maximum: 100 mg)

Adults:

Sedative: 15-30 mg 3-4 times/day

Hypnotic: 50-100 mg

Preop: 50-100 mg 1-1½ hours before surgery

Reference Range Therapeutic: Not established; Toxic: 28-73 µg/mL

Test Interactions ↑ ammonia (B); ↓ bilirubin (S)

Patient Information May cause drowsiness, avoid alcohol or other CNS depressants, may impair judgment and coordination; may cause physical and psychological dependence with prolonged use; do not exceed recommended dose

Nursing Implications Raise bed rails; initiate safety measures; aid with ambulation; monitor for CNS depression

Dosage Forms

Elixir, as sodium, with alcohol 7%: 30 mg/5 mL (480 mL)

Tablet, as sodium: 15 mg, 30 mg, 50 mg, 100 mg

♦ **Butace® Endolor®** see Butalbital Compound on page 59

Butalbital Compound (byoo TAL bi tal KOM pound)

U.S. Brand Names Amaphen®; Anoquan®; Axotal®; B-A-C®; Bancap®; Butace® Endolor®; Esgic®; Femcet®; Fiorgen PF®; Fioricet®; Fiorinal® G-1®; Isollyl® Improved; Lanorinal®; Margesic®; Marnal® Medigesic®; Phrenilin®; Phrenilin® Forte; Repan®; Sedapap-10® Triad®; Triapin®; Two-Dyne®

Pharmacologic Category Barbiturate

Generic Available Yes

Use Relief of symptomatic complex of tension or muscle contraction headache

Restrictions C-III (Fiorinal®)

Pregnancy Risk Factor D

Contraindications Patients with porphyria, known hypersensitivity to butalbital or any component

Warnings/Precautions Children and teenagers should not use for chickenpox or flu symptoms before a physician is consulted about Reye's syndrome (Fiorinal®)

Adverse Reactions

>10%:

Central nervous system: Dizziness, lightheadedness, drowsiness, "hangover" effect

Gastrointestinal: Nausea, heartburn, stomach pains, dyspepsia, epigastric discomfort

1% to 10%:

Central nervous system: Confusion, mental depression, unusual excitement, nervousness, faint feeling, headache, insomnia, nightmares, fatigue

Dermatologic: Rash

Gastrointestinal: Constipation, vomiting, gastrointestinal ulceration

Hematologic: Hemolytic anemia

(Continued)

Butalbital Compound *(Continued)*

Neuromuscular & skeletal: Weakness

Respiratory: Dyspnea

Miscellaneous: Anaphylactic shock

<1%: Agranulocytosis, bronchospasm, exfoliative dermatitis, hallucinations, hepatotoxicity, hypotension, impaired renal function, iron deficiency anemia, jitters, leukopenia, megaloblastic anemia, occult bleeding, prolongation of bleeding time, respiratory depression, Stevens-Johnson syndrome, thrombocytopenia, thrombophlebitis

Overdosage/Toxicology

Symptoms of overdose include slurred speech, confusion, nystagmus, tachycardia, hypotension, tinnitus, headache, dizziness, confusion, metabolic acidosis, hyperpyrexia, hypoglycemia, coma, hepatic necrosis, blood dyscrasias, respiratory depression

Forced alkaline diuresis is of no value in the treatment of intoxications with short-acting barbiturates. Charcoal hemoperfusion or hemodialysis may be useful in the harder to treat intoxications, especially in the presence of very high serum barbiturate levels; see also Acetaminophen for Fioricet® toxicology or Aspirin for Fiorinal® toxicology.

Drug Interactions

Decreased effect: Phenothiazines, haloperidol, quinidine, cyclosporine, TCAs, corticosteroids, theophylline, ethosuximide, warfarin, oral contraceptives, chloramphenicol, griseofulvin, doxycycline, beta-blockers

Increased effect/toxicity: Propoxyphene, benzodiazepines, CNS depressants, valproic acid, methylphenidate, chloramphenicol

Mechanism of Action Butalbital, like other barbiturates, has a generalized depressant effect on the central nervous system (CNS). Barbiturates have little effect on peripheral nerves or muscle at usual therapeutic doses. However, at toxic doses serious effects on the cardiovascular system and other peripheral systems may be observed. These effects may result in hypotension or skeletal muscle weakness. While all areas of the central nervous system are acted on by barbiturates, the mesencephalic reticular activating system is extremely sensitive to their effects. Barbiturates act at synapses where gamma-aminobenzoic acid is a neurotransmitter, but they may act in other areas as well.

Usual Dosage Adults: Oral: 1-2 tablets or capsules every 4 hours; not to exceed 6/day

Dosing interval in renal or hepatic impairment: Should be reduced

Dietary Considerations Alcohol: Additive CNS effects, avoid use

Patient Information Children and teenagers should not use this product; may cause drowsiness, avoid alcohol or other CNS depressants, may impair judgment and coordination; may cause physical and psychological dependence with prolonged use; do not exceed recommended dose

Nursing Implications Raise bed rails; initiate safety measures; aid with ambulation; monitor for CNS depression

Dosage Forms

Capsule, with acetaminophen:

Amaphen®, Anoquan®, Butace®, Endolor®, Esgic®, Femcet®, G-1®, Margesic®, Medigesic®, Repan®, Triad®, Two-Dyne®: Butalbital 50 mg, caffeine 40 mg, and acetaminophen 325 mg

Bancap®, Triapin®: Butalbital 50 mg and acetaminophen 325 mg

Phrenilin® Forte: Butalbital 50 mg and acetaminophen 650 mg

Capsule, with aspirin: (Fiorgen PF®, Fiorinal®, Isollyl® Improved, Lanorinal®, Marnal®): Butalbital 50 mg, caffeine 40 mg, and aspirin 325 mg

Tablet, with acetaminophen:

Esgic®, Fioricet®, Repan®: Butalbital 50 mg, caffeine 40 mg, and acetaminophen 325 mg

Phrenilin®: Butalbital 50 mg and acetaminophen 325 mg

Sedapap-10®: Butalbital 50 mg and acetaminophen 650 mg

Tablet, with aspirin:
Axotal®: Butalbital 50 mg and aspirin 650 mg
B-A-C®: Butalbital 50 mg, caffeine 40 mg, and aspirin 650 mg
Fiorinal®, Isollyl® Improved, Lanorinal®, Marnal®: Butalbital 50 mg, caffeine 40 mg, and aspirin 325 mg

♦ **Butisol (Can)** see Butabarbital Sodium on page 57
♦ **Butisol Sodium®** see Butabarbital Sodium on page 57
♦ **BW-430C** see Lamotrigine on page 187
♦ **Bydramine® Cough Syrup [OTC]** see Diphenhydramine on page 116
♦ **311C90** see Zolmitriptan on page 443
♦ **Cafatine®** see Ergotamine on page 133
♦ **Cafergot®** see Ergotamine on page 133
♦ **C. angustifolia** see Senna on page 373

Carbamazepine (kar ba MAZ e peen)

Related Information
Liquid Compatibility With Antipsychotics and Mood Stabilizers on page 587
Mood Stabilizers on page 588
Patient Information - Mood Stabilizers (Carbamazepine) on page 475
Teratogenic Risks of Psychotropic Medications on page 594

U.S. Brand Names Carbatrol®; Epitol®; Tegretol®; Tegretol®-XR

Canadian Brand Names Apo®-Carbamazepine; Mazepine®; Novo-Carbamaz®; Nu-Carbamazepine®; PMS-Carbamazepine

Synonyms CBZ

Pharmacologic Category Anticonvulsant, Miscellaneous

Generic Available Yes

Use Partial seizures with complex symptomatology (psychomotor, temporal lobe), generalized tonic-clonic seizures (grand mal), mixed seizure patterns; pain relief of trigeminal or glossopharyngeal neuralgia

Unlabeled/Investigational Use Treatment of bipolar disorders and other affective disorders, resistant schizophrenia, alcohol withdrawal, restless leg syndrome, psychotic behavior associated with dementia, post-traumatic stress disorders

Pregnancy Risk Factor D

Pregnancy/Breast-Feeding Implications
Clinical effects on the fetus: Crosses the placenta. Dysmorphic facial features, cranial defects, cardiac defects, spina bifida, IUGR, and multiple other malformations reported. Epilepsy itself, number of medications, genetic factors, or a combination of these probably influence the teratogenicity of anticonvulsant therapy. Benefit:risk ratio usually favors continued use during pregnancy and breast-feeding.
Breast-feeding/lactation: Crosses into breast milk. AAP considers **compatible** with breast-feeding.

Contraindications Hypersensitivity to carbamazepine or any component of the formulation; may have cross-sensitivity with tricyclic antidepressants; marrow depression; MAO inhibitor use; pregnancy (may harm fetus)

Warnings/Precautions MAO inhibitors should be discontinued for a minimum of 14 days before carbamazepine is begun; administer with caution to patients with history of cardiac damage, hepatic or renal disease; potentially fatal blood cell abnormalities have been reported following treatment; patients with a previous history of adverse hematologic reaction to any drug may be at increased risk; early detection of hematologic change is important; advise patients of early signs and symptoms including fever, sore throat, mouth ulcers, infections, easy bruising, petechial or purpuric hemorrhage; carbamazepine is not effective in absence, myoclonic or akinetic seizures; exacerbation of certain seizure types have been seen after initiation of carbamazepine therapy in children with mixed seizure disorders. Elderly may have increased risk of SIADH-like syndrome. Carbamazepine has mild anticholinergic activity; use with caution in patients with increased intraocular pressure (monitor closely), or sensitivity to anticholinergic effects (urinary
(Continued)

Carbamazepine *(Continued)*

retention, constipation). Drug should be discontinued if there are any signs of hypersensitivity.

Adverse Reactions

Cardiovascular: Edema, congestive heart failure, syncope, bradycardia, hypertension or hypotension, AV block, arrhythmias, thrombophlebitis, thromboembolism, lymphadenopathy

Central nervous system: Sedation, dizziness, fatigue, ataxia, confusion, headache, slurred speech, aseptic meningitis (case report)

Dermatologic: Rash, urticaria, toxic epidermal necrolysis, Stevens-Johnson syndrome, photosensitivity reaction, alterations in skin pigmentation, exfoliative dermatitis, erythema multiforme, purpura, alopecia

Endocrine & metabolic: Hyponatremia, SIADH, fever, chills

Gastrointestinal: Nausea, vomiting, gastric distress, abdominal pain, diarrhea, constipation, anorexia, pancreatitis

Genitourinary: Urinary retention, urinary frequency, azotemia, renal failure, impotence

Hematologic: Aplastic anemia, agranulocytosis, eosinophilia, leukopenia, pancytopenia, thrombocytopenia, bone marrow suppression, acute intermittent porphyria, leukocytosis

Hepatic: Hepatitis, abnormal liver function tests, jaundice, hepatic failure

Neuromuscular & skeletal: Peripheral neuritis

Ocular: Blurred vision, nystagmus, lens opacities, conjunctivitis

Otic: Tinnitus, hyperacusis

Miscellaneous: Hypersensitivity (including multi-organ reactions, may include vasculitis, disorders mimicking lymphoma, eosinophilia, hepatosplenomegaly), diaphoresis

Overdosage/Toxicology Symptoms of overdose include dizziness, ataxia, drowsiness, nausea, vomiting, tremor, agitation, nystagmus, urinary retention, dysrhythmias, coma, seizures, twitches, respiratory depression, and neuromuscular disturbances. Activated charcoal is effective at binding certain chemicals and this is especially true for carbamazepine. Other treatment is supportive and symptomatic.

Drug Interactions CYP2C8 and 3A3/4 enzyme substrate; CYP1A2, 2C, and 3A3/4 inducer. **Note:** Carbamazepine (CBZ) is a heteroinducer. It induces its own metabolism as well as the metabolism of other drugs. If CBZ is added to a drug regimen, serum concentrations may decrease. Conversely, if CBZ is part of an ongoing regimen and it is discontinued, elevated concentrations of the other drugs may result.

Acetaminophen: Carbamazepine may enhance hepatotoxic potential of acetaminophen; risk is greater in acetaminophen overdose

Antipsychotics: Carbamazepine may enhance the metabolism (decrease the efficacy) of antipsychotics; monitor for altered response; dose adjustment may be needed

Barbiturates: May reduce serum concentrations of carbamazepine; monitor

Benzodiazepines: Serum concentrations and effect of benzodiazepines may be reduced by carbamazepine; monitor for decreased effect

Calcium channel blockers: Diltiazem and verapamil may increase carbamazepine levels, due to enzyme inhibition (see below); other calcium channel blockers (felodipine) may be decreased by carbamazepine due to enzyme induction

Chlorpromazine: **Note:** Carbamazepine suspension is incompatible with chlorpromazine solution. Schedule carbamazepine suspension at least 1-2 hours apart from other liquid medicinals.

Corticosteroids: Metabolism may be increased by carbamazepine

Cyclosporine (and other immunosuppressants): Carbamazepine may enhance the metabolism of immunosuppressants, decreasing its clinical effect; includes both cyclosporine and tacrolimus

CYP2C8/9 inhibitors: Serum levels and/or toxicity of carbamazepine may be increased; inhibitors include amiodarone, cimetidine, fluvoxamine, some

NSAIDs, metronidazole, ritonavir, sulfonamides, troglitazone, valproic acid, and zafirlukast; monitor for increased effect/toxicity

CYP3A3/4 inhibitors: Serum level and/or toxicity of carbamazepine may be increased; inhibitors include amiodarone, cimetidine, clarithromycin, erythromycin, delavirdine, diltiazem, dirithromycin, disulfiram, fluoxetine, fluvoxamine, grapefruit juice, indinavir, itraconazole, ketoconazole, metronidazole, nefazodone, nevirapine, propoxyphene, quinine, quinupristin-dalfopristin, ritonavir, saquinavir, ticlopidine, verapamil, zafirlukast, zileuton; monitor for altered effects; a decrease in carbamazepine dosage may be required

Danazol: May increase serum concentrations of carbamazepine; monitor

Doxycycline: Carbamazepine may enhance the metabolism of doxycycline, decreasing its clinical effect

Ethosuximide: Serum levels may be reduced by carbamazepine

Felbamate: May increase carbamazepine levels and toxicity (increased epoxide metabolite concentrations); carbamazepine may decrease felbamate levels due to enzyme induction

Immunosuppressants: Carbamazepine may enhance the metabolism of immunosuppressants, decreasing its clinical effect; includes both cyclosporine and tacrolimus

Isoniazid: May increase the serum concentrations and toxicity of carbamazepine; in addition, carbamazepine may increase the hepatic toxicity of isoniazid (INH)

Isotretinoin: May decrease the effect of carbamazepine

Lamotrigine: Increases the epoxide metabolite of carbamazepine resulting in toxicity; carbamazepine increases the metabolism of lamotrigine

Lithium: Neurotoxicity may result in patients receiving concurrent carbamazepine

Loxapine: May increase concentrations of epoxide metabolite and toxicity of carbamazepine

Methadone: Carbamazepine may enhance the metabolism of methadone resulting in methadone withdrawal

Methylphenidate: concurrent use of carbamazepine may reduce the therapeutic effect of methylphenidate; limited documentation; monitor for decreased effect

Neuromuscular blocking agents, nondepolarizing: Effects may be of shorter duration when administered to patients receiving carbamazepine

Oral contraceptives: Metabolism may be increased by carbamazepine, resulting in a loss of efficacy

Phenytoin: Carbamazepine levels may be decreased by phenytoin; metabolism may be altered by carbamazepine

SSRIs: Metabolism may be increased by carbamazepine (due to enzyme induction)

Theophylline: Serum levels may be reduced by carbamazepine

Thioridazine: **Note:** Carbamazepine suspension is incompatible with thioridazine liquid. Schedule carbamazepine suspension at least 1-2 hours apart from other liquid medicinals.

Thyroid: Serum levels may be reduced by carbamazepine

Tramadol: Tramadol's risk of seizures may be increased with TCAs (carbamazepine may be associated with similar risk due to chemical similarity to TCAs)

Tricyclic antidepressants: May increase serum concentrations of carbamazepine; carbamazepine may decrease concentrations of tricyclics due to enzyme induction

Valproic acid: Serum levels may be reduced by carbamazepine; carbamazepine levels may also be altered by valproic acid

Warfarin: Carbamazepine may inhibit the hypoprothrombinemic effects of oral anticoagulants via increased metabolism; this combination should generally be avoided

Ethanol/Nutrition/Herb Interactions

Ethanol: Avoid ethanol (may increase CNS depression).

Food: Carbamazepine serum levels may be increased if taken with food. Carbamazepine serum concentration may be increased if taken with grapefruit juice; avoid concurrent use.

(Continued)

Carbamazepine *(Continued)*

Herb/Nutraceutical: Avoid evening primrose (seizure threshold decreased). Avoid valerian, St John's wort, kava kava, gotu kola (may increase CNS depression).

Mechanism of Action In addition to anticonvulsant effects, carbamazepine has anticholinergic, antineuralgic, antidiuretic, muscle relaxant and antiarrhythmic properties; may depress activity in the nucleus ventralis of the thalamus or decrease synaptic transmission or decrease summation of temporal stimulation leading to neural discharge by limiting influx of sodium ions across cell membrane or other unknown mechanisms; stimulates the release of ADH and potentiates its action in promoting reabsorption of water; chemically related to tricyclic antidepressants

Pharmacodynamics/Kinetics

Absorption: Slowly absorbed from GI tract

Distribution: V_d:

Neonates: 1.5 L/kg

Children: 1.9 L/kg

Adults: 0.59-2 L/kg

Protein binding: 75% to 90%; may be decreased in newborns

Metabolism: In the liver to active epoxide metabolite; induces liver enzymes to increase metabolism and shorten half-life over time

Bioavailability, oral: 85%

Half-life:

Initial: 18-55 hours

Multiple dosing:

Children: 8-14 hours

Adults: 12-17 hours

Time to peak serum concentration: Unpredictable, within 4-8 hours

Elimination: 1% to 3% excreted unchanged in urine

Usual Dosage Oral (dosage must be adjusted according to patient's response and serum concentrations):

Children:

<6 years: Initial: 5 mg/kg/day; dosage may be increased every 5-7 days to 10 mg/kg/day; then up to 20 mg/kg/day if necessary; administer in 2-4 divided doses

6-12 years: Initial: 100 mg twice daily or 10 mg/kg/day in 2 divided doses; increase by 100 mg/day at weekly intervals depending upon response; usual maintenance: 20-30 mg/kg/day in 2-4 divided doses (maximum dose: 1000 mg/day)

Children >12 years and Adults: 200 mg twice daily to start, increase by 200 mg/day at weekly intervals until therapeutic levels achieved; usual dose: 400-1200 mg/day in 2-4 divided doses; maximum dose: 12-15 years: 1000 mg/day, >15 years: 1200 mg/day; some patients have required up to 1.6-2.4 g/day

Trigeminal or glossopharyngeal neuralgia: Initial: 100 mg twice daily with food, gradually increasing in increments of 100 mg twice daily as needed; usual maintenance: 400-800 mg daily in 2 divided doses; maximum dose: 1200 mg/day

Elderly: 100 mg 1-2 times daily, increase in increments of 100 mg/day at weekly intervals until therapeutic level is achieved; usual dose: 400-1000 mg/day

Dosing adjustment in renal impairment: Cl_{cr} <10 mL/minute: Administer 75% of dose

Dietary Considerations Drug may cause GI upset, take with large amount of water or food to decrease GI upset. May need to split doses to avoid GI upset.

Administration

Suspension dosage form must be given on a 3-4 times/day schedule versus tablets which can be given 2-4 times/day. When carbamazepine suspension has been combined with chlorpromazine or thioridazine solutions a precipitate forms which may result in loss of effect. Therefore, it is recommended that the carbamazepine suspension dosage form not be administered at the same time with other liquid medicinal agents or diluents. Since a given dose of suspension will produce higher peak levels than the same dose given as the tablet form, patients given the suspension should be started on lower doses and increased slowly to avoid unwanted side effects.

Extended release tablets should be inspected for damage. Damaged extended release tablets (without release portal) should not be administered.

Monitoring Parameters CBC with platelet count, reticulocytes, serum iron, liver function tests, urinalysis, BUN, serum carbamazepine levels, thyroid function tests, serum sodium; observe patient for excessive sedation, especially when instituting or increasing therapy

Reference Range

Timing of serum samples: Absorption is slow, peak levels occur 6-8 hours after ingestion of the first dose; the half-life ranges from 8-60 hours, therefore, steady-state is achieved in 2-5 days

Therapeutic levels: 4-12 µg/mL (SI: 25-51 µmol/L)

Toxic concentration: >15 µg/mL; patients who require higher levels of 8-12 µg/mL (SI: 34-51 µmol/L) should be watched closely. Side effects including CNS effects occur commonly at higher dosage levels. If other anticonvulsants are given therapeutic range is 4-8 µg/mL.

Test Interactions Increased BUN, AST, ALT, bilirubin, alkaline phosphatase (S); decreased calcium, T_3, T_4, sodium (S)

Patient Information Take with food, may cause drowsiness, periodic blood test monitoring required; notify physician if you observe bleeding, bruising, jaundice, abdominal pain, pale stools, mental disturbances, fever, chills, sore throat, or mouth ulcers

Nursing Implications Observe patient for excessive sedation; suspension dosage form must be given on a 3-4 times/day schedule versus tablets which can be given 2-4 times/day

Additional Information Investigationally, loading doses of the suspension (10 mg/kg for children <12 years of age and 8 mg/kg for children >12 years of age) were given (via NG or ND tubes followed by 5-10 mL of water to flush through tube) to PICU patients with frequent seizures/status. Five of 6 patients attained mean Cp of 4.3 mcg/mL and 7.3 mcg/mL at 1 and 2 hours postload. Concurrent enteral feeding or ileus may delay absorption.

Dosage Forms

Capsule, extended release: 200 mg, 300 mg

Suspension, oral: 100 mg/5 mL (450 mL) [citrus-vanilla flavor]

Tablet: 200 mg

Tablet, chewable: 100 mg

Tablet, extended release: 100 mg, 200 mg, 400 mg

Cevimeline (se vi ME leen)

U.S. Brand Names Evoxac™

Synonyms Cevimeline Hydrochloride

Pharmacologic Category Cholinergic Agonist

Generic Available No

Use Treatment of symptoms of dry mouth in patients with Sjögren's syndrome

(Continued)

Cevimeline *(Continued)*

Pregnancy Risk Factor C

Pregnancy/Breast-Feeding Implications There are no adequate or well-controlled studies in pregnant women. Use only if potential benefit justifies potential risk to the fetus. Excretion in breast milk is unknown/not recommended.

Contraindications Hypersensitivity to cevimeline or any component of the formulation; uncontrolled asthma; narrow-angle glaucoma; acute iritis; other conditions where miosis is undesirable

Warnings/Precautions May alter cardiac conduction and/or heart rate; use caution in patients with significant cardiovascular disease, including angina, myocardial infarction, or conduction disturbances. Cevimeline has the potential to increase bronchial smooth muscle tone, airway resistance, and bronchial secretions; use with caution in patients with controlled asthma, COPD, or chronic bronchitis. May cause decreased visual acuity (particularly at night and in patients with central lens changes) and impaired depth perception. Patients should be cautioned about driving at night or performing hazardous activities in reduced lighting. May cause a variety of parasympathomimetic effects, which may be particularly dangerous in elderly patients; excessive sweating may lead to dehydration in some patients.

Use with caution in patients with a history of biliary stones or nephrolithiasis; cevimeline may induce smooth muscle spasms, precipitating cholangitis, cholecystitis, biliary obstruction, renal colic, or ureteral reflux in susceptible patients. Patients with a known or suspected deficiency of CYP2D6 may be at higher risk of adverse effects. Safety and efficacy has not been established in pediatric patients.

Adverse Reactions

>10%:
  Central nervous system: Headache (14%; placebo 20%)
  Gastrointestinal: Nausea (14%), diarrhea (10%)
  Respiratory: Rhinitis (11%), sinusitis (12%), upper respiratory infection (11%)
  Miscellaneous: Increased diaphoresis (19%)

1% to 10%:
  Cardiovascular: Peripheral edema, chest pain, edema, palpitation
  Central nervous system: Dizziness (4%), fatigue (3%), pain (3%), insomnia (2%), anxiety (1%), fever, depression, migraine, hypoesthesia, vertigo
  Dermatologic: Rash (4%; placebo 6%), pruritus, skin disorder, erythematous rash
  Endocrine & metabolic: Hot flashes (2%)
  Gastrointestinal: Dyspepsia (8%; placebo 9%), abdominal pain (8%), vomiting (5%), excessive salivation (2%), constipation, salivary gland pain, dry mouth, sialoadenitis, gastroesophageal reflux, flatulence, ulcerative stomatitis, eructation, increased amylase, anorexia, tooth disorder
  Genitourinary: Urinary tract infection (6%), vaginitis, cystitis
  Hematologic: Anemia
  Local: Abscess
  Neuromuscular & skeletal: back pain (5%), arthralgia (4%), skeletal pain (3%), rigors (1%), hypertonia, tremor, myalgia, hyporeflexia, leg cramps
  Ocular: Conjunctivitis (4%), abnormal vision, eye pain, eye abnormality, xerophthalmia
  Otic: Ear ache, otitis media
  Respiratory: Coughing (6%), bronchitis (4%), pneumonia, epistaxis
  Miscellaneous: Flu-like syndrome, infection, fungal infection, allergy, hiccups

<1%: Syncope, malaise, substernal chest pain, abnormal ECG, hypertension, hypotension, arrhythmia, T-wave inversion, angina, myocardial infarction, pericarditis, pulmonary embolism, peripheral ischemia, thrombophlebitis, vasculitis, dysphagia, enterocolitis, gastric ulcer, gastrointestinal hemorrhage, ileus, melena, mucositis, esophageal stricture, esophagitis, peptic ulcer, stomatitis, tongue discoloration, tongue ulceration, hypothyroidism, thrombocytopenic purpura, thrombocytopenia, anemia, eosinophilia, granulocytopenia, leukopenia, leukocytosis, lymphadenopathy, cholelithiasis, increased transaminases,

arthropathy, avascular necrosis (femoral head), bursitis, costochondritis, syno-vitis, tendonitis, tenosynovitis, coma, dyskinesia, dysphonia, aggravated multiple sclerosis, neuralgia, neuropathy, paresthesia, agitation, confusion, depersonali-zation, emotional lability, manic reaction, paranoia, somnolence, hyperkinesia, hallucination, fall, sepsis, bronchospasm, nasal ulcer, pleural effusion, pulmonary fibrosis, systemic lupus erythematosus, alopecia, dermatitis, eczema, photosensitivity reaction, dry skin, skin ulceration, bullous eruption, motion sickness, parosmia, taste perversion, blepharitis, cataract, corneal ulcer-ation, diplopia, glaucoma, anterior chamber hemorrhage, retinal disorder, scle-ritis, tinnitus, epididymitis, menstrual disorder, genital pruritus, dysuria, hematuria, renal calculus, abnormal renal function, decreased urine flow, postural hypotension, aphasia, convulsions, paralysis, gingival hyperplasia, intestinal obstruction, bundle branch block, increased CPK, electrolyte abnor-mality, aggressive behavior, delirium, impotence, apnea, oliguria, urinary reten-tion, lymphocytosis

Overdosage/Toxicology Symptoms of toxicity may include headache, visual disturbances, lacrimation, sweating, gastrointestinal spasm, nausea, vomiting, diarrhea, AV block, mental confusion, tremor, cardiac depression, bradycardia, tachycardia, or bronchospasm. Atropine may be of value as an antidote, and epinephrine may be required for bronchoconstriction. Additional treatment is supportive. The effect of hemodialysis is unknown.

Drug Interactions CYP2D6 and CYP3A3/4 substrate

Increased effect: Drugs which inhibit CYP2D6 (including amiodarone, fluoxetine, paroxetine, quinidine, ritonavir) or CYP3A3/4 (including diltiazem, erythromycin, itraconazole, ketoconazole, verapamil) may increase levels of cevimeline. The effects of other cholinergic agents may be increased during concurrent adminis-tration with cevimeline. Concurrent use of cevimeline and beta-blockers may increase the potential for conduction disturbances.

Decreased effect: Anticholinergic agents (atropine, TCAs, phenothiazines) may antagonize the effects of cevimeline

Stability Store at 25°C (77°F)

Mechanism of Action Binds to muscarinic (cholinergic) receptors, causing an increase in secretion of exocrine glands (including salivary glands)

Pharmacodynamics/Kinetics

Distribution: V_d: 6 L/kg

Protein binding: <20%

Metabolism: Hepatic, via CYP2D6 and CYP3A3/4

Half-life: 5 hours

Time to peak: 1.5-2 hours

Elimination: In urine, as metabolites and unchanged drug

Usual Dosage Adults: Oral: 30 mg 3 times/day

Dosage adjustment in renal/hepatic impairment: Not studied; no specific dosage adjustment is recommended

Elderly: No specific dosage adjustment is recommended; however, use caution when initiating due to potential for increased sensitivity

Dietary Considerations Take with or without food.

Patient Information Take exactly as directed; do not alter dosage without consulting prescriber. Take with or without food. You may experience decreased visual acuity (especially at night) (use caution when driving at night or when engaging in other activities in poorly lighted areas until response to medication is known); gastrointestinal distress or nausea (small frequent meals, frequent mouth care, sucking lozenges, or chewing gum may help); headache (mild analgesic may help); or diarrhea (increase dietary fiber and exercise). Report unresolved diarrhea or constipation, abdominal pain, flatulence, anorexia, or excessive salivation; excessive sweating; unresolved respiratory distress, runny nose, cold or flu symp-toms; joint, bone, or muscle weakness, pain, tremor, or cramping; chest pain or palpitations, swelling of extremities, weight gain; or other persistent adverse symp-toms.

Dosage Forms Capsule: 30 mg

- **Cevimeline Hydrochloride** *see* Cevimeline *on page 65*
- **CF100** *see* Ginkgo Biloba *on page 167*

Chamomile

Synonyms *Matricaria chamomilla*; *Matricarta recutita*

Pharmacologic Category Herb

Use Has been used for indigestion and its hypnotic properties; topical anti-inflammatory agent; used for hemorrhoids, irritable bowel, eczema, mastitis and leg ulcers; used to flavor cigarette tobacco

Contraindications Known hypersensitivity to *Asteraceae/Compositae* family

Adverse Reactions Associated with those with severe ragweed allergies
Dermatologic: Contact dermatitis, immunologic contact urticaria
Gastrointestinal: Emesis (from dried flowering heads)
Miscellaneous: Anaphylaxis
While the toxicity of its main chemical constituent (Bisabolol) is low, the tea is essentially prepared from various allergens (ie, pollen-laden flower heads) which can cause hypersensitivity reactions especially in atopic individuals; contains various flavonoids (apigenin, herniarin)

Overdosage/Toxicology Treatment: Supportive therapy; treat allergic reactions with standard therapy (ie, epinephrine, antihistamines, vasopressors, if required)

Drug Interactions
CNS depressants: Sedative effects may be additive with other CNS depressants; includes ethanol, barbiturates, narcotic analgesics, and other sedative agents; monitor for increased effect
Warfarin: Anticoagulant effects may be potentiated (only at very high dosages of chamomile)

Usual Dosage
Tea: ±150 mL H_2O poured over heaping tablespoon (±3 g) of chamomile, covered and steeped 5-10 minutes; tea used 3-4 times/day for G.I. upset
Liquid extract: 1-4 mL 3 times/day

Additional Information Cross-sensitivity may occur in individuals allergic to ragweed pollens, asters, or chrysanthemums

Chaparral

Synonyms *Larrea tridentata*

Pharmacologic Category Herb

Use Herbal medicine to treat acne, bowel cramps, analgesic agent and to "retard aging" (not substantiated)

Adverse Reactions
Dermatologic: Contact dermatitis
Gastrointestinal: Anorexia
Hematologic: Coagulopathy
Hepatic: Lobular necrosis, jaundice
Miscellaneous: Necrosis

Overdosage/Toxicology
Decontamination: Ipecac within 30 minutes or lavage (within 1 hour)/activated charcoal with cathartic
Treatment: Supportive therapy; orthotopic liver transplantation may be required to treat liver failure

Patient Information Considered unsafe by the FDA; large doses and/or prolonged use can cause liver damage

Additional Information A branched bush or shrub that is olive green and can grow to a height of 9 feet in the desert regions of Southwestern U.S. and Mexico. Approximately 200 tons of chaparral were sold in the U.S. for use as teas and herbal dietary supplements in the 20 years from 1973-1993, according to informal herb industry estimates. Few adverse reactions were reported during this period. A medical review by three physicians of patient records obtained from FDA regarding hepatitis associated with chaparral ingestion could not definitively conclude that chaparral was the causative agent. Idiosyncratic reactions were suggested.

Chaste Tree

Synonyms *Vitex agnus-castus*

Pharmacologic Category Herb

Use In herbal medicine, it is used in treatment of menstrual disorders, premenstrual syndrome and mastodynia

Adverse Reactions Dermatologic: Pruritus, rash

Overdosage/Toxicology
Decontamination: Lavage (within 1 hour)/activated charcoal with cathartic
Treatment: Supportive therapy; antihistamines can be used to treat pruritus although there is no data on this modality

Drug Interactions None known per Commission E but may counteract the effectiveness of birth control pills

Usual Dosage
As a concentrated alcoholic extract: ~20 mg/day
Per Commission E: Average daily dose: 3 g herb or equivalent preparations

Additional Information A small deciduous multi-trunk tree which can grow up to 25 feet; native to Mediterranean region with flowers blooming in summer; the dried ripe fruit (which is brown/black with a pepperish flavor or aroma) contains the active chemical ingredients; dried leaves contain some of the active ingredients

♦ **Chloral** *see* Chloral Hydrate *on page 69*

Chloral Hydrate (KLOR al HYE drate)

Related Information
Anxiolytic/Hypnotic Use in Long-Term Care Facilities *on page 562*
Federal OBRA Regulations Recommended Maximum Doses *on page 583*
Nonbenzodiazepine Anxiolytics and Hypnotics *on page 589*

U.S. Brand Names Aquachloral® Supprettes®

Canadian Brand Names Novo-Chlorhydrate®; PMS-Chloral Hydrate

Synonyms Chloral; Hydrated Chloral; Trichloroacetaldehyde Monohydrate

Pharmacologic Category Hypnotic, Miscellaneous

Generic Available Yes

Use Short-term sedative and hypnotic (<2 weeks), sedative/hypnotic for diagnostic procedures; sedative prior to EEG evaluations

Restrictions C-IV

Pregnancy Risk Factor C

Contraindications Hypersensitivity to chloral hydrate or any component of the formulation; hepatic or renal impairment; gastritis or ulcers; severe cardiac disease

Warnings/Precautions Use with caution in patients with porphyria; use with caution in neonates, drug may accumulate with repeated use, prolonged use in neonates associated with hyperbilirubinemia; tolerance to hypnotic effect develops, therefore, not recommended for use >2 weeks; taper dosage to avoid withdrawal with prolonged use; trichloroethanol (TCE), a metabolite of chloral hydrate, is a carcinogen in mice; there is no data in humans. Chloral hydrate is considered a second line hypnotic agent in the elderly. Recent interpretive guidelines from the Health Care Financing Administration (HCFA) discourage the use of chloral hydrate in residents of long-term care facilities.

Adverse Reactions
Central nervous system: Ataxia, disorientation, sedation, excitement (paradoxical), dizziness, fever, headache, confusion, lightheadedness, nightmares, hallucinations, drowsiness, "hangover" effect
Dermatologic: Rash, urticaria
Gastrointestinal: Gastric irritation, nausea, vomiting, diarrhea, flatulence
Hematologic: Leukopenia, eosinophilia, acute intermittent porphyria
(Continued)

Chloral Hydrate (Continued)

Miscellaneous: Physical and psychological dependence may occur with prolonged use of large doses

Overdosage/Toxicology Doses >2 g may produce symptoms of toxicity

Signs and symptoms: Hypotension, respiratory depression, coma, hypothermia, cardiac arrhythmias

Treatment: Supportive and symptomatic; lidocaine or propranolol may be used for ventricular dysrhythmias, while isoproterenol or atropine may be required for torsade de pointes

Drug Interactions CYP2E1 enzyme substrate

CNS depressants: Sedative effects and/or respiratory depression with chloral hydrate may be additive with other CNS depressants; monitor for increased effect; includes ethanol, sedatives, antidepressants, narcotic analgesics, and benzodiazepines

Furosemide: Diaphoresis, flushing, and hypertension have occurred in patients who received I.V. furosemide within 24 hours after administration of chloral hydrate; consider using a benzodiazepine

Phenytoin: Half-life may be decreased by chloral hydrate; limited documentation (small, single-dose study); monitor

Warfarin: Effect of oral anticoagulants may be increased by chloral hydrate; monitor INR; warfarin dosage may require adjustment. Chloral hydrate's metabolite may displace warfarin from its protein binding sites resulting in an increase in the hypoprothrombinemic response to warfarin.

Ethanol/Nutrition/Herb Interactions

Ethanol: Avoid ethanol (may increase CNS depression).

Herb/Nutraceutical: Avoid valerian, St John's wort, kava kava, gotu kola (may increase CNS depression).

Stability Sensitive to light; exposure to air causes volatilization; store in light-resistant, airtight container

Mechanism of Action Central nervous system depressant effects are due to its active metabolite trichloroethanol, mechanism unknown

Pharmacodynamics/Kinetics

Peak effect: Within 0.5-1 hour

Duration: 4-8 hours

Absorption: Oral, rectal: Well absorbed

Distribution: Crosses the placenta; negligible amounts appear in breast milk

Metabolism: Rapidly to trichloroethanol (active metabolite); variable amounts metabolized in liver and kidney to trichloroacetic acid (inactive)

Half-life: Active metabolite: 8-11 hours

Elimination: Metabolites excreted in urine, small amounts excreted in feces via bile

Usual Dosage

Children:

Sedation or anxiety: Oral, rectal: 5-15 mg/kg/dose every 8 hours (maximum: 500 mg/dose)

Prior to EEG: Oral, rectal: 20-25 mg/kg/dose, 30-60 minutes prior to EEG; may repeat in 30 minutes to maximum of 100 mg/kg or 2 g total

Hypnotic: Oral, rectal: 20-40 mg/kg/dose up to a maximum of 50 mg/kg/24 hours or 1 g/dose or 2 g/24 hours

Sedation during nonpainful procedure: Oral: 50-75 mg/kg/dose 30-60 minutes prior to procedure; may repeat 30 minutes after initial dose if needed, to a total maximum dose of 120 mg/kg or 1 g total

Adults: Oral, rectal:

Sedation, anxiety: 250 mg 3 times/day

Hypnotic: 500-1000 mg at bedtime or 30 minutes prior to procedure, not to exceed 2 g/24 hours

Dosing adjustment/comments in renal impairment: Cl_{cr} <50 mL/minute: Avoid use

Hemodialysis: Dialyzable (50% to 100%); supplemental dose is not necessary

Dosing adjustment/comments in hepatic impairment: Avoid use in patients with severe hepatic impairment

Administration Do not crush capsule, contains drug in liquid form

Monitoring Parameters Vital signs, O_2 saturation and blood pressure with doses used for conscious sedation

Test Interactions False-positive urine glucose using Clinitest® method; may interfere with fluorometric urine catecholamine and urinary 17-hydroxycorticosteroid tests

Patient Information Take a capsule with a full glass of water or fruit juice; swallow capsules whole, do not chew; avoid alcohol and other CNS depressants; avoid activities needing good psychomotor coordination until CNS effects are known; drug may cause physical or psychological dependence; avoid abrupt discontinuation after prolonged use; if taking at home prior to a diagnostic procedure, have someone else transport

Nursing Implications Gastric irritation may be minimized by diluting dose in water or other oral liquid

Additional Information Not an analgesic

Dosage Forms
Capsule: 500 mg
Suppository, rectal: 324 mg, 500 mg, 648 mg
Syrup: 500 mg/5 mL (5 mL, 10 mL, 480 mL)

Chlordiazepoxide (klor dye az e POKS ide)

Related Information

Anxiolytic/Hypnotic Use in Long-Term Care Facilities *on page 562*
Benzodiazepines Comparison Chart *on page 566*
Federal OBRA Regulations Recommended Maximum Doses *on page 583*
Patient Information - Anxiolytics & Sedative Hypnotics (Benzodiazepines) *on page 483*

U.S. Brand Names Librium®

Canadian Brand Names Apo®-Chlordiazepoxide; Corax®; Medilium®; Novo-Poxide®; Solium®

Synonyms Methaminodiazepoxide Hydrochloride

Pharmacologic Category Benzodiazepine

Generic Available Yes

Use Management of anxiety disorder or for the short-term relief of symptoms of anxiety; withdrawal symptoms of acute alcoholism; preoperative apprehension and anxiety

Restrictions C-IV

Pregnancy Risk Factor D

Contraindications Hypersensitivity to chlordiazepoxide or any component of the formulation (cross-sensitivity with other benzodiazepines may exist); narrow-angle glaucoma (not in product labeling: however, benzodiazepines are contraindicated); pregnancy

Warnings/Precautions Active metabolites with extended half-lives may lead to delayed accumulation and adverse effects. Use with caution in elderly or debilitated patients, pediatric patients, patients with hepatic disease (including alcoholics) or renal impairment. Use with caution in patients with respiratory disease or impaired gag reflex. Use with caution in patients with porphyria.

Parenteral administration should be avoided in comatose patients or shock. Adequate resuscitative equipment/personnel should be available, and appropriate monitoring should be conducted at the time of injection and for several hours following administration. The parenteral formulation should be diluted for I.M. administration with the supplied diluent only. This diluent should not be used when preparing the drug for intravenous administration.

Causes CNS depression (dose-related) resulting in sedation, dizziness, confusion, or ataxia which may impair physical and mental capabilities. Patients must be cautioned about performing tasks which require mental alertness (ie, operating (Continued)

Chlordiazepoxide (Continued)

machinery or driving). Use with caution in patients receiving other CNS depressants or psychoactive agents (lithium, phenothiazines). Effects with other sedative drugs or ethanol may be potentiated. Benzodiazepines have been associated with falls and traumatic injury and should be used with extreme caution in patients who are at risk of these events (especially the elderly).

Use caution in patients with depression, particularly if suicidal risk may be present. Use with caution in patients with a history of drug dependence. Benzodiazepines have been associated with dependence and acute withdrawal symptoms on discontinuation or reduction in dose. Acute withdrawal, including seizures, may be precipitated in patients after administration of flumazenil to patients receiving long-term benzodiazepine therapy.

Benzodiazepines have been associated with anterograde amnesia. Paradoxical reactions, including hyperactive or aggressive behavior have been reported with benzodiazepines, particularly in adolescent/pediatric or psychiatric patients. Does not have analgesic, antidepressant, or antipsychotic properties.

Adverse Reactions

>10%:
    Central nervous system: Drowsiness, fatigue, ataxia, lightheadedness, memory impairment, dysarthria, irritability
    Dermatologic: Rash
    Endocrine & metabolic: Decreased libido, menstrual disorders
    Gastrointestinal: Xerostomia, decreased salivation, increased or decreased appetite, weight gain/loss
    Genitourinary: Micturition difficulties
1% to 10%:
    Cardiovascular: Hypotension
    Central nervous system: Confusion, dizziness, disinhibition, akathisia, increased libido
    Dermatologic: Dermatitis
    Gastrointestinal: Increased salivation
    Genitourinary: Sexual dysfunction, incontinence
    Neuromuscular & skeletal: Rigidity, tremor, muscle cramps
    Otic: Tinnitus
    Respiratory: Nasal congestion

Overdosage/Toxicology

Signs and symptoms: Hypotension, respiratory depression, coma, hypothermia, cardiac arrhythmias

Treatment: Supportive, rarely is mechanical ventilation required, flumazenil has been shown to selectively block the binding of benzodiazepines to CNS receptors, resulting in a reversal of benzodiazepine- induced CNS depression. Respiratory depression may not be reversed.

Drug Interactions CYP3A3/4 enzyme substrate

CNS depressants: Sedative effects and/or respiratory depression may be additive with CNS depressants; includes ethanol, barbiturates, narcotic analgesics, and other sedative agents; monitor for increased effect

CYP enzyme inducers: Metabolism of some benzodiazepines may be increased, decreasing their therapeutic effect; consider using an alternative sedative/hypnotic agent; potential inducers include phenobarbital, phenytoin, carbamazepine, rifampin, and rifabutin

CYP3A3/4 inhibitors: Serum level and/or toxicity of some benzodiazepines may be increased; inhibitors include amiodarone, cimetidine, clarithromycin, erythromycin, delavirdine, diltiazem, dirithromycin, disulfiram, fluoxetine, fluvoxamine, grapefruit juice, indinavir, itraconazole, ketoconazole, nevirapine, propoxyphene, quinupristin-dalfopristin, ritonavir, saquinavir, verapamil, zafirlukast, zileuton; monitor for altered benzodiazepine response

Levodopa: Therapeutic effects may be diminished in some patients following the addition of a benzodiazepine; limited/inconsistent data

Oral contraceptives: May decrease the clearance of some benzodiazepines (those which undergo oxidative metabolism); monitor for increased benzodiazepine effect

Theophylline: May partially antagonize some of the effects of benzodiazepines; monitor for decreased response; may require higher doses for sedation

Ethanol/Nutrition/Herb Interactions

Ethanol: Avoid ethanol (may increase CNS depression).

Food: Serum concentrations/effects may be increased with grapefruit juice, but unlikely because of high oral bioavailability of chlordiazepoxide.

Herb/Nutraceutical: Avoid valerian, St John's wort, kava kava, gotu kola (may increase CNS depression).

Stability Refrigerate injection; protect from light; **incompatible** when mixed with Ringer's solution, normal saline, ascorbic acid, benzquinamide, heparin, phenytoin, promethazine, secobarbital

Mechanism of Action Binds to stereospecific benzodiazepine receptors on the postsynaptic GABA neuron at several sites within the central nervous system, including the limbic system, reticular formation. Enhancement of the inhibitory effect of GABA on neuronal excitability results by increased neuronal membrane permeability to chloride ions. This shift in chloride ions results in hyperpolarization (a less excitable state) and stabilization.

Pharmacodynamics/Kinetics

Distribution: V_d: 3.3 L/kg; crosses the placenta; appears in breast milk

Protein binding: 90% to 98%

Metabolism: Extensive in the liver to desmethyldiazepam (active and long-acting)

Half-life: 6.6-25 hours

End-stage renal disease: 5-30 hours

Cirrhosis: 30-63 hours

Time to peak serum concentration:

Oral: Within 2 hours

I.M.: Results in lower peak plasma levels than oral

Elimination: Very little excretion in urine as unchanged drug

Usual Dosage

Children:

<6 years: Not recommended

>6 years: Anxiety: Oral, I.M.: 0.5 mg/kg/24 hours divided every 6-8 hours

Adults:

Anxiety:

Oral: 15-100 mg divided 3-4 times/day

I.M., I.V.: Initial: 50-100 mg followed by 25-50 mg 3-4 times/day as needed

Preoperative anxiety: I.M.: 50-100 mg prior to surgery

Ethanol withdrawal symptoms: Oral, I.V.: 50-100 mg to start, dose may be repeated in 2-4 hours as necessary to a maximum of 300 mg/24 hours

Dosing adjustment in renal impairment: Cl_{cr} <10 mL/minute: Administer 50% of dose

Hemodialysis: Not dialyzable (0% to 5%)

Dosing adjustment/comments in hepatic impairment: Avoid use

Administration Up to 300 mg may be given I.M. or I.V. during a 6-hour period, but not more than this in any 24-hour period; do not use diluent provided with parenteral form for I.V. administration; dissolve with normal saline instead; I.V. form is a powder and should be reconstituted with 5 mL of sterile water or saline prior to administration

Monitoring Parameters Respiratory and cardiovascular status, mental status, check for orthostasis

Reference Range Therapeutic: 0.1-3 µg/mL (SI: 0-10 µmol/L); Toxic: >23 µg/mL (SI: >77 µmol/L)

Test Interactions ↓ HDL, ↑ triglycerides (S)

Patient Information Avoid alcohol and other CNS depressants; avoid activities needing good psychomotor coordination until CNS effects are known; drug may (Continued)

Chlordiazepoxide *(Continued)*

cause physical or psychological dependence; avoid abrupt discontinuation after prolonged use, may cause drowsiness, poor balance

Nursing Implications Raise bed rails; initiate safety measures; aid with ambulation

Additional Information Abrupt discontinuation after sustained use (generally >10 days) may cause withdrawal symptoms.

Dosage Forms

Capsule, as hydrochloride: 5 mg, 10 mg, 25 mg

Powder for injection, as hydrochloride: 100 mg

♦ **Chlordiazepoxide and Amitriptyline** *see* Amitriptyline and Chlordiazepoxide *on page 25*

♦ **Chlorprom® (Can)** *see* Chlorpromazine *on page 74*

♦ **Chlorpromanyl® (Can)** *see* Chlorpromazine *on page 74*

Chlorpromazine *(klor PROE ma zeen)*

Related Information

Antipsychotic Agents Comparison Chart *on page 557*

Antipsychotic Medication Guidelines *on page 559*

Discontinuation of Psychotropic Drugs - Withdrawal Symptoms and Recommendations *on page 582*

Federal OBRA Regulations Recommended Maximum Doses *on page 583*

Liquid Compatibility With Antipsychotics and Mood Stabilizers *on page 587*

Patient Information - Antipsychotics (General) *on page 466*

U.S. Brand Names Thorazine®

Canadian Brand Names Apo®-Chlorpromazine; Chlorprom®; Chlorpromanyl®; Largactil®; Novo-Chlorpromazine®

Synonyms Chlorpromazine Hydrochloride; CPZ

Pharmacologic Category Antipsychotic Agent, Phenothiazine, Aliphatic

Generic Available Yes

Use Control of mania; treatment of schizophrenia; control of nausea and vomiting; relief of restlessness and apprehension before surgery; acute intermittent porphyria; adjunct in the treatment of tetanus; intractable hiccups; combativeness and/or explosive hyperexcitable behavior in children 1-12 years of age and in short-term treatment of hyperactive children

Unlabeled/Investigational Use Management of psychotic disorders

Pregnancy Risk Factor C

Contraindications Hypersensitivity to chlorpromazine or any component of the formulation (cross-reactivity between phenothiazines may occur); severe CNS depression; coma

Warnings/Precautions Highly sedating, use with caution in disorders where CNS depression is a feature. Use with caution in Parkinson's disease. Caution in patients with hemodynamic instability; bone marrow suppression; predisposition to seizures; subcortical brain damage; severe cardiac, hepatic, renal, or respiratory disease. Esophageal dysmotility and aspiration have been associated with antipsychotic use - use with caution in patients at risk of aspiration pneumonia (ie, Alzheimer's disease). Caution in breast cancer or other prolactin-dependent tumors (may elevate prolactin levels). May alter temperature regulation or mask toxicity of other drugs due to antiemetic effects. May alter cardiac conduction - life-threatening arrhythmias have occurred with therapeutic doses of neuroleptics. May cause orthostatic hypotension - use with caution in patients at risk of this effect or those who would tolerate transient hypotensive episodes (cerebrovascular disease, cardiovascular disease, or other medications which may predispose). Significant hypotension may occur, particularly with parenteral administration. Injection contains sulfites and benzyl alcohol.

Phenothiazines may cause anticholinergic effects (confusion, agitation, constipation, dry mouth, blurred vision, urinary retention). Therefore, they should be used with caution in patients with decreased gastrointestinal motility, urinary retention, BPH, xerostomia, or visual problems. Conditions which also may be exacerbated by cholinergic blockade include narrow-angle glaucoma (screening is recommended) and worsening of myasthenia gravis. Relative to other neuroleptics, chlorpromazine has a moderate potency of cholinergic blockade.

May cause extrapyramidal reactions, including pseudoparkinsonism, acute dystonic reactions, akathisia, and tardive dyskinesia (risk of these reactions is low-moderate relative to other neuroleptics). May be associated with neuroleptic malignant syndrome (NMS) or pigmentary retinopathy.

Adverse Reactions

Cardiovascular: Postural hypotension, tachycardia, dizziness, nonspecific QT changes

Central nervous system: Drowsiness, dystonias, akathisia, pseudoparkinsonism, tardive dyskinesia, neuroleptic malignant syndrome, seizures

Dermatologic: Photosensitivity, dermatitis, skin pigmentation (slate gray)

Endocrine & metabolic: Lactation, breast engorgement, false-positive pregnancy test, amenorrhea, gynecomastia, hyper- or hypoglycemia

Gastrointestinal: Xerostomia, constipation, nausea

Genitourinary: Urinary retention, ejaculatory disorder, impotence

Hematologic: Agranulocytosis, eosinophilia, leukopenia, hemolytic anemia, aplastic anemia, thrombocytopenic purpura

Hepatic: Jaundice

Ocular: Blurred vision, corneal and lenticular changes, epithelial keratopathy, pigmentary retinopathy

Overdosage/Toxicology

Signs and symptoms: Deep sleep, coma, extrapyramidal symptoms, abnormal involuntary muscle movements, hypotension

Treatment:

Following initiation of essential overdose management, toxic symptom treatment and supportive treatment should be initiated

Hypotension usually responds to I.V. fluids or Trendelenburg positioning. If unresponsive to these measures, the use of a parenteral inotrope may be required

Seizures commonly respond to diazepam (I.V. 5-10 mg bolus in adults every 15 minutes if needed up to a total of 30 mg; I.V. 0.25-0.4 mg/kg/dose up to a total of 10 mg in children) or to phenytoin or phenobarbital

Also critical cardiac arrhythmias often respond to I.V. phenytoin (15 mg/kg up to 1 g), while other antiarrhythmics can be used

Neuroleptics often cause extrapyramidal symptoms (eg, dystonic reactions) requiring management with benztropine mesylate 1-2 mg for adult patients (oral, I.M, I.V.) or diphenhydramine 25-50 mg (oral, I.M., I.V.) may be effective.

Drug Interactions CYP1A2, 2D6, and 3A3/4 enzyme substrate; CYP2D6 enzyme inhibitor

Aluminum salts: May decrease the absorption of phenothiazines; monitor

Amphetamines: Efficacy may be diminished by antipsychotics; in addition, amphetamines may increase psychotic symptoms; avoid concurrent use

Anticholinergics: May inhibit the therapeutic response to phenothiazines and excess anticholinergic effects may occur; includes benztropine, trihexyphenidyl, biperiden, and drugs with significant anticholinergic activity (TCAs, antihistamines, disopyramide)

Antihypertensives: Concurrent use of phenothiazines with an antihypertensive may produce additive hypotensive effects (particularly orthostasis)

Bromocriptine: Phenothiazines inhibit the ability of bromocriptine to lower serum prolactin concentrations

CNS depressants: Sedative effects may be additive with phenothiazines; monitor for increased effect; includes barbiturates, benzodiazepines, narcotic analgesics, ethanol and other sedative agents

(Continued)

Chlorpromazine *(Continued)*

CYP1A2 inhibitors: Metabolism of phenothiazines may be decreased; increasing clinical effect or toxicity. Inhibitors include cimetidine, ciprofloxacin, fluvoxamine, isoniazid, ritonavir, and zileuton

CYP2D6 inhibitors: Metabolism of phenothiazines may be decreased; increasing clinical effect or toxicity; inhibitors include amiodarone, cimetidine, delavirdine, fluoxetine, paroxetine, propafenone, quinidine, and ritonavir; monitor for increased effect/toxicity

CYP3A3/4 inhibitors: Serum level and/or toxicity of chlorpromazine may be increased; inhibitors include amiodarone, cimetidine, clarithromycin, erythromycin, delavirdine, diltiazem, dirithromycin, disulfiram, fluoxetine, fluvoxamine, grapefruit juice, indinavir, itraconazole, ketoconazole, metronidazole, nefazodone, nevirapine, propoxyphene, quinupristin-dalfopristin, ritonavir, saquinavir, verapamil, zafirlukast, zileuton; monitor for increased response

CYP2D6 substrates: Chlorpromazine may decrease the metabolism of drugs metabolized by CYP2D6 (in addition to drugs specifically mentioned in this listing)

Enzyme inducers: May enhance the hepatic metabolism of phenothiazines; larger doses may be required; includes rifampin, rifabutin, barbiturates, phenytoin, and cigarette smoking

Epinephrine: Chlorpromazine (and possibly other low potency antipsychotics) may diminish the pressor effects of epinephrine

Guanethidine and guanadrel: Antihypertensive effects may be inhibited by chlorpromazine

Levodopa: Chlorpromazine may inhibit the antiparkinsonian effect of levodopa; avoid this combination

Lithium: Chlorpromazine may produce neurotoxicity with lithium; this is a rare effect

Phenytoin: May reduce serum levels of phenothiazines; phenothiazines may increase phenytoin serum levels

Propranolol: Serum concentrations of phenothiazines may be increased; propranolol also increases phenothiazine concentrations

Polypeptide antibiotics: Rare cases of respiratory paralysis have been reported with concurrent use of phenothiazines

QT_c-prolonging agents: Effects on QT_c interval may be additive with phenothiazines, increasing the risk of malignant arrhythmias; includes type Ia antiarrhythmics, TCAs, and some quinolone antibiotics (sparfloxacin, moxifloxacin and gatifloxacin)

Sulfadoxine-pyrimethamine: May increase phenothiazine concentrations

Tricyclic antidepressants: Concurrent use may produce increased toxicity or altered therapeutic response

Trazodone: Phenothiazines and trazodone may produce additive hypotensive effects

Valproic acid: Serum levels may be increased by phenothiazines

Ethanol/Nutrition/Herb Interactions

Ethanol: Avoid ethanol (may increase CNS depression).

Herb/Nutraceutical: Avoid St John's wort (may decrease chlorpromazine levels, increase photosensitivity, or enhance sedative effect). Avoid dong quai (may enhance photosensitivity). Avoid kava kava, gotu kola, valerian (may increase CNS depression).

Stability Protect from light; a slightly yellowed solution does not indicate potency loss, but a markedly discolored solution should be discarded; diluted injection (1 mg/mL) with NS and stored in 5 mL vials remains stable for 30 days

Mechanism of Action Blocks postsynaptic mesolimbic dopaminergic receptors in the brain; exhibits a strong alpha-adrenergic blocking effect and depresses the release of hypothalamic and hypophyseal hormones; believed to depress the reticular activating system, thus affecting basal metabolism, body temperature, wakefulness, vasomotor tone, and emesis

Pharmacodynamics/Kinetics

Distribution: Crosses the placenta; appears in breast milk

Metabolism: Extensively in the liver to active and inactive metabolites

Half-life, biphasic:

Initial: 2 hours

Terminal: 30 hours

Elimination: <1% excreted in urine as unchanged drug within 24 hours

Hemodialysis: Not dialyzable (0% to 5%)

Usual Dosage

Children ≥6 months:

Schizophrenia/psychoses:

Oral: 0.5-1 mg/kg/dose every 4-6 hours; older children may require 200 mg/day or higher

I.M., I.V.: 0.5-1 mg/kg/dose every 6-8 hours

<5 years (22.7 kg): Maximum: 40 mg/day

5-12 years (22.7-45.5 kg): Maximum: 75 mg/day

Nausea and vomiting:

Oral: 0.5-1 mg/kg/dose every 4-6 hours as needed

I.M., I.V.: 0.5-1 mg/kg/dose every 6-8 hours

<5 years (22.7 kg): Maximum: 40 mg/day

5-12 years (22.7-45.5 kg): Maximum: 75 mg/day

Rectal: 1 mg/kg/dose every 6-8 hours as needed

Adults:

Schizophrenia/psychoses:

Oral: Range: 30-2000 mg/day in 1-4 divided doses, initiate at lower doses and titrate as needed; usual dose: 400-600 mg/day; some patients may require 1-2 g/day

I.M., I.V.: Initial: 25 mg, may repeat (25-50 mg) in 1-4 hours, gradually increase to a maximum of 400 mg/dose every 4-6 hours until patient is controlled; usual dose: 300-800 mg/day

Intractable hiccups: Oral, I.M.: 25-50 mg 3-4 times/day

Nausea and vomiting:

Oral: 10-25 mg every 4-6 hours

I.M., I.V.: 25-50 mg every 4-6 hours

Rectal: 50-100 mg every 6-8 hours

Elderly: Behavioral symptoms associated with dementia: Initial: 10-25 mg 1-2 times/day; increase at 4- to 7-day intervals by 10-25 mg/day. Increase dose intervals (bid, tid, etc) as necessary to control behavior response or side effects; maximum daily dose: 800 mg; gradual increases (titration) may prevent some side effects or decrease their severity.

Dosing adjustment/comments in hepatic impairment: Avoid use in severe hepatic dysfunction

Administration

Oral: Dilute oral concentrate solution in juice before administration. Chlorpromazine concentrate is not compatible with carbamazepine suspension; schedule dosing at least 1-2 hours apart from each other. **Note:** Avoid skin contact with oral suspension or solution; may cause contact dermatitis.

I.V.: Direct of intermittent infusion: Infuse 1 mg or portion thereof over 1 minute.

Monitoring Parameters Orthostatic blood pressures; tremors, gait changes, abnormal movement in trunk, neck, buccal area, or extremities; monitor target behaviors for which the agent is given; watch for hypotension when administering I.M. or I.V.

Reference Range

Therapeutic: 50-300 ng/mL (SI: 157-942 nmol/L)

Toxic: >750 ng/mL (SI: >2355 nmol/L); serum concentrations poorly correlate with expected response

Test Interactions False-positives for phenylketonuria, amylase, uroporphyrins, urobilinogen

Patient Information Do not stop taking unless informed by your physician; oral concentrate must be diluted in 2-4 oz of liquid (water, fruit juice, carbonated drinks, (Continued)

Chlorpromazine *(Continued)*

milk, or pudding); do not take antacid within 1 hour of taking drug; avoid alcohol; avoid excess sun exposure (use sun block); may cause drowsiness, rise slowly from recumbent position; use of supportive stockings may help prevent orthostatic hypotension

Nursing Implications Avoid contact of oral solution or injection with skin (contact dermatitis)

Additional Information Avoid rectal administration in immunocompromised patients.

Dosage Forms

Capsule, sustained action, as hydrochloride: 30 mg, 75 mg, 150 mg, 200 mg, 300 mg

Injection, as hydrochloride: 25 mg/mL (1 mL, 2 mL, 10 mL)

Solution, oral concentrate, as hydrochloride: 30 mg/mL (120 mL); 100 mg/mL (60 mL, 240 mL)

Suppository, rectal, as base: 25 mg, 100 mg

Syrup, as hydrochloride: 10 mg/5 mL (120 mL)

Tablet, as hydrochloride: 10 mg, 25 mg, 50 mg, 100 mg, 200 mg

♦ **Chlorpromazine Hydrochloride** *see* Chlorpromazine *on page 74*

Chlorprothixene (klor proe THIKS een)

Related Information

Antipsychotic Agents Comparison Chart *on page 557*
Antipsychotic Medication Guidelines *on page 559*
Patient Information - Antipsychotics (General) *on page 466*

Canadian Brand Names Tarasan

Pharmacologic Category Antipsychotic Agent, Thioxanthene Derivative

Generic Available No

Use Management of psychotic disorders

Pregnancy Risk Factor C

Adverse Reactions

>10%:

Cardiovascular: Hypotension, orthostatic hypotension

Central nervous system: Pseudoparkinsonism, akathisia, dystonias, tardive dyskinesia (persistent), dizziness

Gastrointestinal: Constipation

Ocular: Pigmentary retinopathy

Respiratory: Nasal congestion

Miscellaneous: Decreased diaphoresis

1% to 10%:

Dermatologic: Photosensitivity, skin rash

Endocrine & metabolic: Changes in menstrual cycle, changes in libido, pain in breasts

Gastrointestinal: Weight gain, nausea, vomiting, stomach pain

Genitourinary: Dysuria, ejaculatory disturbances

Neuromuscular & skeletal: Trembling of fingers

<1%: Agranulocytosis, cholestatic jaundice, cornea and lens changes, discoloration of skin (blue-gray), galactorrhea, hepatotoxicity, leukopenia, impairment of temperature regulation, lowering of seizures threshold, neuroleptic malignant syndrome (NMS), pigmentary retinopathy, priapism

Drug Interactions

Decreased effect of guanethidine

Increased effect/toxicity: Alcohol, CNS depressants

Ethanol/Nutrition/Herb Interactions Ethanol: Avoid ethanol (may increase CNS depression).

Stability Protect all dosage forms from light, clear or slightly yellow solutions may be used; should be dispensed in amber or opaque vials/bottles. Solutions may be diluted or mixed with fruit juices or other liquids but must be administered immediately after mixing; do not prepare bulk dilutions or store bulk dilutions.

Mechanism of Action The mechanism of action for chlorprothixene, like other thioxanthenes and phenothiazines, is not fully understood. The sites of action appear to be the reticular activating system of the midbrain, the limbic system, the hypothalamus, and the globus pallidus and corpus striatum. The mechanism appears to be one or more of a combination of postsynaptic blockade of adrenergic, dopaminergic, or serotonergic receptor sites, metabolic inhibition of oxidative phosphorylation, or decrease in the excitability of neuronal membranes.

Usual Dosage

Children >6 years: Oral: 10-25 mg 3-4 times/day

Adults:

Oral: 25-50 mg 3-4 times/day, to be increased as needed; doses exceeding 600 mg/day are rarely required

I.M.: 25-50 mg up to 3-4 times/day

Administration I.M. dose is 4-10 times the activity of oral dose

Patient Information May cause drowsiness; avoid alcohol

Dosage Forms

Injection, as hydrochloride: 12.5 mg/mL (2 mL)

Solution, oral concentrate, as lactate and hydrochloride: 100 mg/5 mL (480 mL) [fruit flavor]

Tablet: 10 mg, 25 mg, 50 mg, 100 mg

Chromium

Pharmacologic Category Nutritional Supplement

Use Improves glycemic control; increases lean body mass; reduces obesity; improves lipid profile by decreasing total cholesterol and triglycerides, increasing HDL

Adverse Reactions Gastrointestinal: Nausea, loose stools, flatulence, changes in appetite

Isolated reports of anemia, cognitive impairment, renal failure

Drug Interactions Any medications that may also affect blood sugars; (eg, beta-blockers, thiazides, any medications prescribed to treat diabetes); discuss chromium use prior to initiating

Usual Dosage 50-600 mcg/day

Citalopram (sye TAL oh pram)

Related Information

Antidepressant Agents Comparison Chart on page 553
Discontinuation of Psychotropic Drugs - Withdrawal Symptoms and Recommendations on page 582
Patient Information - Antidepressants (SSRIs) on page 452
Pharmacokinetics of Selective Serotonin-Reuptake Inhibitors (SSRIs) on page 590
Teratogenic Risks of Psychotropic Medications on page 594

U.S. Brand Names Celexa™

Canadian Brand Names Celexa

Synonyms Citalopram Hydrobromide; Nitalapram

Pharmacologic Category Antidepressant, Selective Serotonin Reuptake Inhibitor

Generic Available No

Use Treatment of depression

Unlabeled/Investigational Use Investigational: Treatment of dementia, smoking cessation, ethanol abuse, obsessive-compulsive disorder (OCD) in children, and diabetic neuropathy

Pregnancy Risk Factor C

Pregnancy/Breast-Feeding Implications Animal reproductive studies have revealed adverse effects on fetal and postnatal development (at doses higher than human therapeutic doses). Should be used in pregnancy only if potential benefit *(Continued)*

Citalopram *(Continued)*

justifies potential risk. Citalopram is excreted in human milk; a decision should be made whether to continue or discontinue nursing or discontinue the drug.

Contraindications Hypersensitivity to citalopram or to any component of the formulation; hypersensitivity or other adverse sequelae during therapy with other SSRIs; concomitant use with MAO inhibitors or within 2 weeks of discontinuing MAO inhibitors.

Warnings/Precautions Potential for severe reaction when used with MAO inhibitors - serotonin syndrome (hyperthermia, muscular rigidity, mental status changes/agitation, autonomic instability) may occur. May precipitate a shift to mania or hypomania in patients with bipolar disease. Has a low potential to impair cognitive or motor performance - caution operating hazardous machinery or driving. Use caution in patients with depression, particularly if suicidal risk may be present. Use caution in patients with a previous seizure disorder or condition predisposing to seizures such as brain damage, alcoholism, or concurrent therapy with other drugs which lower the seizure threshold. Use with caution in patients with hepatic or renal dysfunction and in elderly patients. May cause hyponatremia/SIADH. Use with caution in patients with other concurrent illness (due to limited experience). May cause or exacerbate sexual dysfunction.

Adverse Reactions

>10%:
  Central nervous system: Somnolence, insomnia
  Gastrointestinal: Nausea, xerostomia
  Miscellaneous: Diaphoresis
<10%:
  Central nervous system: Anxiety, anorexia, agitation, yawning
  Dermatologic: Rash, pruritus
  Endocrine & metabolic: Sexual dysfunction
  Gastrointestinal: Diarrhea, dyspepsia, vomiting, abdominal pain
  Neuromuscular & skeletal: Tremor, arthralgia, myalgia
  Respiratory: Cough, rhinitis, sinusitis
<1%, postmarketing, and/or case reports: SIADH

Overdosage/Toxicology Signs and symptoms: Dizziness, sweating, nausea, vomiting, tremor, somnolence, tachycardia, EKG changes

Drug Interactions CYP3A3/4 and CYP2C19 enzyme substrate; CYP2D6, 1A2, and 2C19 enzyme inhibitor (weak)

Beta-blockers: Citalopram may increase levels of some beta-blockers (see Carvedilol and Metoprolol); monitor carefully

Buspirone: Concurrent use of citalopram with buspirone may cause serotonin syndrome; avoid concurrent use

Carbamazepine: May enhance the metabolism of citalopram

Carvedilol: Serum concentrations may be increased; monitor carefully for increased carvedilol effect (hypotension and bradycardia)

Cimetidine: May inhibit the metabolism of citalopram

CYP3A3/4 inhibitors: Serum level and/or toxicity of citalopram may be increased; inhibitors include amiodarone, cimetidine, clarithromycin, erythromycin, delavirdine, diltiazem, dirithromycin, disulfiram, fluoxetine, fluvoxamine, grapefruit juice, indinavir, itraconazole, ketoconazole, metronidazole, nefazodone, nevirapine, propoxyphene, quinupristin-dalfopristin, ritonavir, saquinavir, verapamil, zafirlukast, zileuton; monitor for increased response

CYP2C19 inhibitors: Serum levels of citalopram may be increased; inhibitors include cimetidine, felbamate, fluconazole, fluoxetine, fluvoxamine, omeprazole, teniposide, tolbutamide, and troglitazone

Linezolid: Hyperpyrexia, hypertension, tachycardia, confusion, seizures, and **deaths have been reported** with agents which inhibit MAO (serotonin syndrome); this combination should be avoided

MAO inhibitors: Hyperpyrexia, hypertension, tachycardia, confusion, seizures, and **deaths have been reported** with MAO inhibitors (serotonin syndrome); this combination should be avoided

Meperidine: Combined use theoretically may increase the risk of serotonin syndrome

Metoprolol: Citalopram may increase plasma levels of metoprolol; monitor for increased effect

Moclobemide: Concurrent use of citalopram with moclobemide may cause serotonin syndrome; avoid concurrent use

Nefazodone: Concurrent use of citalopram with nefazodone may cause serotonin syndrome

Selegiline: Concurrent use with citalopram has been reported to cause serotonin syndrome; as a MAO type B inhibitor, the risk of serotonin syndrome may be less than with nonselective MAO inhibitors, and reports indicate that this combination has been well tolerated in Parkinson's patients

Serotonin reuptake inhibitors: Concurrent use with other reuptake inhibitors may increase the risk of serotonin syndrome

Sibutramine: May increase the risk of serotonin syndrome with SSRIs

Sumatriptan (and other serotonin agonists): Concurrent use may result in toxicity; weakness, hyper-reflexia, and incoordination have been observed with sumatriptan and SSRIs. In addition, concurrent use may theoretically increase the risk of serotonin syndrome; includes sumatriptan, naratriptan, rizatriptan, and zolmitriptan.

Tramadol: Concurrent use of citalopram with tramadol may cause serotonin syndrome; avoid concurrent use

Trazodone: Concurrent use of citalopram with trazodone may cause serotonin syndrome

Venlafaxine: Combined use with citalopram may increase the risk of serotonin syndrome

Ethanol/Nutrition/Herb Interactions

Ethanol: Avoid ethanol (may increase CNS depression).

Herb/Nutraceutical: Avoid valerian, St John's wort, SAMe, kava kava, and gotu kola (may increase CNS depression).

Stability Store below 25°C

Mechanism of Action A bicyclic phthalane derivative, citalopram selectively inhibits serotonin reuptake in the presynaptic neurons

Pharmacodynamics/Kinetics

Distribution: V_d: 12 L/kg

Protein binding, plasma: ~80%

Metabolism: Extensive hepatic metabolism, including cytochrome P450 oxidase system, to N-demethylated, N-oxide, and deaminated metabolites

Bioavailability: 80%

Half-life: 24-48 hours; average 35 hours (doubled in patients with hepatic impairment)

Time to peak serum concentration: 1-6 hours, average within 4 hours

Elimination: 10% recovered unchanged in urine; systemic clearance: 330 mL/minute (20% renal)

Clearance was decreased, while AUC and half-life were significantly increased in elderly patients and in patients with hepatic impairment. Mild to moderate renal impairment may reduce clearance of citalopram (17% reduction noted in trials). No pharmacokinetic information is available concerning patients with severe renal impairment.

Usual Dosage Oral:

Children and Adolescents: OCD (unlabeled use): 10-40 mg/day

Adults: Depression: Initial: 20 mg/day, generally with an increase to 40 mg/day; doses of more than 40 mg are not usually necessary. Should a dose increase be necessary, it should occur in 20 mg increments at intervals of no less than 1 week. Maximum dose: 60 mg/day; reduce dosage in elderly or those with hepatic impairment.

Child/Adolescent Considerations Twenty-three patients with OCD (9-18 years of age) received 10-40 mg/day (40 mg modal) (Thomsen, 1997).

Dietary Considerations May be taken without regard to food.

(Continued)

Citalopram *(Continued)*

Monitoring Parameters Monitor patient periodically for symptom resolution, heart rate, blood pressure, liver function tests, and CBC with continued therapy

Patient Information Use caution when operating hazardous machinery, including automobiles, until certain how citalopram affects; avoid alcohol

Dosage Forms

Solution, oral: 10 mg/5 mL [peppermint flavor] [sugar free, alcohol free]

Tablet, as hydrobromide: 20 mg, 40 mg

♦ **Citalopram Hydrobromide** *see Citalopram on page 79*

Clomipramine *(kloe MI pra meen)*

Related Information

Antidepressant Agents Comparison Chart *on page 553*

Discontinuation of Psychotropic Drugs - Withdrawal Symptoms and Recommendations *on page 582*

Patient Information - Antidepressants (TCAs) *on page 454*

Teratogenic Risks of Psychotropic Medications *on page 594*

U.S. Brand Names Anafranil®

Canadian Brand Names Apo®-Clomipramine

Synonyms Clomipramine Hydrochloride

Pharmacologic Category Antidepressant, Tricyclic (Tertiary Amine)

Generic Available Yes

Use Treatment of obsessive-compulsive disorder (OCD)

Unlabeled/Investigational Use Depression, panic attacks, chronic pain

Pregnancy Risk Factor C

Contraindications Hypersensitivity to clomipramine, other tricyclic agents, or any component of the formulation; use of MAO inhibitors within 14 days; use in a patient during the acute recovery phase of MI

Warnings/Precautions May cause seizures (relationship to dose and/or duration of therapy) - do not exceed maximum doses. Use caution in patients with a previous seizure disorder or condition predisposing to seizures such as brain damage, alcoholism, or concurrent therapy with other drugs which lower the seizure threshold. Has been associated with a high incidence of sexual dysfunction. Weight gain may occur. May cause sedation, resulting in impaired performance of tasks requiring alertness (ie, operating machinery or driving). Sedative effects may be additive with other CNS depressants and/or ethanol. The degree of sedation is very high relative to other antidepressants. May worsen psychosis in some patients or precipitate a shift to mania or hypomania in patients with bipolar disease. May increase the risks associated with electroconvulsive therapy. This agent should be discontinued, when possible, prior to elective surgery. Therapy should not be abruptly discontinued in patients receiving high doses for prolonged periods.

May cause orthostatic hypotension (risk is moderate-high relative to other antidepressants) - use with caution in patients at risk of hypotension or in patients where transient hypotensive episodes would be poorly tolerated (cardiovascular disease or cerebrovascular disease). The degree of anticholinergic blockade produced by this agent is very high relative to other cyclic antidepressants - use caution in patients with urinary retention, benign prostatic hypertrophy, narrow-angle glaucoma, xerostomia, visual problems, constipation, or history of bowel obstruction.

Use caution in patients with depression, particularly if suicidal risk may be present. Use with caution in patients with a history of cardiovascular disease (including previous MI, stroke, tachycardia, or conduction abnormalities). The risk conduction abnormalities with this agent is high relative to other antidepressants. Use with caution in hyperthyroid patients or those receiving thyroid supplementation. Use with caution in patients with hepatic or renal dysfunction and in elderly patients.

Adverse Reactions

>10%:

Central nervous system: Dizziness, drowsiness, headache, insomnia, nervousness

Endocrine & metabolic: Libido changes

Gastrointestinal: Xerostomia, constipation, increased appetite, nausea, weight gain, dyspepsia, anorexia, abdominal pain

Neuromuscular & skeletal: Fatigue, tremor, myoclonus

Miscellaneous: Increased diaphoresis

1% to 10%:

Cardiovascular: Hypotension, palpitations, tachycardia

Central nervous system: Confusion, hypertonia, sleep disorder, yawning, speech disorder, abnormal dreaming, paresthesia, memory impairment, anxiety, twitching, impaired coordination, agitation, migraine, depersonalization, emotional lability, flushing, fever

Dermatologic: Rash, pruritus, dermatitis

Gastrointestinal: Diarrhea, vomiting

Genitourinary: Difficult urination

Ocular: Blurred vision, eye pain

<1%: Abnormal accommodation, alopecia, breast enlargement, decreased lower esophageal sphincter tone may cause GE reflux, galactorrhea, hyperacusis, increased liver enzymes, marrow depression, photosensitivity, prostatic disorder, seizures, SIADH, trouble with gums

Overdosage/Toxicology

Signs and symptoms: Agitation, confusion, hallucinations, urinary retention, hypothermia, hypotension, tachycardia, ventricular tachycardia, seizures, coma

Treatment: Following initiation of essential overdose management, toxic symptoms should be treated; ventricular arrhythmias often respond to systemic alkalinization (sodium bicarbonate 0.5-2 mEq/kg I.V.) and/or phenytoin 15-20 mg/kg (adults). Arrhythmias unresponsive to this therapy may respond to lidocaine 1 mg/kg I.V. followed by a titrated infusion. Physostigmine (1-2 mg I.V. slowly for adults or 0.5 mg I.V. slowly for children) may be indicated in reversing cardiac arrhythmias that are life-threatening. Seizures usually respond to diazepam I.V. boluses (5-10 mg for adults up to 30 mg or 0.25-0.4 mg/kg/dose for children up to 10 mg/dose). If seizures are unresponsive or recur, phenytoin or phenobarbital may be required.

Drug Interactions
CYP1A2, 2C19, 2D6, and 3A3/4 enzyme substrate; CYP2D6 enzyme inhibitor

Altretamine: Concurrent use may cause orthostatic hypertension

Amphetamines: TCAs may enhance the effect of amphetamines; monitor for adverse CV effects

Anticholinergics: Combined use with TCAs may produce additive anticholinergic effects

Antihypertensives: TCAs inhibit the antihypertensive response to bethanidine, clonidine, debrisoquin, guanadrel, guanethidine, guanabenz, guanfacine; monitor BP; consider alternate antihypertensive agent

Beta-agonists: When combined with TCAs may predispose patients to cardiac arrhythmias

Bupropion: May increase the levels of tricyclic antidepressants; based on limited information; monitor response

Carbamazepine: Tricyclic antidepressants may increase carbamazepine levels; monitor

Cholestyramine and colestipol: May bind TCAs and reduce their absorption; monitor for altered response

Clonidine: Abrupt discontinuation of clonidine may cause hypertensive crisis, amitriptyline may enhance the response

CNS depressants: Sedative effects may be additive with TCAs; monitor for increased effect; includes benzodiazepines, barbiturates, antipsychotics, ethanol, and other sedative medications

(Continued)

Clomipramine *(Continued)*

CYP2C8/9 inhibitors: Serum levels and/or toxicity of some tricyclic antidepressants may be increased; inhibitors include amiodarone, cimetidine, fluvoxamine, some NSAIDs, metronidazole, ritonavir, sulfonamides, troglitazone, valproic acid, and zafirlukast; monitor for increased effect/toxicity

CYP2D6 inhibitors: Serum levels and/or toxicity of some tricyclic antidepressants may be increased; inhibitors include amiodarone, cimetidine, delavirdine, fluoxetine, paroxetine, propafenone, quinidine, and ritonavir; monitor for increased effect/toxicity

CYP3A3/4 inhibitors: Serum level and/or toxicity of some tricyclic antidepressants may be increased; inhibitors include amiodarone, cimetidine, clarithromycin, erythromycin, delavirdine, diltiazem, dirithromycin, disulfiram, fluoxetine, fluvoxamine, grapefruit juice, indinavir, itraconazole, ketoconazole, nefazodone, nevirapine, propoxyphene, quinupristin-dalfopristin, ritonavir, saquinavir, verapamil, zafirlukast, zileuton; monitor for altered effects; a decrease in TCA dosage may be required

Enzyme inducers: May increase the metabolism of TCAs resulting in decreased effect; includes carbamazepine, phenobarbital, phenytoin, and rifampin; monitor for decreased response

Epinephrine (and other direct alpha-agonists): Pressor response to I.V. epinephrine, norepinephrine, and phenylephrine may be enhanced in patients receiving TCAs (**Note:** Effect is unlikely with epinephrine or levonordefrin dosages typically administered as infiltration in combination with local anesthetics)

Fenfluramine: May increase tricyclic antidepressant levels/effects

Hypoglycemic agents (including insulin): TCAs may enhance the hypoglycemic effects of tolazamide, chlorpropamide, or insulin; monitor for changes in blood glucose levels; reported with chlorpropamide, tolazamide, and insulin

Levodopa: Tricyclic antidepressants may decrease the absorption (bioavailability) of levodopa; rare hypertensive episodes have also been attributed to this combination

Linezolid: Hyperpyrexia, hypertension, tachycardia, confusion, seizures, and **deaths have been reported** with agents which inhibit MAO (serotonin syndrome); this combination should be avoided

Lithium: Concurrent use with a TCA may increase the risk for neurotoxicity

MAO inhibitors: Hyperpyrexia, hypertension, tachycardia, confusion, seizures, and **deaths have been reported** (serotonin syndrome); this combination should be avoided

Methylphenidate: Metabolism of some TCAs may be decreased

Olanzapine: When used in combination, clomipramine and olanzapine have been reported to be associated with the development of seizures; limited documentation (case report)

Phenothiazines: Serum concentrations of some TCAs may be increased; in addition, TCAs may increase concentration of phenothiazines; monitor for altered clinical response

QT_c-prolonging agents: Concurrent use of tricyclic agents with other drugs which may prolong QT_c interval may increase the risk of potentially fatal arrhythmias; includes type Ia and type III antiarrhythmics agents, selected quinolones (sparfloxacin, gatifloxacin, moxifloxacin, grepafloxacin), cisapride, and other agents

Sucralfate: Absorption of tricyclic antidepressants may be reduced with coadministration

Sympathomimetics, indirect-acting: Tricyclic antidepressants may result in a decreased sensitivity to indirect-acting sympathomimetics; includes dopamine and ephedrine; also see interaction with epinephrine (and direct-acting sympathomimetics)

Tramadol: Tramadol's risk of seizures may be increased with TCAs

Valproic acid: May increase serum concentrations/adverse effects of some tricyclic antidepressants

Warfarin (and other oral anticoagulants): TCAs may increase the anticoagulant effect in patients stabilized on warfarin; monitor INR

Ethanol/Nutrition/Herb Interactions
    Ethanol: Avoid ethanol (may increase CNS depression).
    Food: Serum concentrations/toxicity may be increased by grapefruit juice.
    Herb/Nutraceutical: Avoid valerian, St John's wort, SAMe, kava kava.

Mechanism of Action Clomipramine appears to affect serotonin uptake while its active metabolite, desmethylclomipramine, affects norepinephrine uptake

Pharmacodynamics/Kinetics
    Absorption: Oral: Rapid
    Metabolism: Extensive first-pass metabolism; metabolized to desmethyl-clomipramine (active) in the liver
    Half-life: 20-30 hours

Usual Dosage Oral: Initial:
    Children: OCD: 25 mg/day; gradually increase, as tolerated, to a maximum of 3 mg/kg/day or 200 mg/day (whichever is smaller)
    Adults: OCD: 25 mg/day and gradually increase, as tolerated, to 100 mg/day the first 2 weeks, may then be increased to a total of 250 mg/day maximum

Monitoring Parameters Pulse rate and blood pressure prior to and during therapy; EKG/cardiac status in older adults and patients with cardiac disease

Test Interactions ↑ glucose

Patient Information May cause seizures; caution should be used in activities that require alertness like driving, operating machinery, or swimming; effect of drug may take several weeks to appear

Nursing Implications Monitor pulse rate and blood pressure prior to and during therapy, evaluate mental status

Dosage Forms Capsule, as hydrochloride: 25 mg, 50 mg, 75 mg

♦ **Clomipramine Hydrochloride** see Clomipramine on page 82

Clonazepam (kloe NA ze pam)

Related Information
    Anxiolytic/Hypnotic Use in Long-Term Care Facilities on page 562
    Benzodiazepines Comparison Chart on page 566
    Patient Information - Anxiolytics & Sedative Hypnotics (Benzodiazepines) on page 483

U.S. Brand Names Klonopin™

Canadian Brand Names PMS-Clonazepam; Rivotril®

Pharmacologic Category Benzodiazepine

Generic Available Yes

Use Alone or as an adjunct in the treatment of petit mal variant (Lennox-Gastaut), akinetic, and myoclonic seizures; petit mal (absence) seizures unresponsive to succimides; panic disorder with or without agoraphobia

Unlabeled/Investigational Use Restless legs syndrome; neuralgia; multifocal tic disorder; parkinsonian dysarthria; bipolar disorder; adjunct therapy for schizophrenia

Restrictions C-IV

Pregnancy Risk Factor D

Pregnancy/Breast-Feeding Implications
    Clinical effects on the fetus: Two reports of cardiac defects; respiratory depression, lethargy, hypotonia may be observed in newborns exposed near time of delivery. Epilepsy itself, number of medications, genetic factors, or a combination of these probably influence the teratogenicity of anticonvulsant therapy. Benefit:risk ratio usually favors continued use during pregnancy and breast-feeding.
    Breast-feeding/lactation: Crosses into breast milk
    Clinical effects on the infant: CNS depression, respiratory depression reported. No recommendation from the AAP.

Contraindications Hypersensitivity to clonazepam or any component of the formulation (cross-sensitivity with other benzodiazepines may exist); significant liver disease; narrow-angle glaucoma; pregnancy
    (Continued)

Clonazepam *(Continued)*

Warnings/Precautions Use with caution in elderly or debilitated patients, patients with hepatic disease (including alcoholics), or renal impairment. Use with caution in patients with respiratory disease or impaired gag reflex or ability to protect the airway from secretions (salivation may be increased). Worsening of seizures may occur when added to patients with multiple seizure types. Concurrent use with valproic acid may result in absence status. Monitoring of CBC and liver function tests has been recommended during prolonged therapy.

Causes CNS depression (dose-related) resulting in sedation, dizziness, confusion, or ataxia which may impair physical and mental capabilities. Patients must be cautioned about performing tasks which require mental alertness (ie, operating machinery or driving). Use with caution in patients receiving other CNS depressants or psychoactive agents. Effects with other sedative drugs or ethanol may be potentiated. Benzodiazepines have been associated with falls and traumatic injury and should be used with extreme caution in patients who are at risk of these events (especially the elderly).

Use caution in patients with depression, particularly if suicidal risk may be present. Use with caution in patients with a history of drug dependence. Benzodiazepines have been associated with dependence and acute withdrawal symptoms, including seizures, on discontinuation or reduction in dose. Acute withdrawal, including seizures, may be precipitated in patients after administration of flumazenil to patients receiving long-term benzodiazepine therapy.

Benzodiazepines have been associated with anterograde amnesia. Paradoxical reactions, including hyperactive or aggressive behavior, have been reported with benzodiazepines, particularly in adolescent/pediatric or psychiatric patients. Does not have analgesic, antidepressant, or antipsychotic properties.

Adverse Reactions

>10%: Central nervous system: Drowsiness

1% to 10%:

Central nervous system: Dizziness, abnormal coordination, ataxia, dysarthria, depression, memory disturbance, fatigue

Dermatologic: Dermatitis, allergic reactions

Endocrine & metabolic: Decreased libido

Gastrointestinal: Anorexia, constipation, diarrhea, xerostomia

Respiratory: Upper respiratory tract infection, sinusitis, rhinitis, coughing

<1%: Blood dyscrasias, menstrual irregularities

Overdosage/Toxicology

Signs and symptoms: Somnolence, confusion, ataxia, diminished reflexes, or coma

Treatment: Supportive. Rarely is mechanical ventilation required.

Flumazenil has been shown to selectively block the binding of benzodiazepines to CNS receptors, resulting in a reversal of benzodiazepine-induced CNS depression, but not respiratory depression

Drug Interactions CYP3A3/4 enzyme substrate

CNS depressants: Sedative effects and/or respiratory depression may be additive with CNS depressants; includes ethanol, barbiturates, narcotic analgesics, and other sedative agents; monitor for increased effect

CYP3A3/4 inhibitors: Serum level and/or toxicity of some benzodiazepines may be increased; inhibitors include amiodarone, cimetidine, clarithromycin, erythromycin, delavirdine, diltiazem, dirithromycin, disulfiram, fluoxetine, fluvoxamine, grapefruit juice, indinavir, itraconazole, ketoconazole, nefazodone, nevirapine, propoxyphene, quinupristin-dalfopristin, ritonavir, saquinavir, verapamil, zafirlukast, zileuton; monitor for altered benzodiazepine response

Disulfiram: Disulfiram may inhibit the metabolism of clonazepam; monitor for increased benzodiazepine effect

Enzyme inducers: Metabolism of some benzodiazepines may be increased, decreasing their therapeutic effect; consider using an alternative sedative/

hypnotic agent; potential inducers include phenobarbital, phenytoin, carbamaze-pine, rifampin, and rifabutin

Levodopa: Therapeutic effects may be diminished in some patients following the addition of a benzodiazepine; limited/inconsistent data

Oral contraceptives: May decrease the clearance of some benzodiazepines (those which undergo oxidative metabolism); monitor for increased benzodiazepine effect

Theophylline: May partially antagonize some of the effects of benzodiazepines; monitor for decreased response; may require higher doses for sedation

Valproic acid: The combined use of clonazepam and valproic acid has been associated with absence seizures

Ethanol/Nutrition/Herb Interactions

Ethanol: Avoid ethanol (may increase CNS depression).

Food: Clonazepam serum concentration is unlikely to be increased by grapefruit juice because of clonazepam's high oral bioavailability.

Herb/Nutraceutical: St John's wort may decrease clonazepam levels. Avoid vale-rian, St John's wort, kava kava, gotu kola (may increase CNS depression).

Mechanism of Action The exact mechanism is unknown, but believed to be related to its ability to enhance the activity of GABA; suppresses the spike-and-wave discharge in absence seizures by depressing nerve transmission in the motor cortex

Pharmacodynamics/Kinetics

Onset of effect: 20-60 minutes

Duration: Up to 6-8 hours in infants and young children, up to 12 hours in adults

Absorption: Oral: Well absorbed

Distribution: Adults: V_d: 1.5-4.4 L/kg

Protein binding: 85%

Metabolism: Extensive; glucuronide and sulfate conjugation

Half-life:
  Children: 22-33 hours
  Adults: 19-50 hours

Time to peak serum concentration: Oral: 1-3 hours
  Steady-state: 5-7 days

Elimination: <2% excreted unchanged in urine; metabolites excreted as glucuro-nide or sulfate conjugates

Usual Dosage Oral:

Children <10 years or 30 kg: Seizure disorders:
  Initial daily dose: 0.01-0.03 mg/kg/day (maximum: 0.05 mg/kg/day) given in 2-3 divided doses; increase by no more than 0.5 mg every third day until seizures are controlled or adverse effects seen
  Usual maintenance dose: 0.1-0.2 mg/kg/day divided 3 times/day, not to exceed 0.2 mg/kg/day

Adults:
  Seizure disorders:
    Initial daily dose not to exceed 1.5 mg given in 3 divided doses; may increase by 0.5-1 mg every third day until seizures are controlled or adverse effects seen (maximum: 20 mg/day)
    Usual maintenance dose: 0.05-0.2 mg/kg; do not exceed 20 mg/day
  Panic disorder: 0.25 mg twice daily; increase in increments of 0.125-0.25 mg twice daily every 3 days; target dose: 1 mg/day (maximum: 4 mg/day)

Elderly: Initiate with low doses and observe closely

Hemodialysis: Supplemental dose is not necessary

Monitoring Parameters CBC, liver function tests

Reference Range Relationship between serum concentration and seizure control is not well established

Timing of serum samples: Peak serum levels occur 1-3 hours after oral ingestion; the half-life is 20-40 hours; therefore, steady-state occurs in 5-7 days

Therapeutic levels: 20-80 ng/mL; Toxic concentration: >80 ng/mL

(Continued)

Clonazepam *(Continued)*

Patient Information Avoid alcohol and other CNS depressants; avoid activities needing good psychomotor coordination until CNS effects are known; drug may cause physical or psychological dependence; avoid abrupt discontinuation after prolonged use

Nursing Implications Observe patient for excess sedation, respiratory depression; raise bed rails, initiate safety measures, assist with ambulation

Additional Information Ethosuximide or valproic acid may be preferred for treatment of absence (petit mal) seizures. Clonazepam-induced behavioral disturbances may be more frequent in mentally handicapped patients. Abrupt discontinuation after sustained use (generally >10 days) may cause withdrawal symptoms. Flumazenil, a competitive benzodiazepine antagonist at the CNS receptor site, reverses benzodiazepine-induced CNS depression.

Dosage Forms Tablet: 0.5 mg, 1 mg, 2 mg

Clonidine *(KLOE ni deen)*

Related Information

Addiction Treatments *on page 550*
Clozapine-Induced Side Effects *on page 568*
Patient Information - Miscellaneous Medications *on page 495*

U.S. Brand Names Catapres®; Catapres-TTS®-1; Catapres-TTS®-2; Catapres-TTS®-3; Duraclon™

Canadian Brand Names Apo®-Clonidine; Dixarit®; Novo-Clonidine®; Nu-Clonidine®

Synonyms Clonidine Hydrochloride

Pharmacologic Category Alpha$_2$ Agonist

Generic Available Yes: Tablet

Use Management of mild to moderate hypertension; either used alone or in combination with other antihypertensives

Orphan drug: Duraclon™: For continuous epidural administration as adjunctive therapy with intraspinal opiates for treatment of cancer pain in patients tolerant to or unresponsive to intraspinal opiates

Unlabeled/Investigational Use Heroin or nicotine withdrawal; severe pain; dysmenorrhea; vasomotor symptoms associated with menopause; ethanol dependence; prophylaxis of migraines; glaucoma; diabetes-associated diarrhea; impulse control disorder, attention-deficit/hyperactivity disorder (ADHD), clozapine-induced sialorrhea

Pregnancy Risk Factor C

Pregnancy/Breast-Feeding Implications

Clinical effects on the fetus: Crosses the placenta. Caution should be used with this drug due to the potential of rebound hypertension with abrupt discontinuation.

Breast-feeding/lactation: Crosses into breast milk. AAP has NO RECOMMENDATION.

Contraindications Hypersensitivity to clonidine hydrochloride or any component

Warnings/Precautions Gradual withdrawal is needed (over 1 week for oral, 2-4 days with epidural) if drug needs to be stopped. Patients should be instructed about abrupt discontinuation (causes rapid increase in BP and symptoms of sympathetic overactivity). In patients on both a beta-blocker and clonidine where withdrawal of clonidine is necessary, withdraw the beta-blocker first and several days before clonidine. Then slowly decrease clonidine.

Use with caution in patients with severe coronary insufficiency; conduction disturbances; recent MI, CVA, or chronic renal insufficiency. Caution in sinus node dysfunction. Continue within 4 hours of surgery then restart as soon as possible after. Clonidine injection should be administered via a continuous epidural infusion device. Epidural clonidine is not recommended for perioperative, obstetrical, or postpartum pain. It is not recommended for use in patients with severe cardiovascular disease or hemodynamic instability. In all cases, the epidural may lead to cardiovascular instability (hypotension, bradycardia). May cause significant CNS depression and xerostomia. Caution in patients with pre-existing CNS disease or depression. Elderly may be at greater risk for CNS depressive effects, favoring other agents in this population.

Adverse Reactions Incidence of adverse events is not always reported.

>10%:

Central nervous system: Drowsiness (35% oral, 12% transdermal), dizziness (16% oral, 2% transdermal)

Dermatologic: Transient localized skin reactions characterized by pruritus, and erythema (15% to 50% transdermal)

Gastrointestinal: Dry mouth (40% oral, 25% transdermal)

1% to 10%:

Cardiovascular: Orthostatic hypotension (3% oral)

Central nervous system: Headache (1% oral, 5% transdermal), sedation (3% transdermal), fatigue (6% transdermal), lethargy (3% transdermal), insomnia (2% transdermal), nervousness (3% oral, 1% transdermal), mental depression (1% oral)

Dermatologic: Rash (1% oral), allergic contact sensitivity (5% transdermal), localized vesiculation (7%), hyperpigmentation (5% at application site), edema (3%), excoriation (3%), burning (3%), throbbing, blanching (1%), papules (1%), and generalized macular rash (1%) has occurred in patients receiving transdermal clonidine.

Endocrine & metabolic: Sodium and water retention, sexual dysfunction (3% oral, 2% transdermal), impotence (3% oral, 2% transdermal), weakness (10% transdermal)

Gastrointestinal: Nausea (5% oral, 1% transdermal), vomiting (5% oral), anorexia and malaise (1% oral), constipation (10% oral, 1% transdermal), dry throat (2% transdermal), taste disturbance (1% transdermal), weight gain (1% oral)

Genitourinary: Nocturia (1% oral)

Hepatic: Liver function test (mild abnormalities, 1% oral)

Miscellaneous: Withdrawal syndrome (1% oral)

<1% (Limited to important or life-threatening symptoms): Hepatitis (oral), difficulty in micturition (oral, transdermal), urinary retention (oral), hives (oral, transdermal), angioedema (oral, transdermal), urticaria (oral, transdermal), alopecia (oral, transdermal), parotid pain (oral), gynecomastia (oral, transdermal), transient elevation of blood glucose (oral), elevation of creatinine phosphokinase (oral), palpitations (oral, transdermal), tachycardia (oral, transdermal), bradycardia (oral), sinus bradycardia (oral, transdermal), atrioventricular block (oral, transdermal), congestive heart failure (oral, transdermal), EKG abnormalities (oral, transdermal), flushing, pallor, Raynaud's phenomenon (oral, transdermal), chest pain (transdermal), increase in blood pressure (transdermal), weakness, muscle or joint pain (0.6% oral), leg cramps (0.3% oral), fever (oral, transdermal), malaise (transdermal), withdrawal syndrome (transdermal), vivid dreams (oral, transdermal), nightmares (oral, transdermal), insomnia (oral), behavioral changes (transdermal), restlessness (oral, transdermal), anxiety (oral, transdermal), mental depression (transdermal), visual and auditory hallucinations (oral, transdermal), delirium (transdermal), CVA (transdermal), irritability (transdermal), weight gain (transdermal), rash (transdermal), orthostatic symptoms (transdermal), syncope (oral, transdermal), agitation (transdermal), contact dermatitis (transdermal), localized hypo- or hyperpigmentation (transdermal), anorexia (transdermal), vomiting (transdermal), loss of libido (transdermal), decreased sexual activity (transdermal), blurred vision (transdermal), burning of the eyes (transdermal), dryness of the eyes (transdermal), weakly positive Coombs' test (oral), increased sensitivity to ethanol (oral), thrombocytopenia (oral), abdominal pain (oral), pseudo-obstruction (oral)

Overdosage/Toxicology

Signs and symptoms: Bradycardia, CNS depression, hypothermia, diarrhea, respiratory depression, apnea

(Continued)

Clonidine *(Continued)*

Treatment: Primarily supportive and symptomatic. Hypotension usually responds to I.V. fluids or Trendelenburg positioning. If unresponsive to these measures, the use of a parenteral vasoconstrictor may be required (eg, norepinephrine 0.1-0.2 mcg/kg/minute titrated to response). Naloxone may be utilized in treating the CNS depression and/or apnea and should be given I.V. 0.4-2 mg, with repeats as needed. Atropine 15 mcg/kg I.V. or may be needed for symptomatic bradycardia.

Drug Interactions

Antipsychotics: Concurrent use with antipsychotics (especially low potency) or nitroprusside may produce additive hypotensive effects

Beta-blockers: May potentiate bradycardia in patients receiving clonidine and may increase the rebound hypertension of withdrawal; discontinue beta-blocker several days before clonidine is tapered

CNS depressants: Sedative effects may be additive; monitor for increased effect; includes barbiturates, benzodiazepines, narcotic analgesics, ethanol, and other sedative agents

Cyclosporine: Clonidine may increase cyclosporine (and perhaps tacrolimus) serum concentrations; cyclosporine dosage adjustment may be needed

Hypoglycemic agents: Clonidine may decrease the symptoms of hypoglycemia; monitor patients receiving antidiabetic agents

Levodopa: Effects may be reduced by clonidine in some patients with Parkinson's disease (limited documentation); monitor

Local anesthetics: Epidural clonidine may prolong the sensory and motor blockade of local anesthetics

Mirtazapine: Antihypertensive effects of clonidine may be antagonized by mirtazapine (hypertensive urgency has been reported following addition of mirtazapine to clonidine); in addition, mirtazapine may potentially enhance the hypertensive response associated with abrupt clonidine withdrawal. Avoid this combination; consider an alternative agent.

Narcotic analgesics: May potentiate hypotensive effects of clonidine

Tricyclic antidepressants: Antihypertensive effects of clonidine may be antagonized by tricyclic antidepressants; in addition, tricyclic antidepressants may enhance the hypertensive response associated with abrupt clonidine withdrawal; avoid this combination; consider an alternative agent

Verapamil: Concurrent administration may be associated with hypotension and AV block in some patients (limited documentation); monitor

Ethanol/Nutrition/Herb Interactions

Ethanol: Avoid ethanol (may increase CNS depression).

Herb/Nutraceutical: Avoid dong quai if using for hypertension (has estrogenic activity). Avoid ephedra, yohimbe, ginseng (may worsen hypertension). Avoid valerian, St John's wort, kava kava, gotu kola (may increase CNS depression).

Mechanism of Action

Stimulates alpha$_2$-adrenoceptors in the brain stem, thus activating an inhibitory neuron, resulting in reduced sympathetic outflow from the CNS, producing a decrease in peripheral resistance, renal vascular resistance, heart rate, and blood pressure; epidural clonidine may produce pain relief at spinal presynaptic and postjunctional alpha$_2$-adrenoceptors by preventing pain signal transmission; pain relief occurs only for the body regions innervated by the spinal segments where analgesic concentrations of clonidine exist

Pharmacodynamics/Kinetics

Onset of effect: Oral: 0.5-1 hour; T_{max}: 2-4 hours

Duration: 6-10 hours

Distribution: V_d: 2.1 L/kg (adults); highly lipid soluble; distributes readily into extravascular sites; protein binding: 20% to 40%

Metabolism: Hepatic (enterohepatic recirculation); extensively metabolized to inactive metabolites

Bioavailability: 75% to 95%

Half-life: Adults:

Normal renal function: 6-20 hours

Renal impairment: 18-41 hours

Elimination: 65% excreted in urine, 32% unchanged, and 22% excreted in feces; not removed significantly by hemodialysis

Usual Dosage

Children:

Oral:

Hypertension: Initial: 5-10 mcg/kg/day in divided doses every 8-12 hours; increase gradually at 5- to 7-day intervals to 25 mcg/kg/day in divided doses every 6 hours; maximum: 0.9 mg/day

Clonidine tolerance test (test of growth hormone release from pituitary): 0.15 mg/m^2 or 4 mcg/kg as single dose

ADHD (unlabeled use): Initial: 0.05 mg/day; increase every 3-7 days by 0.05 mg/day to 3-5 mcg/kg/day given in divided doses 3-4 times/day (maximum dose: 0.3-0.4 mg/day)

Epidural infusion: Pain management: Reserved for patients with severe intractable pain, unresponsive to other analgesics or epidural or spinal opiates: Initial: 0.5 mcg/kg/hour; adjust with caution, based on clinical effect

Adults:

Oral:

Acute hypertension (urgency): Initial 0.1-0.2 mg; may be followed by additional doses of 0.1 mg every hour, if necessary, to a maximum total dose of 0.6 mg

Hypertension: Initial dose: 0.1 mg twice daily, usual maintenance dose: 0.2-1.2 mg/day in 2-4 divided doses; maximum recommended dose: 2.4 mg/day

Nicotine withdrawal symptoms: 0.1 mg twice daily to maximum of 0.4 mg/day for 3-4 weeks

Transdermal: Hypertension: Apply once every 7 days; for initial therapy start with 0.1 mg and increase by 0.1 mg at 1- to 2-week intervals; dosages >0.6 mg do not improve efficacy

Epidural infusion: Pain management: Starting dose: 30 mcg/hour; titrate as required for relief of pain or presence of side effects; minimal experience with doses >40 mcg/hour; should be considered an adjunct to intraspinal opiate therapy

Elderly: Initial: 0.1 mg once daily at bedtime, increase gradually as needed

Dosing adjustment in renal impairment: Cl_{cr} <10 mL/minute: Administer 50% to 75% of normal dose initially

Dialysis: Not dialyzable (0% to 5%) via hemo- or peritoneal dialysis; supplemental dose not necessary

Dietary Considerations Hypertensive patients may need to decrease sodium and calories in diet.

Administration

Oral: Do not discontinue clonidine abruptly. if needed, gradually reduce dose over 2-4 days to avoid rebound hypertension

Transdermal patch: Patches should be applied weekly at bedtime to a clean, hairless area of the upper outer arm or chest. Rotate patch sites weekly. Redness under patch may be reduced if a topical corticosteroid spray is applied to the area before placement of the patch.

Monitoring Parameters Blood pressure, standing and sitting/supine, mental status, heart rate

Reference Range Therapeutic: 1-2 ng/mL (SI: 4.4-8.7 nmol/L)

Test Interactions ↑ sodium (S); ↓ catecholamines (U)

Patient Information Do not discontinue drug except on instruction of physician; check daily to be sure patch is present; may cause drowsiness, impaired coordination, and judgment

Nursing Implications Patches should be applied weekly at bedtime to a clean, hairless area of the upper outer arm or chest; rotate patch sites weekly; redness under patch may be reduced if a topical corticosteroid spray is applied to the area before placement of the patch; if needed, gradually reduce dose over 2-4 days to avoid rebound hypertension; during epidural administration, monitor cardiovascular and respiratory status carefully

(Continued)

Clonidine *(Continued)*

Additional Information Transdermal clonidine should only be used in patients unable to take oral medication. The transdermal product is much more expensive than oral clonidine and produces no better therapeutic effects.

Dosage Forms

Injection, as hydrochloride [preservative free]: 100 mcg/mL (10 mL); 500 mcg/mL (10 mL)

Patch, transdermal, as hydrochloride [7-day duration]:
Catapres-TTS®-1: 0.1 mg/day (4s)
Catapres-TTS®-2: 0.2 mg/day (4s)
Catapres-TTS®-3: 0.3 mg/day (4s)

Tablet, as hydrochloride: 0.1 mg, 0.2 mg, 0.3 mg

♦ **Clonidine Hydrochloride** *see* Clonidine *on page 88*

Clorazepate *(klor AZ e pate)*

Related Information

Anxiolytic/Hypnotic Use in Long-Term Care Facilities *on page 562*
Benzodiazepines Comparison Chart *on page 566*
Federal OBRA Regulations Recommended Maximum Doses *on page 583*
Patient Information - Anxiolytics & Sedative Hypnotics (Benzodiazepines) *on page 483*

U.S. Brand Names Tranxene®

Canadian Brand Names Apo®-Clorazepate; Novo-Clopate®

Synonyms Clorazepate Dipotassium

Pharmacologic Category Benzodiazepine

Generic Available Yes

Use Treatment of generalized anxiety disorder; management of alcohol withdrawal; adjunct anticonvulsant in management of partial seizures

Restrictions C-IV

Pregnancy Risk Factor D

Contraindications Hypersensitivity to this drug or any component of the formulation (cross-sensitivity with other benzodiazepines may exist); narrow-angle glaucoma; pregnancy

Warnings/Precautions Not recommended for use in patients <9 years of age or patients with depressive or psychotic disorders. Use with caution in elderly or debilitated patients, patients with hepatic disease (including alcoholics), or renal impairment. Active metabolites with extended half-lives may lead to delayed accumulation and adverse effects. Use with caution in patients with respiratory disease or impaired gag reflex. Use is not recommended in patients with depressive disorders or psychoses. Avoid use in patients with sleep apnea.

Causes CNS depression (dose-related) resulting in sedation, dizziness, confusion, or ataxia which may impair physical and mental capabilities. Patients must be cautioned about performing tasks which require mental alertness (ie, operating machinery or driving). Use with caution in patients receiving other CNS depressants or psychoactive agents. Effects with other sedative drugs or ethanol may be potentiated. Benzodiazepines have been associated with falls and traumatic injury and should be used with extreme caution in patients who are at risk of these events (especially the elderly).

Use caution in patients with depression, particularly if suicidal risk may be present. Use with caution in patients with a history of drug dependence. Benzodiazepines have been associated with dependence and acute withdrawal symptoms on discontinuation or reduction in dose. Acute withdrawal, including seizures, may be precipitated in patients after administration of flumazenil to patients receiving long-term benzodiazepine therapy.

Benzodiazepines have been associated with anterograde amnesia. Paradoxical reactions, including hyperactive or aggressive behavior, have been reported with benzodiazepines, particularly in adolescent/pediatric or psychiatric patients. Does not have analgesic, antidepressant, or antipsychotic properties.

Adverse Reactions

Cardiovascular: Hypotension

Central nervous system: Drowsiness, fatigue, ataxia, lightheadedness, memory impairment, insomnia, anxiety, headache, depression, slurred speech, confusion, nervousness, dizziness, irritability

Dermatologic: Rash

Endocrine & metabolic: Decreased libido

Gastrointestinal: Xerostomia, constipation, diarrhea, decreased salivation, nausea, vomiting, increased or decreased appetite

Neuromuscular & skeletal: Dysarthria, tremor

Ocular: Blurred vision, diplopia

Overdosage/Toxicology

Signs and symptoms: Somnolence, confusion, ataxia, diminished reflexes, coma

Treatment: Supportive; rarely is mechanical ventilation required

Flumazenil has been shown to selectively block the binding of benzodiazepines to CNS receptors, resulting in a reversal of benzodiazepine- induced CNS depression, but not respiratory depression

Drug Interactions CYP3A3/4 enzyme substrate

CNS depressants: Sedative effects and/or respiratory depression may be additive with CNS depressants; includes ethanol, barbiturates, narcotic analgesics, and other sedative agents; monitor for increased effect

Enzyme inducers: Metabolism of some benzodiazepines may be increased, decreasing their therapeutic effect; consider using an alternative sedative/hypnotic agent; potential inducers include phenobarbital, phenytoin, carbamazepine, rifampin, and rifabutin

CYP3A3/4 inhibitors: Serum level and/or toxicity of some benzodiazepines may be increased; inhibitors include amiodarone, cimetidine, clarithromycin, erythromycin, delavirdine, diltiazem, dirithromycin, disulfiram, fluoxetine, fluvoxamine, grapefruit juice, indinavir, itraconazole, ketoconazole, nefazodone, nevirapine, propoxyphene, quinupristin-dalfopristin, ritonavir, saquinavir, verapamil, zafirlukast, zileuton; monitor for altered benzodiazepine response

Levodopa: Therapeutic effects may be diminished in some patients following the addition of a benzodiazepine; limited/inconsistent data

Oral contraceptives: May decrease the clearance of some benzodiazepines (those which undergo oxidative metabolism); monitor for increased benzodiazepine effect

Theophylline: May partially antagonize some of the effects of benzodiazepines; monitor for decreased response; may require higher doses for sedation

Ethanol/Nutrition/Herb Interactions

Ethanol: Avoid ethanol (may increase CNS depression).

Food: Serum concentrations/toxicity may be increased by grapefruit juice.

Herb/Nutraceutical: Avoid valerian, St John's wort, kava kava, gotu kola (may increase CNS depression).

Stability Unstable in water

Mechanism of Action Binds to stereospecific benzodiazepine receptors on the postsynaptic GABA neuron at several sites within the central nervous system, including the limbic system, reticular formation. Enhancement of the inhibitory effect of GABA on neuronal excitability results by increased neuronal membrane permeability to chloride ions. This shift in chloride ions results in hyperpolarization (a less excitable state) and stabilization.

Pharmacodynamics/Kinetics

Distribution: Crosses the placenta; appears in urine

Metabolism: Rapidly decarboxylated to desmethyldiazepam (active) in acidic stomach prior to absorption; metabolized in the liver to oxazepam (active)

Half-life: Adults:

Desmethyldiazepam: 48-96 hours

Oxazepam: 6-8 hours

(Continued)

Clorazepate *(Continued)*

Time to peak serum concentration: Oral: Within 1 hour
Elimination: Primarily in urine

Usual Dosage Oral:

Children 9-12 years: Anticonvulsant: Initial: 3.75-7.5 mg/dose twice daily; increase dose by 3.75 mg at weekly intervals, not to exceed 60 mg/day in 2-3 divided doses

Children >12 years and Adults: Anticonvulsant: Initial: Up to 7.5 mg/dose 2-3 times/day; increase dose by 7.5 mg at weekly intervals, not to exceed 90 mg/day

Adults:

Anxiety:

Regular release tablets (Tranxene® T-Tab™): 7.5-15 mg 2-4 times/day
Sustained release (Tranxene®-SD): 11.25 or 22.5 mg once daily at bedtime

Alcohol withdrawal: Initial: 30 mg, then 15 mg 2-4 times/day on first day; maximum daily dose: 90 mg; gradually decrease dose over subsequent days

Monitoring Parameters Respiratory and cardiovascular status, excess CNS depression

Reference Range Therapeutic: 0.12-1 µg/mL (SI: 0.36-3.01 µmol/L)

Test Interactions ↓ hematocrit, abnormal liver and renal function tests

Patient Information Avoid alcohol and other CNS depressants; avoid activities needing good psychomotor coordination until CNS effects are known; drug may cause physical or psychological dependence; avoid abrupt discontinuation after prolonged use

Nursing Implications Observe patient for excess sedation, respiratory depression; raise bed rails, initiate safety measures, assist with ambulation

Additional Information Abrupt discontinuation after sustained use (generally >10 days) may cause withdrawal symptoms.

Dosage Forms

Tablet, as dipotassium:
Tranxene®-SD™: 22.5 mg [once daily]
Tranxene®-SD™ Half Strength: 11.25 mg [once daily]
Tranxene® T-Tab™: 3.75 mg, 7.5 mg, 15 mg

♦ **Clorazepate Dipotassium** *see* Clorazepate *on page 92*

Clozapine *(KLOE za peen)*

Related Information
Antipsychotic Agents Comparison Chart *on page 557*
Antipsychotic Medication Guidelines *on page 559*
Atypical Antipsychotics *on page 565*
Clozapine-Induced Side Effects *on page 568*
Discontinuation of Psychotropic Drugs - Withdrawal Symptoms and Recommendations *on page 582*
Federal OBRA Regulations Recommended Maximum Doses *on page 583*
Patient Information - Antipsychotics (Clozapine) *on page 469*
Patient Information - Antipsychotics (General) *on page 466*
Teratogenic Risks of Psychotropic Medications *on page 594*

U.S. Brand Names Clozaril®

Canadian Brand Names Clozaril

Pharmacologic Category Antipsychotic Agent, Dibenzodiazepine

Generic Available Yes

Use Treatment of refractory schizophrenia

Unlabeled/Investigational Use Schizoaffective disorder, bipolar disorder, childhood psychosis

Pregnancy Risk Factor B

Contraindications Hypersensitivity to clozapine or any component of the formulation; history of agranulocytosis or granulocytopenia with clozapine; uncontrolled epilepsy; severe central nervous system depression or comatose state; myeloproliferative disorders or use with other agents which have a well-known risk of agranulocytosis or bone marrow suppression

In patients with WBC ≤3500 cells/mm^3 before therapy; if WBC falls to <3000 cells/mm^3 during therapy the drug should be withheld until signs and symptoms of infection disappear and WBC rises to >3000 cells/mm^3

Warnings/Precautions Medication should not be stopped abruptly; taper off over 1-2 weeks. WBC testing should occur weekly for the first 6 months of therapy; thereafter, if acceptable, WBC counts are maintained (WBC >3000/mm^3, ANC >1500/mm^3) then WBC counts can be monitored every other week. WBCs must be monitored weekly for the first 4 weeks after therapy discontinuation. Significant risk of agranulocytosis, potentially life-threatening. Use with caution in patients receiving other marrow suppressive agents. Elderly patients are more susceptible to adverse effects (including cardiovascular, anticholinergic, and tardive dyskinesia).

Cognitive and/or motor impairment (sedation) is common with clozapine, resulting in impaired performance of tasks requiring alertness (ie, operating machinery or driving).

May cause orthostatic hypotension and tachycardia; use with caution in patients at risk of hypotension or in patients where transient hypotensive episodes would be poorly tolerated (cardiovascular disease or cerebrovascular disease). Concurrent use of psychotropics and benzodiazepines may increase the risk of severe cardiopulmonary reactions. Use with caution in patients at risk of seizures, including those with a history of seizures, head trauma, brain damage, alcoholism, or concurrent therapy with medications which may lower seizure threshold.

Has been associated with benign, self-limiting fever (<100.4 F, usually within first three weeks). However, clozapine may also be associated with severe febrile reactions, including neuroleptic malignant syndrome (NMS). Clozapine's potential for extrapyramidal reactions appears to be extremely low.

May cause anticholinergic effects; use with caution in patients with urinary retention, benign prostatic hypertrophy, narrow-angle glaucoma, xerostomia, visual problems, constipation, or history of bowel obstruction.

Eosinophilia has been reported to occur with clozapine and may require temporary or permanent interruption of therapy. Pulmonary embolism has been associated with clozapine therapy. May cause hyperglycemia - use with caution in patients with diabetes or other disorders of glucose regulation. Use with caution in patients with hepatic disease or impairment - hepatitis has been reported as a consequence of therapy.

Rare cases of thromboembolism, including pulmonary embolism and stroke resulting in fatalities, have been associated with clozapine.

Adverse Reactions
>10%:
    Cardiovascular: Tachycardia
    Central nervous system: Drowsiness, dizziness
    Gastrointestinal: Constipation, weight gain, diarrhea, sialorrhea
    Genitourinary: Urinary incontinence
1% to 10%:
    Cardiovascular: EKG changes, hypertension, hypotension, syncope
    Central nervous system: Akathisia, seizures, headache, nightmares, akinesia, confusion, insomnia, fatigue, myoclonic jerks
    Dermatologic: Rash
    Gastrointestinal: Abdominal discomfort, heartburn, xerostomia, nausea, vomiting
    Hematologic: Eosinophilia, leukopenia
    Neuromuscular & skeletal: Tremor
    Miscellaneous: Diaphoresis (increased), fever
<1%: Agranulocytosis, arrhythmias, blurred vision, congestive heart failure, difficult urination, granulocytopenia, impotence, myocardial infarction, myocarditis, (Continued)

Clozapine *(Continued)*

neuroleptic malignant syndrome, pericardial effusion, pericarditis, rigidity, tardive dyskinesia, thrombocytopenia, thromboembolism, pulmonary embolism, stroke

Overdosage/Toxicology

Signs and symptoms: Altered states of consciousness, tachycardia, hypotension, hypersalivation, respiratory depression

Treatment:

Following initiation of essential overdose management, toxic symptom treatment and supportive treatment should be initiated

Hypotension usually responds to I.V. fluids or Trendelenburg positioning. If unresponsive to these measures, the use of a parenteral inotrope may be required

Seizures commonly respond to diazepam (I.V. 5-10 mg bolus in adults every 15 minutes if needed up to a total of 30 mg; I.V. 0.25-0.4 mg/kg/dose up to a total of 10 mg in children) or to phenytoin or phenobarbital; in situations where clozapine is to be continued, valproate is the anticonvulsant of choice

Also critical cardiac arrhythmias often respond to I.V. phenytoin (15 mg/kg up to 1 g), while other antiarrhythmics can be used

Drug Interactions

CYP1A2, 2C (minor), 2D6 (minor), 2E1, 3A3/4 enzyme substrate

Benzodiazepines: In combination with clozapine may produce respiratory depression and hypotension, especially during the first few weeks of therapy; monitor for altered response

Carbamazepine: A case of neuroleptic malignant syndrome has been reported in combination with clozapine; in addition, carbamazepine may alter clozapine levels (see enzyme inducers); monitor

CYP enzyme inducers: Metabolism of clozapine may be increased, decreasing its therapeutic effect; potential inducers include phenobarbital, phenytoin, carbamazepine, rifampin, rifabutin, and cigarette smoking

CYP1A2 inhibitors: Serum level and/or toxicity of clozapine may be increased; inhibitors include cimetidine, ciprofloxacin, fluvoxamine, isoniazid, ritonavir, and zileuton; monitor for altered effects; a decrease in clozapine dosage may be required

CYP2E1 inhibitors: Serum level and/or toxicity of clozapine may be increased; inhibitors include disulfiram and ritonavir; monitor for altered effects; a decrease in clozapine dosage may be required

CYP3A4 inhibitors: Serum level and/or toxicity of clozapine may be increased; inhibitors include amiodarone, cimetidine, clarithromycin, erythromycin, delavirdine, diltiazem, dirithromycin, disulfiram, fluoxetine, fluvoxamine, grapefruit juice, indinavir, itraconazole, ketoconazole, metronidazole, nefazodone, nevirapine, propoxyphene, quinupristin-dalfopristin, ritonavir, saquinavir, verapamil, zafirlukast, zileuton; monitor for altered effects; a decrease in clozapine dosage may be required

Epinephrine: Clozapine may reverse the pressor effect of epinephrine

Risperidone: Effects and/or toxicity may be increased when combined with clozapine; monitor

Valproic acid: May cause reductions in clozapine concentrations; monitor for altered response

Ethanol/Nutrition/Herb Interactions

Ethanol: Avoid ethanol (may increase CNS depression).

Herb/Nutraceutical: St John's wort may decrease clozapine levels. Avoid kava kava, gotu kola, valerian, St John's wort (may increase CNS depression).

Stability Dispensed in "clozapine patient system" packaging

Mechanism of Action Clozapine is a weak dopamine$_1$ and dopamine$_2$ receptor blocker, but blocks D$_1$-D$_5$ receptors; in addition, it blocks the serotonin$_2$, alpha-adrenergic, histamine H$_1$, and cholinergic receptors

Pharmacodynamics/Kinetics

Protein binding: 95% bound to serum proteins

Metabolism: Extensively metabolized prior to excretion with only a trace amount of unchanged drug in the urine and feces

Half-life: 12 hours (range: 4-66 hours)

Time to peak: 2.5 hours

Elimination: ~50% of the administered dose is excreted in urine, 30% in feces

Usual Dosage Oral: If dosing is interrupted for >48 hours, therapy must be re-initiated at 12.5-25 mg/day; may be increased more rapidly than with initial titration:

Children and Adolescents: Childhood psychosis (unlabeled use): Initial: 25 mg/day; increase to a target dose of 25-400 mg/day

Adults: Schizophrenia: Initial: 25 mg once or twice daily; increased, as tolerated to a target dose of 300-450 mg/day after 2-4 weeks, but may require doses as high as 600-900 mg/day

Elderly: Schizophrenia: Dose selection and titration should be cautious

Child/Adolescent Considerations Eleven adolescents with childhood-onset schizophrenia who failed a 6-week trial of haloperidol were treated with clozapine (mean 6-week daily dose: 370 mg) (Frazier, 1994). Twenty-one patients (mean age: 14 ± 2.3 years) with schizophrenia (DSM-III-R) who had been nonresponsive to typical antipsychotics received clozapine 176 ± 149 mg/day (final dose) (Kumra, 1996). Clozapine was evaluated in 11 neuroleptic-resistant children (<13 years of age) mean dosage: 227 mg/day (Turetz, 1997). A 15 year old boy with severe treatment-refractory bipolar disorder type I was treated successfully with clozapine 300 mg/day (Masi, 1998).

Dietary Considerations May be taken without regard to food.

Monitoring Parameters Complete blood count weekly for 6 months then every other week thereafter, if clozapine is discontinued, continue monitoring for 1 month; EKG, liver function tests

Patient Information Report any lethargy, fever, sore throat, flu-like symptoms, or any other signs or symptoms of infection; may cause drowsiness; frequent blood samples must be taken; do not stop taking even if you think it is not working

Nursing Implications Benign, self-limiting temperature elevations sometimes occur during the first 3 weeks of treatment, weekly CBC mandatory for first 6 months

Dosage Forms Tablet: 25 mg, 100 mg

Cyproheptadine (si proe HEP ta deen)

U.S. Brand Names Periactin®

Canadian Brand Names PMS-Cyproheptadine

Synonyms Cyproheptadine Hydrochloride

Pharmacologic Category Antihistamine

(Continued)

Cyproheptadine *(Continued)*

Generic Available Yes

Use Perennial and seasonal allergic rhinitis and other allergic symptoms including urticaria

Unlabeled/Investigational Use Appetite stimulation, blepharospasm, cluster headaches, migraine headaches, Nelson's syndrome, pruritus, schizophrenia, spinal cord damage associated spasticity, and tardive dyskinesia

Pregnancy Risk Factor B

Contraindications Hypersensitivity to cyproheptadine or any component of the formulation; narrow-angle glaucoma; bladder neck obstruction; acute asthmatic attack; stenosing peptic ulcer; GI tract obstruction; concurrent use of MAO inhibitors; avoid use in premature and term newborns due to potential association with SIDS

Warnings/Precautions Do not use in neonates, safety and efficacy have not been established in children <2 years of age; symptomatic prostate hypertrophy; antihistamines are more likely to cause dizziness, excessive sedation, syncope, toxic confusion states, and hypotension in the elderly. In case reports, cyproheptadine has promoted weight gain in anorexic adults, though it has not been specifically studied in the elderly. All cases of weight loss or decreased appetite should be adequately assessed.

Adverse Reactions

>10%:

Central nervous system: Slight to moderate drowsiness

Respiratory: Thickening of bronchial secretions

1% to 10%:

Central nervous system: Headache, fatigue, nervousness, dizziness

Gastrointestinal: Appetite stimulation, nausea, diarrhea, abdominal pain, xerostomia

Neuromuscular & skeletal: Arthralgia

Respiratory: Pharyngitis

<1%: Tachycardia, palpitations, edema, sedation, CNS stimulation, seizures, depression, photosensitivity, rash, angioedema, hemolytic anemia, leukopenia, thrombocytopenia, hepatitis, myalgia, paresthesia, bronchospasm, epistaxis, allergic reactions

Overdosage/Toxicology

Signs and symptoms: CNS depression or stimulation, dry mouth, flushed skin, fixed and dilated pupils, apnea

Treatment: There is no specific treatment for an antihistamine overdose, however, most of its clinical toxicity is due to anticholinergic effects. Anticholinesterase inhibitors may be useful by reducing acetylcholinesterase. Anticholinesterase inhibitors include physostigmine, neostigmine, pyridostigmine, and edrophonium. For anticholinergic overdose with severe life-threatening symptoms, physostigmine 1-2 mg (0.5 or 0.02 mg/kg for children) I.V., slowly may be given to reverse these effects.

Drug Interactions Increased toxicity: MAO inhibitors → hallucinations

Ethanol/Nutrition/Herb Interactions Ethanol: Avoid ethanol (may increase CNS sedation).

Mechanism of Action A potent antihistamine and serotonin antagonist, competes with histamine for H_1-receptor sites on effector cells in the gastrointestinal tract, blood vessels, and respiratory tract

Usual Dosage Oral:

Children:

Allergic conditions: 0.25 mg/kg/day or 8 mg/m²/day in 2-3 divided doses **or**

2-6 years: 2 mg every 8-12 hours (not to exceed 12 mg/day)

7-14 years: 4 mg every 8-12 hours (not to exceed 16 mg/day)

Migraine headaches: 4 mg 2-3 times/day

Children ≥12 years and Adults: Spasticity associated with spinal cord damage: 4 mg at bedtime; increase by a 4 mg dose every 3-4 days; average daily dose: 16 mg in divided doses; not to exceed 36 mg/day

Children >13 years and Adults: Appetite stimulation (anorexia nervosa): 2 mg 4 times/day; may be increased gradually over a 3-week period to 8 mg 4 times/day

Adults:

Allergic conditions: 4-20 mg/day divided every 8 hours (not to exceed 0.5)

Cluster headaches: 4 mg 4 times/day

Migraine headaches: 4-8 mg 3 times/day

Dosage adjustment in hepatic impairment: Reduce dosage in patients with significant hepatic dysfunction

Test Interactions Diagnostic antigen skin tests, ↑ amylases (S), ↓ fasting glucose (S)

Patient Information Take as directed; do not exceed recommended dose. Avoid use of other depressants, alcohol, or sleep-inducing medications unless approved by prescriber. You may experience drowsiness or dizziness (use caution when driving or engaging in tasks requiring alertness until response to drug is known); or dry mouth, nausea, or abdominal pain (frequent small meals, frequent mouth care, chewing gum, or sucking hard candy may help). Report persistent sedation, confusion, or agitation; changes in urinary pattern; blurred vision; chest pain or palpitations; sore throat difficulty breathing or expectorating (thick secretions); or lack of improvement or worsening or condition.

Nursing Implications Raise bed rails, institute safety measures, assist with ambulation

Additional Information May stimulate appetite; in case reports, cyproheptadine has promoted weight gain in anorexic adults.

Dosage Forms

Syrup, as hydrochloride: 2 mg/5 mL with alcohol 5% (473 mL)

Tablet, as hydrochloride: 4 mg

- **Cyproheptadine Hydrochloride** *see* Cyproheptadine *on page 97*
- **Cytochrome P450 Enzymes and and Drug Metabolism** *see page 570*
- **Cytomel**® *see* Liothyronine *on page 202*
- **Dalmane**® *see* Flurazepam *on page 155*
- ***d*-Alpha Tocopherol** *see* Vitamin E *on page 433*
- **Dantrium**® *see* Dantrolene *on page 99*

Dantrolene (DAN troe leen)

U.S. Brand Names Dantrium®

Canadian Brand Names Dantrium

Synonyms Dantrolene Sodium

Pharmacologic Category Skeletal Muscle Relaxant

Generic Available No

Use Treatment of spasticity associated with spinal cord injury, stroke, cerebral palsy, or multiple sclerosis; treatment of malignant hyperthermia

Unlabeled/Investigational Use Neuroleptic malignant syndrome (NMS)

Pregnancy Risk Factor C

Contraindications Active hepatic disease; should not be used where spasticity is used to maintain posture or balance

Warnings/Precautions Use with caution in patients with impaired cardiac function or impaired pulmonary function; has potential for hepatotoxicity; overt hepatitis has been most frequently observed between the third and twelfth month of therapy; hepatic injury appears to be greater in females and in patients >35 years of age

Adverse Reactions

>10%:

Central nervous system: Drowsiness, dizziness, lightheadedness, fatigue

Dermatologic: Rash

Gastrointestinal: Diarrhea (mild), nausea, vomiting

Neuromuscular & skeletal: Muscle weakness

(Continued)

Dantrolene *(Continued)*

1% to 10%:
  Cardiovascular: Pleural effusion with pericarditis
  Central nervous system: Chills, fever, headache, insomnia, nervousness, mental depression
  Gastrointestinal: Diarrhea (severe), constipation, anorexia, stomach cramps
  Ocular: Blurred vision
  Respiratory: Respiratory depression
<1%: Seizures, confusion, hepatitis

Overdosage/Toxicology

Signs and symptoms: CNS depression, hypotension, nausea, vomiting
Treatment: For decontamination, lavage/activated charcoal with cathartic; do not use ipecac; hypotension can be treated with isotonic I.V. fluids with the patient placed in the Trendelenburg position; dopamine or norepinephrine can be given if hypotension is refractory to above therapy

Drug Interactions

Increased toxicity: Estrogens (hepatotoxicity), CNS depressants (sedation), MAO inhibitors, phenothiazines, clindamycin (increased neuromuscular blockade), verapamil (hyperkalemia and cardiac depression), warfarin, clofibrate and tolbutamide

Ethanol/Nutrition/Herb Interactions

Ethanol: Avoid ethanol (may increase CNS depression).
Herb/Nutraceutical: Avoid valerian, St John's wort, kava kava, gotu kola (may increase CNS depression).

Stability Reconstitute vial by adding 60 mL of sterile water for injection USP (**not bacteriostatic water for injection**); protect from light; use within 6 hours; avoid glass bottles for I.V. infusion

Mechanism of Action Acts directly on skeletal muscle by interfering with release of calcium ion from the sarcoplasmic reticulum; prevents or reduces the increase in myoplasmic calcium ion concentration that activates the acute catabolic processes associated with malignant hyperthermia

Usual Dosage

Spasticity: Oral:
  Children: Initial: 0.5 mg/kg/dose twice daily, increase frequency to 3-4 times/day at 4- to 7-day intervals, then increase dose by 0.5 mg/kg to a maximum of 3 mg/kg/dose 2-4 times/day up to 400 mg/day
  Adults: 25 mg/day to start, increase frequency to 2-4 times/day, then increase dose by 25 mg every 4-7 days to a maximum of 100 mg 2-4 times/day or 400 mg/day

Malignant hyperthermia: Children and Adults:
  Preoperative prophylaxis:
    Oral: 4-8 mg/kg/day in 4 divided doses, begin 1-2 days prior to surgery with last dose 3-4 hours prior to surgery
    I.V.: 2.5 mg/kg ~1¼ hours prior to anesthesia and infused over 1 hour with additional doses as needed and individualized
  Crisis: I.V.: 2.5 mg/kg; may repeat dose up to cumulative dose of 10 mg/kg; if physiologic and metabolic abnormalities reappear, repeat regimen
  Postcrisis follow-up: Oral: 4-8 mg/kg/day in 4 divided doses for 1-3 days; I.V. dantrolene may be used when oral therapy is not practical; individualize dosage beginning with 1 mg/kg or more as the clinical situation dictates
Neuroleptic malignant syndrome (unlabeled use): I.V.: 1 mg/kg; may repeat dose up to maximum cumulative dose of 10 mg/kg, then switch to oral dosage

Administration I.V.: Therapeutic or emergency dose can be administered with rapid continuous I.V. push. Follow-up doses should be administered over 2-3 minutes.

Monitoring Parameters Motor performance should be monitored for therapeutic outcomes; nausea, vomiting, and liver function tests should be monitored for potential hepatotoxicity; intravenous administration requires cardiac monitor and blood pressure monitor

Test Interactions ↑ serum AST (SGOT), ALT (SGPT), alkaline phosphatase, LDH, BUN, and total serum bilirubin

Patient Information Take exactly as directed. Do not increase dose or discontinue without consulting prescriber. Do not use alcohol, prescriptive or OTC antidepressants, sedatives, or pain medications without consulting prescriber. You may experience drowsiness, dizziness, lightheadedness (avoid driving or engaging in tasks that require alertness until response to drug is known); nausea or vomiting (small, frequent meals, frequent mouth care, or sucking hard candy may help); or diarrhea (buttermilk, boiled milk, or yogurt may help). Report excessive confusion; drowsiness or mental agitation; chest pain, palpitations, or difficulty breathing; skin rash; or vision disturbances.

Nursing Implications Exercise caution at meals on the day of administration because difficulty swallowing and choking has been reported; avoid extravasation as is a tissue irritant

Dosage Forms
Capsule, as sodium: 25 mg, 50 mg, 100 mg
Powder for injection, as sodium: 20 mg

Desipramine (des IP ra meen)

Related Information
Antidepressant Agents Comparison Chart *on page 553*
Discontinuation of Psychotropic Drugs - Withdrawal Symptoms and Recommendations *on page 582*
Federal OBRA Regulations Recommended Maximum Doses *on page 583*
Patient Information - Antidepressants (TCAs) *on page 454*
Teratogenic Risks of Psychotropic Medications *on page 594*

U.S. Brand Names Norpramin®

Canadian Brand Names PMS-Desipramine

Synonyms Desipramine Hydrochloride; Desmethylimipramine Hydrochloride

Pharmacologic Category Antidepressant, Tricyclic (Secondary Amine)

Generic Available Yes

Use Treatment of depression

Unlabeled/Investigational Use Analgesic adjunct in chronic pain; peripheral neuropathies; substance-related disorders

Pregnancy Risk Factor C

Contraindications Hypersensitivity to desipramine and drugs of similar chemical class; use of MAO inhibitors within 14 days; use in a patient during the acute recovery phase of MI

Warnings/Precautions May cause sedation, resulting in impaired performance of tasks requiring alertness (ie, operating machinery or driving). Sedative effects may be additive with other CNS depressants and/or ethanol. The degree of sedation is low-moderate relative to other antidepressants. May worsen psychosis in some patients or precipitate a shift to mania or hypomania in patients with bipolar disease. May cause hyponatremia/SIADH. May increase the risks associated with electroconvulsive therapy. This agent should be discontinued, when possible, prior to elective surgery. Therapy should not be abruptly discontinued in patients receiving high doses for prolonged periods.
(Continued)

Desipramine *(Continued)*

May cause orthostatic hypotension (risk is moderate relative to other antidepressants) - use with caution in patients at risk of hypotension or in patients where transient hypotensive episodes would be poorly tolerated (cardiovascular disease or cerebrovascular disease). The degree of anticholinergic blockade produced by this agent is low relative to other cyclic antidepressants - however, caution should be used in patients with urinary retention, benign prostatic hypertrophy, narrow-angle glaucoma, xerostomia, visual problems, constipation, or a history of bowel obstruction.

Use caution in patients with depression, particularly if suicidal risk may be present. Use with caution in patients with a history of cardiovascular disease (including previous MI, stroke, tachycardia, or conduction abnormalities). The risk conduction abnormalities with this agent is moderate relative to other antidepressants. Use caution in patients with a previous seizure disorder or condition predisposing to seizures such as brain damage, alcoholism, or concurrent therapy with other drugs which lower the seizure threshold. Use with caution in hyperthyroid patients or those receiving thyroid supplementation. Use with caution in patients with hepatic or renal dysfunction and in elderly patients.

Adverse Reactions

Cardiovascular: Arrhythmias, hypotension, hypertension, palpitations, heart block, tachycardia

Central nervous system: Dizziness, drowsiness, headache, confusion, delirium, hallucinations, nervousness, restlessness, parkinsonian syndrome, insomnia, disorientation, anxiety, agitation, hypomania, exacerbation of psychosis, incoordination, seizures, extrapyramidal symptoms

Dermatologic: Alopecia, photosensitivity, skin rash, urticaria

Endocrine & metabolic: Breast enlargement, galactorrhea, SIADH

Gastrointestinal: Xerostomia, decreased lower esophageal sphincter tone may cause GE reflux, constipation, nausea, unpleasant taste, weight gain/loss, anorexia, abdominal cramps, diarrhea, heartburn

Genitourinary: Difficult urination, sexual dysfunction, testicular edema

Hematologic: Agranulocytosis, eosinophilia, purpura, thrombocytopenia

Hepatic: Cholestatic jaundice, increased liver enzyme

Neuromuscular & skeletal: Fine muscle tremors, weakness, numbness, tingling, paresthesia of extremities, ataxia

Ocular: Blurred vision, disturbances of accommodation, mydriasis, increased intraocular pressure

Miscellaneous: Diaphoresis (excessive), allergic reactions

Overdosage/Toxicology

Signs and symptoms: Agitation, confusion, hallucinations, hyperthermia, urinary retention, CNS depression, cyanosis, dry mucous membranes, cardiac arrhythmias, seizures

Treatment:

Following initiation of essential overdose management, toxic symptoms should be treated

Ventricular arrhythmias often respond with concurrent systemic alkalinization (sodium bicarbonate 0.5-2 mEq/kg I.V.). Arrhythmias unresponsive to phenytoin 15-20 mg/kg (adults) may respond to lidocaine 1 mg/kg I.V. followed by a titrated infusion. Physostigmine (1-2 mg I.V. slowly for adults or 0.5 mg I.V. slowly for children) may be indicated in reversing cardiac arrhythmias that are life-threatening.

Seizures usually respond to diazepam I.V. boluses (5-10 mg for adults up to 30 mg or 0.25-0.4 mg/kg/dose for children up to 10 mg/dose). If seizures are unresponsive or recur, phenytoin or phenobarbital may be required.

Drug Interactions CYP1A2 and 2D6 enzyme substrate; CYP2D6 inhibitor

Altretamine: Concurrent use may cause orthostatic hypertension

Amphetamines: TCAs may enhance the effect of amphetamines; monitor for adverse CV effects

Anticholinergics: Combined use with TCAs may produce additive anticholinergic effects

Antihypertensives: TCAs inhibit the antihypertensive response to bethanidine, clonidine, debrisoquin, guanadrel, guanethidine, guanabenz, guanfacine; monitor BP; consider alternate antihypertensive agent

Beta-agonists: When combined with TCAs may predispose patients to cardiac arrhythmias

Bupropion: May increase the levels of tricyclic antidepressants; based on limited information; monitor response

Carbamazepine: Tricyclic antidepressants may increase carbamazepine levels; monitor

Cholestyramine and colestipol: May bind TCAs and reduce their absorption; monitor for altered response

Clonidine: Abrupt discontinuation of clonidine may cause hypertensive crisis; amitriptyline may enhance the response

CNS depressants: Sedative effects may be additive with TCAs; monitor for increased effect; includes benzodiazepines, barbiturates, antipsychotics, ethanol, and other sedative medications

CYP2C8/9 inhibitors: Serum levels and/or toxicity of some tricyclic antidepressants may be increased; inhibitors include amiodarone, cimetidine, fluvoxamine, some NSAIDs, metronidazole, ritonavir, sulfonamides, troglitazone, valproic acid, and zafirlukast; monitor for increased effect/toxicity

CYP2D6 inhibitors: Serum levels and/or toxicity of some tricyclic antidepressants may be increased; inhibitors include amiodarone, cimetidine, delavirdine, fluoxetine, paroxetine, propafenone, quinidine, and ritonavir; monitor for increased effect/toxicity

CYP3A3/4 inhibitors: Serum level and/or toxicity of some tricyclic antidepressants may be increased; inhibitors include amiodarone, cimetidine, clarithromycin, erythromycin, delavirdine, diltiazem, dirithromycin, disulfiram, fluoxetine, fluvoxamine, grapefruit juice, indinavir, itraconazole, ketoconazole, nevirapine, propoxyphene, quinupristin-dalfopristin, ritonavir, saquinavir, verapamil, zafirlukast, zileuton; monitor for altered effects; a decrease in TCA dosage may be required

Enzyme inducers: May increase the metabolism of TCAs resulting in decreased effect; includes carbamazepine, phenobarbital, phenytoin, and rifampin; monitor for decreased response

Epinephrine (and other direct alpha-agonists): Pressor response to I.V. epinephrine, norepinephrine, and phenylephrine may be enhanced in patients receiving TCAs (**Note:** Effect is unlikely with epinephrine or levonordefrin dosages typically administered as infiltration in combination with local anesthetics)

Fenfluramine: May increase tricyclic antidepressant levels/effects

Hypoglycemic agents (including insulin): TCAs may enhance the hypoglycemic effects of tolazamide, chlorpropamide, or insulin; monitor for changes in blood glucose levels; reported with chlorpropamide, tolazamide, and insulin

Levodopa: Tricyclic antidepressants may decrease the absorption (bioavailability) of levodopa; rare hypertensive episodes have also been attributed to this combination

Linezolid: Hyperpyrexia, hypertension, tachycardia, confusion, seizures, and **deaths have been reported** with agents which inhibit MAO (serotonin syndrome); this combination should be avoided

Lithium: Concurrent use with a TCA may increase the risk for neurotoxicity

MAO inhibitors: Hyperpyrexia, hypertension, tachycardia, confusion, seizures, and **deaths have been reported** (serotonin syndrome); this combination should be avoided

Methylphenidate: Metabolism of TCAs may be decreased

Phenothiazines: Serum concentrations of some TCAs may be increased; in addition, TCAs may increase concentration of phenothiazines; monitor for altered clinical response

QT_c-prolonging agents: Concurrent use of tricyclic agents with other drugs which may prolong QT_c interval may increase the risk of potentially fatal arrhythmias; (Continued)

Desipramine *(Continued)*

includes type Ia and type III antiarrhythmics agents, selected quinolones (sparfloxacin, gatifloxacin, moxifloxacin, grepafloxacin), cisapride, and other agents

Sucralfate: Absorption of tricyclic antidepressants may be reduced with coadministration

Sympathomimetics, indirect-acting: Tricyclic antidepressants may result in a decreased sensitivity to indirect-acting sympathomimetics; includes dopamine and ephedrine; also see interaction with epinephrine (and direct-acting sympathomimetics)

Tramadol: Tramadol's risk of seizures may be increased with TCAs

Valproic acid: May increase serum concentrations/adverse effects of some tricyclic antidepressants

Warfarin (and other oral anticoagulants): TCAs may increase the anticoagulant effect in patients stabilized on warfarin; monitor INR

Ethanol/Nutrition/Herb Interactions

Ethanol: Avoid ethanol (may increase CNS depression).

Food: Grapefruit juice may inhibit the metabolism of some TCAs and clinical toxicity may result.

Herb/Nutraceutical: Avoid valerian, St John's wort, SAMe, kava kava (may increase risk of serotonin syndrome and/or excessive sedation).

Mechanism of Action Traditionally believed to increase the synaptic concentration of norepinephrine (and to a lesser extent, serotonin) in the central nervous system by inhibition of its reuptake by the presynaptic neuronal membrane. However, additional receptor effects have been found including desensitization of adenyl cyclase, down regulation of beta-adrenergic receptors, and down regulation of serotonin receptors.

Pharmacodynamics/Kinetics

Onset of action: 1-3 weeks

Absorption: Well absorbed from GI tract

Metabolism: In the liver

Half-life: Adults: 7-60 hours

Peak plasma levels occur within 4-6 hours

Elimination: 70% excreted in urine

Usual Dosage Oral:

Children 6-12 years: Depression: 10-30 mg/day or 1-3 mg/kg/day in divided doses; do not exceed 5 mg/kg/day

Adolescents: Depression: Initial: 25-50 mg/day; gradually increase to 100 mg/day in single or divided doses (maximum: 150 mg/day)

Adults: Depression: Initial: 75 mg/day in divided doses; increase gradually to 150-200 mg/day in divided or single dose (maximum: 300 mg/day)

Elderly: Depression: Initial dose: 10-25 mg/day; increase by 10-25 mg every 3 days for inpatients and every week for outpatients if tolerated; usual maintenance dose: 75-100 mg/day, but doses up to 150 mg/day may be necessary

Hemodialysis/peritoneal dialysis: Supplemental dose is not necessary

Monitoring Parameters Monitor blood pressure and pulse rate prior to and during initial therapy evaluate mental status; monitor weight; EKG in older adults and those patients with cardiac disease

Reference Range

Plasma levels do not always correlate with clinical effectiveness

Timing of serum samples: Draw trough just before next dose

Therapeutic: 50-300 ng/mL

In elderly patients the response rate is greatest with steady-state plasma concentrations >115 ng/mL

Possible toxicity: >300 ng/mL

Toxic: >1000 ng/mL

Patient Information Avoid alcohol ingestion; do not discontinue medication abruptly; may cause urine to turn blue-green; may cause drowsiness; avoid unnecessary exposure to sunlight; sugarless hard candy or gum can help with dry mouth; full effect may not occur for 4-6 weeks

Nursing Implications
May increase appetite

Monitor blood pressure and pulse rate prior to and during initial therapy; evaluate mental status; monitor weight

Additional Information Less sedation and anticholinergic effects than with amitriptyline or imipramine

Dosage Forms Tablet, as hydrochloride: 10 mg, 25 mg, 50 mg, 75 mg, 100 mg, 150 mg

- ◆ **Desipramine Hydrochloride** *see Desipramine on page 101*
- ◆ **Desmethylimipramine Hydrochloride** *see Desipramine on page 101*
- ◆ **Desoxyephedrine Hydrochloride** *see Methamphetamine on page 230*
- ◆ **Desoxyn®** *see Methamphetamine on page 230*
- ◆ **Desoxyn® Gradumet®** *see Methamphetamine on page 230*
- ◆ **Desoxyphenobarbital** *see Primidone on page 325*
- ◆ **Desyrel®** *see Trazodone on page 408*
- ◆ **Detensol® (Can)** *see Propranolol on page 340*
- ◆ **Dexedrine®** *see Dextroamphetamine on page 105*

Dextroamphetamine (deks troe am FET a meen)
Related Information
Patient Information - Stimulants *on page 481*

Stimulant Agents Used for ADHD *on page 593*

U.S. Brand Names Dexedrine®

Canadian Brand Names Dexedrine

Synonyms Dextroamphetamine Sulfate

Pharmacologic Category Stimulant

Generic Available Yes

Use Narcolepsy; attention-deficit/hyperactivity disorder (ADHD)

Unlabeled/Investigational Use Exogenous obesity; depression; abnormal behavioral syndrome in children (minimal brain dysfunction)

Restrictions C-II

Pregnancy Risk Factor C

Contraindications Hypersensitivity or idiosyncrasy to dextroamphetamine or other sympathomimetic amines. Patients with advanced arteriosclerosis, symptomatic cardiovascular disease, moderate to severe hypertension (stage II or III), hyperthyroidism, glaucoma, diabetes mellitus, agitated states, patients with a history of drug abuse, and during or within 14 days following MAO inhibitor therapy. Stimulant medications are contraindicated for use in children with attention-deficit/hyperactivity disorders and concomitant Tourette's syndrome or tics.

Warnings/Precautions Use with caution in patients with bipolar disorder, cardiovascular disease, seizure disorders, insomnia, porphyria, mild hypertension (stage I), or history of substance abuse. May exacerbate symptoms of behavior and thought disorder in psychotic patients. Stimulants may unmask tics in individuals with coexisting Tourette's syndrome. Potential for drug dependency exists - avoid abrupt discontinuation in patients who have received for prolonged periods. Use in weight reduction programs only when alternative therapy has been ineffective. Products may contain tartrazine - use with caution in potentially sensitive individuals. Stimulant use in children has been associated with growth suppression.

Adverse Reactions
Cardiovascular: Palpitations, tachycardia, hypertension, cardiomyopathy

Central nervous system: Overstimulation, euphoria, dyskinesia, dysphoria, exacerbation of motor and phonic tics, restlessness, insomnia, dizziness, headache, psychosis, Tourette's syndrome

Dermatologic: Rash, urticaria

Endocrine & metabolic: Changes in libido

Gastrointestinal: Diarrhea, constipation, anorexia, weight loss, xerostomia, unpleasant taste

(Continued)

105

Dextroamphetamine *(Continued)*

Genitourinary: Impotence

Neuromuscular & skeletal: Tremor

Overdosage/Toxicology

Signs and symptoms: Restlessness, tremor, confusion, hallucinations, panic, dysrhythmias, nausea, vomiting

Treatment:

There is no specific antidote for dextroamphetamine intoxication and the bulk of the treatment is supportive

Hyperactivity and agitation usually respond to reduced sensory input; however, with extreme agitation, haloperidol (2-5 mg I.M. for adults) may be required

Hyperthermia is best treated with external cooling measures, or when severe or unresponsive, muscle paralysis with pancuronium may be needed

Hypertension is usually transient and generally does not require treatment unless severe. For diastolic blood pressures >110 mm Hg, a nitroprusside infusion should be initiated.

Seizures usually respond to diazepam I.V. and/or phenytoin maintenance regimens

Drug Interactions

Acidifiers: Very large doses of potassium acid phosphate or ammonium chloride may increase the renal elimination of amphetamines due to urinary acidification

Alkalinizers: Large doses of sodium bicarbonate or other alkalinizers may increase renal tubular reabsorption (decreased elimination) and diminish the effect of amphetamine; includes potassium or sodium citrate and acetate

Antipsychotics: Efficacy of amphetamines may be decreased by antipsychotics; in addition, amphetamines may induce an increase in psychotic symptoms in some patients

CYP2D6 inhibitors: Serum levels and/or toxicity of amphetamine may be increased; inhibitors include amiodarone, cimetidine, delavirdine, fluoxetine, paroxetine, propafenone, quinidine, and ritonavir; monitor for increased effect/toxicity

Enzyme inducers: Metabolism of amphetamine may be increased; decreasing clinical effect; inducers include barbiturates, carbamazepine, phenytoin, and rifampin

Furazolidone: Amphetamines may induce hypertensive episodes in patients receiving furazolidone

Guanethidine: Amphetamines inhibit the antihypertensive response to guanethidine; probably also may occur with guanadrel

MAO inhibitors: Severe hypertensive episodes have occurred with amphetamine when used in patients receiving MAO inhibitors; concurrent use or use within 14 days is contraindicated.

Norepinephrine: Amphetamines enhance the pressor response to norepinephrine

Sibutramine: Concurrent use of sibutramine and amphetamines may cause severe hypertension and tachycardia; use is contraindicated with SSRIs; amphetamines may increase the potential for serotonin syndrome when used concurrently with selective serotonin re-uptake inhibitors (including fluoxetine, fluvoxamine, paroxetine, and sertraline)

Tricyclic antidepressants: Concurrent of amphetamines with TCAs may result in hypertension and CNS stimulation; avoid this combination

Ethanol/Nutrition/Herb Interactions

Ethanol: Avoid ethanol (may increase CNS depression).

Food: Dextroamphetamine serum levels may be altered if taken with acidic food, juices, or vitamin C.

Herb/Nutraceutical: Avoid ephedra (may cause hypertension or arrhythmias).

Stability Protect from light

Mechanism of Action Blocks reuptake of dopamine and norepinephrine from the synapse, thus increases the amount of circulating dopamine and norepinephrine in cerebral cortex to reticular activating system; inhibits the action of monoamine oxidase and causes catecholamines to be released. Peripheral actions include elevated blood pressure, weak bronchodilator, and respiratory stimulant action.

Pharmacodynamics/Kinetics
Onset of action: 1-1.5 hours
Metabolism: In the liver
Half-life: Adults: 34 hours (pH dependent)
Time to peak serum concentration: Oral: Within 3 hours
Elimination: In urine as unchanged drug and inactive metabolites after oral dose

Usual Dosage Oral:
Children:
Narcolepsy: 6-12 years: Initial: 5 mg/day; may increase at 5 mg increments in weekly intervals until side effects appear (maximum dose: 60 mg/day)
ADHD:
3-5 years: Initial: 2.5 mg/day given every morning; increase by 2.5 mg/day in weekly intervals until optimal response is obtained; usual range: 0.1-0.5 mg/kg/dose every morning with maximum of 40 mg/day
≥6 years: 5 mg once or twice daily; increase in increments of 5 mg/day at weekly intervals until optimal response is obtained; usual range: 0.1-0.5 mg/kg/dose every morning (5-20 mg/day) with maximum of 40 mg/day
Children >12 years and Adults:
Narcolepsy: Initial: 10 mg/day, may increase at 10 mg increments in weekly intervals until side effects appear; maximum: 60 mg/day
Exogenous obesity (unlabeled use): 5-30 mg/day in divided doses of 5-10 mg 30-60 minutes before meals

Dietary Considerations Should be administered 30 minutes before meals and at least 6 hours before bedtime.

Administration Administer as single dose in morning or as divided doses with breakfast and lunch

Monitoring Parameters Growth in children and CNS activity in all

Patient Information Take during day to avoid insomnia; do not discontinue abruptly, may cause physical and psychological dependence with prolonged use

Nursing Implications Last daily dose should be given 6 hours before retiring; do not crush sustained release drug product

Dosage Forms
Capsule, sustained release, as sulfate: 5 mg, 10 mg, 15 mg
Tablet, as sulfate: 5 mg, 10 mg (5 mg tablets contain tartrazine)

Dextroamphetamine and Amphetamine
(deks troe am FET a meen & am FET a meen)

Related Information
Patient Information - Stimulants *on page 481*
Stimulant Agents Used for ADHD *on page 593*

U.S. Brand Names Adderall®

Synonyms Amphetamine and Dextroamphetamine

Pharmacologic Category Stimulant

Generic Available No

Use Attention-deficit/hyperactivity disorder (ADHD); narcolepsy

Unlabeled/Investigational Use Short-term adjunct to exogenous obesity

Restrictions C-II

Pregnancy Risk Factor C

Pregnancy/Breast-Feeding Implications Use during pregnancy may lead to increased risk of premature delivery and low birth weight. Infants may experience symptoms of withdrawal. Teratogenic effects were reported when taken during the 1st trimester.

Contraindications Hypersensitivity to dextroamphetamine, amphetamine, of any component of the formulation; advanced arteriosclerosis; symptomatic cardiovascular disease; moderate to severe hypertension; hyperthyroidism; hypersensitivity or idiosyncrasy to the sympathomimetic amines; glaucoma; agitated states; (Continued)

Dextroamphetamine and Amphetamine *(Continued)*

patients with a history of drug abuse; during or within 14 days following MAO inhibitor (hypertensive crisis); breast-feeding

Warnings/Precautions Use caution in mildly hypertensive patients; amphetamines may impair the ability to engage in potentially hazardous activities. In psychotic children, amphetamines may exacerbate symptoms of behavior disturbance and thought disorder. Stimulants may unmask tics in individuals with coexisting Tourette's syndrome. Not recommended for children <3 years of age. Avoid abrupt discontinuation.

Adverse Reactions

Cardiovascular: Palpitations, tachycardia, hypertension, cardiomyopathy

Central nervous system: Overstimulation, euphoria, dyskinesia, dysphoria, exacerbation of motor and phonic tics, restlessness, insomnia, dizziness, headache, psychosis, exacerbation of Tourette's syndrome

Dermatologic: Rash, urticaria

Endocrine & metabolic: Changes in libido

Gastrointestinal: Diarrhea, constipation, anorexia, weight loss, xerostomia, unpleasant taste

Genitourinary: Impotence

Neuromuscular & skeletal: Tremor

Overdosage/Toxicology Manifestations of overdose vary widely. Symptoms of central stimulation are usually followed by fatigue and depression. Cardiovascular and gastrointestinal symptoms are also reported. Treatment is symptomatic and supportive. Chlorpromazine may be used to antagonize CNS effects.

Drug Interactions

Acidifiers (urinary): Very large doses of potassium acid phosphate or ammonium chloride may increase the renal elimination of amphetamines due to urinary acidification. Acidification of the urine may increase risk of acute renal failure in the presence of myoglobinuria.

Alkalinizers (urinary): Large doses of sodium bicarbonate or other alkalinizers may increase renal tubular reabsorption (decreased elimination) and potentiate the effect of amphetamine; includes potassium or sodium citrate and acetate

Antihypertensive agents: Amphetamines may antagonize the hypotensive effect.

Antipsychotics: Efficacy of amphetamines may be decreased by antipsychotics; in addition, amphetamines may induce an increase in psychotic symptoms in some patients

CYP2D6 inhibitors: Serum levels and/or toxicity of amphetamine may be increased; inhibitors include amiodarone, cimetidine, delavirdine, fluoxetine, paroxetine, propafenone, quinidine, and ritonavir; monitor for increased effect/toxicity

Enzyme inducers: Metabolism of amphetamine may be increased; decreasing clinical effect; inducers include barbiturates, carbamazepine, phenytoin, and rifampin

Ethosuximide: Absorption of ethosuximide may de delayed.

Furazolidone: Amphetamines may induce hypertensive episodes in patients receiving furazolidone

Guanethidine: Amphetamines inhibit the antihypertensive response to guanethidine; probably also may occur with guanadrel

Haloperidol: Inhibits CNS stimulant effects of amphetamines.

Lithium: Inhibits anorectic and stimulant effects of amphetamines.

MAO inhibitors: Severe hypertensive episodes have occurred with amphetamine when used in patients receiving MAO inhibitors; concurrent use or use within 14 days is contraindicated

Meperidine: Analgesic effects of meperidine may be potentiated.

Norepinephrine: Amphetamines enhance the pressor response to norepinephrine

Phenobarbital: Absorption of phenobarbital may be delayed; may have synergistic anticonvulsant action.

Phenytoin: Absorption of phenytoin may be delayed; may have synergistic anticonvulsant action.

Propoxyphene: Fatal convulsions may occur in cases of propoxyphene overdose.

Sibutramine: Concurrent use of sibutramine and amphetamines may cause severe hypertension and tachycardia; use is contraindicated with SSRIs; amphetamines may increase the potential for serotonin syndrome when used concurrently with selective serotonin reuptake inhibitors (including fluoxetine, fluvoxamine, paroxetine, and sertraline)

SSRIs: Increase sensitivity to amphetamines; amphetamines may increase risk of serotonin syndrome.

Tricyclic antidepressants: Concurrent of amphetamines with TCAs may result in hypertension and CNS stimulation; avoid this combination

Ethanol/Nutrition/Herb Interactions

Ethanol: Avoid ethanol (may increase CNS depression).

Food: Dextroamphetamine serum levels may be altered if taken with acidic food, juices, or vitamin C. Avoid caffeine.

Herb/Nutraceutical: Avoid ephedra (may cause hypertension or arrhythmias).

Stability Store at controlled room temperature of 15°C to 30°C (59°F to 86°F)

Mechanism of Action Blocks reuptake of dopamine and norepinephrine from the synapse, thus increases the amount of circulating dopamine and norepinephrine in cerebral cortex to reticular activating system; inhibits the action of monoamine oxidase and causes catecholamines to be released. Peripheral actions include elevated blood pressure, weak bronchodilator, and respiratory stimulant action.

Pharmacodynamics/Kinetics

Onset: 30-60 minutes

Duration: 4-6 hours

Absorption: Well-absorbed

Distribution: V_d: Adults: 3.5-4.6 L/kg; concentrates in breast milk (avoid breast-feeding); distributes into CNS, mean CSF concentrations are 80% of plasma

Metabolism: In the liver by cytochrome P450 monooxygenase and glucuronidation

Elimination: 70% of a single dose is eliminated within 24 hours; excreted as unchanged amphetamine (30%), benzoic acid, hydroxyamphetamine, hippuric acid, norephedrine, and p-hydroxynorephedrine

Usual Dosage Oral: **Note:** Use lowest effective individualized dose; administer first dose as soon as awake; use intervals of 4-6 hours between additional doses

ADHD:

Children: <3 years: Not recommended

Children: 3-5 years: Initial 2.5 mg/day given every morning; increase daily dose by 2.5 mg at weekly intervals until optimal response is obtained (maximum dose: 40 mg/day given in 1-3 divided doses)

Children: ≥6 years: Initial: 5 mg 1-2 times/day; increase daily dose by 5 mg at weekly intervals until optimal response is obtained (usual maximum dose: 40 mg/day given in 1-3 divided doses)

Narcolepsy:

Children: 6-12 years: Initial: 5 mg/day; increase daily dose by 5 mg at weekly intervals until optimal response is obtained (maximum dose: 60 mg/day given in 1-3 divided doses)

Children >12 years and Adults: Initial: 10 mg/day; increase daily dose by 10 mg at weekly intervals until optimal response is obtained (maximum dose: 60 mg/day given in 1-3 divided doses)

Short-term adjunct to exogenous obesity (unlabeled use): Children >12 years and Adults: 5-30 mg/day in divided doses

Administration Oral: To avoid insomnia, last daily dose should be administered no less than 6 hours before retiring

Monitoring Parameters CNS activity, blood pressure, height, weight

Test Interactions Increased corticosteroid levels (greatest in evening); may interfere with urinary steroid testing

Patient Information May impair ability to perform potentially hazardous activities; do not discontinue abruptly; limit caffeine; avoid alcohol

Additional Information Treatment of ADHD should include "drug holidays" or periodic discontinuation of medication in order to assess the patient's requirments, (Continued)

Dextroamphetamine and Amphetamine *(Continued)*

decrease tolerance, and limit suppression of linear growth and weight; the combination of equal parts of *d*, *l*-amphetamine aspartate, *d*, *l*-amphetamine sulfate, dextroamphetamine saccharate and dextroamphetamine sulfate results in a 75:25 ratio of the dextro- and levo isomers of amphetamine.

The duration of action of Adderall® is longer than methylphenidate; behavioral effects of a single morning dose of Adderall® may last throughout the school day; a single morning dose of Adderall® has been shown in several studies to be as effective as twice daily dosing of methylphenidate for the treatment of ADHD (see Pelham et al, *Pediatrics*, 1999, 104(6):1300-11; Manos 1999, Pliszka 2000).

Dosage Forms
Tablet:
5 mg [dextroamphetamine sulfate 1.25 mg, dextroamphetamine saccharate 1.25 mg and amphetamine aspartate 1.25 mg, amphetamine sulfate 1.25 mg]
7.5 mg [dextroamphetamine sulfate 1.875 mg, dextroamphetamine saccharate 1.875 mg and amphetamine aspartate 1.875 mg, amphetamine sulfate 1.875 mg]
10 mg [dextroamphetamine sulfate 2.5 mg, dextroamphetamine saccharate 2.5 mg and amphetamine aspartate 2.5 mg, amphetamine sulfate 2.5 mg]
12.5 mg [dextroamphetamine sulfate 3.125 mg, dextroamphetamine saccharate 3.125 mg and amphetamine aspartate 3.125 mg, amphetamine sulfate 3.125 mg]
15 mg [dextroamphetamine sulfate 3.75 mg, dextroamphetamine saccharate 3.75 mg and amphetamine aspartate 3.75 mg, amphetamine sulfate 3.75 mg]
20 mg [dextroamphetamine sulfate 5 mg, dextroamphetamine saccharate 5 mg and amphetamine aspartate 5 mg, amphetamine sulfate 5 mg]
30 mg [dextroamphetamine sulfate 7.5 mg, dextroamphetamine saccharate 7.5 mg and amphetamine aspartate 7.5 mg, amphetamine sulfate 7.5 mg]

♦ **Dextroamphetamine Sulfate** *see Dextroamphetamine on page 105*
♦ **Diagnostic and Statistical Manual of Mental Disorders (DSM-IV)** *see page 531*
♦ **Diastat® Rectal Delivery System** *see Diazepam on page 110*
♦ **Diazemuls® (Can)** *see Diazepam on page 110*

Diazepam *(dye AZ e pam)*

Related Information
Anxiolytic/Hypnotic Use in Long-Term Care Facilities *on page 562*
Benzodiazepines Comparison Chart *on page 566*
Federal OBRA Regulations Recommended Maximum Doses *on page 583*
Patient Information - Anxiolytics & Sedative Hypnotics (Benzodiazepines) *on page 483*

U.S. Brand Names Diastat® Rectal Delivery System; Diazepam Intensol®; Valium®
Canadian Brand Names Apo®-Diazepam; Diazemuls®; E Pam®; Meval®; Novo-Dipam®; PMS-Diazepam; Vivol®
Pharmacologic Category Benzodiazepine
Generic Available Yes

Use Management of anxiety disorders, alcohol withdrawal symptoms; skeletal muscle relaxant; treatment of convulsive disorders
Orphan drug: Viscous solution for rectal administration: Management of selected, refractory epilepsy patients on stable regimens of antiepileptic drugs (AEDs) requiring intermittent use of diazepam to control episodes of increased seizure activity

Unlabeled/Investigational Use Panic disorders; preoperative sedation, light anesthesia, amnesia
Restrictions C-IV
Pregnancy Risk Factor D
Pregnancy/Breast-Feeding Implications
Clinical effects on the fetus: Crosses the placenta. Oral clefts reported, however, more recent data does not support an association between drug and oral clefts;

inguinal hernia, cardiac defects, spina bifida, dysmorphic facial features, skeletal defects, multiple other malformations reported; hypotonia and withdrawal symptoms reported following use near time of delivery

Breast-feeding/lactation: Crosses into breast milk

Clinical effects on the infant: Sedation; AAP reports that USE MAY BE OF CONCERN.

Contraindications Hypersensitivity to diazepam or any component of the formulation (cross-sensitivity with other benzodiazepines may exist); narrow-angle glaucoma; not for use in children <6 months of age (oral) or <30 days of age (parenteral); pregnancy

Warnings/Precautions Diazepam has been associated with increasing the frequency of grand mal seizures. Withdrawal has also been associated with an increase in the seizure frequency. Use with caution with drugs which may decrease diazepam metabolism. Use with caution in elderly or debilitated patients, patients with hepatic disease (including alcoholics), or renal impairment. Active metabolites with extended half-lives may lead to delayed accumulation and adverse effects. Use with caution in patients with respiratory disease or impaired gag reflex.

Acute hypotension, muscle weakness, apnea, and cardiac arrest have occurred with parenteral administration. Acute effects may be more prevalent in patients receiving concurrent barbiturates, narcotics, or ethanol. Appropriate resuscitative equipment and qualified personnel should be available during administration and monitoring. Avoid use of the injection in patients with shock, coma, or acute ethanol intoxication. Intra-arterial injection or extravasation of the parenteral formulation should be avoided. Parenteral formulation contains propylene glycol, which has been associated with toxicity when administered in high dosages.

Causes CNS depression (dose-related) resulting in sedation, dizziness, confusion, or ataxia which may impair physical and mental capabilities. Patients must be cautioned about performing tasks which require mental alertness (ie, operating machinery or driving). Use with caution in patients receiving other CNS depressants or psychoactive agents. Effects with other sedative drugs or ethanol may be potentiated. The dosage of narcotics should be reduced by approximately 1/3 when diazepam is added. Benzodiazepines have been associated with falls and traumatic injury and should be used with extreme caution in patients who are at risk of these events (especially the elderly).

Use caution in patients with depression, particularly if suicidal risk may be present. Use with caution in patients with a history of drug dependence. Benzodiazepines have been associated with dependence and acute withdrawal symptoms on discontinuation or reduction in dose. Acute withdrawal, including seizures, may be precipitated in patients after administration of flumazenil to patients receiving long-term benzodiazepine therapy.

Diazepam has been associated with anterograde amnesia. Paradoxical reactions, including hyperactive or aggressive behavior, have been reported with benzodiazepines, particularly in adolescent/pediatric or psychiatric patients. Does not have analgesic, antidepressant, or antipsychotic properties.

Adverse Reactions

Cardiovascular: Hypotension

Central nervous system: Drowsiness, ataxia, amnesia, slurred speech, paradoxical excitement or rage, fatigue, insomnia, memory impairment, headache, anxiety, depression, vertigo, confusion

Dermatologic: Rash

Endocrine & metabolic: Changes in libido

Gastrointestinal: Changes in salivation, constipation, nausea

Genitourinary: Incontinence, urinary retention

Hepatic: Jaundice

Local: Phlebitis, pain with injection

Neuromuscular & skeletal: Dysarthria, tremor

Ocular: Blurred vision, diplopia

(Continued)

Diazepam *(Continued)*

Respiratory: Decrease in respiratory rate, apnea

Overdosage/Toxicology

Signs and symptoms: Somnolence, confusion, coma, hypoactive reflexes, dyspnea, hypotension, slurred speech, impaired coordination

Treatment: Treatment for benzodiazepine overdose is supportive. Rarely is mechanical ventilation required. Flumazenil has been shown to selectively block the binding of benzodiazepines to CNS receptors, resulting in a reversal of benzodiazepine-induced CNS depression, but not respiratory depression.

Drug Interactions CYP2B6, 2C8/9, 2C19, 3A3/4, 3A5-7 enzyme substrate; CYP2C19 and 3A3/4 enzyme inhibitor

CNS depressants: Sedative effects and/or respiratory depression may be additive with CNS depressants; includes ethanol, barbiturates, narcotic analgesics, and other sedative agents; monitor for increased effect

CYP1A2 inhibitors: Metabolism of diazepam may be decreased; increasing clinical effect or toxicity; inhibitors include cimetidine, ciprofloxacin, fluvoxamine, isoniazid, ritonavir, and zileuton.

CYP2C8/9 inhibitors: Serum levels and/or toxicity of diazepam may be increased; inhibitors include amiodarone, cimetidine, fluvoxamine, some NSAIDs, metronidazole, ritonavir, sulfonamides, troglitazone, valproic acid, and zafirlukast; monitor for increased sedation

Enzyme inducers: Metabolism of some benzodiazepines may be increased, decreasing their therapeutic effect; consider using an alternative sedative/hypnotic agent; potential inducers include phenobarbital, phenytoin, carbamazepine, rifampin, and rifabutin

Levodopa: Therapeutic effects may be diminished in some patients following the addition of a benzodiazepine; limited/inconsistent data

Oral contraceptives: May decrease the clearance of some benzodiazepines (those which undergo oxidative metabolism); monitor for increased benzodiazepine effect

Theophylline: May partially antagonize some of the effects of benzodiazepines; monitor for decreased response; may require higher doses for sedation

Ethanol/Nutrition/Herb Interactions

Ethanol: Avoid ethanol (may increase CNS depression).

Food: Diazepam serum levels may be increased if taken with food. Diazepam effect/toxicity may be increased by grapefruit juice; avoid concurrent use.

Herb/Nutraceutical: St John's wort may decrease diazepam levels. Avoid valerian, St John's wort, kava kava, gotu kola (may increase CNS depression).

Stability

Protect parenteral dosage form from light; potency is retained for up to 3 months when kept at room temperature; most stable at pH 4-8, hydrolysis occurs at pH <3; do not mix I.V. product with other medications

Rectal gel: Store at 25°C (77°F); excursion permitted to 15°C to 30°C (59°F to 86°F).

Mechanism of Action Binds to stereospecific benzodiazepine receptors on the postsynaptic GABA neuron at several sites within the central nervous system, including the limbic system, reticular formation. Enhancement of the inhibitory effect of GABA on neuronal excitability results by increased neuronal membrane permeability to chloride ions. This shift in chloride ions results in hyperpolarization (a less excitable state) and stabilization.

Pharmacodynamics/Kinetics

I.V. for status epilepticus:

Onset of action: Almost immediate

Duration: Short, 20-30 minutes

Absorption: Oral: 85% to 100%, more reliable than I.M.

Protein binding: 98%

Metabolism: In the liver

Half-life:
  Parent drug: Adults: 20-50 hours, increased half-life in neonates, elderly, and those with severe hepatic disorders
  Active major metabolite (desmethyldiazepam): 50-100 hours, can be prolonged in neonates

Usual Dosage Oral absorption is more reliable than I.M.

Children:
  Conscious sedation for procedures: Oral: 0.2-0.3 mg/kg (maximum: 10 mg) 45-60 minutes prior to procedure
  Sedation/muscle relaxant/anxiety:
    Oral: 0.12-0.8 mg/kg/day in divided doses every 6-8 hours
    I.M., I.V.: 0.04-0.3 mg/kg/dose every 2-4 hours to a maximum of 0.6 mg/kg within an 8-hour period if needed
  Status epilepticus:
    Infants 30 days to 5 years: I.V.: 0.05-0.3 mg/kg/dose given over 2-3 minutes, every 15-30 minutes to a maximum total dose of 5 mg; repeat in 2-4 hours as needed **or** 0.2-0.5 mg/dose every 2-5 minutes to a maximum total dose of 5 mg
    >5 years: I.V.: 0.05-0.3 mg/kg/dose given over 2-3 minutes every 15-30 minutes to a maximum total dose of 10 mg; repeat in 2-4 hours as needed **or** 1 mg/dose given over 2-3 minutes, every 2-5 minutes to a maximum total dose of 10 mg
    Rectal: 0.5 mg/kg, then 0.25 mg/kg in 10 minutes if needed
  Anticonvulsant (acute treatment): Rectal gel formulation:
    Infants <6 months: Not recommended
    Children <2 years: Safety and efficacy have not been studied
    Children 2-5 years: 0.5 mg/kg
    Children 6-11 years: 0.3 mg/kg
    Children ≥12 years and Adults: 0.2 mg/kg
    Note: Dosage should be rounded upward to the next available dose, 2.5, 5, 10, 15, and 20 mg/dose; dose may be repeated in 4-12 hours if needed; do not use more than 5 times per month or more than once every 5 days
Adolescents: Conscious sedation for procedures:
  Oral: 10 mg
  I.V.: 5 mg, may repeat with ½ dose if needed
Adults:
  Anxiety/sedation/skeletal muscle relaxant:
    Oral: 2-10 mg 2-4 times/day
    I.M., I.V.: 2-10 mg, may repeat in 3-4 hours if needed
  Status epilepticus: I.V.: 5-10 mg every 10-20 minutes, up to 30 mg in an 8-hour period; may repeat in 2-4 hours if necessary
  Rapid tranquilization of agitated patient (administer every 30-60 minutes): Oral: 5-10 mg; average total dose for tranquilization: 20-60 mg
Elderly: Oral: Initial:
  Anxiety: 1-2 mg 1-2 times/day; increase gradually as needed, rarely need to use >10 mg/day (watch for hypotension and excessive sedation)
  Skeletal muscle relaxant: 2-5 mg 2-4 times/day
Hemodialysis: Not dialyzable (0% to 5%); supplemental dose is not necessary
Dosing adjustment in hepatic impairment: Reduce dose by 50% in cirrhosis and avoid in severe/acute liver disease

Administration Intensol® should be diluted before use; diazepam does not have any analgesic effects
  In children, do not exceed 1-2 mg/minute IVP; adults 5 mg/minute

Monitoring Parameters Respiratory, cardiovascular, and mental status; check for orthostasis

Reference Range Therapeutic: Diazepam: 0.2-1.5 µg/mL (SI: 0.7-5.3 µmol/L); N-desmethyldiazepam (nordiazepam): 0.1-0.5 µg/mL (SI: 0.35-1.8 µmol/L)

Test Interactions False-negative urinary glucose determinations when using Clinistix® or Diastix®
(Continued)

Diazepam *(Continued)*

Patient Information Avoid alcohol and other CNS depressants; avoid activities needing good psychomotor coordination until CNS effects are known; drug may cause physical or psychological dependence; avoid abrupt discontinuation after prolonged use

Nursing Implications Provide safety measures (ie, side rails, night light, and call button); supervise ambulation

Additional Information Intensol® should be diluted before use; diazepam does not have any analgesic effects.

Dosage Forms

Gel, rectal delivery system (Diastat®):

Adult rectal tip (6 cm): 5 mg/mL (10 mg, 15 mg, 20 mg) [twin packs]

Pediatric rectal tip (4.4 cm): 5 mg/mL (2.5 mg, 5 mg, 10 mg) [twin packs]

Injection: 5 mg/mL (1 mL, 2 mL, 5 mL, 10 mL)

Solution, oral: 5 mg/5 mL (5 mL, 10 mL, 500 mL) [wintergreen-spice flavor]

Solution, oral concentrate (Diazepam Intensol®): 5 mg/mL (30 mL)

Tablet: 2 mg, 5 mg, 10 mg

- ♦ **Diazepam Intensol®** *see Diazepam on page 110*
- ♦ **Dichloralphenazone, Acetaminophen, and Isometheptene** *see Acetaminophen, Isometheptene, and Dichloralphenazone on page 14*
- ♦ **Dichloralphenazone, Isometheptene, and Acetaminophen** *see Acetaminophen, Isometheptene, and Dichloralphenazone on page 14*
- ♦ **Didrex®** *see Benzphetamine on page 43*

Diethylpropion *(dye eth il PROE pee on)*

Related Information

Phentermine *on page 307*

U.S. Brand Names Tenuate®; Tenuate® Dospan®

Canadian Brand Names Nobesine®

Synonyms Amfepramone; Diethylpropion Hydrochloride

Pharmacologic Category Anorexiant

Generic Available Yes

Use Short-term adjunct in a regimen of weight reduction based on exercise, behavioral modification, and caloric reduction in the management of exogenous obesity for patients with an initial body mass index ≥30 kg/m^2 or ≥27 kg/m^2 in the presence of other risk factors (diabetes, hypertension); see Body Mass Index *on page 569* in the Appendix)

Unlabeled/Investigational Use Migraine

Restrictions C-IV

Pregnancy Risk Factor B

Contraindications Hypersensitivity or idiosyncrasy to sympathomimetic amines. Patients with advanced arteriosclerosis, symptomatic cardiovascular disease, moderate to severe hypertension (stage II or III), hyperthyroidism, glaucoma, agitated states, patients with a history of drug abuse, and during or within 14 days following MAO inhibitor therapy. Concurrent use with other anorectic agents; stimulant medications are contraindicated for use in children with attention-deficit/hyperactivity disorders and concomitant Tourette's syndrome or tics.

Warnings/Precautions Use with caution in patients with bipolar disorder, diabetes mellitus, cardiovascular disease, seizure disorders, insomnia, porphyria, or mild hypertension (stage I). May exacerbate symptoms of behavior and thought disorder in psychotic patients. Stimulants may unmask tics in individuals with coexisting Tourette's syndrome. Potential for drug dependency exists - avoid abrupt discontinuation in patients who have received for prolonged periods. Stimulant use in children has been associated with growth suppression. Not recommended for use in patients <12 years of age.

Adverse Reactions

Cardiovascular: Hypertension, palpitations, tachycardia, chest pain, T-wave changes, arrhythmias, pulmonary hypertension, valvulopathy

Central nervous system: Euphoria, nervousness, insomnia, restlessness, dizziness, anxiety, headache, agitation, confusion, mental depression, psychosis, CVA, seizure

Dermatologic: Alopecia, urticaria, skin rash, ecchymosis, erythema

Endocrine & metabolic: Changes in libido, gynecomastia, menstrual irregularities, porphyria

Gastrointestinal: Nausea, vomiting, abdominal cramps, constipation, xerostomia, metallic taste

Genitourinary: Impotence

Hematologic: Bone marrow depression, agranulocytosis, leukopenia

Neuromuscular & skeletal: Tremor

Ocular: Blurred vision, mydriasis

Overdosage/Toxicology Treatment: There is no specific antidote for amphetamine intoxication and the bulk of the treatment is supportive. Hyperactivity and agitation usually respond to reduced sensory input; however, with extreme agitation, haloperidol (2-5 mg I.M. for adults) may be required. Hyperthermia is best treated with external cooling measures, or when severe or unresponsive, muscle paralysis with pancuronium may be needed. Hypertension is usually transient and generally does not require treatment unless severe. For diastolic blood pressures >110 mm Hg, a nitroprusside infusion should be initiated. Seizures usually respond to diazepam I.V. and/or phenytoin maintenance regimens.

Drug Interactions

Anorectic agents: Concurrent use with other anorectic agents may cause serious cardiac problems and is contraindicated

Furazolidone: May induce a hypertensive episode in patients receiving furazolidone

Guanethidine: Diethylpropion may inhibit the antihypertensive response to guanethidine; probably also may occur with guanadrel

MAO inhibitors: Severe hypertensive episodes have occurred with amphetamine when used in patients receiving MAO inhibitors; concurrent use or use within 14 days is contraindicated

Norepinephrine: Diethylpropion may enhance the pressor response to norepinephrine

Sibutramine: Concurrent use of sibutramine and diethylpropion may cause severe hypertension and tachycardia; use is contraindicated

Tricyclic antidepressants: Concurrent use with tricyclic antidepressants may result in hypertension and CNS stimulation; avoid this combination

Ethanol/Nutrition/Herb Interactions Ethanol: Avoid ethanol (may increase CNS depression).

Mechanism of Action Diethylpropion is used as an anorexiant agent possessing pharmacological and chemical properties similar to those of amphetamines. The mechanism of action of diethylpropion in reducing appetite appears to be secondary to CNS effects, specifically stimulation of the hypothalamus to release catecholamines into the central nervous system; anorexiant effects are mediated via norepinephrine and dopamine metabolism. An increase in physical activity and metabolic effects (inhibition of lipogenesis and enhancement of lipolysis) may also contribute to weight loss.

Usual Dosage Adults: Oral:

Tablet: 25 mg 3 times/day before meals or food

Tablet, controlled release: 75 mg at midmorning

Monitoring Parameters Monitor CNS

Patient Information Avoid alcoholic beverages; take during day to avoid insomnia; do not discontinue abruptly, may cause physical and psychological dependence with prolonged use

Nursing Implications Do not crush 75 mg controlled release tablets; dose should not be given in evening or at bedtime

(Continued)

Diethylpropion *(Continued)*

Dosage Forms
Tablet, as hydrochloride: 25 mg
Tablet, controlled release, as hydrochloride: 75 mg

- **Diethylpropion** *see Phentermine on page 307*
- **Diethylpropion Hydrochloride** *see Diethylpropion on page 114*
- **Dihydrex®** *see Diphenhydramine on page 116*
- **Dihydroergotoxine** *see Ergoloid Mesylates on page 133*
- **Dihydrogenated Ergot Alkaloids** *see Ergoloid Mesylates on page 133*
- **Dilantin®** *see Phenytoin on page 308*
- **Diphenacen-50®** *see Diphenhydramine on page 116*
- **Diphen® Cough [OTC]** *see Diphenhydramine on page 116*
- **Diphenhist [OTC]** *see Diphenhydramine on page 116*

Diphenhydramine *(dye fen HYE dra meen)*

Related Information
Antiparkinsonian Agents Comparison Chart *on page 556*
Anxiolytic/Hypnotic Use in Long-Term Care Facilities *on page 562*
Discontinuation of Psychotropic Drugs - Withdrawal Symptoms and Recommendations *on page 582*
Federal OBRA Regulations Recommended Maximum Doses *on page 583*
Nonbenzodiazepine Anxiolytics and Hypnotics *on page 589*
Patient Information - Agents for Treatment of Extrapyramidal Symptoms *on page 493*

U.S. Brand Names AllerMax® [OTC]; Banophen® [OTC]; Benadryl® [OTC]; Bydramine® Cough Syrup [OTC]; Compoz® Gel Caps [OTC]; Compoz® Nighttime Sleep Aid [OTC]; Dihydrex®; Diphenacen-50®; Diphen® Cough [OTC]; Diphenhist [OTC]; Dormin® [OTC]; Genahist®; Hyrexin-50®; Maximum Strength Nytol® [OTC]; Miles Nervine® [OTC]; Nordryl® [OTC]; Nytol® [OTC]; Siladryl® [OTC]; Silphen® Cough [OTC]; Sleep-eze 3® Oral [OTC]; Sleepinal® [OTC]; Sleepwell 2-nite® [OTC]; Sominex® [OTC]; Tusstat®; Twilite® [OTC]; Uni-Bent® Cough Syrup; 40 Winks® [OTC]

Canadian Brand Names Allerdryl®; Allernix®

Synonyms Diphenhydramine Hydrochloride

Pharmacologic Category Antihistamine; Hypnotic, Miscellaneous

Generic Available Yes

Use Symptomatic relief of allergic symptoms caused by histamine release which include nasal allergies and allergic dermatosis; can be used for mild nighttime sedation; prevention of motion sickness and as an antitussive; has antinauseant and topical anesthetic properties; treatment of antipsychotic-induced extrapyramidal reactions

Pregnancy Risk Factor B

Contraindications Hypersensitivity to diphenhydramine or any component of the formulation; acute asthma; not for use in neonates

Warnings/Precautions Causes sedation, caution must be used in performing tasks which require alertness (ie, operating machinery or driving). Sedative effects of CNS depressants or ethanol are potentiated. Use with caution in patients with angle-closure glaucoma, pyloroduodenal obstruction (including stenotic peptic ulcer), urinary tract obstruction (including bladder neck obstruction and symptomatic prostatic hypertrophy), hyperthyroidism, increased intraocular pressure, and cardiovascular disease (including hypertension and tachycardia). Diphenhydramine has high sedative and anticholinergic properties, so it may not be considered the antihistamine of choice for prolonged use in the elderly. May cause paradoxical excitation in pediatric patients, and can result in hallucinations, coma, and death in overdose. Some preparations contain sodium bisulfite; syrup formulations may contain alcohol.

Adverse Reactions
Cardiovascular: Hypotension, palpitations, tachycardia

Central nervous system: Sedation, sleepiness, dizziness, disturbed coordination, headache, fatigue, nervousness, paradoxical excitement, insomnia, euphoria, confusion

Dermatologic: Photosensitivity, rash, angioedema, urticaria

Gastrointestinal: Nausea, vomiting, diarrhea, abdominal pain, xerostomia, appetite increase, weight gain, dry mucous membranes, anorexia

Genitourinary: Urinary retention, urinary frequency, difficult urination

Hematologic: Hemolytic anemia, thrombocytopenia, agranulocytosis

Neuromuscular & skeletal: Tremor, paresthesia

Ocular: blurred vision

Respiratory: Thickening of bronchial secretions

Overdosage/Toxicology
Signs and symptoms: CNS stimulation or depression; overdose may result in death in infants and children

Treatment: There is no specific treatment for an antihistamine overdose, however, most of its clinical toxicity is due to anticholinergic effects. Anticholinesterase inhibitors (eg, physostigmine, neostigmine, pyridostigmine, or edrophonium) may be useful by reducing acetylcholinesterase. For anticholinergic overdose with severe life-threatening symptoms, physostigmine 1-2 mg (0.5 or 0.02 mg/kg for children) I.V., slowly may be given to reverse these effects.

Drug Interactions CYP2D6 enzyme substrate
Amantadine, rimantadine: Central and/or peripheral anticholinergic syndrome can occur when administered with amantadine or rimantadine

Anticholinergic agents: Central and/or peripheral anticholinergic syndrome can occur when administered with narcotic analgesics, phenothiazines and other antipsychotics (especially with high anticholinergic activity), tricyclic antidepressants, quinidine and some other antiarrhythmics, and antihistamines

Atenolol: Drugs with high anticholinergic activity may increase the bioavailability of atenolol (and possibly other beta-blockers); monitor for increased effect

Cholinergic agents: Drugs with high anticholinergic activity may antagonize the therapeutic effect of cholinergic agents; includes donepezil, rivastigmine, and tacrine

CNS depressants: Sedative effects may be additive with CNS depressants; includes ethanol, benzodiazepines, barbiturates, narcotic analgesics, and other sedative agents; monitor for increased effect

Digoxin: Drugs with high anticholinergic activity may decrease gastric degradation and increase the amount of digoxin absorbed by delaying gastric emptying

Ethanol: Syrup should not be given to patients taking drugs that can cause disulfiram reactions (ie, metronidazole, chlorpropamide) due to high alcohol content

Levodopa: Drugs with high anticholinergic activity may increase gastric degradation and decrease the amount of levodopa absorbed by delaying gastric emptying

Neuroleptics: Drugs with high anticholinergic activity may antagonize the therapeutic effects of neuroleptics

Ethanol/Nutrition/Herb Interactions
Ethanol: Avoid ethanol (may increase CNS depression).

Herb/Nutraceutical: Avoid valerian, St John's wort, kava kava, gotu kola (may increase CNS depression).

Stability Protect from light; the following drugs are **incompatible** with diphenhydramine when mixed in the same syringe: Amobarbital, amphotericin B, cephalothin, diatrizoate, foscarnet, heparin, hydrocortisone, hydroxyzine, pentobarbital, phenobarbital, phenytoin, prochlorperazine, promazine, promethazine, tetracycline, thiopental

Mechanism of Action Competes with histamine for H_1-receptor sites on effector cells in the gastrointestinal tract, blood vessels, and respiratory tract; anticholinergic and sedative effects are also seen

Pharmacodynamics/Kinetics
Maximum sedative effect: 1-3 hours

(Continued)

Diphenhydramine *(Continued)*

Duration of action: 4-7 hours

Absorption: Oral: 40% to 60% reaches systemic circulation due to first-pass metabolism

Metabolism: Extensive in the liver and, to smaller degrees, in the lung and kidney

Half-life: 2-8 hours; elderly: 13.5 hours

Protein binding: 78%

Time to peak serum concentration: 2-4 hours

Usual Dosage

Children:

Oral, I.M., I.V.:

Treatment of moderate to severe allergic reactions: 5 mg/kg/day or 150 mg/m^2/day in divided doses every 6-8 hours, not to exceed 300 mg/day

Minor allergic rhinitis or motion sickness:

2 to <6 years: 6.25 mg every 4-6 hours; maximum: 37.5 mg/day

6 to <12 years: 12.5-25 mg every 4-6 hours; maximum: 150 mg/day

≥12 years: 25-50 mg every 4-6 hours; maximum: 300 mg/day

Night-time sleep aid: 30 minutes before bedtime:

2 to <12 years: 1 mg/kg/dose; maximum: 50 mg/dose

≥12 years: 50 mg

Oral: Antitussive:

2 to <6 years: 6.25 mg every 4 hours; maximum 37.5 mg/day

6 to <12 years: 12.5 mg every 4 hours; maximum 75 mg/day

≥12 years: 25 mg every 4 hours; maximum 150 mg/day

I.M., I.V.: Treatment of dystonic reactions: 0.5-1 mg/kg/dose

Adults:

Oral: 25-50 mg every 6-8 hours

Minor allergic rhinitis or motion sickness: 25-50 mg every 4-6 hours; maximum: 300 mg/day

Moderate to severe allergic reactions: 25-50 mg every 4 hours, not to exceed 400 mg/day

Nighttime sleep aid: 50 mg at bedtime

I.M., I.V.: 10-50 mg in a single dose every 2-4 hours, not to exceed 400 mg/day

Dystonic reaction: 50 mg in a single dose; may repeat in 20-30 minutes if necessary

Topical: For external application, not longer than 7 days

Monitoring Parameters Relief of symptoms, mental alertness

Reference Range

Antihistamine effects at levels >25 ng/mL

Drowsiness at levels 30-40 ng/mL

Mental impairment at levels >60 ng/mL

Therapeutic: Not established

Toxic: >0.1 µg/mL

Test Interactions May suppress the wheal and flare reactions to skin test antigens

Patient Information May cause drowsiness; swallow whole, do not crush or chew sustained release product; avoid alcohol, may impair coordination and judgment

Nursing Implications Raise bed rails, institute safety measures, assist with ambulation

Additional Information Its use as a sleep aid is discouraged due to its anticholinergic effects.

Dosage Forms

Capsule, as hydrochloride: 25 mg, 50 mg

Cream, as hydrochloride: 1%, 2%

Elixir, as hydrochloride: 12.5 mg/5 mL (5 mL, 10 mL, 20 mL, 120 mL, 480 mL, 3780 mL)

Injection, as hydrochloride: 10 mg/mL (10 mL, 30 mL); 50 mg/mL (1 mL, 10 mL)

Liquid, as hydrochloride: 6.25/5 mL

Lotion, as hydrochloride: 1% (75 mL)

Solution, topical, as hydrochloride [spray]: 1% (60 mL), 2%

Syrup, as hydrochloride: 12.5 mg/5 mL (5 mL, 120 mL, 240 mL, 480 mL, 3780 mL)
Tablet, as hydrochloride: 25 mg, 50 mg
Tablet, chewable, as hydrochloride: 12.5 mg

◆ **Diphenhydramine Hydrochloride** *see* Diphenhydramine *on page 116*
◆ **Diphenylhydantoin** *see* Phenytoin *on page 308*
◆ **Dipropylacetic Acid** *see* Valproic Acid and Derivatives *on page 425*
◆ **Discontinuation of Psychotropic Drugs - Withdrawal Symptoms and Recommendations** *see page 582*

Disulfiram (dye SUL fi ram)

Related Information
Addiction Treatments *on page 550*
Patient Information - Miscellaneous Medications *on page 495*

U.S. Brand Names Antabuse®

Canadian Brand Names Antabuse

Pharmacologic Category Aldehyde Dehydrogenase Inhibitor

Generic Available Yes

Use Management of chronic alcoholism

Pregnancy Risk Factor C

Contraindications Hypersensitivity to disulfiram and related compounds or any component of the formulation; patients receiving or using alcohol, metronidazole, paraldehyde, or alcohol-containing preparations like cough syrup or tonics; psychosis; severe myocardial disease and coronary occlusion

Warnings/Precautions Use with caution in patients with diabetes, hypothyroidism, seizure disorders, nephritis (acute or chronic); hepatic cirrhosis or insufficiency; should never be administered to a patient when he/she is in a state of alcohol intoxication, or without his/her knowledge. Patient must receive appropriate counseling, including information on "disguised" forms of alcohol (tonics, mouthwashes, etc) and the duration of the drug's activity (up to 14 days).

Severe (sometimes fatal) hepatitis and/or hepatic failure have been associated with disulfiram. May occur in patients with or without prior history of abnormal hepatic function.

Adverse Reactions
Central nervous system: Drowsiness, headache, fatigue, psychosis
Dermatologic: Rash, acneiform eruptions, allergic dermatitis
Gastrointestinal: Metallic or garlic-like aftertaste
Genitourinary: Impotence
Hepatic: Hepatitis (cholestatic and fulminant), hepatic failure (multiple case reports)
Neuromuscular & skeletal: Peripheral neuritis, polyneuritis, peripheral neuropathy
Ocular: Optic neuritis

Overdosage/Toxicology Treatment: Management of disulfiram reaction: Institute support measures to restore blood pressure (pressors and fluids); monitor for hypokalemia

Drug Interactions CYP2C9 and 2E1 enzyme inhibitor, both disulfiram and diethyldithiocarbamate (disulfiram metabolite) are CYP3A3/4 inhibitors
Benzodiazepines: Disulfiram may increase serum concentrations of benzodiazepines; includes only benzodiazepines which undergo oxidative metabolism (all but oxazepam, lorazepam, temazepam)
Cocaine: Disulfiram may increase serum concentrations of cocaine; avoid concurrent use
Co-trimoxazole: Intravenous trimethoprim-sulfamethoxazole contains 10% ethanol as a solubilizing agent and may interact with disulfiram; monitor for Antabuse® reaction
CYP2C9 substrates: Potentially, disulfiram may inhibit the metabolism of drugs metabolized by this isoenzyme system, increasing the serum levels/effect; use caution
(Continued)

Disulfiram *(Continued)*

CYP3A3/4 substrates: Potentially, disulfiram may inhibit the metabolism of drugs metabolized by this isoenzyme system, increasing the serum levels/effect. Some drugs metabolized by this system have been associated with significant toxicity when dosed with inhibitors (including astemizole, benzodiazepines, cisapride, cyclosporine, erythromycin, and statins). Review potential for this interaction and avoid combination when significant toxicity may result from increased levels.

Diphenhydramine: Syrup contains ethanol, avoid use of syrup; monitor for Antabuse® reaction

Ethanol: Disulfiram results in severe ethanol intolerance (Antabuse® reaction) secondary to disulfiram's ability to inhibit aldehyde dehydrogenase; this combination should be avoided. Pharmaceutical products should be evaluated for possible inclusion of ethanol (ie, elixirs, etc).

Isoniazid: Concurrent use with disulfiram may result in adverse CNS effects; this combination should be avoided

MAO inhibitors: Concurrent use with disulfiram may result in adverse CNS effects; this combination should be avoided

Metronidazole: Concurrent use with disulfiram may result in adverse CNS effects; this combination should be avoided

Omeprazole: May cause CNS adverse effects (limited documentation); monitor

Phenytoin: Disulfiram may increase theophylline serum concentrations; toxicity may occur

Theophylline: Disulfiram may increase theophylline serum concentrations; toxicity may occur

Tricyclic antidepressants: Disulfiram may increase adverse CNS effects; monitor for acute changes in mental status

Warfarin: Disulfiram inhibits the metabolism of warfarin resulting in an increased hypoprothrombinemic response; avoid when possible or monitor INR closely and adjust warfarin dosage

Ethanol/Nutrition/Herb Interactions Ethanol: Disulfiram inhibits ethanol's usual metabolism. Avoid all ethanol. Patients can have a disulfiram reaction (headache, nausea, vomiting, chest, or abdominal pain) if they drink ethanol concurrently. Avoid cough syrups and elixirs containing ethanol. Avoid vinegars, cider, extracts, and foods containing ethanol.

Mechanism of Action Disulfiram is a thiuram derivative which interferes with aldehyde dehydrogenase. When taken concomitantly with alcohol, there is an increase in serum acetaldehyde levels. High acetaldehyde causes uncomfortable symptoms including flushing, nausea, thirst, palpitations, chest pain, vertigo, and hypotension. This reaction is the basis for disulfiram use in postwithdrawal long-term care of alcoholism.

Pharmacodynamics/Kinetics

Absorption: Rapid from GI tract

Full effect: 12 hours

Metabolism: To diethylthiocarbamate

Duration: May persist for 1-2 weeks after last dose

Usual Dosage Adults: Oral: Do not administer until the patient has abstained from alcohol for at least 12 hours

Initial: 500 mg/day as a single dose for 1-2 weeks; maximum daily dose is 500 mg

Average maintenance dose: 250 mg/day; range: 125-500 mg; duration of therapy is to continue until the patient is fully recovered socially and a basis for permanent self control has been established; maintenance therapy may be required for months or even years

Monitoring Parameters Hypokalemia; liver function tests at baseline and after 10-14 days of treatment; CBC, serum chemistries, liver function tests should be monitored during therapy

Patient Information Do not drink any alcohol, including products containing alcohol (such as cough and cold syrups or some mouthwashes), or use alcohol-containing skin products for at least 3 days and preferably 14 days after stopping this medication or while taking this medication; not for treatment of alcohol intoxication; may cause drowsiness; tablets can be crushed or mixed with water

Nursing Implications Administration of any medications containing alcohol including topicals is contraindicated

Dosage Forms Tablet: 250 mg, 500 mg

♦ **Divalproex Sodium** *see* Valproic Acid and Derivatives *on page 425*

♦ **Dixarit® (Can)** *see* Clonidine *on page 88*

♦ ***dl*-Alpha Tocopherol** *see* Vitamin E *on page 433*

♦ **Dolophine®** *see* Methadone *on page 228*

Donepezil (don EH pa zil)

Related Information

Patient Information - Agents for the Treatment of Alzheimer's Disease *on page 491*

U.S. Brand Names Aricept®

Canadian Brand Names Aricept

Synonyms E2020

Pharmacologic Category Acetylcholinesterase Inhibitor (Central)

Generic Available No

Use Treatment of mild to moderate dementia of the Alzheimer's type

Unlabeled/Investigational Use Attention-deficit/hyperactivity disorder (ADHD)

Pregnancy Risk Factor C

Contraindications Hypersensitivity to donepezil, piperidine derivatives, or any component of the formulation

Warnings/Precautions Cholinesterase inhibitors may have vagotonic effects. May cause bradycardia and/or heart block; syncopal episodes have been associated with donepezil. Use with caution in patients with sick sinus syndrome or other supraventricular cardiac conduction abnormalities, in patients with seizures, COPD, or asthma; avoid use in nursing mothers. Use with caution in patients at risk of ulcer disease (ie, previous history or NSAID use), or in patients with bladder outlet obstruction. May cause diarrhea, nausea, and/or vomiting, which may be dose-related.

Adverse Reactions

>10%:

Central nervous system: Headache

Gastrointestinal: Nausea, diarrhea

1% to 10%:

Cardiovascular: Syncope, chest pain, hypertension, atrial fibrillation, hypotension, hot flashes

Central nervous system: Abnormal dreams, depression, dizziness, fatigue, insomnia, somnolence

Dermatologic: Bruising

Gastrointestinal: Anorexia, vomiting, weight loss, fecal incontinence, GI bleeding, bloating, epigastric pain

Genitourinary: Frequent urination

Neuromuscular & skeletal: Muscle cramps, arthritis, body pain

<1%: CHF, delusions, dysarthria, dysphasia, dyspnea, eosinophilia, intracranial hemorrhage, paresthesia, pruritus, thrombocytopenia, tremor

Postmarketing and/or case reports: Abdominal pain, agitation, cholecystitis, confusion, convulsions, hallucinations, heart block, hemolytic anemia, hyponatremia, neuroleptic malignant syndrome, pancreatitis, rash

Overdosage/Toxicology Implement general supportive measures. Donepezil can cause a cholinergic crisis characterized by severe nausea, vomiting, salivation, sweating, bradycardia, hypotension, collapse, and convulsions. Increased muscle weakness is a possibility and may result in death if respiratory muscles are involved.

Tertiary anticholinergics, such as atropine, may be used as an antidote for overdose. I.V. atropine sulfate titrated to effect is recommended with an initial dose of

(Continued)

Donepezil *(Continued)*

1-2 mg I.V., with subsequent doses based upon clinical response. Atypical increases in blood pressure and heart rate have been reported with other cholinomimetics when coadministered with quaternary anticholinergics such as glycopyrrolate.

Drug Interactions CYP2D6 and 3A3/4 enzyme substrate

Anticholinergic agents: Effects of donepezil may be inhibited by anticholinergic agents (benztropine)

Cholinergic agents: A synergistic effect may be seen with concurrent administration of succinylcholine or cholinergic agonists (bethanechol); excessive cholinergic stimulation and toxicity may occur; use caution

CYP2D6 inhibitors: Serum level and/or toxicity of donepezil may be increased; inhibitors include amiodarone, cimetidine, delavirdine, fluoxetine, paroxetine, propafenone, quinidine, and ritonavir; monitor for increased effect/toxicity

CYP3A3/4 inhibitors: Serum level and/or toxicity of donepezil may be increased; inhibitors include amiodarone, cimetidine, clarithromycin, erythromycin, delavirdine, diltiazem, dirithromycin, disulfiram, fluoxetine, fluvoxamine, grapefruit juice, indinavir, itraconazole, ketoconazole, metronidazole, nefazodone, nevirapine, propoxyphene, quinupristin-dalfopristin, ritonavir, saquinavir, verapamil, zafirlukast, zileuton; ketoconazole and quinidine inhibit donepezil's metabolism *in vitro*; monitor for altered clinical response

Enzyme inducers: Inducers of cytochrome P450 enzymes may increase the rate of elimination of donepezil; monitor for altered clinical response; includes phenytoin, carbamazepine, dexamethasone, rifampin, and phenobarbital

Ethanol/Nutrition/Herb Interactions Herb/Nutraceutical: St John's wort may decrease donepezil levels.

Mechanism of Action Alzheimer's disease is characterized by cholinergic deficiency in the cortex and basal forebrain, which contributes to cognitive deficits. Donepezil reversibly and noncompetitively inhibits centrally-active acetylcholinesterase, the enzyme responsible for hydrolysis of acetylcholine. This appears to result in increased concentrations of acetylcholine available for synaptic transmission in the central nervous system.

Pharmacodynamics/Kinetics

Absorption: Well absorbed

Protein binding: 96% mainly to albumin (75%) and alpha$_1$ acid glycoprotein (21%)

Metabolism: By CYP450 isoenzymes 2D6 and 3A4 and undergoes glucuronidation

Bioavailability: 100%

Half-life: 70 hours

Steady-state: 15 days

Time to peak plasma concentration: 3-4 hours

Elimination: Unchanged in urine and extensively metabolized to four major metabolites, two of which are active

Usual Dosage Oral:

Children: ADHD (unlabeled use): 5 mg/day

Adults: Dementia of Alzheimer's type: Initial: 5 mg/day at bedtime; may increase to 10 mg/day at bedtime after 4-6 weeks

Child/Adolescent Considerations Five children (8-17 years of age) with ADHD showed improvement when treated with donepezil.

Monitoring Parameters Behavior, mood, bowel function

Patient Information May be taken with or without food; donepezil is not a cure for Alzheimer's disease, but may slow the progression of symptoms

Additional Information Donepezil does not significantly elevate liver enzymes.

Dosage Forms Tablet: 5 mg, 10 mg

♦ **Dopar**® *see* Levodopa *on page 190*

♦ **Doral**® *see* Quazepam *on page 347*

♦ **Dormin**® [OTC] *see* Diphenhydramine *on page 116*

Doxepin (DOKS e pin)

Related Information

Antidepressant Agents Comparison Chart *on page 553*

Discontinuation of Psychotropic Drugs - Withdrawal Symptoms and Recommendations *on page 582*

Federal OBRA Regulations Recommended Maximum Doses *on page 583*

Patient Information - Antidepressants (TCAs) *on page 454*

Teratogenic Risks of Psychotropic Medications *on page 594*

U.S. Brand Names Sinequan®; Zonalon® Cream

Canadian Brand Names Apo®-Doxepin; Novo-Doxepin®; Triadapin®

Synonyms Doxepin Hydrochloride

Pharmacologic Category Antidepressant, Tricyclic (Tertiary Amine); Topical Skin Product

Generic Available Yes: Oral

Use

Oral: Depression

Topical: Short-term (<8 days) management of moderate pruritus in adults with atopic dermatitis or lichen simplex chronicus

Unlabeled/Investigational Use Analgesic for certain chronic and neuropathic pain; anxiety

Pregnancy Risk Factor C

Contraindications Hypersensitivity to doxepin and drugs from similar chemical class; narrow-angle glaucoma; urinary retention; use of monoamine oxidase inhibitors within 14 days; use in a patient during the acute recovery phase of MI

Warnings/Precautions Often causes sedation, which may result in impaired performance of tasks requiring alertness (ie, operating machinery or driving). Sedative effects may be additive with other CNS depressants and/or ethanol. The degree of sedation is very high relative to other antidepressants. May worsen psychosis in some patients or precipitate a shift to mania or hypomania in patients with bipolar disease. May increase the risks associated with electroconvulsive therapy. This agent should be discontinued, when possible, prior to elective surgery. Therapy should not be abruptly discontinued in patients receiving high doses for prolonged periods.

May cause orthostatic hypotension (risk is moderate relative to other antidepressants) - use with caution in patients at risk of hypotension or in patients where transient hypotensive episodes would be poorly tolerated (cardiovascular disease or cerebrovascular disease). The degree of anticholinergic blockade produced by this agent is high relative to other cyclic antidepressants - use caution in patients with benign prostatic hypertrophy, xerostomia, visual problems, constipation, or history of bowel obstruction.

Use caution in patients with depression, particularly if suicidal risk may be present. Use with caution in patients with a history of cardiovascular disease (including previous MI, stroke, tachycardia, or conduction abnormalities). The risk conduction abnormalities with this agent is moderate relative to other antidepressants. Use caution in patients with a previous seizure disorder or condition predisposing to seizures such as brain damage, alcoholism, or concurrent therapy with other drugs which lower the seizure threshold. Use with caution in hyperthyroid patients or those receiving thyroid supplementation. Use with caution in patients with hepatic or renal dysfunction and in elderly patients. Use in children <12 years of age has not been established.

Adverse Reactions

Cardiovascular: Hypotension, hypertension, tachycardia

Central nervous system: Drowsiness, dizziness, headache, disorientation, ataxia, confusion, seizure

Dermatologic: Alopecia, photosensitivity, rash, pruritus

Endocrine & metabolic: Breast enlargement, galactorrhea, SIADH, increase or decrease in blood sugar, increased or decreased libido

(Continued)

Doxepin (Continued)

Gastrointestinal: Xerostomia, constipation, vomiting, indigestion, anorexia, aphthous stomatitis, nausea, unpleasant taste, weight gain, diarrhea, trouble with gums, decreased lower esophageal sphincter tone may cause GE reflux

Genitourinary: Urinary retention, testicular edema

Hematologic: Agranulocytosis, leukopenia, eosinophilia, thrombocytopenia, purpura

Neuromuscular & skeletal: Weakness, tremors, numbness, paresthesia, extrapyramidal symptoms, tardive dyskinesia

Ocular: Blurred vision

Otic: Tinnitus

Miscellaneous: Diaphoresis (excessive), allergic reactions

Overdosage/Toxicology

Signs and symptoms: Confusion, hallucinations, seizures, urinary retention, hypothermia, hypotension, tachycardia, cyanosis

Treatment:

Following initiation of essential overdose management, toxic symptoms should be treated

Ventricular arrhythmias often respond to systemic alkalinization with or without phenytoin 15-20 mg/kg (adults) (sodium bicarbonate 0.5-2 mEq/kg I.V.). Arrhythmias unresponsive to this therapy may respond to lidocaine 1 mg/kg I.V. followed by a titrated infusion. Physostigmine (1-2 mg I.V. slowly for adults or 0.5 mg I.V. slowly for children) may be indicated in reversing cardiac arrhythmias that are life-threatening,

Seizures usually respond to diazepam I.V. boluses (5-10 mg for adults up to 30 mg or 0.25-0.4 mg/kg/dose for children up to 10 mg/dose). If seizures are unresponsive or recur, phenytoin or phenobarbital may be required.

Drug Interactions CYP2D6 enzyme substrate

Altretamine: Concurrent use may cause orthostatic hypertension

Amphetamines: TCAs may enhance the effect of amphetamines; monitor for adverse CV effects

Anticholinergics: Combined use with TCAs may produce additive anticholinergic effects

Antihypertensives: TCAs may inhibit the antihypertensive response to bethanidine, clonidine, debrisoquin, guanadrel, guanethidine, guanabenz, guanfacine; monitor BP; consider alternate antihypertensive agent

Beta-agonists (nonselective): When combined with TCAs may predispose patients to cardiac arrhythmias

Bupropion: May increase the levels of tricyclic antidepressants; based on limited information; monitor response

Carbamazepine: Tricyclic antidepressants may increase carbamazepine levels; monitor

Cholestyramine and colestipol: May bind TCAs and reduce their absorption; monitor for altered response

Clonidine: Abrupt discontinuation of clonidine may cause hypertensive crisis, amitriptyline may enhance the response

CNS depressants: Sedative effects may be additive with TCAs; monitor for increased effect; includes benzodiazepines, barbiturates, antipsychotics, ethanol and other sedative medications

CYP2D6 inhibitors: Serum levels and/or toxicity of some tricyclic antidepressants may be increased; inhibitors include amiodarone, cimetidine, delavirdine, fluoxetine, paroxetine, propafenone, quinidine, and ritonavir; monitor for increased effect/toxicity

Enzyme inducers: May increase the metabolism of TCAs resulting in decreased effect; includes carbamazepine, phenobarbital, phenytoin, and rifampin; monitor for decreased response

Epinephrine (and other direct alpha-agonists): Pressor response to I.V. epinephrine, norepinephrine, and phenylephrine may be enhanced in patients receiving

TCAs (**Note:** Effect is unlikely with epinephrine or levonordefrin dosages typically administered as infiltration in combination with local anesthetics)

Fenfluramine: May increase tricyclic antidepressant levels/effects

Hypoglycemic agents (including insulin): TCAs may enhance the hypoglycemic effects of tolazamide, chlorpropamide, or insulin; monitor for changes in blood glucose levels; reported with chlorpropamide, tolazamide, and insulin

Levodopa: Tricyclic antidepressants may decrease the absorption (bioavailability) of levodopa; rare hypertensive episodes have also been attributed to this combination

Linezolid: Hyperpyrexia, hypertension, tachycardia, confusion, seizures, and **deaths have been reported** with agents which inhibit MAO (serotonin syndrome); this combination should be avoided

Lithium: Concurrent use with a TCA may increase the risk for neurotoxicity

MAO inhibitors: Hyperpyrexia, hypertension, tachycardia, confusion, seizures, and **deaths have been reported** (serotonin syndrome); this combination should be avoided

Methylphenidate: Metabolism of TCAs may be decreased

Phenothiazines: Serum concentrations of some TCAs may be increased; in addition, TCAs may increase concentration of phenothiazines; monitor for altered clinical response

QT_c-prolonging agents: Concurrent use of tricyclic agents with other drugs which may prolong QT_c interval may increase the risk of potentially fatal arrhythmias; includes type Ia and type III antiarrhythmics agents, selected quinolones (sparfloxacin, gatifloxacin, moxifloxacin, grepafloxacin), cisapride, and other agents

Sucralfate: Absorption of tricyclic antidepressants may be reduced with coadministration

Sympathomimetics, indirect-acting: Tricyclic antidepressants may result in a decreased sensitivity to indirect-acting sympathomimetics; includes dopamine and ephedrine; also see interaction with epinephrine (and direct-acting sympathomimetics)

Tramadol: Tramadol's risk of seizures may be increased with TCAs

Valproic acid: May increase serum concentrations/adverse effects of some tricyclic antidepressants

Warfarin (and other oral anticoagulants): TCAs may increase the anticoagulant effect in patients stabilized on warfarin; monitor INR

Ethanol/Nutrition/Herb Interactions

Ethanol: Avoid ethanol (may increase CNS depression).

Food: Grapefruit juice may inhibit the metabolism of some TCAs and clinical toxicity may result.

Herb/Nutraceutical: Avoid valerian, St John's wort, SAMe, kava kava (may increase risk of serotonin syndrome and/or excessive sedation).

Stability Protect from light

Mechanism of Action Increases the synaptic concentration of serotonin and norepinephrine in the central nervous system by inhibition of their reuptake by the presynaptic neuronal membrane

Pharmacodynamics/Kinetics

Peak effect (antidepressant): Usually more than 2 weeks; anxiolytic effects may occur sooner

Distribution: Crosses the placenta; appears in breast milk

Protein binding: 80% to 85%

Metabolism: Hepatic; metabolites include desmethyldoxepin (active)

Half-life: Adults: 6-8 hours

Elimination: Renal

Usual Dosage Oral (entire daily dose may be given at bedtime):

Depression or anxiety (unlabeled use):

Children: 1-3 mg/kg/day in single or divided doses

Adolescents: Initial: 25-50 mg/day in single or divided doses; gradually increase to 100 mg/day

(Continued)

Doxepin *(Continued)*

Adults: Initial: 30-150 mg/day at bedtime or in 2-3 divided doses; may gradually increase up to 300 mg/day; single dose should not exceed 150 mg; select patients may respond to 25-50 mg/day

Elderly: Use a lower dose and adjust gradually

Dosing adjustment in hepatic impairment: Use a lower dose and adjust gradually

Topical: Adults: Apply a thin film 4 times/day with at least 3- to 4-hour interval between applications. **Note:** Low-dose (25-50 mg) oral administration has also been used to treat pruritus, but systemic effects are increased.

Monitoring Parameters Monitor blood pressure and pulse rate prior to and during initial therapy; monitor mental status, weight; EKG in older adults

Reference Range Therapeutic: 30-150 ng/mL; Toxic: >500 ng/mL; utility of serum level monitoring is controversial

Test Interactions ↑ glucose

Patient Information Avoid unnecessary exposure to sunlight; avoid alcohol ingestion; do not discontinue medication abruptly; may cause urine to turn blue-green; may cause drowsiness; can use sugarless gum or hard candy for dry mouth; full effect may not occur for 4-6 weeks

Nursing Implications May increase appetite; may cause drowsiness, raise bed rails, institute safety precautions

Dosage Forms

Capsule, as hydrochloride (Sinequan®): 10 mg, 25 mg, 50 mg, 75 mg, 100 mg, 150 mg

Cream (Zonalon®): 5% (30 g, 45 g)

Solution, oral concentrate, as hydrochloride (Sinequan®): 10 mg/mL (120 mL)

◆ **Doxepin Hydrochloride** *see Doxepin on page 123*

◆ **DPA** *see Valproic Acid and Derivatives on page 425*

◆ **DPH** *see Phenytoin on page 308*

Droperidol *(droe PER i dole)*

Related Information

Discontinuation of Psychotropic Drugs - Withdrawal Symptoms and Recommendations *on page 582*

Patient Information - Antipsychotics (General) *on page 466*

U.S. Brand Names Inapsine®

Canadian Brand Names Inapsine

Pharmacologic Category Antiemetic

Generic Available Yes

Use Tranquilizer and antiemetic in surgical and diagnostic procedures; preoperative medication; induction and adjunct in the maintenance of general and regional anesthesia; neuroleptanalgesia, in which droperidol is given concurrently with a narcotic analgesic (fentanyl) to aid in producing tranquility and decreasing anxiety and pain

Unlabeled/Investigational Use Agitation in psychiatric emergencies; antiemetic for cancer chemotherapy

Pregnancy Risk Factor C

Pregnancy/Breast-Feeding Implications

Clinical effects on the fetus: Crosses the placenta

Breast-feeding/lactation: No data available

Contraindications Hypersensitivity to droperidol or any component of the formulation

Warnings/Precautions Safety in children <6 months of age has not been established; use with caution in patients with seizures, bone marrow suppression, or severe liver disease

Significant hypotension may occur, especially when the drug is administered parenterally; injection contains benzyl alcohol; injection also contains sulfites which may cause allergic reaction

May be sedating, use with caution in disorders where CNS depression is a feature. Caution in patients with hemodynamic instability, predisposition to seizures, subcortical brain damage, renal or respiratory disease. Esophageal dysmotility and aspiration have been associated with antipsychotic use - use with caution in patients at risk of pneumonia (ie, Alzheimer's disease). Caution in breast cancer or other prolactin-dependent tumors (may elevate prolactin levels). May alter temperature regulation or mask toxicity of other drugs due to antiemetic effects. May alter cardiac conduction - life-threatening arrhythmias have occurred with therapeutic doses of antipsychotics. May cause orthostatic hypotension - use with caution in patients at risk of this effect or those who would tolerate transient hypotensive episodes (cerebrovascular disease, cardiovascular disease, or other medications which may predispose).

May cause anticholinergic effects (confusion, agitation, constipation, dry mouth, blurred vision, urinary retention). Therefore, they should be used with caution in patients with decreased gastrointestinal motility, urinary retention, BPH, xerostomia, or visual problems. Conditions which also may be exacerbated by cholinergic blockade include narrow-angle glaucoma (screening is recommended) and worsening of myasthenia gravis. Relative to other neuroleptics, droperidol has a low potency of cholinergic blockade.

May cause extrapyramidal reactions, including pseudoparkinsonism, acute dystonic reactions, akathisia, and tardive dyskinesia (risk of these reactions is high relative to other neuroleptics). May be associated with neuroleptic malignant syndrome (NMS) or pigmentary retinopathy.

Adverse Reactions EKG changes, retinal pigmentation are more common than with chlorpromazine.

>10%:
Central nervous system: Restlessness, anxiety, extrapyramidal reactions, dystonic reactions, pseudoparkinsonian signs and symptoms, tardive dyskinesia, neuroleptic malignant syndrome (NMS), seizures, altered central temperature regulation, akathisia
Endocrine & metabolic: Swelling of breasts
Gastrointestinal: Weight gain, constipation

1% to 10%:
Cardiovascular: Hypotension (especially orthostatic), tachycardia, arrhythmias, abnormal T waves with prolonged ventricular repolarization
Central nervous system: Hallucinations, sedation, drowsiness, persistent tardive dyskinesia
Gastrointestinal: Nausea, vomiting
Genitourinary: Dysuria

<1%: Tardive dystonia, hyperpigmentation, pruritus, rash, contact dermatitis, alopecia, photosensitivity (rare), amenorrhea, galactorrhea, gynecomastia, sexual dysfunction, adynamic ileus, xerostomia, urinary retention, overflow incontinence, priapism, agranulocytosis, leukopenia (usually with large doses for prolonged periods), cholestatic jaundice, obstructive jaundice, blurred vision, retinal pigmentation, decreased visual acuity (may be irreversible), laryngospasm, respiratory depression, heat stroke

Overdosage/Toxicology
Signs and symptoms: Hypotension, tachycardia, hallucinations, extrapyramidal symptoms
Treatment: Following initiation of essential overdose management, toxic symptom treatment and supportive treatment should be initiated. Hypotension usually responds to I.V. fluids or Trendelenburg positioning. If unresponsive to these measures, the use of a parenteral inotrope may be required (eg, norepinephrine 0.1-0.2 mcg/kg/minute titrated to response). Seizures commonly respond to diazepam (I.V. 5-10 mg bolus in adults every 15 minutes if needed up to a total
(Continued)

Droperidol *(Continued)*

of 30 mg; I.V. 0.25-0.4 mg/kg/dose up to a total of 10 mg in children) or to phenytoin or phenobarbital. Also critical cardiac arrhythmias often respond to I.V. phenytoin (15 mg/kg up to 1 g), while other antiarrhythmics can be used. Neuroleptics often cause extrapyramidal symptoms (eg, dystonic reactions) requiring management with diphenhydramine 1-2 mg/kg (adults) up to a maximum of 50 mg I.M. or I.V. slow push followed by a maintenance dose for 48-72 hours. Alternatively, benztropine mesylate I.V. 1-2 mg (adults) may be effective. These agents are generally effective within 2-5 minutes.

Drug Interactions

CNS depressants: Sedative effects may be additive with other CNS depressants; monitor for increased effect; includes benzodiazepines, barbiturates, antipsychotics, ethanol, and other sedative medications

Cyclobenzaprine: Droperidol and cyclobenzaprine may have an additive effect on prolonging the QT interval; based on limited documentation; monitor

Inhalation anesthetics: Droperidol in combination with certain forms of induction anesthesia may produce peripheral vasodilitation and hypotension

Propofol: An increased incidence of postoperative nausea and vomiting have been reported following coadministration

Stability

Droperidol ampuls/vials should be stored at room temperature and protected from light

Stability of parenteral admixture at room temperature (25°C): 7 days

Standard diluent: 2.5 mg/50 mL D_5W

Incompatible with barbiturates

Mechanism of Action Butyrophenone derivative that produces tranquilization, sedation, and an antiemetic effect; other effects include alpha-adrenergic blockade, peripheral vascular dilation, and reduction of the pressor effect of epinephrine resulting in hypotension and decreased peripheral vascular resistance; may also reduce pulmonary artery pressure

Pharmacodynamics/Kinetics

Following parenteral administration:

Peak effect: Within 30 minutes

Duration: 2-4 hours, may extend to 12 hours

Metabolism: In the liver

Half-life: Adults: 2.3 hours

Elimination: In urine (75%) and feces (22%)

Usual Dosage Titrate carefully to desired effect

Children 2-12 years:

Premedication: I.M.: 0.1-0.15 mg/kg; smaller doses may be sufficient for control of nausea or vomiting

Adjunct to general anesthesia: I.V. induction: 0.088-0.165 mg/kg

Nausea and vomiting: I.M., I.V.: 0.05-0.06 mg/kg/dose every 4-6 hours as needed

Adults:

Premedication: I.M.: 2.5-10 mg 30 minutes to 1 hour preoperatively

Adjunct to general anesthesia: I.V. induction: 0.22-0.275 mg/kg; maintenance: 1.25-2.5 mg/dose

Alone in diagnostic procedures: I.M.: Initial: 2.5-10 mg 30 minutes to 1 hour before; then 1.25-2.5 mg if needed

Nausea and vomiting: I.M., I.V.: 2.5-5 mg/dose every 3-4 hours as needed

Rapid tranquilization of agitated patient (unlabeled use): I.M.: Administered every 30-60 minutes: 2.5-5 mg; average total dose for tranquilization: 5-20 mg

Administration Administer I.M. or I.V.; I.V. should be administered slow IVP (over 2-5 minutes) or IVPB

Monitoring Parameters Blood pressure, heart rate, respiratory rate; observe for dystonias, extrapyramidal side effects, and temperature changes

Patient Information Avoid alcoholic beverages

Nursing Implications
Parenteral: I.V. over 2-5 minutes
Monitor blood pressure, heart rate, respiratory rate
Additional Information Does not possess analgesic effects; has little or no amnesic properties.
Dosage Forms Injection: 2.5 mg/mL (1 mL, 2 mL, 5 mL, 10 mL)

♦ **Duraclon™** *see* Clonidine *on page 88*
♦ **Duralith® (Can)** *see* Lithium *on page 205*
♦ **E2020** *see* Donepezil *on page 121*

Echinacea

Synonyms Black Susans; Comb Flower; *Echinacea angustifolia*; Indian Head; Purple Coneflower; Scury Root, American Coneflower; Snakeroot
Pharmacologic Category Herb
Use Prophylaxis and treatment of cold and flu; also used as an immunostimulant in herbal medicine; used to treat minor upper respiratory tract infections, urinary tract infections, wound/skin infections, arthritis, vaginal yeast infections
Contraindications Autoimmune diseases, such as collagen vascular disease (Lupus, RA), multiple sclerosis; allergy to sunflowers, daisies, ragweed; tuberculosis, HIV, AIDS, pregnancy, breast-feeding; parenteral administration only contraindicated per Commission E; oral use of Echinacea not contraindicated during pregnancy by Commission E
Adverse Reactions May become immunosuppressive with continuous use over 6-8 weeks
Gastrointestinal: Tingling sensation of tongue
Miscellaneous: Allergic reactions (rarely)
Per Commission E: None known for oral and external use
Overdosage/Toxicology Treatment: Supportive therapy; can treat allergic manifestations with an antihistamine
Drug Interactions Theoretically may alter response to immunosuppressive therapy
Usual Dosage Continuous use should not exceed 8 weeks
Per Commission E: Expressed juice (of fresh herb): 6-9 mL/day
Capsule/tablet or tea form: 500 mg to 2 g 3 times/day
Liquid extract: 0.25-1 mL 3 times/day
Tincture: 1-2 mL 3 times/day
May be applied topically
Additional Information Persons allergic to sunflowers may display cross-allergy potential with this herb; a perennial daisy-like flowering plant 2-5 feet high usually found in the midwest and southeastern United States

♦ *Echinacea angustifolia* *see* Echinacea *on page 129*
♦ **E-Complex-600® [OTC]** *see* Vitamin E *on page 433*
♦ **Effexor®** *see* Venlafaxine *on page 430*
♦ **Effexor® XR** *see* Venlafaxine *on page 430*
♦ **Elavil®** *see* Amitriptyline *on page 22*
♦ **Elavil Plus® (Can)** *see* Amitriptyline and Perphenazine *on page 28*
♦ **Eldepryl®** *see* Selegiline *on page 370*
♦ **Eltroxin® (Can)** *see* Levothyroxine *on page 198*
♦ **ENA 713** *see* Rivastigmine *on page 357*
♦ **Endantadine® (Can)** *see* Amantadine *on page 19*
♦ **Endo®-Levodopa/Carbidopa (Can)** *see* Levodopa and Carbidopa *on page 193*
♦ **English Hawthorn** *see* Hawthorn *on page 175*

Entacapone (en TA ka pone)

U.S. Brand Names Comtan®
Pharmacologic Category Anti-Parkinson's Agent (COMT Inhibitor)
Generic Available No
(Continued)

Entacapone *(Continued)*

Use Adjunct to levodopa/carbidopa therapy in patients with idiopathic Parkinson's disease who experience "wearing-off" symptoms at the end of a dosing interval

Pregnancy Risk Factor C

Pregnancy/Breast-Feeding Implications Not recommended

Contraindications Hypersensitivity to entacapone or any of component of the formulation

Warnings/Precautions Patient should not be treated concomitantly with entacapone and a nonselective MAO inhibitor. Orthostatic hypotension may be increased in patients on dopaminergic therapy in Parkinson's disease.

Adverse Reactions

>10%:
    Gastrointestinal: Nausea (14%)
    Neuromuscular & skeletal: Dyskinesia (25%), placebo (15%)

1% to 10%:
    Cardiovascular: Orthostatic hypotension (4%), syncope (1%)
    Central nervous system: Dizziness (8%), fatigue (6%), hallucinations (4%), anxiety (2%), somnolence (2%), agitation (1%)
    Dermatologic: Purpura (2%)
    Gastrointestinal: Diarrhea (10%), abdominal pain (8%), constipation (6%), vomiting (4%), dry mouth (3%), dyspepsia (2%), flatulence (2%), gastritis (1%), taste perversion (1%)
    Genitourinary: Brown-orange urine discoloration (10%)
    Neuromuscular & skeletal: Hyperkinesia (10%), hypokinesia (9%), back pain (4%), weakness (2%)
    Respiratory: Dyspnea (3%)
    Miscellaneous: Increased diaphoresis (2%), bacterial infection (1%)

<1%: Hyperpyrexia and confusion (resembling neuroleptic malignant syndrome), pulmonary fibrosis, rhabdomyolysis, retroperitoneal fibrosis

Note: Approximately 14% of the 603 patients given entacapone in the double-blind, placebo-controlled trials discontinued treatment due to adverse events compared to 9% of the 400 patients who received placebo.

Overdosage/Toxicology There have been no reported cases of intentional or accidental overdose with this drug. COMT inhibition by entacapone treatment is dose-dependent.

Drug Interactions CYP1A2, 2A6, 2C9, 2C19, 2D6, 2E1, and 3A3/4 enzyme inhibitor, but only at high concentrations; not believed to be important clinically. These effects are seen only at concentrations higher than those achieved at recommended dosing.

    Bromocriptine: Fibrotic complications (retroperitoneal or pulmonary fibrosis) have been associated with combinations of entacapone and bromocriptine
    Catecholamines (and other drugs metabolized by COMT): Significant increases in cardiac effects or arrhythmias with drugs metabolized by COMT (eg, alpha-methyldopa, apomorphine, bitolterol, dobutamine, dopamine, epinephrine, isoproterenol, isoetharine, methyldopa, norepinephrine)
    CNS depressants: Effects on mental status may be additive with other CNS depressants; includes barbiturates, benzodiazepines, TCAs, antipsychotics, ethanol, narcotic analgesics, and other sedative-hypnotics
    Iron: Entacapone chelates iron and absorption may be limited; an iron supplement should not be administered at the same time as this agent
    Levodopa: Therapeutic effects may be enhanced by entacapone
    Linezolid: Due to MAO inhibition (see note on MAO inhibitors): this combination should be avoided
    MAO inhibitors: Concurrent use of nonselective MAO inhibitors with entacapone is contraindicated
    Pergolide: Fibrotic complications (retroperitoneal or pulmonary fibrosis) have been associated with combinations of entacapone and pergolide

Selegiline: At low doses of selegiline, a selective MAO type B inhibitor, there does not appear to be an interaction with entacapone

Note: Caution with drugs that interfere with glucuronidation, intestinal, biliary excretion, intestinal beta-glucuronidase (eg, probenecid, cholestyramine, erythromycin, chloramphenicol, rifampicin, ampicillin)

Ethanol/Nutrition/Herb Interactions

Ethanol: Avoid ethanol (may increase CNS adverse effects). ©

Mechanism of Action Entacapone is a reversible and selective inhibitor of catechol-O-methyltransferase (COMT). When entacapone is taken with levodopa, the pharmacokinetics are altered, resulting in more sustained levodopa serum levels compared to levodopa taken alone. The resulting levels of levodopa provide for increased concentrations available for absorption across the blood-brain barrier, thereby providing for increased CNS levels of dopamine, the active metabolite of levodopa.

Pharmacodynamics/Kinetics

Onset of action: Rapid

Peak effect: 1 hour

Absorption: Rapid

Distribution: V_d: 20 L after an I.V. dose at steady-state

Protein binding: 98% mainly to albumin

Metabolism: Isomerization to the cis-isomer, followed by direct glucuronidation of the parent and cis-isomer

Bioavailability: 35%

Half-life: 0.4-0.7 hours based on B-phase; 2.4 hours based on Y-phase

Time to peak serum concentration: 1 hour

Elimination: 10% in urine, 90% in feces

Usual Dosage

Adults: Oral: 200 mg dose, up to a maximum of 8 times/day; maximum daily dose: 1600 mg/day. Always administer with levodopa/carbidopa. To optimize therapy, the levodopa/carbidopa dosage must be reduced, usually by 25%. This reduction is usually necessary when the patient is taking more than 800 mg of levodopa daily.

Dosage adjustment in hepatic impairment: Treat with caution and monitor carefully; AUC and C_{max} can be possibly doubled

Dietary Considerations Can take with or without food.

Administration Always administer in association with levodopa/carbidopa; can be combined with both the immediate and sustained release formulations of levodopa/carbidopa. Can be taken with or without food. Should not be abruptly withdrawn from patient's therapy due to significant worsening of symptoms.

Monitoring Parameters Signs and symptoms of Parkinson's disease; liver function tests, blood pressure, patient's mental status

Patient Information Take only as prescribed; can be taken with or without food. Possible nausea, hallucinations, and change in color of urine (not clinically relevant) may occur. Do not drive a car or operate other complex machinery until there is sufficient experience with entacapone. Do not withdraw medication unless advised by healthcare professional.

Dosage Forms Tablet: 200 mg

♦ **E Pam®️ (Can)** *see Diazepam on page 110*

Ephedra

Synonyms *Ephedra sinica*; Ma-Huang; Mormon Tea; Poptillo; Sea Grape; Squaw Tea

Pharmacologic Category Herb

Use Herbal medicinal uses include treatment for asthma, bronchitis, edema, arthritis, headache, fever, urticaria; also used for weight reduction and for euphoria

Restrictions Limit daily consumption to 120 mg total ephedra alkaloids in 4 equal doses

Pregnancy Risk Factor Contraindicated

(Continued)

Ephedra *(Continued)*

Contraindications Per Commission E: Anxiety, restlessness, hypertension, glaucoma, impaired cerebral circulation, prostate adenoma with residual urine accumulation, pheochromocytoma, thyrotoxicosis

Adverse Reactions

>10%: Central nervous system: Nervousness, restlessness, insomnia

<10%:

Cardiovascular: Hypertension, cardiomyopathy, vasculitis, cardiomegaly, palpitations, vasoconstriction

Central nervous system: CNS-stimulating effects, anxiety, fear, psychosis, tension, agitation, excitation, irritability, auditory and visual hallucinations, sympathetic storm

Gastrointestinal: Nausea, anorexia

Neuromuscular & skeletal: Tremors, weakness

Overdosage/Toxicology

Signs and symptoms: Dysrhythmias, CNS depression, depression, insomnia, dry skin, respiratory depression, vomiting, respiratory alkalosis, seizures, mydriasis

Decontamination: Lavage (within 1 hour)/activated charcoal with cathartic

Treatment: Supportive therapy; there is no specific antidote for ephedrine intoxication and the bulk of the treatment is supportive. Hyperactivity and agitation usually respond to reduced sensory input, however with extreme agitation haloperidol (2-5 mg I.M. for adults) may be required. Hyperthermia is best treated with external cooling measures, or when severe or unresponsive, muscle paralysis with pancuronium may be needed. Hypertension is usually transient and generally does not require treatment unless severe. For diastolic blood pressures >110 mm Hg, a nitroprusside infusion should be initiated. Seizures usually respond to diazepam or lorazepam I.V. and/or phenytoin maintenance regimens.

Drug Interactions

Antihypertensives (including calcium channel blockers and beta-blockers): Effects may be decreased by ephedra; contraindicated

Cardiac glycosides (digoxin): May precipitate arrhythmias; contraindicated

CNS stimulants: Effects/toxicity may be potentiated by ephedra

Guanethidine: Enhancement of sympathomimetic effect by ephedra

Halothane: May precipitate arrhythmias; contraindicated

Linezolid: Effect/toxicity may be enhanced and the sympathomimetic effect of ephedrine is potentiated; avoid concurrent administration

MAO inhibitors: Effect/toxicity may be enhanced and the sympathomimetic effect of ephedrine is potentiated; avoid concurrent administration

Usual Dosage

E. sinica extracts (with 10% alkaloid content): 125-250 mg 3 times/day

As a tea: Steeping 1 heaping teaspoon in 240 mL of boiling water for 10 minutes (equivalent to 15-30 mg of ephedrine)

Per Commission E: Single dose: Herb preparation corresponds to 15-30 mg total alkaloid (calculation as ephedrine)

Patient Information Considered unsafe by the FDA

Additional Information Erect evergreen shrubs growing up to 6 feet in height with rounded flowers blooming in early spring; while the fruits are nearly alkaloid free, the green stems and twigs contain the highest amount of ephedrine and pseudoephedrine; Mormon tea (*Ephedra nevadensis*) contains large amount of tannin, no ephedrine (but possibly t-norpseudoephedrine, a CNS stimulant) and can produce a mild diuresis along with constipation; in fact North and Central American ephedra species lack sympathomimetic alkaloids

♦ **Ephedra sinica** *see* Ephedra *on page 131*

♦ **Epitol**® *see* Carbamazepine *on page 61*

♦ **Epival**® **(Can)** *see* Valproic Acid and Derivatives *on page 425*

♦ **Equanil**® *see* Meprobamate *on page 223*

♦ **Ercaf**® *see* Ergotamine *on page 133*

Ergoloid Mesylates (ER goe loid MES i lates)

U.S. Brand Names Germinal®; Hydergine®; Hydergine® LC

Canadian Brand Names Hydergine

Synonyms Dihydroergotoxine; Dihydrogenated Ergot Alkaloids

Pharmacologic Category Ergot Derivative

Generic Available Yes

Use Treatment of cerebrovascular insufficiency in primary progressive dementia, Alzheimer's dementia, and senile onset

Pregnancy Risk Factor C

Contraindications Hypersensitivity to ergot or any component of the formulation; acute or chronic psychosis; concurrent use of amprenavir, ritonavir, nelfinavir

Adverse Reactions 1% to 10%:

Gastrointestinal: Transient nausea

Miscellaneous: Sublingual irritation

Overdosage/Toxicology

Signs and symptoms: Sinus bradycardia, blurred vision, headache, stomach cramps

Treatment: Chronic overdose usually manifests as signs and symptoms of extremity or organ ischemia; nitroprusside has been shown to reverse the vasoconstriction associated with ergot toxicity

Drug Interactions

Dopamine: Increased toxicity with dopamine

5-HT$_1$ receptor antagonists (sumatriptan): Avoid use within 24 hours (per manufacturer)

Macrolide antibiotics: Erythromycin, clarithromycin, and troleandomycin may increase levels of ergot alkaloids, resulting in toxicity (ischemia, vasospasm)

Propranolol: Rare toxicity (peripheral vasoconstriction) reported; monitor

Ritonavir, amprenavir, and nelfinavir increase blood levels of ergot alkaloids; avoid concurrent use

Sibutramine: May cause serotonin syndrome; avoid concurrent use

SSRIs: Rarely, weakness and incoordination have been noted when used concurrently with 5-HT$_1$ agonists; monitor

Vasoconstrictors: Effects may be increased

Mechanism of Action Ergoloid mesylates do not have the vasoconstrictor effects of the natural ergot alkaloids; exact mechanism in dementia is unknown; originally classed as peripheral and cerebral vasodilator, now considered a "metabolic enhancer"; there is no specific evidence which clearly establishes the mechanism by which ergoloid mesylate preparations produce mental effects, nor is there conclusive evidence that the drug particularly affects cerebral arteriosclerosis or cerebrovascular insufficiency

Usual Dosage Adults: Oral: 1 mg 3 times/day up to 4.5-12 mg/day; up to 6 months of therapy may be necessary

Dietary Considerations Should not eat or drink while tablet dissolves under tongue.

Patient Information Do not chew or crush sublingual tablets, allow to dissolve under tongue

Nursing Implications Monitor blood pressure, heart rate

Dosage Forms

Capsule, liquid (Hydergine® LC): 1 mg

Liquid (Hydergine®): 1 mg/mL (100 mL)

Tablet (Hydergine®): 1 mg

Tablet, sublingual (Gerimal®, Hydergine®): 0.5 mg, 1 mg

♦ **Ergomar**® see Ergotamine on page 133

Ergotamine (er GOT a meen)

U.S. Brand Names Cafatine®; Cafergot®; Ercaf®; Ergomar®; Migranal®; Wigraine®

Canadian Brand Names Ergomar®; Gynergen®

Synonyms Ergotamine Tartrate; Ergotamine Tartrate and Caffeine

(Continued)

Ergotamine *(Continued)*

Pharmacologic Category Ergot Derivative

Generic Available Yes

Use Abort or prevent vascular headaches, such as migraine or cluster

Pregnancy Risk Factor X

Pregnancy/Breast-Feeding Implications Prolonged constriction of the uterine vessels and/or increased myometrial tone may lead to reduced placental blood flow. This has contributed to fetal growth retardation in animals. Excreted in breast milk, breast-feeding is not recommended.

Contraindications Hypersensitivity to ergotamine, caffeine, or any component of the formulation; peripheral vascular disease; hepatic or renal disease; coronary artery disease; hypertension; peptic ulcer disease; sepsis; concurrent use with ritonavir, nelfinavir, and amprenavir; pregnancy

Warnings/Precautions Avoid prolonged administration or excessive dosage because of the danger of ergotism (intense vasoconstriction) and gangrene; patients who take ergotamine for extended periods of time may become dependent on it. May be harmful due to reduction in cerebral blood flow; may precipitate angina, myocardial infarction, or aggravate intermittent claudication; therefore, not considered a drug of choice in the elderly.

Adverse Reactions

>10%:

Cardiovascular: Tachycardia, bradycardia, arterial spasm, claudication and vasoconstriction; rebound headache may occur with sudden withdrawal of the drug in patients on prolonged therapy; localized edema, peripheral vascular effects (numbness and tingling of fingers and toes)

Central nervous system: Drowsiness, dizziness

Gastrointestinal: Nausea, vomiting, diarrhea, xerostomia

1% to 10%:

Cardiovascular: Transient tachycardia or bradycardia

Neuromuscular & skeletal: Weakness in the legs, abdominal or muscle pain, muscle pains in the extremities, paresthesia

<1%: Cyanosis, gangrene, precordial distress, EKG changes, itching, paresthesia, numbness, vertigo

Case reports: Rectal or anal ulcer (suppositories, associated with excessive dose or continual use), retroperitoneal and/or pleuropulmonary fibrosis, thickening of cardiac valves (long-term, continuous use)

Overdosage/Toxicology

Signs and symptoms: Vasospastic effects, nausea, vomiting, lassitude, impaired mental function, hypotension, hypertension, unconsciousness, seizures, shock, and death

Treatment: General supportive therapy, gastric lavage, or induction of emesis, activated charcoal, saline cathartic; keep extremities warm. Activated charcoal is effective at binding certain chemicals, and this is especially true for ergot alkaloids; treatment is symptomatic with heparin, vasodilators (nitroprusside); vasodilators should be used with caution to avoid exaggerating any pre-existing hypotension.

Drug Interactions

5-HT$_1$ receptor antagonists (sumatriptan): Avoid use within 24 hours (per manufacturer)

Macrolide antibiotics: Erythromycin, clarithromycin, and troleandomycin may increase levels of ergot alkaloids, resulting in toxicity (ischemia, vasospasm)

Propranolol: Rare toxicity (peripheral vasoconstriction) reported; monitor

Ritonavir, amprenavir, and nelfinavir increase blood levels of ergot alkaloids; avoid concurrent use

Sibutramine: May cause serotonin syndrome; avoid concurrent use

SSRIs: Rarely, weakness and incoordination have been noted when used concurrently with 5-HT$_1$ agonists; monitor

Vasoconstrictors: Effects may be increased

Ethanol/Nutrition/Herb Interactions Food: Avoid tea, cola, and coffee (caffeine may increase GI absorption of ergotamine).

Mechanism of Action Has partial agonist and/or antagonist activity against tryptaminergic, dopaminergic and alpha-adrenergic receptors depending upon their site; is a highly active uterine stimulant; it causes constriction of peripheral and cranial blood vessels and produces depression of central vasomotor centers

Usual Dosage

Oral:

Cafergot®: 2 tablets at onset of attack; then 1 tablet every 30 minutes as needed; maximum: 6 tablets per attack; do not exceed 10 tablets/week.

Ergostat®: 1 tablet under tongue at first sign, then 1 tablet every 30 minutes, 3 tablets/24 hours, 5 tablets/week

Rectal (Cafergot® suppositories, Wigraine® suppositories, Cafatine® suppositories): 1 at first sign of an attack; follow with second dose after 1 hour, if needed; maximum: 2 per attack; do not exceed 5/week.

Patient Information Take this drug as directed; do not increase dose or use more often than prescribed. If relief is not obtained, contact your prescriber. Avoid caffeine-containing products (eg, tea, coffee, colas, cocoa); caffeine increases GI absorption of ergotamines. May cause drowsiness (avoid activities requiring alertness until effects of medication are known). You may experience mild nausea/ vomiting (you may have an antiemetic prescribed), mild weakness or numbness of extremities (avoid injury). Inspect your extremities for coldness, numbness, or injury. Report immediately extreme numbness, pain, tingling or weakness in extremities (toes, fingers), severe unresolved nausea or vomiting, difficulty breathing or irregular heartbeat.

Nursing Implications Do not crush sublingual drug product

Dosage Forms

Solution, intranasal [spray] (Migranal®): 4 mg/mL (1 mL)

Suppository, rectal (Cafatine®, Cafergot®, Wigraine®): Ergotamine tartrate 2 mg and caffeine 100 mg (12s)

Tablet (Ercaf®, Wigraine®): Ergotamine tartrate 1 mg and caffeine 100 mg

Tablet, sublingual (Ergomar®): Ergotamine tartrate 2 mg

♦ **Ergotamine Tartrate** see Ergotamine on page 133

♦ **Ergotamine Tartrate and Caffeine** see Ergotamine on page 133

♦ **Esgic®** see Butalbital Compound on page 59

♦ **Eskalith®** see Lithium on page 205

♦ **Eskalith CR®** see Lithium on page 205

Estazolam (es TA zoe lam)

Related Information

Anxiolytic/Hypnotic Use in Long-Term Care Facilities on page 562

Benzodiazepines Comparison Chart on page 566

Patient Information - Anxiolytics & Sedative Hypnotics (Benzodiazepines) on page 483

U.S. Brand Names ProSom™

Canadian Brand Names Prosom

Pharmacologic Category Benzodiazepine

Generic Available Yes

Use Short-term management of insomnia

Restrictions C-IV

Pregnancy Risk Factor X

Contraindications Hypersensitivity to estazolam or any component of the formulation (cross-sensitivity with other benzodiazepines may exist); pregnancy

Warnings/Precautions Use with caution in elderly or debilitated patients, patients with hepatic disease (including alcoholics), or renal impairment. Use with caution in patients with respiratory disease or impaired gag reflex. Avoid use in patients with sleep apnea. As a hypnotic, should be used only after evaluation of potential causes of sleep disturbance. Failure of sleep disturbance to resolve after 7-10 (Continued)

Estazolam *(Continued)*

days may indicate psychiatric or medical illness. A worsening of insomnia or the emergence of new abnormalities of thought or behavior may represent unrecognized psychiatric or medical illness and requires immediate and careful evaluation.

Causes CNS depression (dose-related) resulting in sedation, dizziness, confusion, or ataxia which may impair physical and mental capabilities. Patients must be cautioned about performing tasks which require mental alertness (ie, operating machinery or driving). Use with caution in patients receiving other CNS depressants or psychoactive agents. Effects with other sedative drugs or ethanol may be potentiated. Benzodiazepines have been associated with falls and traumatic injury and should be used with extreme caution in patients who are at risk of these events (especially the elderly).

Benzodiazepines have been associated with anterograde amnesia. Paradoxical reactions, including hyperactive or aggressive behavior, have been reported with benzodiazepines, particularly in adolescent/pediatric or psychiatric patients. Does not have analgesic, antidepressant, or antipsychotic properties.

Use caution in patients with depression, particularly if suicidal risk may be present. Use with caution in patients with a history of drug dependence. Benzodiazepines have been associated with dependence and acute withdrawal symptoms on discontinuation or reduction in dose. Acute withdrawal, including seizures, may be precipitated in patients after administration of flumazenil to patients receiving long-term benzodiazepine therapy.

Adverse Reactions

>10%:

Central nervous system: Somnolence

Neuromuscular & skeletal: Weakness

1% to 10%:

Cardiovascular: Flushing, palpitations

Central nervous system: Anxiety, confusion, dizziness, hypokinesia, abnormal coordination, hangover effect, agitation, amnesia, apathy, emotional lability, euphoria, hostility, seizure, sleep disorder, stupor, twitch

Dermatologic: Dermatitis, pruritus, rash, urticaria

Gastrointestinal: Xerostomia, constipation, decreased appetite, flatulence, gastritis, increased appetite, perverse taste

Genitourinary: Frequent urination, menstrual cramps, urinary hesitancy, urinary frequency, vaginal discharge/itching

Neuromuscular & skeletal: Paresthesia

Otic: Photophobia, eye pain, eye swelling

Respiratory: Cough, dyspnea, asthma, rhinitis, sinusitis

Miscellaneous: Diaphoresis

<1%: Allergic reactions, chills, drug dependence, fever, muscle spasm, myalgia, neck pain

Overdosage/Toxicology

Signs and symptoms: Respiratory depression, hypoactive reflexes, unsteady gait, hypotension

Treatment: Supportive; rarely is mechanical ventilation required

Flumazenil has been shown to selectively block the binding of benzodiazepines to CNS receptors, resulting in a reversal of benzodiazepine-induced CNS depression

Drug Interactions CYP3A3/4 enzyme substrate

CNS depressants: Sedative effects and/or respiratory depression may be additive with CNS depressants; includes ethanol, barbiturates, narcotic analgesics, and other sedative agents; monitor for increased effect

Enzyme inducers: Metabolism of some benzodiazepines may be increased, decreasing their therapeutic effect; consider using an alternative sedative/hypnotic agent; potential inducers include phenobarbital, phenytoin, carbamazepine, rifampin, and rifabutin

CYP3A3/4 inhibitors: Serum level and/or toxicity of some benzodiazepines may be increased; inhibitors include amiodarone, cimetidine, clarithromycin, erythromycin, delavirdine, diltiazem, dirithromycin, disulfiram, fluoxetine, fluvoxamine, grapefruit juice, indinavir, itraconazole, ketoconazole, nefazodone, nevirapine, propoxyphene, quinupristin-dalfopristin, ritonavir, saquinavir, verapamil, zafirlukast, zileuton; monitor for altered benzodiazepine response

Levodopa: Therapeutic effects may be diminished in some patients following the addition of a benzodiazepine; limited/inconsistent data

Oral contraceptives: May decrease the clearance of some benzodiazepines (those which undergo oxidative metabolism); monitor for increased benzodiazepine effect

Theophylline: May partially antagonize some of the effects of benzodiazepines; monitor for decreased response; may require higher doses for sedation

Ethanol/Nutrition/Herb Interactions
Ethanol: Avoid ethanol (may increase CNS depression).
Food: Serum levels and/or toxicity may be increased by grapefruit juice.

Mechanism of Action Binds to stereospecific benzodiazepine receptors on the postsynaptic GABA neuron at several sites within the central nervous system, including the limbic system, reticular formation. Enhancement of the inhibitory effect of GABA on neuronal excitability results by increased neuronal membrane permeability to chloride ions. This shift in chloride ions results in hyperpolarization (a less excitable state) and stabilization.

Pharmacodynamics/Kinetics
Studies have shown that the elderly are more sensitive to the effects of benzodiazepines as compared to younger adults
Metabolism: Rapid and extensive in the liver to inactive metabolites
Half-life: 10-24 hours (no significant changes in the elderly)
Peak serum levels: 0.5-1.6 hours
Elimination: <5% excreted unchanged in urine

Usual Dosage Adults: Oral: 1 mg at bedtime, some patients may require 2 mg; start at doses of 0.5 mg in debilitated or small elderly patients

Dosing adjustment in hepatic impairment: May be necessary

Monitoring Parameters Respiratory and cardiovascular status

Patient Information May cause daytime drowsiness, avoid alcohol and drugs with CNS depressant effects; avoid activities needing good psychomotor coordination until CNS effects are known; drug may cause physical or psychological dependence; avoid abrupt discontinuation after prolonged use

Nursing Implications Provide safety measures (ie, side rails, night light, and call button); remove smoking materials from area; supervise ambulation; avoid abrupt discontinuance in patients with prolonged therapy or seizure disorders

Additional Information Abrupt discontinuation after sustained use (generally >10 days) may cause withdrawal symptoms.

Dosage Forms Tablet: 1 mg, 2 mg

Ethchlorvynol (eth klor VI nole)

Related Information
Anxiolytic/Hypnotic Use in Long-Term Care Facilities *on page 562*
Federal OBRA Regulations Recommended Maximum Doses *on page 583*

U.S. Brand Names Placidyl®

Canadian Brand Names Placidyl

Pharmacologic Category Hypnotic, Miscellaneous

Generic Available No

Use Short-term management of insomnia

Restrictions C-IV

Pregnancy Risk Factor C

Contraindications Hypersensitivity to ethchlorvynol or any component of the formulation; porphyria
(Continued)

Ethchlorvynol *(Continued)*

Warnings/Precautions Administer with caution to depressed or suicidal patients or to patients with a history of drug abuse; intoxication symptoms may appear with prolonged daily doses of as little as 1 g; withdrawal symptoms may be seen upon abrupt discontinuation; use with caution in the elderly and in patients with hepatic or renal dysfunction; use with caution in patients who have a history of paradoxical restlessness to barbiturates or alcohol; some products may contain tartrazine

Adverse Reactions

Cardiovascular: Hypotension, syncope

Central nervous system: Dizziness, facial numbness, mild hangover, excitement, ataxia, hysteria, prolonged hypnosis, mild stimulation, giddiness

Dermatologic: Rash, urticaria

Gastrointestinal: Indigestion, nausea, stomach pain, unpleasant aftertaste, vomiting

Hematologic: Thrombocytopenia

Hepatic: Cholestatic jaundice

Neuromuscular & skeletal: Weakness (severe)

Ocular: Blurred vision

Overdosage/Toxicology

Signs and symptoms: Prolonged deep coma, respiratory depression, hypothermia, bradycardia, hypotension, nystagmus

Treatment: Supportive in nature; hemoperfusion may be helpful in enhancing elimination

Drug Interactions

CNS depressants: Sedative effects may be additive with other CNS depressants; monitor for increased effect; includes benzodiazepines, barbiturates, antipsychotics, ethanol, and other sedative medications

Warfarin: May inhibit the hypoprothrombinemic response to warfarin via an unknown mechanism; monitor for altered anticoagulant effect or consider using a benzodiazepine

Ethanol/Nutrition/Herb Interactions

Ethanol: Avoid ethanol (may increase CNS depression).

Herb/Nutraceutical: Avoid valerian, St John's wort, kava kava, gotu kola (may increase CNS depression).

Stability Capsules should not be crushed and should not be refrigerated

Mechanism of Action Unknown; causes nonspecific depression of the reticular activating system

Pharmacodynamics/Kinetics

Onset of action: 15-60 minutes

Duration: 5 hours

Absorption: Rapid from GI tract

Metabolism: In the liver

Half-life: 10-20 hours

Time to peak serum concentration: 2 hours

Usual Dosage Adults: Oral: 500-1000 mg at bedtime

Dosing adjustment in renal impairment: Cl_{cr} <50 mL/minute: Avoid use

Monitoring Parameters Cardiac and respiratory function and abuse potential

Reference Range Therapeutic: 2-9 µg/mL; Toxic: >20 µg/mL

Patient Information May cause drowsiness, can impair judgment and coordination; avoid alcohol and other CNS depressants; ataxia can be reduced if taken with food, do not crush or refrigerate capsules

Nursing Implications Raise bed rails, institute safety measures, assist with ambulation

Dosage Forms Capsule: 200 mg, 500 mg, 750 mg

Ethosuximide *(eth oh SUKS i mide)*

U.S. Brand Names Zarontin®

Canadian Brand Names Zarontin

Pharmacologic Category Anticonvulsant, Succinimide

Generic Available Yes

Use Management of absence (petit mal) seizures

Pregnancy Risk Factor C

Contraindications Hypersensitivity to succinimides or any component of the formulation

Warnings/Precautions Use with caution in patients with hepatic or renal disease; abrupt withdrawal of the drug may precipitate absence status; ethosuximide may increase tonic-clonic seizures in patients with mixed seizure disorders; ethosuximide must be used in combination with other anticonvulsants in patients with both absence and tonic-clonic seizures. Succinimides have been associated with severe blood dyscrasias and cases of systemic lupus erythematosus. Consider evaluation of blood counts in patients with signs/symptoms of infection. Safety and efficacy in patients <3 years of age have not been established.

Adverse Reactions

Central nervous system: Ataxia, drowsiness, sedation, dizziness, lethargy, euphoria, headache, irritability, hyperactivity, fatigue, night terrors, disturbance in sleep, inability to concentrate, aggressiveness, mental depression (with cases of overt suicidal intentions), paranoid psychosis

Dermatologic: Stevens-Johnson syndrome, SLE, rash, hirsutism

Endocrine & metabolic: Increased libido

Gastrointestinal: Weight loss, gastric upset, cramps, epigastric pain, diarrhea, nausea, vomiting, anorexia, abdominal pain, gum hypertrophy, tongue swelling

Genitourinary: Vaginal bleeding, microscopic hematuria

Hematologic: Leukopenia, agranulocytosis, pancytopenia, eosinophilia

Ocular: Myopia

Miscellaneous: Hiccups

Overdosage/Toxicology

Signs and symptoms: Acute overdosage can cause CNS depression, ataxia, stupor, coma, hypotension; chronic overdose can cause skin rash, confusion, ataxia, proteinuria, hepatic dysfunction, hematuria

Treatment: Supportive; hemoperfusion and hemodialysis may be useful

Drug Interactions CYP3A3/4 enzyme substrate; CYP3A3/4 enzyme inducer

CNS depressants: Sedative effects and/or respiratory depression may be additive with CNS depressants; includes ethanol, benzodiazepines, barbiturates, narcotic analgesics, and other sedative agents; monitor for increased effect

CYP3A3/4 inhibitors: Serum level and/or toxicity of ethosuximide may be increased; inhibitors include amiodarone, cimetidine, clarithromycin, erythromycin, delavirdine, diltiazem, dirithromycin, disulfiram, fluoxetine, fluvoxamine, grapefruit juice, indinavir, itraconazole, ketoconazole, nefazodone, nevirapine, propoxyphene, quinupristin-dalfopristin, ritonavir, saquinavir, verapamil, zafirlukast, zileuton; monitor for altered benzodiazepine response

Enzyme inducers: Metabolism of ethosuximide may be increased, decreasing its therapeutic effect; consider using an alternative sedative/hypnotic agent; potential inducers include phenobarbital, phenytoin, carbamazepine, rifampin, and rifabutin

Isoniazid: May inhibit hepatic metabolism of ethosuximide with a resultant increase in ethosuximide serum concentrations

Phenytoin: Ethosuximide may elevate phenytoin levels; phenytoin may decrease ethosuximide levels (see enzyme inducers)

Valproate acid: Has been reported to both increase and decrease ethosuximide levels

Ethanol/Nutrition/Herb Interactions

Ethanol: Avoid ethanol (may increase CNS depression).

Herb/Nutraceutical: St John's wort may decrease ethosuximide levels.

Mechanism of Action Increases the seizure threshold and suppresses paroxysmal spike-and-wave pattern in absence seizures; depresses nerve transmission in the motor cortex

(Continued)

Ethosuximide *(Continued)*

Pharmacodynamics/Kinetics
Time to peak serum concentration:
Capsule: Within 2-4 hours
Syrup: <2-4 hours
Distribution: Adults: V_d: 0.62-0.72 L/kg
Metabolism: ~80% metabolized in the liver to three inactive metabolites
Half-life:
Children: 30 hours
Adults: 50-60 hours
Elimination: Slowly excreted in urine as metabolites (50%) and as unchanged drug (10% to 20%); small amounts excreted in feces

Usual Dosage Oral:
Children 3-6 years: Initial: 250 mg/day (or 15 mg/kg/day) in 2 divided doses; increase every 4-7 days; usual maintenance dose: 15-40 mg/kg/day in 2 divided doses

Children >6 years and Adults: Initial: 250 mg twice daily; increase by 250 mg as needed every 4-7 days, up to 1.5 g/day in 2 divided doses; usual maintenance dose: 20-40 mg/kg/day in 2 divided doses

Dosing comment in renal/hepatic dysfunction: Use with caution.

Dietary Considerations Increase dietary intake of folate; may be administered with food or milk.

Administration Administer with food or milk to avoid GI upset

Monitoring Parameters Seizure frequency, trough serum concentrations; CBC, platelets, liver enzymes, urinalysis

Patient Information Take with food; do not discontinue abruptly; may cause drowsiness and impair judgment

Nursing Implications Monitor CBC, platelets, liver enzymes; observe patient for excess sedation; maintain serum levels; monitor for bruising and bleeding

Dosage Forms
Capsule: 250 mg
Syrup: 250 mg/5 mL (473 mL) [raspberry flavor]

♦ **Etrafon**® *see* Amitriptyline and Perphenazine *on page 28*
♦ **E-Vitamin**® **[OTC]** *see* Vitamin E *on page 433*
♦ **Evoxac**™ *see* Cevimeline *on page 65*
♦ **Exelon**® *see* Rivastigmine *on page 357*
♦ **Eye Balm** *see* Golden Seal *on page 169*
♦ **Eye Root** *see* Golden Seal *on page 169*
♦ **Fastin (Can)** *see* Phentermine *on page 307*
♦ **Featherfew** *see* Feverfew *on page 143*
♦ **Featherfoil** *see* Feverfew *on page 143*
♦ **Federal OBRA Regulations Recommended Maximum Doses** *see page 583*

Felbamate *(FEL ba mate)*

U.S. Brand Names Felbatol®

Pharmacologic Category Anticonvulsant, Miscellaneous

Generic Available No

Use Not as a first-line antiepileptic treatment; only in those patients who respond inadequately to alternative treatments and whose epilepsy is so severe that a substantial risk of aplastic anemia and/or liver failure is deemed acceptable in light of the benefits conferred by its use. Patient must be fully advised of risk and has signed written informed consent. Felbamate can be used as either monotherapy or adjunctive therapy in the treatment of partial seizures (with and without generalization) and in adults with epilepsy.

Orphan drug: Adjunctive therapy in the treatment of partial and generalized seizures associated with Lennox-Gastaut syndrome in children

Pregnancy Risk Factor C

Contraindications Hypersensitivity to felbamate or any component of the formulation; use with caution in those patients who have demonstrated hypersensitivity reactions to other carbamates

Warnings/Precautions Use with caution in patients allergic to other carbamates (eg, meprobamate); antiepileptic drugs should not be suddenly discontinued because of the possibility of increasing seizure frequency; **ten cases of aplastic anemia reported in the U.S. after 2½ to 6 months of therapy**; Carter Wallace and the FDA recommended the use of this agent be suspended unless withdrawal of the product would place a patient at greater risk as compared to the frequently fatal form of anemia

Adverse Reactions

>10%:

Central nervous system: Somnolence, headache, fatigue, dizziness

Gastrointestinal: Nausea, anorexia, vomiting, constipation

1% to 10%:

Cardiovascular: Chest pain, palpitations, tachycardia

Central nervous system: Depression or behavior changes, nervousness, anxiety, ataxia, stupor, malaise, agitation, psychological disturbances, aggressive reaction

Dermatologic: Skin rash, acne, pruritus

Gastrointestinal: Xerostomia, diarrhea, abdominal pain, weight gain, taste perversion

Neuromuscular & skeletal: Tremor, abnormal gait, paresthesia, myalgia

Ocular: Diplopia, abnormal vision

Respiratory: Sinusitis, pharyngitis

Miscellaneous: ALT increase

<1%: Euphoria, hallucinations, leukocytosis, leukopenia, lymphadenopathy, migraine, suicide attempts, thrombocytopenia, urticaria, aplastic anemia

Overdosage/Toxicology

Signs and symptoms: No serious adverse reactions have been reported

Treatment: Symptomatic

Drug Interactions CYP2C19 enzyme inhibitor

Carbamazepine: Felbamate may decrease carbamazepine levels and increase levels of the active metabolite of carbamazepine (10,11-epoxide) resulting in carbamazepine toxicity; monitor for signs of carbamazepine toxicity (dizziness, ataxia, nystagmus, drowsiness)

Enzyme inducers: May decrease serum felbamate concentrations; includes carbamazepine, phenytoin, and rifampin

Gabapentin: May increase serum concentrations of felbamate; monitor for increased effect

Oral contraceptives: Serum levels have been noted to decrease modestly in some patients receiving felbamate; clinical significance in terms of contraceptive failure has not been established

Phenytoin: Felbamate may increase serum concentrations, consider decreasing phenytoin dosage by 25%

Phenobarbital: Felbamate may increase serum concentrations, consider decreasing phenobarbital dosage by 25%

Valproic acid: Felbamate may increase serum concentrations; a decrease in valproic acid dosage may be necessary; monitor for valproic acid toxicity (confusion, irritability, restlessness)

Ethanol/Nutrition/Herb Interactions

Ethanol: Avoid ethanol (may increase CNS depression).

Food: Food does not affect absorption.

Herb/Nutraceutical: Avoid evening primrose (seizure threshold decreased).

Stability Store medication in tightly closed container at room temperature away from excessive heat.

Mechanism of Action Mechanism of action is unknown but has properties in common with other marketed anticonvulsants; has weak inhibitory effects on
(Continued)

Felbamate *(Continued)*

GABA-receptor binding, benzodiazepine receptor binding, and is devoid of activity at the MK-801 receptor binding site of the NMDA receptor-ionophore complex.

Pharmacodynamics/Kinetics

Absorption: Oral: Rapidly and almost completely absorbed after oral administration, food has no effect upon the tablet's absorption

Peak serum concentrations: Within 3 hours

V_d: 0.7-1 L/kg

Protein binding: 22% to 25%

Half-life: 20-23 hours average

Elimination: Cleared renally 40% to 50% as unchanged drug and 40% as inactive metabolites in the urine

Usual Dosage Anticonvulsant:

Monotherapy: Children >14 years and Adults:

Initial: 1200 mg/day in divided doses 3 or 4 times/day; titrate previously untreated patients under close clinical supervision, increasing the dosage in 600 mg increments every 2 weeks to 2400 mg/day based on clinical response and thereafter to 3600 mg/day as clinically indicated

Conversion to monotherapy: Initiate at 1200 mg/day in divided doses 3 or 4 times/day, reduce the dosage of the concomitant anticonvulsant(s) by 20% to 33% at the initiation of felbamate therapy; at week 2, increase the felbamate dosage to 2400 mg/day while reducing the dosage of the other anticonvulsant(s) up to an additional 33% of their original dosage; at week 3, increase the felbamate dosage up to 3600 mg/day and continue to reduce the dosage of the other anticonvulsant(s) as clinically indicated

Adjunctive therapy: Children with Lennox-Gastaut and ages 2-14 years:

Week 1:

Felbamate: 15 mg/kg/day divided 3-4 times/day

Concomitant anticonvulsant(s): Reduce original dosage by 20% to 30%

Week 2:

Felbamate: 30 mg/kg/day divided 3-4 times/day

Concomitant anticonvulsant(s): Reduce original dosage up to an additional 33%

Week 3:

Felbamate: 45 mg/kg/day divided 3-4 times/day

Concomitant anticonvulsant(s): Reduce dosage as clinically indicated

Adjunctive therapy: Children >14 years and Adults:

Week 1:

Felbamate: 1200 mg/day initial dose

Concomitant anticonvulsant(s): Reduce original dosage by 20% to 33%

Week 2:

Felbamate: 2400 mg/day (therapeutic range)

Concomitant anticonvulsant(s): Reduce original dosage by up to an additional 33%

Week 3:

Felbamate: 3600 mg/day (therapeutic range)

Concomitant anticonvulsant(s): Reduce original dosage as clinically indicated

Dietary Considerations May be taken without regard to meals.

Administration Administer on an empty stomach for best absorption.

Monitoring Parameters Monitor serum levels of concomitant anticonvulsant therapy; monitor AST, ALT, and bilirubin weekly. Hematologic evaluations before therapy begins, frequently during therapy, and for a significant period after discontinuation.

Reference Range Not necessary to routinely monitor serum drug levels, since dose should be titrated to clinical response

Patient Information Shake oral suspension well before using

Nursing Implications Monitor serum levels of concomitant anticonvulsant therapy.

Additional Information Monotherapy has not been associated with gingival hyperplasia, impaired concentration, weight gain, or abnormal thinking. Because felbamate is the only drug shown effective in Lennox-Gastaut syndrome, it is considered an orphan drug for this indication.

Dosage Forms
Suspension, oral: 600 mg/5 mL (240 mL, 960 mL)
Tablet: 400 mg, 600 mg

♦ **Felbatol**® *see Felbamate on page 140*

♦ **Femcet**® *see Butalbital Compound on page 59*

Feverfew

Synonyms Altamisa; Bachelor's Buttons; Featherfew; Featherfoil; Nosebleed; *Tanacetum parthenium*; Wild Quinine

Pharmacologic Category Herb

Use Prophylaxis and treatment of migraine headaches; menstrual complaints and fever

Contraindications Pregnancy, breast-feeding; children <2 years of age; allergies to feverfew and other members of the Asteraceae, daisy, ragweed, chamomile

Adverse Reactions
>10%: Gastrointestinal: Mouth ulcerations
<10%:
Dermatologic: Contact dermatitis
Gastrointestinal: Swelling of tongue, lips, abdominal pain, nausea, vomiting, loss of taste
Post-feverfew syndrome: Nervousness, insomnia, stiff joints, headache

Overdosage/Toxicology
Signs and symptoms: Nausea, vomiting, loss of taste, abdominal pain
Decontamination:
Oral: Do **not** induce emesis; dilute with milk or water
Dermal: Wash skin with soap and water
Treatment: Supportive therapy; treat contact dermatitis with diphenhydramine and/ or steroids

Drug Interactions Use with caution in patients taking aspirin or anticoagulants due to increased potential for bleeding

Usual Dosage 125 mg of a preparation standardized to 0.2% parthenolide (250 mcg) once or twice daily

Additional Information Perennial bush which grows up to 3 feet tall with daisy-like yellow or white flowers; leaves are bitter tasting; contraindications in pregnancy and children <2 years of age

♦ **Fiorgen PF**® *see Butalbital Compound on page 59*

♦ **Fioricet**® *see Butalbital Compound on page 59*

♦ **Fiorinal**® **G-1**® *see Butalbital Compound on page 59*

Flumazenil *(FLO may ze nil)*

U.S. Brand Names Romazicon™
Canadian Brand Names Anexate®
Pharmacologic Category Antidote
Generic Available No

Use Benzodiazepine antagonist - reverses sedative effects of benzodiazepines used in general anesthesia; for management of benzodiazepine overdose; flumazenil does **not** antagonize the CNS effects of other GABA agonists (eg, ethanol, barbiturates, or general anesthetics), **does not** reverse narcotics

Pregnancy Risk Factor C

Contraindications Hypersensitivity to flumazenil or benzodiazepines; patients given benzodiazepines for control of potentially life-threatening conditions (eg, control of intracranial pressure or status epilepticus); patients who are showing signs of serious cyclic-antidepressant overdosage

Warnings/Precautions
Risk of seizures = high-risk patients:
Patients on benzodiazepines for long-term sedation
(Continued)

Flumazenil *(Continued)*

Tricyclic antidepressant overdose patients
Concurrent major sedative-hypnotic drug withdrawal
Recent therapy with repeated doses of parenteral benzodiazepines
Myoclonic jerking or seizure activity prior to flumazenil administration

Hypoventilation: Does not reverse respiratory depression/hypoventilation or cardiac depression

Resedation: Occurs more frequently in patients where a large single dose or cumulative dose of a benzodiazepine is administered along with a neuromuscular blocking agent and multiple anesthetic agents

Flumazenil should be used with caution in the intensive care unit because of increased risk of unrecognized benzodiazepine dependence in such settings.

Does **not** antagonize the CNS effects of other GABA agonists (such as ethanol, barbiturates, or general anesthetics), nor does it reverse narcotics

Adverse Reactions
>10%: Gastrointestinal: Vomiting, nausea
1% to 10%:
   Cardiovascular: Palpitations
   Central nervous system: Headache, anxiety, nervousness, insomnia, abnormal crying, euphoria, depression, agitation, dizziness, emotional lability, ataxia, depersonalization, increased tears, dysphoria, paranoia
   Endocrine & metabolic: Hot flashes
   Gastrointestinal: Xerostomia
   Local: Pain at injection site
   Neuromuscular & skeletal: Tremor, weakness, paresthesia
   Ocular: Abnormal vision, blurred vision
   Respiratory: Dyspnea, hyperventilation
   Miscellaneous: Diaphoresis
<1%: Abnormal hearing, altered blood pressure (increases and decreases), anxiety and sensation of coldness, bradycardia, chest pain, generalized convulsions, hiccups, hypertension, shivering, somnolence, tachycardia, thick tongue, ventricular extrasystoles, withdrawal syndrome

Overdosage/Toxicology Treatment: Management of suspected benzodiazepine overdose: 0.2 mg (2 mL) administered I.V. over 30 seconds; if desired level of consciousness is not obtained after 30 seconds, give 0.3 mg (3 mL) over another 30 seconds; further doses of 0.5 mg (5 mL) can be administered over 30 seconds at 1-minute intervals up to a cumulative dose of 3 mg (30 mL); on rare occasions, patients with partial response at 3 mg may require additional titration up to a total dose of 5 mg; if patient has not responded 5 minutes after cumulative dose of 5 mg, the major cause of sedation is likely not due to benzodiazepines.

Drug Interactions Note: Use with caution in overdose involving mixed drug overdose; toxic effects may emerge (especially with cyclic antidepressants) with the reversal of the benzodiazepine effect by flumazenil
Benzodiazepines: Flumazenil may precipitate acute withdrawal reaction, including seizures, in patients who are habituated

Stability For I.V. use only; **compatible** with D_5W, lactated Ringer's, or normal saline; once drawn up in the syringe or mixed with solution use within 24 hours; discard any unused solution after 24 hours

Mechanism of Action Competitively inhibits the activity at the benzodiazepine recognition site on the GABA/benzodiazepine receptor complex. Flumazenil does not antagonize the CNS effect of drugs affecting GABA-ergic neurons by means other than the benzodiazepine receptor (ethanol, barbiturates, general anesthetics) and does not reverse the effects of opioids

Pharmacodynamics/Kinetics
Onset of action: 1-3 minutes; 80% response within 3 minutes
Peak effect: 6-10 minutes

Duration: Resedation occurs usually within 1 hour; duration is related to dose given and benzodiazepine plasma concentrations; reversal effects of flumazenil may wear off before effects of benzodiazepine

Distribution: 0.63-1.06 L/kg

Initial V_d: 0.5 L/kg

V_{dss} 0.77-1.6 L/kg

Protein binding: 40% to 50%

Half-life, adults:

Alpha: 7-15 minutes

Terminal: 41-79 minutes

Elimination: Clearance dependent upon hepatic blood flow; hepatically eliminated, 0.2% unchanged in urine

Usual Dosage Children and Adults: I.V.: See table.

Pediatric Dosage	
Further studies are needed	
Pediatric dosage for **reversal of conscious sedation:** Intravenously through a freely running intravenous infusion into a large vein to minimize pain at the injection site	
Initial dose	0.01 mg/kg over 15 seconds (maximum dose of 0.2 mg)
Repeat doses	0.005-0.01 mg/kg (maximum dose of 0.2 mg) repeated at 1-minute intervals
Maximum total cumulative dose	1 mg
Pediatric dosage for **management of benzodiazepine overdose:** Intravenously through a freely running intravenous infusion into a large vein to minimize pain at the injection site	
Initial dose	0.01 mg/kg (maximum dose: 0.2 mg)
Repeat doses	0.01 mg/kg (maximum dose of 0.2 mg) repeated at 1-minute intervals
Maximum total cumulative dose	1 mg
In place of repeat bolus doses, follow-up continuous infusions of 0.005-0.01 mg/kg/h have been used; further studies are needed.	
Adult Dosage	
Adult dosage for **reversal of conscious sedation:** Intravenously through a freely running intravenous infusion into a large vein to minimize pain at the injection site	
Initial dose	0.2 mg intravenously over 15 seconds
Repeat doses	If desired level of consciousness is not obtained, 0.2 mg may be repeated at 1-minute intervals.
Maximum total cumulative dose	1 mg (usual dose 0.6-1 mg) **In the event of resedation:** Repeat doses may be given at 20-minute intervals with maximum of 1 mg/dose and 3 mg/h.
Adult dosage for **suspected benzodiazepine overdose:** Intravenously through a freely running intravenous infusion into a large vein to minimize pain at the injection site	
Initial dose	0.2 mg intravenously over 30 seconds
Repeat doses	0.5 mg over 30 seconds repeated at 1-minute intervals
Maximum total cumulative dose	3 mg (usual dose 1-3 mg) Patients with a partial response at 3 mg may require additional titration up to a total dose of 5 mg. If a patient has not responded 5 minutes after cumulative dose of 5 mg, the major cause of sedation is not likely due to benzodiazepines. **In the event of resedation:** May repeat doses at 20-minute intervals with maximum of 1 mg/dose and 3 mg/h.

(Continued)

Flumazenil *(Continued)*

Resedation: Repeated doses may be given at 20-minute intervals as needed; repeat treatment doses of 1 mg (at a rate of 0.5 mg/minute) should be given at any time and no more than 3 mg should be given in any hour. After intoxication with high doses of benzodiazepines, the duration of a single dose of flumazenil is not expected to exceed 1 hour; if desired, the period of wakefulness may be prolonged with repeated low intravenous doses of flumazenil, or by an infusion of 0.1-0.4 mg/hour. Most patients with benzodiazepine overdose will respond to a cumulative dose of 1-3 mg and doses >3 mg do not reliably produce additional effects. Rarely, patients with a partial response at 3 mg may require additional titration up to a total dose of 5 mg. **If a patient has not responded 5 minutes after receiving a cumulative dose of 5 mg, the major cause of sedation is not likely to be due to benzodiazepines.**

Elderly: No differences in safety or efficacy have been reported. However, increased sensitivity may occur in some elderly patients.

Dosing in renal impairment: Not significantly affected by renal failure (Cl_{cr} <10 mL/minute) or hemodialysis beginning 1 hour after drug administration

Dosing in hepatic impairment: Initial dose of flumazenil used for initial reversal of benzodiazepine effects is not changed; however, subsequent doses in liver disease patients should be reduced in size or frequency

Monitoring Parameters Monitor patients for return of sedation or respiratory depression

Patient Information Flumazenil does not consistently reverse amnesia; do not engage in activities requiring alertness for 18-24 hours after discharge; resedation may occur in patients on long-acting benzodiazepines (such as diazepam)

Nursing Implications Parenteral: For I.V. use only; administer via freely running I.V. infusion into larger vein to decrease chance of pain, phlebitis

Dosage Forms Injection: 0.1 mg/mL (5 mL, 10 mL)

Fluoxetine *(floo OKS e teen)*

Related Information

Antidepressant Agents Comparison Chart *on page 553*

Discontinuation of Psychotropic Drugs - Withdrawal Symptoms and Recommendations *on page 582*

Patient Information - Antidepressants (SSRIs) *on page 452*

Pharmacokinetics of Selective Serotonin-Reuptake Inhibitors (SSRIs) *on page 590*

Teratogenic Risks of Psychotropic Medications *on page 594*

U.S. Brand Names Prozac®; Prozac® Weekly™; Sarafem™

Canadian Brand Names Prozac

Synonyms Fluoxetine Hydrochloride

Pharmacologic Category Antidepressant, Selective Serotonin Reuptake Inhibitor

Generic Available No (except 20 mg capsule)

Use Treatment of major depression; geriatric depression; treatment of binge-eating and vomiting in patients with moderate-to-severe bulimia nervosa; obsessive-compulsive disorder (OCD); premenstrual dysphoric disorder (PMDD)

Unlabeled/Investigational Use Selective mutism

Pregnancy Risk Factor C

Pregnancy/Breast-Feeding Implications Fluoxetine crosses the placenta

Contraindications Hypersensitivity to fluoxetine or any component of the formulation; patients receiving MAO inhibitors, thioridazine, or mesoridazine currently or within prior 14 days; an MAO inhibitor, thioridazine, or mesoridazine should not be initiated until 5 weeks after the discontinuation of fluoxetine

Warnings/Precautions Potential for severe reaction when used with MAO inhibitors - serotonin syndrome (hyperthermia, muscular rigidity, mental status changes/agitation, autonomic instability) may occur. Fluoxetine may elevate plasma levels of thioridazine and increase the risk of QT_c interval prolongation. This may lead to serious ventricular arrhythmias such as torsade de pointe-type arrhythmias and sudden death. Fluoxetine use has been associated with occurrences of significant rash and allergic events, including vasculitis, lupus-like syndrome, laryngospasm, anaphylactoid reactions, and pulmonary inflammatory disease. May precipitate a shift to mania or hypomania in patients with bipolar disease. May cause insomnia, anxiety, nervousness or anorexia. Use with caution in patients where weight loss is undesirable. May impair cognitive or motor performance - caution operating hazardous machinery or driving. Use caution in patients with depression, particularly if suicidal risk may be present. Use caution in patients with a previous seizure disorder or condition predisposing to seizures such as brain damage, alcoholism, or concurrent therapy with other drugs which lower the seizure threshold. Use with caution in patients with hepatic or renal dysfunction and in elderly patients. May cause hyponatremia/SIADH. May increase the risks associated with electroconvulsive treatment. Use with caution in patients at risk of bleeding or receiving concurrent anticoagulant therapy - may cause impairment in platelet function. May alter glycemic control in patients with diabetes. Due to the long half-life of fluoxetine and its metabolites, the effects and interactions noted may persist for prolonged periods following discontinuation. May cause or exacerbate sexual dysfunction.

Adverse Reactions Predominant adverse effects are CNS and GI

>10%:

Central nervous system: Headache, nervousness (7% to 14%), insomnia (9% to 24%), anxiety, drowsiness

Gastrointestinal: Nausea, diarrhea, xerostomia, anorexia

Neuromuscular & skeletal: Weakness, tremor

1% to 10%:

Cardiovascular: Vasodilation, palpitation, hypertension

Central nervous system: Amnesia, confusion, emotional lability, sleep disorder, dizziness, agitation, yawning, pain, fever, abnormal dreams

Dermatologic: Rash, pruritus

Systemic events, possibly related to vasculitis (including lupus-like syndrome), have occurred rarely in patients with rash; may include lung, kidney, and/or hepatic involvement. Death has been reported.

Endocrine & metabolic: SIADH, hypoglycemia, hyponatremia (elderly or volume-depleted patients)

Gastrointestinal: Dyspepsia, increased appetite, constipation, vomiting, flatulence, weight gain/loss, abdominal pain, dyspepsia

Genitourinary: Sexual dysfunction, urinary frequency

Ocular: Abnormal vision

Respiratory: Pharyngitis

Miscellaneous: Diaphoresis, fever, flu syndrome, infection, abnormal thinking

<1%, postmarketing and/or case reports: Acne, agitation, albuminuria, allergies, alopecia, amenorrhea, anaphylactoid reactions, anemia, angina, aphthous stomatitis, arrhythmia, arthritis, asthma, bone pain, bruising, bursitis, cataract, CHF, chills, cholelithiasis, cholestatic jaundice, colitis, confusion, dehydration, dyskinesia, dysphagia, ecchymosis, edema, eosinophilic pneumonia, epistaxis, erythema nodosum, esophagitis, euphoria, exfoliative dermatitis, extrapyramidal reactions (rare), gastritis, glossitis, gout, gynecomastia, hallucinations, heart arrest, hepatic failure/necrosis, hemorrhage, hiccup, hostility, hypercholesteremia, hyperprolactinemia, hyperventilation, hypoglycemia, hypokalemia, hypotension, hypothyroidism, immune-related hemolytic anemia, kidney failure, laryngospasm, leg cramps, liver function test abnormalities, lupus-like syndrome, malaise, migraine, misuse/abuse, myocardial infarction, neuroleptic malignant syndrome (NMS), optic neuritis, pancreatitis, pancytopenia, photosensitivity reaction, postural hypotension, priapism, pulmonary embolism, pulmonary hypertension, QT prolongation, serotonin syndrome, Stevens-Johnson syndrome, suicidal ideation, syncope, tachycardia, taste perversion, tinnitus, (Continued)

Fluoxetine *(Continued)*

thrombocytopenia, thrombocytopenic purpura, vasculitis, ventricular tachycardia (including torsade de pointes), vomiting

Overdosage/Toxicology Symptoms of overdose include ataxia, sedation, coma, and EKG abnormalities (QT prolongation, torsade de pointes). Respiratory depression may occur, especially with coingestion of alcohol or other drugs. Seizures rarely occur. Treatment is supportive.

Drug Interactions CYP2D6 (minor) and CYP3A3/4 enzyme substrate; CYP2C9 enzyme inducer; CYP1A2 (high dose), 2C9, 2C19, 2D6, and 3A3/4 enzyme inhibitor

Amphetamines: SSRIs may increase the sensitivity to amphetamines, and amphetamines may increase the risk of serotonin syndrome

Benzodiazepines: Fluoxetine may inhibit the metabolism of alprazolam and diazepam resulting in elevated serum levels; monitor for increased sedation and psychomotor impairment

Beta-blockers: Fluoxetine may inhibit the metabolism of metoprolol and propranolol resulting in cardiac toxicity; monitor for bradycardia, hypotension, and heart failure if combination is used; not established for all beta-blockers (unlikely with atenolol or nadolol due to renal elimination)

Buspirone: Fluoxetine inhibits the reuptake of serotonin; combined use with a serotonin agonist (buspirone) may cause serotonin syndrome

Carbamazepine: Fluoxetine may inhibit the metabolism of carbamazepine resulting in increased carbamazepine levels and toxicity; monitor for altered carbamazepine response

Carvedilol: Serum concentrations may be increased; monitor carefully for increased carvedilol effect (hypotension and bradycardia)

Clozapine: Fluoxetine may increase serum levels of clozapine; levels may increase by 76%; monitor for increased effect/toxicity

Cyclosporine: Fluoxetine may increase serum levels of cyclosporine (and possibly tacrolimus); monitor

Cyproheptadine: May inhibit the effects of serotonin reuptake inhibitors (fluoxetine); monitor for altered antidepressant response; cyproheptadine acts as a serotonin agonist

Dextromethorphan: Fluoxetine inhibits the metabolism of dextromethorphan; visual hallucinations occurred in a patient receiving this combination; monitor for serotonin syndrome

Digoxin: Fluoxetine may increase serum levels of digoxin; monitor

Haloperidol: Fluoxetine may inhibit the metabolism of haloperidol and cause extrapyramidal symptoms (EPS); monitor patients for EPS if combination is utilized

HMG-CoA reductase inhibitors: Fluoxetine may inhibit the metabolism of lovastatin and simvastatin resulting in myositis and rhabdomyolysis; these combinations are best avoided

Lithium: Patients receiving fluoxetine and lithium have developed neurotoxicity; if combination is used; monitor for neurotoxicity

Loop diuretics: Fluoxetine may cause hyponatremia; additive hyponatremic effects may be seen with combined use of a loop diuretic (bumetanide, furosemide, torsemide); monitor for hyponatremia

MAO inhibitors: Fluoxetine should not be used with nonselective MAO inhibitors (isocarboxazid, phenelzine); fatal reactions have been reported; wait 5 weeks after stopping fluoxetine before starting an MAO inhibitor and 2 weeks after stopping an MAO inhibitor before starting fluoxetine

Meperidine: Combined use with fluoxetine theoretically may increase the risk of serotonin syndrome

Mesoridazine: Fluoxetine may inhibit the metabolism of mesoridazine, resulting in increased plasma levels and increasing the risk of QT_c interval prolongation. This may lead to serious ventricular arrhythmias, such as torsade de pointe-type arrhythmias and sudden death. Do not use concurrently. Wait at least 5 weeks after discontinuing fluoxetine prior to starting mesoridazine.

Nefazodone: May increase the risk of serotonin syndrome with SSRIs; monitor

Phenytoin: Fluoxetine inhibits the metabolism of phenytoin and may result in phenytoin toxicity; monitor for phenytoin toxicity (ataxia, confusion, dizziness, nystagmus, involuntary muscle movement)

Propafenone: Serum concentrations and/or toxicity may be increased by fluoxetine; avoid concurrent administration

Selegiline: Fluoxetine has been reported to cause mania or hypertension when combined with selegiline; this combination is best avoided. Concurrent use with SSRIs has also been reported to cause serotonin syndrome. As a MAO type-B inhibitor, the risk of serotonin syndrome may be less than with nonselective MAO inhibitors.

Sibutramine: May increase the risk of serotonin syndrome with SSRIs; avoid coadministration

SSRIs: Fluoxetine inhibits the reuptake of serotonin; combined use with other drugs which inhibit the reuptake may cause serotonin syndrome

Sumatriptan (and other serotonin agonists): Concurrent use may result in toxicity; weakness, hyper-reflexia, and incoordination have been observed with sumatriptan and SSRIs. In addition, concurrent use may theoretically increase the risk of serotonin syndrome; includes sumatriptan, naratriptan, rizatriptan, and zolmitriptan.

Sympathomimetics: May increase the risk of serotonin syndrome with SSRIs

Thioridazine: Fluoxetine may inhibit the metabolism of thioridazine, resulting in increased plasma levels and increasing the risk of QT_c interval prolongation. This may lead to serious ventricular arrhythmias, such as torsade de pointe-type arrhythmias and sudden death. Do not use together. Wait at least 5 weeks after discontinuing fluoxetine prior to starting thioridazine.

Tramadol: Fluoxetine combined with tramadol (serotonergic effects) may cause serotonin syndrome; monitor

Trazodone: Fluoxetine may inhibit the metabolism of trazodone resulting in increased toxicity; monitor

Tricyclic antidepressants: Fluoxetine inhibits the metabolism of tricyclic antidepressants (amitriptyline, desipramine, imipramine, nortriptyline) resulting is elevated serum levels; if combination is warranted, a low dose of TCA (10-25 mg/day) should be utilized

Tryptophan: Fluoxetine inhibits the reuptake of serotonin; combination with tryptophan, a serotonin precursor, may cause agitation and restlessness; this combination is best avoided

Valproic acid: Fluoxetine may increase serum levels of valproic acid; monitor

Venlafaxine: Fluoxetine may increase the risk of serotonin syndrome

Warfarin: Fluoxetine may alter the hypoprothrombinemic response to warfarin; monitor

Ethanol/Nutrition/Herb Interactions

Ethanol: Avoid ethanol (may increase CNS depression). Depressed patients should avoid/limit intake.

Herb/Nutraceutical: Avoid valerian, St John's wort, kava kava, gotu kola (may increase CNS depression).

Stability All dosage forms should be stored at controlled room temperature of 15°C to 30°C (50°F to 86°F); oral liquid should be dispensed in a light-resistant container

Mechanism of Action Inhibits CNS neuron serotonin reuptake; minimal or no effect on reuptake of norepinephrine or dopamine; does not significantly bind to alpha-adrenergic, histamine, or cholinergic receptors

Pharmacodynamics/Kinetics

Absorption: Oral: well absorbed; delayed 1-2 hours with weekly formulation

Protein binding: 95%

Metabolism: Hepatic, to norfluoxetine (active; equal to fluoxetine)

Half-life: Adults: 2-3 days for parent drug, 4-16 days for metabolite (norfluoxetine); due to long half-life, resolution of adverse reactions after discontinuation may be slow

Time to peak: Within 4-8 hours

Excretion: In urine as fluoxetine (2.5% to 5%) and norfluoxetine (10%)

(Continued)

Fluoxetine *(Continued)*

Note: Weekly formulation results in greater fluctuations between peak and trough concentrations of fluoxetine and norfluoxetine compared to once-daily dosing (24% daily/164% weekly; 17% daily/43% weekly, respectively). Trough concentrations are 76% lower for fluoxetine and 47% lower for norfluoxetine than the concentrations maintained by 20 mg once-daily dosing. Steady-state fluoxetine concentrations are ~50% lower following the once-weekly regimen compared to 20 mg once daily.

Usual Dosage Oral:

Children: Selective mutism (unlabeled use):

<5 years: No dosing information available

5-18 years: Initial: 5-10 mg/day; titrate upwards as needed (usual maximum dose: 60 mg/day)

Adults: 20 mg/day in the morning; may increase after several weeks by 20 mg/day increments; maximum: 80 mg/day; doses >20 mg should be divided into morning and noon doses. **Note:** Lower doses of 5-10 mg/day have been used for initial treatment.

Usual dosage range:

Bulimia nervosa: 60-80 mg/day

Depression: 20-40 mg/day; patients maintained on Prozac® 20 mg/day may be changed to Prozac® Weekly™ 90 mg/week, starting dose 7 days after the last 20 mg/day dose

Obesity: 20-60 mg/day

OCD: 40-80 mg/day

PMDD (Sarafem™): 20 mg/day

Elderly: Depression: Some patients may require an initial dose of 10 mg/day with dosage increases of 10 and 20 mg every several weeks as tolerated; should not be taken at night unless patient experiences sedation

Dosing adjustment in renal impairment:

Single dose studies: Pharmacokinetics of fluoxetine and norfluoxetine were similar among subjects with all levels of impaired renal function, including anephric patients on chronic hemodialysis

Chronic administration: Additional accumulation of fluoxetine or norfluoxetine may occur in patients with severely impaired renal function

Hemodialysis: Not removed by hemodialysis

Dosing adjustment in hepatic impairment: Elimination half-life of fluoxetine is prolonged in patients with hepatic impairment; a lower or less frequent dose of fluoxetine should be used in these patients

Cirrhosis patients: Administer a lower dose or less frequent dosing interval

Compensated cirrhosis without ascites: Administer 50% of normal dose

Child/Adolescent Considerations A study in children 8-15 years of age with obsessive compulsive disorder (n=14) used a fixed dose of 20 mg/day (Riddle, 1992). A study of children 10-18 years of age with obsessive compulsive symptoms and Tourette's syndrome (n=5) used 20-40 mg/day (Kurlan, 1993). Six children 6-12 years of age with selective mutism were treated with initial doses of 0.2 mg/kg/day for 1 week, then 0.4 mg/kg/day for 1 week, then 0.6 mg/kg/day for 10 weeks (Black, 1994). Twenty-one children (mean age: 8.2 years) with selective mutism received a mean end dose of 28.1 mg (10-60 mg) in a 9 week open trial (Dummit, 1996). Ninety-six outpatients 7-17 years of age with nonpsychotic major depression received 20 mg/day (Emslie, 1997); further studies are needed.

Dietary Considerations May be taken with or without food.

Monitoring Parameters Signs and symptoms of depression, anxiety, sleep

Reference Range Therapeutic levels have not been well established

Therapeutic: Fluoxetine: 100-800 ng/mL (SI: 289-2314 nmol/L); Norfluoxetine: 100-600 ng/mL (SI: 289-1735 nmol/L)

Toxic: Fluoxetine plus norfluoxetine: >2000 ng/mL

Test Interactions Increased albumin in urine

Patient Information Take exactly as directed (do not increase dose or frequency); may take 2-3 weeks to achieve desired results; may cause physical and/or psychological dependence. Take once-a-day dose in the morning to reduce incidence of insomnia. Avoid excessive alcohol, caffeine, and other prescription or OTC medications not approved by prescriber. Maintain adequate hydration (2-3 L/day of fluids unless instructed to restrict fluid intake). You may experience drowsiness, lightheadedness, impaired coordination, dizziness, or blurred vision (use caution when driving or engaging in tasks requiring alertness until response to drug is known); constipation (increased exercise, fluids, or dietary fruit and fiber may help); anorexia (maintain regular dietary intake to avoid excessive weight loss); or postural hypotension (use caution when climbing stairs or changing position from lying or sitting to standing). If diabetic, monitor serum glucose closely (may cause hypoglycemia). Report persistent CNS effects (nervousness, restlessness, insomnia, anxiety, excitation, headache, sedation); rash or skin irritation; muscle cramping, tremors, or change in gait; respiratory depression or difficulty breathing; or worsening of condition.

Nursing Implications Offer patient sugarless hard candy for dry mouth

Additional Information EKG may reveal S-T segment depression; not shown to be teratogenic in rodents; 15-60 mg/day, buspirone and cyproheptadine, may be useful in treatment of sexual dysfunction during treatment with a selective serotonin reuptake inhibitor.

Weekly capsules are a delayed release formulation containing enteric-coated pellets of fluoxetine hydrochloride, equivalent to 90 mg fluoxetine. Therapeutic equivalence of weekly formulation with daily formulation for delaying time to relapse has not been established.

Dosage Forms
Capsule, as hydrochloride:
Prozac®: 10 mg, 20 mg, 40 mg
Sarafem™: 10 mg, 20 mg
Capsule, sustained release, as hydrochloride (Prozac® Weekly™): 90 mg
Solution, oral, as hydrochloride (Prozac®): 20 mg/5 mL (120 mL) [contains 0.23% alcohol] [mint flavor]
Tablet, scored, as hydrochloride (Prozac®): 10 mg

♦ **Fluoxetine Hydrochloride** see Fluoxetine on page 146

Fluphenazine (floo FEN a zeen)

Related Information
Antipsychotic Agents Comparison Chart on page 557
Antipsychotic Medication Guidelines on page 559
Discontinuation of Psychotropic Drugs - Withdrawal Symptoms and Recommendations on page 582
Federal OBRA Regulations Recommended Maximum Doses on page 583
Liquid Compatibility With Antipsychotics and Mood Stabilizers on page 587
Patient Information - Antipsychotics (General) on page 466

U.S. Brand Names Permitil®; Prolixin®; Prolixin Decanoate®; Prolixin Enanthate®

Canadian Brand Names Apo®-Fluphenazine [Hydrochloride]; Modecate® [Fluphenazine Decanoate]; Modecate Enanthate [Fluphenazine Enanthate]; Moditen Hydrochloride; PMS-Fluphenazine [Hydrochloride]

Synonyms Fluphenazine Decanoate; Fluphenazine Enanthate; Fluphenazine Hydrochloride

Pharmacologic Category Antipsychotic Agent, Phenothiazine, Piperazine

Generic Available Yes

Use Management of manifestations of psychotic disorders and schizophrenia; depot formulation may offer improved outcome in individuals with psychosis who are nonadherent with oral antipsychotics

Unlabeled/Investigational Use Pervasive developmental disorder

Pregnancy Risk Factor C
(Continued)

Fluphenazine (Continued)

Contraindications Hypersensitivity to fluphenazine or any component (cross-reactivity between phenothiazines may occur); severe CNS depression; coma; subcortical brain damage; blood dyscrasias; hepatic disease

Warnings/Precautions May be sedating, use with caution in disorders where CNS depression is a feature. Use with caution in Parkinson's disease. Caution in patients with hemodynamic instability; bone marrow suppression; predisposition to seizures; severe cardiac, renal, or respiratory disease. Esophageal dysmotility and aspiration have been associated with antipsychotic use - use with caution in patients at risk of pneumonia (ie, Alzheimer's disease). Caution in breast cancer or other prolactin-dependent tumors (may elevate prolactin levels). May alter temperature regulation or mask toxicity of other drugs due to antiemetic effects. May alter cardiac conduction; life-threatening arrhythmias have occurred with therapeutic doses of phenothiazines. Hypotension may occur, particularly with I.M. administration. May cause orthostatic hypotension - use with caution in patients at risk of this effect or those who would tolerate transient hypotensive episodes (cerebrovascular disease, cardiovascular disease, or other medications which may predispose). Adverse effects of depot injections may be prolonged.

Phenothiazines may cause anticholinergic effects (confusion, agitation, constipation, dry mouth, blurred vision, urinary retention). Therefore, they should be used with caution in patients with decreased gastrointestinal motility, urinary retention, BPH, xerostomia, or visual problems. Conditions which also may be exacerbated by cholinergic blockade include narrow-angle glaucoma (screening is recommended) and worsening of myasthenia gravis. Relative to other antipsychotics, fluphenazine has a low potency of cholinergic blockade.

May cause extrapyramidal reactions, including pseudoparkinsonism, acute dystonic reactions, akathisia and tardive dyskinesia (risk of these reactions is high relative to other antipsychotics). May be associated with neuroleptic malignant syndrome (NMS) or pigmentary retinopathy.

Adverse Reactions

Cardiovascular: Hypotension, tachycardia, fluctuations in blood pressure, hypertension, arrhythmias, edema

Central nervous system: Parkinsonian symptoms, akathisia, dystonias, tardive dyskinesia, dizziness, hyper-reflexia, headache, cerebral edema, drowsiness, lethargy, restlessness, excitement, bizarre dreams, EEG changes, depression, seizures, NMS, altered central temperature regulation

Dermatologic: Increased sensitivity to sun, rash, skin pigmentation, itching, erythema, urticaria, seborrhea, eczema, dermatitis

Endocrine & metabolic: Changes in menstrual cycle, breast pain, amenorrhea, galactorrhea, gynecomastia, changes in libido, elevated prolactin, SIADH

Gastrointestinal: Weight gain, loss of appetite, salivation, xerostomia, constipation, paralytic ileus, laryngeal edema

Genitourinary: Ejaculatory disturbances, impotence, polyuria, bladder paralysis, enuresis

Hematologic: Agranulocytosis, leukopenia, thrombocytopenia, nonthrombocytopenic purpura, eosinophilia, pancytopenia

Hepatic: Cholestatic jaundice, hepatotoxicity

Neuromuscular & skeletal: Trembling of fingers, SLE, facial hemispasm

Ocular: Pigmentary retinopathy, cornea and lens changes, blurred vision, glaucoma

Respiratory: Nasal congestion, asthma

Overdosage/Toxicology

Signs and symptoms: Deep sleep, hypotension or hypertension, dystonia, seizures, extrapyramidal symptoms, respiratory failure

Treatment: Following initiation of essential overdose management, toxic symptom treatment and supportive treatment should be initiated. Hypotension usually responds to I.V. fluids or Trendelenburg positioning. If unresponsive to these measures, the use of a parenteral inotrope may be required. Seizures commonly respond to diazepam (I.V. 5-10 mg bolus in adults every 15 minutes if needed up to a total of 30 mg; I.V. 0.25-0.4 mg/kg/dose up to a total of 10 mg in children) or to phenytoin or phenobarbital. Cardiac arrhythmias often respond to I.V. lidocaine while other antiarrhythmics can be used. Neuroleptics often cause extrapyramidal symptoms (eg, dystonic reactions) requiring management; benztropine mesylate I.V. 1-2 mg (adults) may be effective. These agents are generally effective within 2-5 minutes.

Drug Interactions CYP2D6 enzyme substrate; CYP2D6 enzyme inhibitor

Aluminum salts: May decrease the absorption of phenothiazines; monitor

Amphetamines: Efficacy may be diminished by antipsychotics; in addition, amphetamines may increase psychotic symptoms. Avoid concurrent use

Anticholinergics: May inhibit the therapeutic response to phenothiazines and excess anticholinergic effects may occur; includes benztropine, trihexyphenidyl, biperiden, and drugs with significant anticholinergic activity (TCAs, antihistamines, disopyramide)

Antihypertensives: Concurrent use of phenothiazines with an antihypertensive may produce additive hypotensive effects (particularly orthostasis)

Bromocriptine: Phenothiazines inhibit the ability of bromocriptine to lower serum prolactin concentrations

CNS depressants: Sedative effects may be additive with phenothiazines; monitor for increased effect; includes barbiturates, benzodiazepines, narcotic analgesics, ethanol, and other sedative agents

CYP2D6 inhibitors: Metabolism of phenothiazines may be decreased; increasing clinical effect or toxicity; inhibitors include amiodarone, cimetidine, delavirdine, fluoxetine, paroxetine, propafenone, quinidine, and ritonavir; monitor for increased effect/toxicity

Enzyme inducers: May enhance the hepatic metabolism of phenothiazines; larger doses may be required; includes rifampin, rifabutin, barbiturates, phenytoin, and cigarette smoking

Epinephrine: Chlorpromazine (and possibly other low potency antipsychotics) may diminish the pressor effects of epinephrine

Guanethidine and guanadrel: Antihypertensive effects may be inhibited by phenothiazines

Levodopa: Phenothiazines may inhibit the antiparkinsonian effect of levodopa; avoid this combination

Lithium: Phenothiazines may produce neurotoxicity with lithium; this is a rare effect

Phenytoin: May reduce serum levels of phenothiazines; phenothiazines may increase phenytoin serum levels

Propranolol: Serum concentrations of phenothiazines may be increased; propranolol also increases phenothiazine concentrations

Polypeptide antibiotics: Rare cases of respiratory paralysis have been reported with concurrent use of phenothiazines

QT_c-prolonging agents: Effects on QT_c interval may be additive with phenothiazines, increasing the risk of malignant arrhythmias; includes type Ia antiarrhythmics, TCAs, and some quinolone antibiotics (sparfloxacin, moxifloxacin and gatifloxacin)

Sulfadoxine-pyrimethamine: May increase phenothiazine concentrations

Tricyclic antidepressants: Concurrent use may produce increased toxicity or altered therapeutic response

Trazodone: Phenothiazines and trazodone may produce additive hypotensive effects

Valproic acid: Serum levels may be increased by phenothiazines

Ethanol/Nutrition/Herb Interactions

Ethanol: Avoid ethanol (may increase CNS depression).

Herb/Nutraceutical: Avoid dong quai, St John's wort (may also cause photosensitization). Avoid kava kava, gotu kola, valerian, St John's wort (may increase CNS depression).

Stability Avoid freezing; protect all dosage forms from light; clear or slightly yellow solutions may be used; should be dispensed in amber or opaque vials/bottles. Solutions may be diluted or mixed with fruit juices or other liquids but must be
(Continued)

Fluphenazine *(Continued)*

administered immediately after mixing; do not prepare bulk dilutions or store bulk dilutions.

Mechanism of Action Blocks postsynaptic mesolimbic dopaminergic D_1 and D_2 receptors in the brain; depresses the release of hypothalamic and hypophyseal hormones; believed to depress the reticular activating system thus affecting basal metabolism, body temperature, wakefulness, vasomotor tone, and emesis

Pharmacodynamics/Kinetics

Following I.M. or S.C. administration (derivative dependent):

Decanoate (lasts the longest and requires more time for onset):
Onset of action: 24-72 hours
Peak neuroleptic effect: Within 48-96 hours

Hydrochloride salt (acts quickly and persists briefly):
Onset of activity: Within 1 hour
Duration: 6-8 hours

Distribution: Crosses the placenta; appears in breast milk

Metabolism: In the liver

Half-life: Derivative dependent:
Enanthate: 84-96 hours
Hydrochloride: 33 hours
Decanoate: 163-232 hours

Usual Dosage

Children: Childhood-onset pervasive developmental disorder (unlabeled use): 0.04 mg/kg/day

Adults: Psychoses:

Oral: 0.5-10 mg/day in divided doses at 6- to 8-hour intervals; some patients may require up to 40 mg/day

I.M.: 2.5-10 mg/day in divided doses at 6- to 8-hour intervals (parenteral dose is $^1/_3$ to $^1/_2$ the oral dose for the hydrochloride salts)

I.M. (decanoate): 12.5 mg every 2 weeks
Conversion from hydrochloride to decanoate I.M. 0.5 mL (12.5 mg) decanoate every 3 weeks is approximately equivalent to 10 mg hydrochloride/day

I.M. (enanthate): 12.5-25 mg every 2 weeks

Hemodialysis: Not dialyzable (0% to 5%)

Child/Adolescent Considerations Twelve hospitalized children 7-11 years of age with childhood-onset pervasive developmental disorder received haloperidol or fluphenazine at an average dose of 0.04 mg/kg/day (Joshi, 1988).

Monitoring Parameters EKG monitoring for 48 hours

Reference Range Therapeutic: 5-20 ng/mL; correlation of serum concentrations and efficacy is controversial; most often dosed to best response

Test Interactions ↑ cholesterol (S), ↑ glucose; ↓ uric acid (S)

Patient Information Avoid alcoholic beverages, may cause drowsiness, do not discontinue without consulting physician

Nursing Implications Avoid contact of oral solution or injection with skin (contact dermatitis); watch for hypotension when administering I.M. or I.V.; oral liquid to be diluted in the following **only**: water, saline, 7-UP®, homogenized milk, carbonated orange beverages, pineapple, apricot, prune, orange, V8® juice, tomato, and grapefruit juices

Additional Information Less sedative and hypotensive effects than chlorpromazine

Dosage Forms

Elixir, as hydrochloride (Prolixin®): 2.5 mg/5 mL with alcohol 14% (60 mL, 473 mL)

Injection, as decanoate (Prolixin Decanoate®): 25 mg/mL (1 mL, 5 mL)

Injection, as enanthate (Prolixin Enanthate®): 25 mg/mL (5 mL)

Injection, as hydrochloride (Prolixin®): 2.5 mg/mL (10 mL)

Solution, oral concentrate, as hydrochloride:
Permitil®: 5 mg/mL with alcohol 1% (118 mL)
Prolixin®: 5 mg/mL with alcohol 14% (120 mL)

Tablet, as hydrochloride:
Permitil®: 2.5 mg, 5 mg, 10 mg
Prolixin®: 1 mg, 2.5 mg, 5 mg, 10 mg

♦ **Fluphenazine Decanoate** *see Fluphenazine on page 151*

♦ **Fluphenazine Enanthate** *see Fluphenazine on page 151*

♦ **Fluphenazine Hydrochloride** *see Fluphenazine on page 151*

Flurazepam (flure AZ e pam)

Related Information

Anxiolytic/Hypnotic Use in Long-Term Care Facilities *on page 562*
Benzodiazepines Comparison Chart *on page 566*
Federal OBRA Regulations Recommended Maximum Doses *on page 583*
Patient Information - Anxiolytics & Sedative Hypnotics (Benzodiazepines) *on page 483*

U.S. Brand Names Dalmane®

Canadian Brand Names Apo®-Flurazepam; Novo-Flupam®; PMS-Flupam; Somnol®; Som Pam®

Synonyms Flurazepam Hydrochloride

Pharmacologic Category Benzodiazepine

Generic Available Yes

Use Short-term treatment of insomnia

Restrictions C-IV

Pregnancy Risk Factor X

Contraindications Hypersensitivity to flurazepam or any component of the formulation (cross-sensitivity with other benzodiazepines may exist); narrow-angle glaucoma; pregnancy

Warnings/Precautions Use with caution in elderly or debilitated patients, patients with hepatic disease (including alcoholics), or renal impairment. Active metabolites with extended half-lives may lead to delayed accumulation and adverse effects. Use with caution in patients with respiratory disease, or impaired gag reflex. Avoid use in patients with sleep apnea.

Causes CNS depression (dose-related) resulting in sedation, dizziness, confusion, or ataxia which may impair physical and mental capabilities. Patients must be cautioned about performing tasks which require mental alertness (ie, operating machinery or driving). Use with caution in patients receiving other CNS depressants or psychoactive agents. Effects with other sedative drugs or ethanol may be potentiated. Benzodiazepines have been associated with falls and traumatic injury and should be used with extreme caution in patients who are at risk of these events (especially the elderly).

Use caution in patients with depression, particularly if suicidal risk may be present. Use with caution in patients with a history of drug dependence. Benzodiazepines have been associated with dependence and acute withdrawal symptoms on discontinuation or reduction in dose (may occur after as little as 10 days of use). Acute withdrawal, including seizures, may be precipitated in patients after administration of flumazenil to patients receiving long-term benzodiazepine therapy.

As a hypnotic, should be used only after evaluation of potential causes of sleep disturbance. Failure of sleep disturbance to resolve after 7-10 days may indicate psychiatric or medical illness. A worsening of insomnia or the emergence of new abnormalities of thought or behavior may represent unrecognized psychiatric or medical illness and requires immediate and careful evaluation.

Benzodiazepines have been associated with anterograde amnesia. Paradoxical reactions, including hyperactive or aggressive behavior have been reported with benzodiazepines, particularly in adolescent/pediatric or psychiatric patients. Does not have analgesic, antidepressant, or antipsychotic properties.

Adverse Reactions

Cardiovascular: Palpitations, chest pain
(Continued)

Flurazepam *(Continued)*

Central nervous system: Drowsiness, ataxia, lightheadedness, memory impairment, depression, headache, hangover effect, confusion, nervousness, dizziness, falling, apprehension, irritability, euphoria, slurred speech, restlessness, hallucinations, paradoxical reactions, talkativeness

Dermatologic: Rash, pruritus

Gastrointestinal: Xerostomia, constipation, increased/excessive salivation, heartburn, upset stomach, nausea, vomiting, diarrhea, increased or decreased appetite, bitter taste, weight gain/loss

Hematologic: Granulocytopenia

Hepatic: Elevated AST/ALT, total bilirubin, alkaline phosphatase, cholestatic jaundice

Neuromuscular & skeletal: Dysarthria, body/joint pain, reflex slowing, weakness

Ocular: Blurred vision, burning eyes, difficulty focusing

Otic: Tinnitus

Respiratory: Apnea, dyspnea

Miscellaneous: Diaphoresis, drug dependence

Overdosage/Toxicology

Signs and symptoms: Respiratory depression, hypoactive reflexes, unsteady gait, hypotension

Treatment: Supportive; rarely is mechanical ventilation required. Flumazenil has been shown to selectively block the binding of benzodiazepines to CNS receptors, resulting in a reversal of benzodiazepine-induced CNS depression.

Drug Interactions CYP3A3/4 enzyme substrate

CNS depressants: Sedative effects and/or respiratory depression may be additive with CNS depressants; includes ethanol, barbiturates, narcotic analgesics, and other sedative agents; monitor for increased effect

Enzyme inducers: Metabolism of some benzodiazepines may be increased, decreasing their therapeutic effect; consider using an alternative sedative/hypnotic agent; potential inducers include phenobarbital, phenytoin, carbamazepine, rifampin, and rifabutin

CYP3A3/4 inhibitors: Serum level and/or toxicity of some benzodiazepines may be increased; inhibitors include amiodarone, cimetidine, clarithromycin, erythromycin, delavirdine, diltiazem, dirithromycin, disulfiram, fluoxetine, fluvoxamine, grapefruit juice, indinavir, itraconazole, ketoconazole, nefazodone, nevirapine, propoxyphene, quinupristin-dalfopristin, ritonavir, saquinavir, verapamil, zafirlukast, zileuton; monitor for altered benzodiazepine response

Levodopa: Therapeutic effects may be diminished in some patients following the addition of a benzodiazepine; limited/inconsistent data

Oral contraceptives: May decrease the clearance of some benzodiazepines (those which undergo oxidative metabolism); monitor for increased benzodiazepine effect

Theophylline: May partially antagonize some of the effects of benzodiazepines; monitor for decreased response; may require higher doses for sedation

Ethanol/Nutrition/Herb Interactions

Ethanol: Avoid ethanol (may increase CNS depression).

Food: Serum levels and response to flurazepam may be increased by grapefruit juice, but unlikely because of flurazepam's high oral bioavailability.

Herb/Nutraceutical: Avoid valerian, St John's wort, kava kava, gotu kola (may increase CNS depression).

Stability Store in light-resistant containers

Mechanism of Action Binds to stereospecific benzodiazepine receptors on the postsynaptic GABA neuron at several sites within the central nervous system, including the limbic system, reticular formation. Enhancement of the inhibitory effect of GABA on neuronal excitability results by increased neuronal membrane permeability to chloride ions. This shift in chloride ions results in hyperpolarization (a less excitable state) and stabilization.

Pharmacodynamics/Kinetics

Onset of hypnotic effect: 15-20 minutes

Peak: 3-6 hours
Duration of action: 7-8 hours
Metabolism: In the liver to N-desalkylflurazepam (active)
Half-life: Adults: 40-114 hours
Usual Dosage Oral:
Children: Insomnia:
≤15 years: Dose not established
>15 years: 15 mg at bedtime
Adults: Insomnia: 15-30 mg at bedtime
Elderly: Insomnia: Oral: 15 mg at bedtime; avoid use if possible
Monitoring Parameters Respiratory and cardiovascular status
Reference Range Therapeutic: 0-4 ng/mL (SI: 0-9 nmol/L); Metabolite N-desalkyl-flurazepam: 20-110 ng/mL (SI: 43-240 nmol/L); Toxic: >0.12 µg/mL
Patient Information Avoid alcohol and other CNS depressants; avoid activities needing good psychomotor coordination until CNS effects are known; drug may cause physical or psychological dependence; avoid abrupt discontinuation after prolonged use
Nursing Implications Provide safety measures (ie, side rails, night light, and call button); remove smoking materials from area; supervise ambulation; avoid abrupt discontinuance in patients with prolonged therapy or seizure disorders
Dosage Forms Capsule, as hydrochloride: 15 mg, 30 mg

♦ **Flurazepam Hydrochloride** *see Flurazepam on page 155*

Fluvoxamine (floo VOKS ah meen)
Related Information
Antidepressant Agents Comparison Chart *on page 553*
Discontinuation of Psychotropic Drugs - Withdrawal Symptoms and Recommendations *on page 582*
Patient Information - Antidepressants (SSRIs) *on page 452*
Pharmacokinetics of Selective Serotonin-Reuptake Inhibitors (SSRIs) *on page 590*
Teratogenic Risks of Psychotropic Medications *on page 594*
U.S. Brand Names Luvox®
Canadian Brand Names Apo®-Fluvoxamine
Pharmacologic Category Antidepressant, Selective Serotonin Reuptake Inhibitor
Generic Available Yes
Use Treatment of obsessive-compulsive disorder (OCD) in children ≥8 years of age and adults
Unlabeled/Investigational Use Treatment of major depression; panic disorder; anxiety disorders in children
Pregnancy Risk Factor C
Contraindications Hypersensitivity to fluvoxamine or any component of the formulation; concurrent use with terfenadine, astemizole, pimozide, thioridazine, mesoridazine, or cisapride; use of MAO inhibitors within 14 days
Warnings/Precautions Potential for severe reaction when used with MAO inhibitors - serotonin syndrome (hyperthermia, muscular rigidity, mental status changes/ agitation, autonomic instability) may occur. May precipitate a shift to mania or hypomania in patients with bipolar disease. Has a low potential to impair cognitive or motor performance - caution when operating hazardous machinery or driving. Use caution in patients with depression, particularly if suicidal risk may be present. Use caution in patients with a previous seizure disorder or condition predisposing to seizures such as brain damage, alcoholism, or concurrent therapy with other drugs which lower the seizure threshold. Use with caution in patients with hepatic or dysfunction and in elderly patients. May cause hyponatremia/SIADH. Use with caution in patients with renal insufficiency or other concurrent illness (cardiovascular disease). Use with caution in patients at risk of bleeding or receiving concurrent anticoagulant therapy, although not consistently noted, fluvoxamine may cause impairment in platelet function. May cause or exacerbate sexual dysfunction.
(Continued)

Fluvoxamine *(Continued)*

Adverse Reactions

>10%:

Central nervous system: Headache (22%), somnolence (22%), insomnia (21%), nervousness (12%), dizziness (11%)

Gastrointestinal: Nausea (40%), diarrhea (11%), xerostomia (14%)

Neuromuscular & skeletal: Weakness (14%)

1% to 10%:

Cardiovascular: Palpitations

Central nervous system: Somnolence, mania, hypomania, vertigo, abnormal thinking, agitation, anxiety, malaise, amnesia, yawning, hypertonia, CNS stimulation, depression

Endocrine & metabolic: Decreased libido

Gastrointestinal: Abdominal pain, vomiting, dyspepsia, constipation, abnormal taste, anorexia, flatulence

Genitourinary: Delayed ejaculation, impotence, anorgasmia, urinary frequency, urinary retention

Neuromuscular & skeletal: Tremors

Ocular: Blurred vision

Respiratory: Dyspnea

Miscellaneous: Diaphoresis

<1%: Acne, alopecia, anemia, angina, ataxia, bradycardia, delayed menstruation, dermatitis, dry skin, dysuria, elevated liver transaminases, extrapyramidal reactions, hyponatremia, lactation, leukocytosis, nocturia, priapism, seizures, serotonin syndrome, SIADH, thrombocytopenia, urticaria

Postmarketing and/or case reports (causal relationship not established): Agranulocytosis, akinesia with fever, anaphylaxis, angioedema, aplastic anemia, Henoch-Schönlein purpura, hepatitis, neuropathy, pancreatitis, Stevens-Johnson syndrome, torsade de pointes, toxic epidermal necrolysis, vasculitis, ventricular tachycardia

Overdosage/Toxicology

Signs and symptoms: Drowsiness, vomiting, diarrhea, dizziness, coma, tachycardia, bradycardia, hypotension, EKG abnormalities, liver function abnormalities, convulsions

Treatment: Primarily symptomatic and supportive; administration of activated charcoal may be as effective as emesis or lavage and should be considered; no specific antidotes for fluvoxamine; dialysis is not believed to be beneficial

Drug Interactions CYP1A2 enzyme substrate; CYP1A2, 2C9, 2C19, 2D6, and 3A3/4 enzyme inhibitor

Amphetamines: SSRIs may increase the sensitivity to amphetamines, and amphetamines may increase the risk of serotonin syndrome

Astemizole: Concurrent use is contraindicated

Benzodiazepines: Fluvoxamine may inhibit the metabolism of alprazolam, diazepam, and triazolam resulting in elevated serum levels; monitor for increased sedation and psychomotor impairment

Beta-blockers: Fluvoxamine may inhibit the metabolism of metoprolol and propranolol resulting in cardiac toxicity; monitor for bradycardia, hypotension, and heart failure if combination is used; not established for all beta-blockers (unlikely with atenolol or nadolol due to renal elimination)

Buspirone: Fluvoxamine inhibits the reuptake of serotonin; combined use with a serotonin agonist (buspirone) may cause serotonin syndrome; fluvoxamine may also increase serum concentrations of buspirone

Carbamazepine: Fluvoxamine may inhibit the metabolism of carbamazepine resulting in increased carbamazepine levels and toxicity; monitor for altered carbamazepine response

Carvedilol: Serum concentrations may be increased; monitor carefully for increased carvedilol effect (hypotension and bradycardia)

Cisapride: Concurrent use is contraindicated

Clozapine: Fluvoxamine inhibits the metabolism of clozapine; adjust clozapine dosage downward or use an alternative SSRI

Cyproheptadine: May inhibit the effects of serotonin reuptake inhibitors (fluvoxamine); monitor for altered antidepressant response; cyproheptadine acts as a serotonin agonist

Dextromethorphan: Fluvoxamine inhibits the metabolism of dextromethorphan; visual hallucinations occurred in a patient receiving this combination; monitor for serotonin syndrome

Haloperidol: Fluvoxamine may inhibit the metabolism of haloperidol and cause extrapyramidal symptoms (EPS); monitor patients for EPS if combination is utilized

HMG-CoA reductase inhibitors: Fluvoxamine may inhibit the metabolism of lovastatin and simvastatin resulting in myositis and rhabdomyolysis; these combinations are best avoided

Lithium: Patients receiving SSRIs and lithium have developed neurotoxicity; if combination is used, monitor for neurotoxicity

Loop diuretics: Fluvoxamine may cause hyponatremia; additive hyponatremic effects may be seen with combined use of a loop diuretic (bumetanide, furosemide, torsemide); monitor for hyponatremia

MAO inhibitors: Fluvoxamine should not be used with nonselective MAO inhibitors (isocarboxazid, phenelzine); fatal reactions have been reported; this combination should be avoided

Meperidine: Combined use with fluvoxamine theoretically may increase the risk of serotonin syndrome

Methadone: Fluvoxamine may increase serum concentrations of methadone; monitor for increased effect

Nefazodone: May increase the risk of serotonin syndrome with SSRIs

Pimozide: Concurrent use is contraindicated

Phenothiazines: Fluvoxamine may inhibit metabolism of phenothiazines; **concurrent use of agents associated with QT prolongation (thioridazine, mesoridazine) is contraindicated**

Phenytoin: Fluvoxamine inhibits the metabolism of phenytoin and may result in phenytoin toxicity; monitor for phenytoin toxicity (ataxia, confusion, dizziness, nystagmus, involuntary muscle movement)

Propafenone: Serum concentrations and/or toxicity may be increased by fluoxetine; avoid concurrent administration

Quinidine: Serum concentrations may be increased with fluvoxamine; avoid concurrent use

Selegiline: SSRIs have been reported to cause mania or hypertension when combined with selegiline; this combination is best avoided. In addition, use with some SSRIs has been reported to cause serotonin syndrome. As a MAO type-B inhibitor, the risk of serotonin syndrome may be less than with nonselective MAO inhibitors.

Serotonin reuptake inhibitors: Combined use with other drugs which inhibit the reuptake may cause serotonin syndrome; monitor patient for altered response with nefazodone; avoid sibutramine combination

Sibutramine: May increase the risk of serotonin syndrome with SSRIs

Sumatriptan (and other serotonin agonists): Concurrent use may result in toxicity; weakness, hyper-reflexia, and incoordination have been observed with sumatriptan and SSRIs. In addition, concurrent use may theoretically increase the risk of serotonin syndrome; includes sumatriptan, naratriptan, rizatriptan, and zolmitriptan.

Sympathomimetics: May increase the risk of serotonin syndrome with SSRIs

Tacrine: Fluvoxamine inhibits the metabolism of tacrine; use alternative SSRI

Tacrolimus: Fluvoxamine may inhibit the metabolism of tacrolimus; monitor for adverse effects; consider an alternative SSRI

Theophylline: Fluvoxamine inhibits the metabolism of theophylline; monitor for theophylline toxicity or use alternative SSRI

Tramadol: Fluvoxamine combined with tramadol (serotonergic effects) may cause serotonin syndrome; monitor

(Continued)

Fluvoxamine *(Continued)*

Trazodone: Fluvoxamine may inhibit the metabolism of trazodone resulting in increased toxicity; monitor

Tricyclic antidepressants Fluvoxamine inhibits the metabolism of tricyclic antidepressants (amitriptyline, desipramine, imipramine, nortriptyline) resulting is elevated serum levels; if combination is warranted, a low dose of TCA (10-25 mg/day) should be utilized

Tryptophan: Fluvoxamine inhibits the reuptake of serotonin; combination with tryptophan, a serotonin precursor, may cause agitation and restlessness; this combination is best avoided

Venlafaxine: Combined use with fluvoxamine may increase the risk of serotonin syndrome

Warfarin: Fluvoxamine may alter the hypoprothrombinemic response to warfarin; monitor

Ethanol/Nutrition/Herb Interactions

Ethanol: Avoid ethanol. Depressed patients should avoid/limit intake.

Food: The bioavailability of melatonin has been reported to be increased by fluvoxamine.

Herb/Nutraceutical: Avoid valerian, St John's wort, SAMe, kava kava (may increase risk of serotonin syndrome and/or excessive sedation).

Stability Protect from high humidity and store at controlled room temperature 15°C to 30°C (59°F to 86°F); dispense in tight containers

Mechanism of Action Inhibits CNS neuron serotonin uptake; minimal or no effect on reuptake of norepinephrine or dopamine; does not significantly bind to alpha-adrenergic, histamine or cholinergic receptors

Pharmacodynamics/Kinetics

Distribution: V_d: ~25 L/kg

Protein binding: ~80% (mostly albumin)

Metabolism: In liver

Bioavailability: 53%; not significantly affected by food

Half-life: 16 hours

Time to peak plasma concentration: 3-8 hours

Elimination: Excreted in urine

Usual Dosage Oral:

Children 8-17 years: Initial: 25 mg at bedtime; adjust in 25 mg increments at 4- to 7-day intervals, as tolerated, to maximum therapeutic benefit: Range: 50-200 mg/day

Maximum: Children: 8-11 years: 200 mg/day, adolescents: 300 mg/day; lower doses may be effective in female versus male patients

Adults: Initial: 50 mg at bedtime; adjust in 50 mg increments at 4- to 7-day intervals; usual dose range: 100-300 mg/day; divide total daily dose into 2 doses; administer larger portion at bedtime

Elderly: Reduce dose, titrate slowly

Dosage adjustment in hepatic impairment: Reduce dose, titrate slowly

Child/Adolescent Considerations Children 8-17 years of age with obsessive-compulsive disorder (OCD) received 50-200 mg/day for 10 weeks (Riddle, 2001). One hundred twenty-eight children 6-17 years of age with social phobia, separation anxiety disorder, or generalized anxiety disorder, who had received psychological treatment for 3 weeks without improvement, received fluvoxamine up to 300 mg/day for 8 weeks (Research Unit, 2001).

Monitoring Parameters Signs and symptoms of depression, anxiety, weight gain or loss, nutritional intake, sleep

Patient Information Avoid alcoholic beverages; its favorable side effect profile makes it a useful alternative to the traditional agents; use sugarless hard candy for dry mouth; avoid alcoholic beverages, may cause drowsiness; improvement may take several weeks; rise slowly to prevent dizziness. As with all psychoactive drugs, fluvoxamine may impair judgment, thinking, or motor skills, so use caution when operating hazardous machinery, including automobiles, especially early on into therapy. Inform your physician of any concurrent medications you may be taking.

Dosage Forms Tablet: 25 mg, 50 mg, 100 mg

Gabapentin (GA ba pen tin)
Related Information
Mood Stabilizers *on page 588*
Patient Information - Mood Stabilizers (Gabapentin) *on page 477*
U.S. Brand Names Neurontin®
Canadian Brand Names Neurontin
Pharmacologic Category Anticonvulsant, Miscellaneous
Generic Available No
Use Adjunct for treatment of partial seizures with and without secondary generalized seizures in patients >12 years of age with epilepsy; adjunct for treatment of partial seizures in pediatric patients 3-12 years of age
Unlabeled/Investigational Use Bipolar disorder, chronic pain, social phobia
Pregnancy Risk Factor C
Pregnancy/Breast-Feeding Implications Clinical effects on the fetus: No data on crossing the placenta; there have been reports of normal pregnancy outcomes, as well as respiratory distress, pyloric stenosis, and inguinal hernia following 1st trimester exposure to gabapentin plus carbamazepine; epilepsy itself, number of medications, genetic factors, or a combination of these probably influence the teratogenicity of anticonvulsant therapy. Use during pregnancy only if the potential benefit to the mother outweighs the potential risk to the fetus. Gabapentin is excreted in human breast milk. A nursed infant could be exposed to ~1 mg/kg/day of gabapentin; the effect on the child is not known. Use in breast-feeding women only if the benefits to the mother outweigh the potential risk to the infant.
Contraindications Hypersensitivity to gabapentin or any component of the formulation
Warnings/Precautions Avoid abrupt withdrawal, may precipitate seizures; may be associated with a slight incidence (0.6%) of status epilepticus and sudden deaths (0.0038 deaths/patient year); use cautiously in patients with severe renal dysfunction; rat studies demonstrated an association with pancreatic adenocarcinoma in male rats; clinical implication unknown. May cause CNS depression, which may impair physical or mental abilities. Patients must be cautioned about performing tasks which require mental alertness (ie, operating machinery or driving). Effects with other sedative drugs or ethanol may be potentiated. Pediatric patients (3-12 years of age) have shown increased incidence of CNS-related adverse effects, including emotional lability, hostility, thought disorder, and hyperkinesia. Safety and efficacy in children <3 years of age have not been established.
Adverse Reactions As reported in patients >12 years of age, unless otherwise noted
>10%:
 Central nervous system: Somnolence (20%), dizziness (17%), ataxia (12%), fatigue (11% in adults)
 Miscellaneous: Viral infection (11% in children 3-12 years)
1% to 10%:
 Cardiovascular: Peripheral edema (2%)
 Central nervous system: Fever (10% in children 3-12 years), hostility (8% in children 3-12 years), somnolence (8% in children 3-12 years), emotional lability (4% to 6% in children 3-12 years), fatigue (3% in children 3-12 years), abnormal thinking (2% in children and adults), amnesia (2%), depression (2%), dizziness (2% in children 3-12 years), dysarthria (2%), nervousness (2%), abnormal coordination (1%), twitching (1%)
 Dermatologic: Pruritus (1%)
 Gastrointestinal: Nausea/vomiting (8% in children 3-12 years), weight gain (3% in adults and children), dyspepsia (2%), dry throat (2%), xerostomia (2%), appetite stimulation (1%), constipation (1%), dental abnormalities (1%)
 Genitourinary: Impotence (1%)
(Continued)

Gabapentin *(Continued)*

Hematologic: Leukopenia (1%), decreased WBC (1%)

Neuromuscular & skeletal: Tremor (7%), hyperkinesia (3% to 5% in children 3-12 years), back pain (2%), myalgia (2%)

Ocular: Nystagmus (8%), diplopia (6%), blurred vision (4%)

Respiratory: Rhinitis (4%), bronchitis (3% in children 3-12 years), pharyngitis (3%), coughing (2%), respiratory infection (2% in children 3-12 years)

Postmarketing and additional clinical reports (limited): Alcohol intolerance, allergy, alopecia, angina pectoris, angioedema, anorexia, coagulation defect, erythema multiforme, facial edema, flatulence, gingivitis, blood glucose fluctuation, subdural hematoma, hepatitis, hypercholesterolemia, hyperlipidemia, hypertension, hyponatremia, intracranial hemorrhage, jaundice, elevated liver function tests, malaise, palpitation, pancreatitis, peripheral vascular disorder, pneumonia, purpura, Stevens-Johnson syndrome, new tumor formation/worsening of existing tumors, vertigo, weakness

Overdosage/Toxicology Acute oral overdoses of up to 49 g have been reported; double vision, slurred speech, drowsiness, lethargy, and diarrhea were observed. Patients recovered with supportive care. Decontaminate using lavage/activated charcoal with cathartic. Multiple dosing of activated charcoal may be useful; hemodialysis may be useful.

Drug Interactions

Antacids: Antacids may reduce the bioavailability of gabapentin by ~20%; gabapentin should be taken at least 2 hours following antacid administration

Cimetidine: Cimetidine may increase gabapentin serum concentrations; clearance of gabapentin is decreased by 14%

Felbamate: Serum concentrations may be increased by gabapentin; monitor for increased felbamate effect/toxicity

Norethindrone: Gabapentin may increase C_{max} of norethindrone by 13%

Phenytoin: Phenytoin serum concentrations may be increased by gabapentin; limited documentation; monitor. **Note:** Valproic acid, carbamazepine, and phenobarbital do not seem to be affected by gabapentin.

Ethanol/Nutrition/Herb Interactions

Ethanol: Avoid ethanol (may increase CNS depression).

Food: Does not change rate or extent of absorption.

Herb/Nutraceutical: Avoid evening primrose (seizure threshold decreased). Avoid valerian, St John's wort, kava kava, gotu kola (may increase CNS depression).

Stability Store capsules and tablets at controlled room temperature. Oral solution should be stored under refrigeration, 2°C to 8°C (59°F to 86°F).

Mechanism of Action Exact mechanism of action is not known, but does have properties in common with other anticonvulsants; although structurally related to GABA, it does not interact with GABA receptors

Pharmacodynamics/Kinetics

Absorption: Oral: 50% to 60%

Distribution: V_d: 0.6-0.8 L/kg

Protein binding: 0%

Half-life: 5-6 hours

Elimination: Renal, 56% to 80%

Usual Dosage Oral:

Children: Anticonvulsant:

3-12 years: Initial: 10-15 mg/kg/day in 3 divided doses; titrate to effective dose over ~3 days; dosages of up to 50 mg/kg/day have been tolerated in clinical studies

3-4 years: Effective dose: 40 mg/kg/day in 3 divided doses

≥5-12 years: Effective dose: 25-35 mg/kg/day in 3 divided doses

Note: If gabapentin is discontinued or if another anticonvulsant is added to therapy, it should be done slowly over a minimum of 1 week

Children >12 years and Adults:

Anticonvulsant: Initial: 300 mg 3 times/day; if necessary the dose may be increased using 300 mg or 400 mg capsules 3 times/day up to 1800 mg/day

Dosage range: 900-1800 mg administered in 3 divided doses at 8-hour intervals

Pain (unlabeled use): 300-1800 mg/day given in 3 divided doses has been the most common dosage range

Bipolar disorder (unlabeled use): 300-3000 mg/day given in 3 divided doses; **Note:** Does not appear to be effective as an adjunctive treatment for bipolar disorder (Pande AC, 2000)

Elderly: Studies in elderly patients have shown a decrease in clearance as age increases. This is most likely due to age-related decreases in renal function; dose reductions may be needed.

Dosing adjustment in renal impairment: Children ≥12 years and Adults:
Cl_{cr} >60 mL/minute: Administer 1200 mg/day (400 mg 3 times/day)
Cl_{cr} 30-60 mL/minute: Administer 600 mg/day (300 mg 2 times/day)
Cl_{cr} 15-30 mL/minute: Administer 300 mg/day (300 mg/day)
Cl_{cr} <15 mL/minute: Administer 150 mg/day (300 mg every other day)
Hemodialysis: 200-300 mg after each 4-hour dialysis following a loading dose of 300-400 mg

Dietary Considerations May take without regard to meals.

Administration Maximum time interval between multiple daily doses should not exceed 12 hours; administer first dose on first day at bedtime to avoid somnolence and dizziness

Monitoring Parameters Monitor serum levels of concomitant anticonvulsant therapy

Reference Range Minimum effective serum concentration may be 2 µg/mL

Test Interactions False positives have been reported with the Ames N-Multistix SG® dipstick test for urine protein

Patient Information Take only as prescribed; may cause dizziness, somnolence, and other symptoms and signs of CNS depression; do not operate machinery or drive a car until you have experience with the drug; may be administered without regard to meals

Nursing Implications Dosage must be adjusted for reduced renal function and elderly often have reduced renal function

Dosage Forms
Capsule: 100 mg, 300 mg, 400 mg
Solution, oral: 250 mg/5 mL
Tablet: 600 mg, 800 mg

♦ **Gabitril**® *see* Tiagabine *on page 399*

Galantamine (ga LAN ta meen)

Related Information
Patient Information - Agents for the Treatment of Alzheimer's Disease *on page 491*

U.S. Brand Names Reminyl®

Synonyms Galantamine Hydrobromide

Pharmacologic Category Acetylcholinesterase Inhibitor (Central)

Generic Available No

Use Treatment of mild to moderate dementia of Alzheimer's disease

Pregnancy Risk Factor B

Pregnancy/Breast-Feeding Implications In animal studies, there was a slight increased in the incident of skeletal variations when given during organogenesis. Adequate, well-controlled studies in pregnant women do not exist. Should be used in pregnancy only if benefit outweighs potential risk to the fetus. Excretion in breast milk unknown/not recommended.

Contraindications Hypersensitivity to galantamine or any component of the formulation; severe liver dysfunction (Child-Pugh score 10-15); severe renal dysfunction (Cl_{cr} <9 mL/minute)

Warnings/Precautions May exaggerate neuromuscular blockade effects of depolarizing neuromuscular-blocking agents like succinylcholine. Vagotonic effects on
(Continued)

Galantamine *(Continued)*

the SA and AV nodes may lead to bradycardia or AV block. Use caution in patients with supraventricular cardiac conduction delays (without a functional pacemaker in place) or patients taking concurrent medications that slow conduction through the SA or AV node. Use caution in peptic ulcer disease (or in patients at risk of ulcer disease); seizure disorder; asthma; COPD; mild to moderate liver dysfunction; moderate renal dysfunction. May cause bladder outflow obstruction. Safety and efficacy in children have not been established.

Adverse Reactions

>10%: Gastrointestinal: Nausea (6% to 24%), vomiting (4% to 13%), diarrhea (6% to 12%)

1% to 10%:

Cardiovascular: Bradycardia (2% to 3%), syncope (0.4% to 2.2%: dose-related), chest pain (≥1%)

Central nervous system: Dizziness (9%), headache (8%), depression (7%), fatigue (5%), insomnia (5%), somnolence (4%), tremor (3%)

Gastrointestinal: Anorexia (7% to 9%), weight loss (5% to 7%), abdominal pain (5%), dyspepsia (5%), flatulence (≥1%)

Genitourinary: Urinary tract infection (8%), hematuria (<1% to 3%), incontinence (≥1%)

Hematologic: Anemia (3%)

Respiratory: Rhinitis (4%)

<1%: Alkaline phosphatase increase, apathy, aphasia, apraxia, ataxia, atrial fibrillation, AV block, bundle branch block, convulsions, cystitis, delirium, dependent edema, diverticulitis, dysphagia, epistaxis, esophageal perforation, gastritis, gastroenteritis, heart failure, hiccups, hyperglycemia, hypertonia, hypokinesia, hypotension, involuntary muscle contractions, libido increase, melena, increased micturition frequency, muscle weakness, nocturia, palpitations, paranoid reaction, paresthesia, paroniria, postural hypotension, purpura, QT prolongation, rectal hemorrhage, renal calculi, saliva increased, supraventricular tachycardia, T-wave inversion, thrombocytopenia, urinary retention, ventricular tachycardia, vertigo, xerostomia

Overdosage/Toxicology Symptoms of overdose may include: bradycardia, collapse, convulsions, defecation, gastrointestinal cramping, hypotension, lacrimation, muscle fasciculations, muscle weakness, respiratory depression, salivation, severe nausea, sweating, urination, vomiting. Treatment is symptom-directed and supportive. Atropine may be used as an antidote; initial dose 0.5-1 mg I.V. and titrate to effect. An atypical response in blood pressure and heart rate has been reported. Effects of hemodialysis are unknown.

Drug Interactions CYP3A4, CYP2D6 enzyme substrates

Amiodarone: Concurrent use may lead to bradycardia

Anticholinergic agents (eg. atropine, benztropine, tolterodine): Galantamine may antagonize anticholinergic actions

Beta blockers without ISA activity: Concurrent use may lead to bradycardia

Cimetidine: Increased bioavailability of galantamine by 16%

Cholinergic agonists: May have synergistic effects

CYP2D6 inhibitors: Metabolism of galantamine may be decreased; increasing clinical effect or toxicity. Inhibitors include amiodarone, amitriptyline, cimetidine, delavirdine, fluoxetine, paroxetine, propafenone, quinidine, and ritonavir; monitor for increased effect/toxicity.

CYP3A4 inhibitors: Metabolism of galantamine may be decreased; increasing clinical effect or toxicity. Inhibitors include clarithromycin, erythromycin, fluvoxamine, itraconazole, ketoconazole, nefazodone, ritonavir; monitor for increased effect/toxicity.

Digoxin: Concurrent use may lead to AV block

Diltiazem: Concurrent use may lead to bradycardia

Enzyme inducers: May enhance the hepatic metabolism of galantamine; larger doses of galantamine may be required. Inducers include rifampin, rifabutin, barbiturates, phenytoin, and cigarette smoking.

Ketoconazole: Increased galantamine levels (AUC increased by 30%)

NSAIDs: Concurrent use may increase risk of gastrointestinal ulcer because of increased gastric acid secretion.

Paroxetine: Increased galantamine levels (AUC increased by 40%)

Succinylcholine: Concurrent use may lead to enhanced neuromuscular blockade

Verapamil: Concurrent use may lead to bradycardia

Ethanol/Nutrition/Herb Interactions

Ethanol: Avoid ethanol (may increase CNS adverse events).

Herb/Nutraceutical: St John's wort may decrease galantamine serum levels; avoid concurrent use.

Stability Store at 15°C to 30°C (59°F to 86°F). Do not freeze oral solution; protect from light.

Mechanism of Action Centrally-acting cholinesterase inhibitor (competitive and reversible). It elevates acetylcholine in cerebral cortex by slowing the degradation of acetylcholine. Modulates nicotinic acetylcholine receptor to increase acetylcholine from surviving presynaptic nerve terminals. May increase glutamate and serotonin levels.

Pharmacodynamics/Kinetics

Duration: 3 hours; maximum inhibition of erythrocyte acetylcholinesterase approximately 40% at 1 hour post 10 mg oral dose; levels return to baseline at 30 hours

Absorption: Rapidly and completely absorbed

Distribution: 1.8-2.6 L/kg; levels in the brain are 2-3 times higher than in plasma

Protein binding: 18%

Metabolism: Linear, CYP2D6 and 3A4; metabolized to epigalanthaminone and galanthaminone both of which have acetylcholinesterase inhibitory activity 130 times less than galantamine

Bioavailability: 80% to 100%

Half-life: 6-8 hours

Time to peak: 45-120 minutes

Elimination: Renal (25%)

Usual Dosage Note: Take with breakfast and dinner. If therapy is interrupted for ≥3 days, restart at the lowest dose and increase to current dose.

Oral: Adults: Mild to moderate dementia of Alzheimer's: Initial: 4 mg twice a day for 4 weeks

If 8 mg per day tolerated, increase to 8 mg twice daily for ≥4 weeks

If 16 mg per day tolerated, increase to 12 mg twice daily

Range: 16-24 mg/day in 2 divided doses

Elderly: No dosage adjustment needed

Dosage adjustment in renal impairment:

Moderate renal impairment: Maximum dose: 16 mg/day.

Severe renal dysfunction (Cl_{cr} <9 mL/minute): Use is not recommended

Dosage adjustment in hepatic impairment:

Moderate liver dysfunction (Child-Pugh score 7-9): Maximum dose: 16 mg/day

Severe liver dysfunction (Child-Pugh score 10-15): Use is not recommended

Dietary Considerations Take with breakfast and dinner.

Administration Take with breakfast and dinner. If therapy is interrupted for ≥3 days, restart at the lowest dose and increase to current dose. If using oral solution, mix dose with 3-4 ounces of any nonalcoholic beverage; mix well and drink immediately.

Monitoring Parameters Mental status

Nursing Implications Have patient take with breakfast and dinner. If therapy is interrupted for ≥3 days, restart at the lowest dose and increase to current dose as per patient tolerance.

Dosage Forms

Solution, oral, as hydrobromide: 4 mg/mL (100 mL) [with calibrated pipette]

Tablet, as hydrobromide: 4 mg, 8 mg, 12 mg

♦ **Galantamine Hydrobromide** *see* Galantamine *on page 163*

Garlic

Synonyms *Allium savitum*; Comphor of the Poor; Nectar of the Gods; Poor Mans Treacle; Rustic Treacle; Stinking Rose

Pharmacologic Category Herb

Use Herbal medicine used for lowering LDL cholesterol and triglycerides, and raising HDL cholesterol; protection against atherosclerosis, hypertension, antiseptic agent; may lower blood glucose and decrease thrombosis; potential anti-inflammatory and antitumor effects

Adverse Reactions

Dermatologic: Skin blistering, eczema, systemic contact dermatitis, immunologic contact urticaria

Gastrointestinal: G.I. upset and changes in intestinal flora (in rare cases) per Commission E

Ocular: Lacrimation

Respiratory: Asthma (upon inhalation of garlic dust)

Miscellaneous: Allergic reactions (in rare cases); change in odor of skin and breath per Commission E

Overdosage/Toxicology

Signs and symptoms: Dizziness, lightheadedness, burning sensation of mouth, hematoma, nausea, sweating, leukocytosis; at doses >50 g daily - anorexia, diarrhea, emesis, and menorrhagia may develop

Decontamination:

Oral: Ipecac within 30 minutes or lavage within 1 hour acute ingestions >25 mL of garlic extract; dilute with milk or water; activated charcoal may prevent absorption

Ocular: Irrigate with saline

Drug Interactions Iodine uptake may be reduced with garlic ingestion; can exacerbate bleeding in patients taking aspirin or anticoagulant agents; may increase risk of hypoglycemia, may increase response to antihypertensives

Usual Dosage Adult dose: 4-12 mg allicin/day

Average daily dose for cardiovascular benefits: 0.25-1 g/kg or 1-4 cloves daily in an 80 kg individual in divided doses

Toxic dose: >5 cloves or >25 mL of extract can cause gastrointestinal symptoms

Additional Information 1% as active as penicillin as an antibiotic; number one over-the-counter medication in Germany; enteric-coated products may demonstrate best results

♦ **Genahist®** *see* Diphenhydramine *on page 116*

♦ **Gen-Pindolol® (Can)** *see* Pindolol *on page 319*

♦ **Gen-Triazolam® (Can)** *see* Triazolam *on page 410*

♦ **Geodon®** *see* Ziprasidone *on page 439*

Germander

Synonyms *Teucrium chamaedrys*

Pharmacologic Category Herb

Use In folk medicine to treat obesity; digestive aid; gout; gall bladder conditions

Adverse Reactions Hepatic: Jaundice, liver function tests (elevated), hepatic necrosis (centrilobular)

Overdosage/Toxicology

Decontamination: Ipecac within 30 minutes or lavage (within 1 hour)/activated charcoal with cathartic

Treatment: Supportive therapy; although there are no human or animal data, due to the fact that glutathione depletion can result in increased hepatotoxicity in mice, there exists a rational to use N-acetylcysteine

Usual Dosage Daily dose: 600 mg to 1.62 g

Patient Information Considered unsafe

Additional Information Not reviewed by Commission E; not generally sold in the United States, mainly in Europe; plant is found in Eastern Europe and Mediterranean; dexamethasone or clotrimazole may increase hepatotoxicity; hepatotoxicity usually presents 3-18 hours after ingestion; blossoms are used in folk medicine in Europe, not in U.S.

Dosage Forms
Capsules: 200-275 mg (no longer marketed)
Herbal teas: ~1 g/bag of germander (no longer marketed)

♦ **Germinal**® *see* Ergoloid Mesylates *on page 133*

Ginger

Synonyms *Zingiber officinale*

Pharmacologic Category Herb

Use In herbal medicine as a digestive aid; for treatment of nausea (antiemetic) and motion sickness; also used as a menstruation promoter in Chinese herbal medicine; headaches, colds and flu; ginger oil is used as a flavoring agent in beverages and mouthwashes; may be useful in some forms of arthritis

Contraindications Gallstones per Commission E

Overdosage/Toxicology
Signs and symptoms: May cause central nervous system depression in large doses
Decontamination: Lavage (within 1 hour)/activated charcoal with cathartic

Drug Interactions May alter response to cardiotonic, hypoglycemia, anticoagulant, antiplatelet agents

Usual Dosage
For preventing motion sickness or digestive aid: 1-4 g/day (250 mg of ginger root powder 4 times/day)
Per Commission E: 2-4 g/day or equivalent preparations

Additional Information Density of ginger oil is ~0.9; ginger is a perennial plant with green-purple flowers similar to orchids which grows in India, the Orient, and Jamaica; 8 oz of ginger ale contains ~1 g of ginger; ginger tea (1 cup) contains ~250 mg of ginger

Ginkgo Biloba

Synonyms CF100

Pharmacologic Category Herb

Use Dilates blood vessels; plant/leaf extract has been used in Europe for intermittent claudication, arterial insufficiency, and cerebral vascular disease (dementia); tinnitus, visual disorders, traumatic brain injury, vertigo of vascular origin
Per Commission E: Demential syndromes including memory deficits, etc (tinnitus, headache); depressive emotional conditions, primary degenerative dementia, vascular dementia, or both

Unlabeled/Investigational Use Asthma, impotence (male)

Contraindications Pregnancy, patients with clotting disorders; hypersensitivity to ginkgo biloba preparations per Commission E

Adverse Reactions
Cardiovascular: Palpitations, bilateral subdural hematomas
Central nervous system: Headache (very seldom per Commission E), dizziness, seizures (in children), restlessness
Dermatologic: Urticaria, cheilitis
Gastrointestinal: Nausea, diarrhea, vomiting, stomatitis, proctitis; very seldom stomach or intestinal upsets (per Commission E)
Ocular: Hyphema
Miscellaneous: Allergic skin reactions (very seldom per Commission E)

Overdosage/Toxicology
Decontamination:
Dermal: Washing skin within 10 minutes may prevent dermal allergic contact dermatitis; remove all clothing
Oral: Lavage (within 1 hour)/activated charcoal (laxative not needed)
Treatment: Supportive therapy; although human data are lacking, since the central nervous system effects may be due to 4-o-methylpyridoxine (an antipyridoxine (Continued)

167

Ginkgo Biloba *(Continued)*

compound), pyridoxine may be useful after ingestion of ginkgo seeds or kernels in children; topical corticosteroids can be used for skin reactions

Drug Interactions

Acetylcholinesterase inhibitors: Effect and/or toxicity may be increased with concurrent administration

Antiplatelet agents: Effects on platelet aggregation may be potentiated by ginkgo

MAO inhibitors: Effect/toxicity may be enhanced by ginkgo

Linezolid: Effect/toxicity may be enhanced by ginkgo

Warfarin: Anticoagulant effects may be potentiated by antiplatelet activity of ginkgo

Usual Dosage Beneficial effects for cerebral ischemia in the elderly occur after one month of use

Usual dosage: ~40 mg 3 times/day with meals; 60-80 mg twice daily to 3 times/day depending on indication; maximum dose: 360 mg/day

Cerebral ischemia: 120 mg/day in 2-3 divided doses (24% flavonoid-glycoside extract, 6% terpene glycosides)

Additional Information Seeds and pulp are poisonous; beneficial effects for cerebral ischemia in the elderly occur after one month of use. Grown on plantations, leaves are extracted with organic solvent (acetone) to a potency of 24% flavonoids and 6% terpenoids. Can increase alpha waves and decrease slow potentials in EEG. An Oriental deciduous tree with plum-like fruits (in autumn) and flowers in spring. May reach a height of 125' (20' girth) and is found in the U.S., Europe, China, and Japan. Cross-reactivity for contact dermatitis due to the fruit pulp exists with poison ivy and poison oak; the dermatological symptoms may last for 10 days, inner bark is used as a whitish brown cloth dye. Leaf extract has been used in herbal medicine to treat dementia, chronic tinnitus, vertigo, cochlear deafness, and impotence.

Ginseng

Synonyms *P. quinquefolium* L.; *P. trifolius* L.

Pharmacologic Category Herb

Use A popular ingredient in herbal teas; has been advocated for its antistress and adaptogenic effects although these effects have not been scientifically confirmed, there's much "suggestive" scientific literature

Contraindications Estrogen-receptor positive breast cancer

Adverse Reactions

Cardiovascular: Tachycardia, hypertension, sinus tachycardia

Central nervous system: Nervousness, agitation, mania, headache, sciatic nerve inflammation

Dermatologic: Stevens Johnson syndrome

Endocrine & metabolic: Hypoglycemia, vaginal bleeding, breast nodules

Overdosage/Toxicology

Signs and symptoms: Ginseng abuse syndrome (noted in patients ingesting 3-15 g/day for up to 2 years) is characterized by morning diarrhea, insomnia, euphoria, edema, nervousness, and skin eruptions

Decontamination: Usually decontamination is not required for ingestions <3 g; lavage (within 1 hour)/activated charcoal can be utilized

Drug Interactions

Note: Drug interaction potential may vary by species (Panax vs Siberian ginseng)

Antihypertensives: Effect on blood pressure may be antagonized or potentiated (orthostasis); monitor BP

Antiplatelet agents: Effects on platelet aggregation may be potentiated by ginseng

Barbiturates: Effects may be potentiated by Siberian ginseng

CNS stimulants: Effects may be potentiated by ginseng

Digoxin: Serum levels may be increased by Siberian ginseng

Estrogens: Effects may be potentiated by Siberian ginseng

Hypoglycemics (including insulin): Effects may be potentiated by Siberian ginseng (not Panax)

Sympathomimetics: Effects may be potentiated by ginseng

Warfarin: Anticoagulant effects may be potentiated by antiplatelet activity of ginseng

Usual Dosage Avoid long-term use
Herbal tea: Usually about 1.75 g; 0.5-2 g/day
Dried root: 0.6-3 g/day of dried root or equivalent preparations
Ethanolic extract: 0.5-6 mL 1-3 times/day
Root: 1-2 g/day
Extract: (7% ginsenosides) 100-300 mg 3 times/day

Additional Information There are three forms of ginseng (American, Asian, and Siberian); each has slightly different properties. In the U.S., the root crop of ginseng is obtained from *Panax quinquefolius* L (American ginseng) or *Panax trifolius* L (Dwarf ginseng). The plants are found in woody areas and are about 3 feet tall with yellow-green flowers and red/yellow fruits (from June to July). Additional information can be obtained from:

Ginseng Board of Wisconsin
16-H Menard Plaza
Wausau, Wisconsin 54401
(715) 845-7300

Capsules: 100-200 mg ginseng claimed per capsule (0.4-23.2 mg of ginsenoside noted per capsule). Most brands contain <8% concentration of ginsenoside/capsule.

Glucosamine

Pharmacologic Category Nutritional Supplement
Use Osteoarthritis, rheumatoid arthritis, tendonitis, gout, bursitis
Adverse Reactions Gastrointestinal: Very few effects (eg, flatulence, nausea)
Drug Interactions None known
Usual Dosage 500 mg of the sulfate form 3 times/day
Additional Information Both a sulfate and a hydrochloride salt are available. Glucosamine appears more highly absorbed when administered in the sulfate form, and sulfate is also an important mineral in cartilage.

♦ *Glycyrrhiza glabra* see Licorice *on page 201*
♦ **Goatweed** see St John's Wort *on page 382*

Golden Seal

Synonyms Eye Balm; Eye Root; *Hydrastis canadensis*; Indian Eye: Orange Root; Jaundice Root; Tumeric Root; Yellow Indian Paint; Yellow Root
Pharmacologic Category Herb
Use Gastrointestinal and peripheral vascular activity; also used in sterile eye washes, as a mouthwash, laxative, hemorrhoids, and to stop postpartum hemorrhage. Efficacy not established in clinical studies; has been used to treat mucosal inflammation/gastritis
Contraindications Pregnancy, breast-feeding
Adverse Reactions Generally high doses:
Central nervous system: Stimulation/agitation
Gastrointestinal: Nausea, vomiting, diarrhea, mouth and throat irritation
Neuromuscular & skeletal: Extremity numbness
Respiratory: Respiratory failure
Overdosage/Toxicology
Signs and symptoms: Hypotension, respiratory depression, seizures, nausea, vomiting, diarrhea, uterine contractions, brown discoloration of urine, mydriasis, paresthesia
Decontamination: activated charcoal with cathartic
Treatment: Supportive therapy; benzodiazepines can be utilized for seizure control
Drug Interactions May interfere with vitamin B absorption
Usual Dosage
Root: 0.5-1 g 3 times/day
Solid form: Usual dosage: 5-10 grains
(Continued)

Golden Seal *(Continued)*

Additional Information Perennial with green-white flowers and dark red berries (from April to May) that is found from Vermont to Arkansas

- ◆ **GP 47680** *see* Oxcarbazepine *on page 278*
- ◆ **G. palidiflora** *see* Licorice *on page 201*
- ◆ **Green Ginger** *see* Wormwood *on page 435*
- ◆ **G. uralensis** *see* Licorice *on page 201*
- ◆ **Gynergen® (Can)** *see* Ergotamine *on page 133*
- ◆ **Habitrol™ Patch** *see* Nicotine *on page 264*

Halazepam *(hal AZ e pam)*

Related Information

Anxiolytic/Hypnotic Use in Long-Term Care Facilities *on page 562*
Benzodiazepines Comparison Chart *on page 566*
Federal OBRA Regulations Recommended Maximum Doses *on page 583*
Patient Information - Anxiolytics & Sedative Hypnotics (Benzodiazepines) *on page 483*

U.S. Brand Names Paxipam®

Pharmacologic Category Benzodiazepine

Generic Available No

Use Management of anxiety disorders

Unlabeled/Investigational Use Hostility; alcohol withdrawal

Restrictions C-IV

Pregnancy Risk Factor D

Contraindications Hypersensitivity to halazepam or any component of the formulation (cross-sensitivity with other benzodiazepines may exist); narrow-angle glaucoma; pregnancy

Warnings/Precautions Use with caution in elderly or debilitated patients, patients with hepatic disease (including alcoholics), or renal impairment. Active metabolites with extended half-lives may lead to delayed accumulation and adverse effects. Use with caution in patients with respiratory disease, or impaired gag reflex. Avoid use in patients with sleep apnea.

Causes CNS depression (dose-related) resulting in sedation, dizziness, confusion, or ataxia which may impair physical and mental capabilities. Patients must be cautioned about performing tasks which require mental alertness (ie, operating machinery or driving). Use with caution in patients receiving other CNS depressants or psychoactive agents. Effects with other sedative drugs or ethanol may be potentiated. Benzodiazepines have been associated with falls and traumatic injury and should be used with extreme caution in patients who are at risk of these events (especially the elderly).

Use caution in patients with depression, particularly if suicidal risk may be present. Use with caution in patients with a history of drug dependence. Benzodiazepines have been associated with dependence and acute withdrawal symptoms on discontinuation or reduction in dose. Acute withdrawal, including seizures, may be precipitated after administration of flumazenil to patients receiving long-term benzodiazepine therapy.

Benzodiazepines have been associated with anterograde amnesia. Paradoxical reactions, including hyperactive or aggressive behavior, have been reported with benzodiazepines, particularly in adolescent/pediatric or psychiatric patients. Does not have analgesic, antidepressant, or antipsychotic properties.

Adverse Reactions

>10%: Central nervous system: Drowsiness
1% to 10%:
  Cardiovascular: Tachycardia, hypotension, bradycardia
  Central nervous system: Confusion, headache, apathy, euphoria, disorientation
  Dermatologic: Dermatitis, rash

Gastrointestinal: Increased salivation, xerostomia, nausea, sense of seasickness, constipation

Ocular: Blurred vision

<1%: Blood dyscrasias, drug dependence menstrual irregularities, reflex slowing

Overdosage/Toxicology Treatment: Supportive; rarely is mechanical ventilation required; flumazenil has been shown to selectively block the binding of benzodiazepines to CNS receptors, resulting in a reversal of benzodiazepine-induced sedation; however, its use may not alter the course of overdose

Drug Interactions CYP3A3/4 enzyme substrate

CNS depressants: Sedative effects and/or respiratory depression may be additive with CNS depressants; includes ethanol, barbiturates, narcotic analgesics, and other sedative agents; monitor for increased effect

Enzyme inducers: Metabolism of some benzodiazepines may be increased, decreasing their therapeutic effect; consider using an alternative sedative/hypnotic agent; potential inducers include phenobarbital, phenytoin, carbamazepine, rifampin, and rifabutin

CYP3A3/4 inhibitors: Serum level and/or toxicity of some benzodiazepines may be increased; inhibitors include amiodarone, cimetidine, clarithromycin, erythromycin, delavirdine, diltiazem, dirithromycin, disulfiram, fluoxetine, fluvoxamine, grapefruit juice, indinavir, itraconazole, ketoconazole, nefazodone, nevirapine, propoxyphene, quinupristin-dalfopristin, ritonavir, saquinavir, verapamil, zafirlukast, zileuton; monitor for altered benzodiazepine response

Levodopa: Therapeutic effects may be diminished in some patients following the addition of a benzodiazepine; limited/inconsistent data

Oral contraceptives: May decrease the clearance of some benzodiazepines (those which undergo oxidative metabolism); monitor for increased benzodiazepine effect

Theophylline: May partially antagonize some of the effects of benzodiazepines; monitor for decreased response; may require higher doses for sedation

Ethanol/Nutrition/Herb Interactions Ethanol: Avoid ethanol (may increase CNS depression).

Mechanism of Action Binds to stereospecific benzodiazepine receptors on the postsynaptic GABA neuron at several sites within the central nervous system, including the limbic system, reticular formation. Enhancement of the inhibitory effect of GABA on neuronal excitability results by increased neuronal membrane permeability to chloride ions. This shift in chloride ions results in hyperpolarization (a less excitable state) and stabilization.

Pharmacodynamics/Kinetics

Half-life:

Parent: 14 hours

Active metabolite (desmethyldiazepam): 50-100 hours

Peak level: 1-3 hours

Elimination: <1% excreted unchanged in urine

Usual Dosage Oral:

Adults: 20-40 mg 3-4 times/day; optimal dosage usually ranges from 80-160 mg/day. If side effects occur with the starting dose, lower the dose.

Elderly ≥70 years or debilitated patients: 20 mg 1-2 times/day and adjust dose accordingly

Monitoring Parameters Respiratory, cardiovascular and mental status, symptoms of anxiety

Patient Information Avoid alcohol and other CNS depressants; may cause drowsiness; avoid activities needing good psychomotor coordination until CNS effects are known; may cause physical or psychological dependence; avoid abrupt discontinuation after prolonged use

Nursing Implications Assist patient with ambulation; monitor for alertness

Additional Information Halazepam offers no significant advantage over other benzodiazepines. Abrupt discontinuation after sustained use (generally >10 days) may cause withdrawal symptoms.

Dosage Forms Tablet: 20 mg, 40 mg

- ♦ **Halcion**® *see* Triazolam *on page 410*
- ♦ **Haldol**® *see* Haloperidol *on page 172*
- ♦ **Haldol**® **Decanoate** *see* Haloperidol *on page 172*
- ♦ **Hallucinogenic Drugs** *see page 585*

Haloperidol (ha loe PER i dole)

Related Information

Antipsychotic Agents Comparison Chart *on page 557*
Antipsychotic Medication Guidelines *on page 559*
Discontinuation of Psychotropic Drugs - Withdrawal Symptoms and Recommendations *on page 582*
Federal OBRA Regulations Recommended Maximum Doses *on page 583*
Liquid Compatibility With Antipsychotics and Mood Stabilizers *on page 587*
Patient Information - Antipsychotics (General) *on page 466*

U.S. Brand Names Haldol®; Haldol® Decanoate

Canadian Brand Names Peridol

Synonyms Haloperidol Decanoate; Haloperidol Lactate

Pharmacologic Category Antipsychotic Agent, Butyrophenone

Generic Available Yes

Use Treatment of psychoses; control of tics and vocal utterances of Tourette's disorder in children and adults; severe behavioral problems in children

Unlabeled/Investigational Use May be used for the emergency sedation of severely agitated or delirious patients; adjunctive treatment of alcohol dependence; antiemetic

Pregnancy Risk Factor C

Contraindications Hypersensitivity to haloperidol or any component of the formulation; Parkinson's disease; severe CNS depression; bone marrow suppression; severe cardiac or hepatic disease; coma

Warnings/Precautions Hypotension may occur, particularly with parenteral administration. Decanoate form should never be administered I.V. Avoid in thyrotoxicosis. May be sedating, use with caution in disorders where CNS depression is a feature. Caution in patients with hemodynamic instability, predisposition to seizures, subcortical brain damage, renal or respiratory disease. Esophageal dysmotility and aspiration have been associated with antipsychotic use - use with caution in patients at risk of pneumonia (ie, Alzheimer's disease). Caution in breast cancer or other prolactin-dependent tumors (may elevate prolactin levels). May alter temperature regulation or mask toxicity of other drugs due to antiemetic effects. May alter cardiac conduction - life-threatening arrhythmias have occurred with therapeutic doses of antipsychotics. Adverse effects of decanoate may be prolonged. May cause orthostatic hypotension - use with caution in patients at risk of this effect or those who would tolerate transient hypotensive episodes (cerebrovascular disease, cardiovascular disease, or other medications which may predispose). Some tablets contain tartrazine.

May cause anticholinergic effects (confusion, agitation, constipation, dry mouth, blurred vision, urinary retention). Therefore, they should be used with caution in patients with decreased gastrointestinal motility, urinary retention, BPH, xerostomia, or visual problems. Conditions which also may be exacerbated by cholinergic blockade include narrow-angle glaucoma (screening is recommended) and worsening of myasthenia gravis. Relative to other neuroleptics, haloperidol has a low potency of cholinergic blockade.

May cause extrapyramidal reactions, including pseudoparkinsonism, acute dystonic reactions, akathisia, and tardive dyskinesia (risk of these reactions is high relative to other neuroleptics). May be associated with neuroleptic malignant syndrome (NMS) or pigmentary retinopathy.

Adverse Reactions

Cardiovascular: Hypotension, hypertension, tachycardia, arrhythmias, abnormal T waves with prolonged ventricular repolarization

Central nervous system: Restlessness, anxiety, extrapyramidal reactions, dystonic reactions, pseudoparkinsonian signs and symptoms, tardive dyskinesia, neuroleptic malignant syndrome (NMS), altered central temperature regulation, akathisia, tardive dystonia, insomnia, euphoria, agitation, drowsiness, depression, lethargy, headache, confusion, vertigo, seizures

Dermatologic: Hyperpigmentation, pruritus, rash, contact dermatitis, alopecia, photosensitivity (rare)

Endocrine & metabolic: Amenorrhea, galactorrhea, gynecomastia, sexual dysfunction, lactation, breast engorgement, mastalgia, menstrual irregularities, hyperglycemia, hypoglycemia, hyponatremia

Gastrointestinal: Nausea, vomiting, anorexia, constipation, diarrhea, hypersalivation, dyspepsia, xerostomia

Genitourinary: Urinary retention, priapism

Hematologic: Cholestatic jaundice, obstructive jaundice

Ocular: Blurred vision

Respiratory: Laryngospasm, bronchospasm

Miscellaneous: Heat stroke, diaphoresis

Overdosage/Toxicology

Signs and symptoms: deep sleep, dystonia, agitation, dysrhythmias, extrapyramidal symptoms

Treatment: Following initiation of essential overdose management, toxic symptom treatment and supportive treatment should be initiated. Also critical cardiac arrhythmias often respond to I.V. lidocaine, while other antiarrhythmics can be used. Neuroleptics often cause extrapyramidal symptoms (eg, dystonic reactions) requiring management with benztropine mesylate I.V. 1-2 mg (adult) may be effective. These agents are generally effective within 2-5 minutes.

Drug Interactions CYP1A2 (minor), CYP2D6 (minor), and CYP3A3/4 enzyme substrate; CYP2C enzyme inducer; CYP2D6 and CYP3A3/4 enzyme inhibitor

Anticholinergics: May inhibit the therapeutic response to haloperidol and excess anticholinergic effects may occur; tardive dyskinesias have also been reported; includes benztropine and trihexyphenidyl

Antihypertensives: Concurrent use of haloperidol with an antihypertensive may produce additive hypotensive effects (particularly orthostasis)

Bromocriptine: Antipsychotics inhibit the ability of bromocriptine to lower serum prolactin concentrations

Chloroquine: Serum concentrations of haloperidol may be increased by chloroquine

CNS depressants: Sedative effects may be additive; monitor for increased effect; includes barbiturates, benzodiazepines, narcotic analgesics, ethanol and other sedative agents

CYP3A3/4 inhibitors: Serum level and/or toxicity of haloperidol may be increased; inhibitors include amiodarone, cimetidine, clarithromycin, erythromycin, delavirdine, diltiazem, dirithromycin, disulfiram, fluoxetine, fluvoxamine, grapefruit juice, indinavir, itraconazole, ketoconazole, metronidazole, nefazodone, nevirapine, propoxyphene, ritonavir, saquinavir, verapamil, zafirlukast, zileuton; monitor for increased response

Enzyme inducers: May enhance the hepatic metabolism of haloperidol, decreasing its effects; larger doses of haloperidol may be required; includes barbiturates, carbamazepine, phenytoin, rifampin, and rifabutin

Indomethacin: Haloperidol in combination with indomethacin may result in drowsiness, tiredness, and confusion; monitor for adverse effects

Inhalation anesthetics: Haloperidol in combination with certain forms of induction anesthesia may produce peripheral vasodilitation and hypotension

Levodopa: Haloperidol may inhibit the antiparkinsonian effect of levodopa; avoid this combination

Lithium: Haloperidol may produce neurotoxicity with lithium; this is a rare effect

Methyldopa: Effect of haloperidol may be altered; enhanced effects, as well as reduced efficacy have been reported

Nefazodone: Haloperidol and nefazodone may produce additive CNS toxicity, including sedation

(Continued)

Haloperidol *(Continued)*

Propranolol: Serum concentrations of haloperidol may be increased

Quinidine: May increase haloperidol concentrations; monitor for EPS and/or QT_c prolongation

SSRIs: Fluoxetine, fluvoxamine, and paroxetine may inhibit the metabolism of haloperidol resulting in EPS; monitor for EPS

Sulfadoxine-pyrimethamine: May increase fluphenazine concentrations

Tricyclic antidepressants: Concurrent use may produce increased toxicity or altered therapeutic response

Trazodone: Haloperidol and trazodone may produce additive hypotensive effects

Ethanol/Nutrition/Herb Interactions

Ethanol: Avoid ethanol (may increase CNS depression).

Herb/Nutraceutical: Avoid valerian, St John's wort, kava kava, gotu kola (may increase CNS depression).

Stability

Protect oral dosage forms from light

Haloperidol lactate injection should be stored at controlled room temperature and protected from light, freezing and temperatures >40°C; exposure to light may cause discoloration and the development of a grayish-red precipitate over several weeks

Haloperidol lactate may be administered IVPB or I.V. infusion in D_5W solutions; NS solutions should not be used due to reports of decreased stability and incompatibility

Standardized dose: 0.5-100 mg/50-100 mL D_5W

Stability of standardized solutions is 38 days at room temperature (24°C)

Mechanism of Action Blocks postsynaptic mesolimbic dopaminergic D_1 and D_2 receptors in the brain; depresses the release of hypothalamic and hypophyseal hormones; believed to depress the reticular activating system thus affecting basal metabolism, body temperature, wakefulness, vasomotor tone, and emesis

Pharmacodynamics/Kinetics

Onset of sedation: I.V.: Within 1 hour

Duration of action: ~3 weeks for decanoate form

Distribution: Crosses the placenta; appears in breast milk

Protein binding: 90%

Metabolism: In the liver to inactive compounds

Bioavailability: Oral: 60%

Half-life: 20 hours

Time to peak serum concentration: 20 minutes

Elimination: 33% to 40% excreted in urine within 5 days; an additional 15% excreted in feces

Usual Dosage

Children: 3-12 years (15-40 kg): Oral:

Initial: 0.05 mg/kg/day or 0.25-0.5 mg/day given in 2-3 divided doses; increase by 0.25-0.5 mg every 5-7 days; maximum: 0.15 mg/kg/day

Usual maintenance:

Agitation or hyperkinesia: 0.01-0.03 mg/kg/day once daily

Nonpsychotic disorders: 0.05-0.075 mg/kg/day in 2-3 divided doses

Psychotic disorders: 0.05-0.15 mg/kg/day in 2-3 divided doses

Children 6-12 years: Sedation/psychotic disorders: I.M. (as lactate): 1-3 mg/dose every 4-8 hours to a maximum of 0.15 mg/kg/day; change over to oral therapy as soon as able

Adults:

Psychosis:

Oral: 0.5-5 mg 2-3 times/day; usual maximum: 30 mg/day

I.M. (as lactate): 2-5 mg every 4-8 hours as needed

I.M. (as decanoate): Initial: 10-20 times the daily oral dose administered at 4-week intervals

Maintenance dose: 10-15 times initial oral dose; used to stabilize psychiatric symptoms

Sedation in the intensive care unit:
I.M., IVP, IVPB: May repeat bolus doses after 30 minutes until calm achieved then administer 50% of the maximum dose every 6 hours
Mild agitation: 0.5-2 mg
Moderate agitation: 2.5-5 mg
Severe agitation: 10-20 mg
Oral: Agitation: 5-10 mg
Continuous intravenous infusion (100 mg/100 mL D$_5$W): Rates of 1-40 mg/hour have been used
Rapid tranquilization of severely-agitated patient (unlabeled use): Administer every 30-60 minutes:
Oral: 5-10 mg
I.M.: 5 mg
Average total dose (oral or I.M.) for tranquilization: 10-20 mg
Elderly: Initial: Oral: 0.25-0.5 mg 1-2 times/day; increase dose at 4- to 7-day intervals by 0.25-0.5 mg/day; increase dosing intervals (twice daily, 3 times/day, etc) as necessary to control response or side effects
Hemodialysis/peritoneal dialysis: Supplemental dose is not necessary

Administration The decanoate injectable formulation should be administered I.M. only, **do not administer decanoate I.V.** Dilute the oral concentrate with water or juice before administration

Monitoring Parameters Monitor orthostatic blood pressures after initiation of therapy or a dose increase; observe for tremor and abnormal movement or posturing (extrapyramidal symptoms)

Reference Range
Therapeutic: 5-15 ng/mL (SI: 10-30 nmol/L) (psychotic disorders - less for Tourette's and mania)
Toxic: >42 ng/mL (SI: >84 nmol/L)

Test Interactions ↓ cholesterol (S)

Patient Information May cause drowsiness, restlessness, avoid alcohol and other CNS depressants, rise slowly from recumbent position; use of supportive stockings may help prevent orthostatic hypotension; do not alter dosage or discontinue without consulting physician; oral concentrate must be diluted in 2-4 oz of liquid (water, fruit juice, carbonated drinks, milk, or pudding)

Nursing Implications Avoid skin contact with oral suspension or solution; may cause contact dermatitis

Additional Information May be used for the emergency sedation of severely agitated or delirious patients.

Dosage Forms
Injection, as decanoate: 50 mg/mL (1 mL, 5 mL); 100 mg/mL (1 mL, 5 mL)
Injection, as lactate: 5 mg/mL (1 mL, 2 mL, 2.5 mL, 10 mL)
Solution, oral concentrate, as lactate: 2 mg/mL (5 mL, 10 mL, 15 mL, 120 mL, 240 mL)
Tablet: 0.5 mg, 1 mg, 2 mg, 5 mg, 10 mg, 20 mg

♦ **Haloperidol Decanoate** *see* Haloperidol *on page 172*
♦ **Haloperidol Lactate** *see* Haloperidol *on page 172*
♦ **Haw** *see* Hawthorn *on page 175*

Hawthorn

Synonyms *Crataegus laevigata*; *Crataegus monogyna*; *Crataegus oxyacantha*; *Crataegus pinnatifida*; English Hawthorn; Haw; Maybush; Whitehorn

Pharmacologic Category Herb

Use In herbal medicine to treat cardiovascular abnormalities (arrhythmia, angina), increased cardiac output, increased contractility of heart muscle; also used as a sedative

Contraindications Pregnancy and breast-feeding

Adverse Reactions
Cardiovascular: Hypotension, bradycardia, hypertension
(Continued)

Hawthorn (Continued)

Central nervous system: Depression, fatigue, sedation

Dermatologic: Rash

Gastrointestinal: Nausea

Overdosage/Toxicology

Signs and symptoms: Hypotension, CNS depression, syncope

Decontamination: Lavage (within 1 hour)/activated charcoal with cathartic

Treatment: Supportive therapy; treat hypotension with I.V. crystalloid infusion and placement in Trendelenburg position; vasopressor agents can be used in refractory cases

Drug Interactions Antihypertensives (effect enhanced), digoxin; effects with Viagra® unknown

Usual Dosage Daily dose of total flavonoids: ~10 mg

Per Commission E: 160-900 mg native water-ethanol extract (ethanol 45% v/v or methanol 70% v/v, drug-extract ratio: 4-7:1, with defined flavonoid or procyanidin content), corresponding to 30-168.7 mg procyanidins, calculated as epicatechin, or 3.5-19.8 mg flavonoids, calculated as hyperoside in accordance with DAB 10 [German pharmacopoeia #10] in 2 or 3 individual doses; duration of administration: 6 weeks minimum

Additional Information A small deciduous tree which can grow up to 25 feet; its white, strongly aromatic flowers bloom in mid to late spring; tincture has a bitter taste

♦ **Herb-of-Grace** see Rue on page 365

Hexobarbital (hex oh BAR bi tal)

Related Information

Patient Information - Anxiolytics & Sedative Hypnotics (Barbiturates) on page 485

U.S. Brand Names Pre-Sed®

Pharmacologic Category Barbiturate

Use Preoperative medication; short-term sedation for diagnostic and minor surgical procedures; potentiating agent for analgesic; postoperative medication; patients suffering from mental and emotional stress that cannot fall asleep

Restrictions C-III

Pregnancy Risk Factor D

Contraindications Hypersensitivity to barbiturates or any component of the formulation; marked hepatic impairment; dyspnea or airway obstruction; porphyria

Drug Interactions CYP2C9 and 2C19 enzyme substrate

Note: Barbiturates are enzyme inducers; patients should be monitored when these drugs are started or stopped for a decreased or increased therapeutic effect respectively

Acetaminophen: Barbiturates may enhance the hepatotoxic potential of acetaminophen overdoses

Antiarrhythmics: Barbiturates may increase the metabolism of antiarrhythmics, decreasing their clinical effect; includes disopyramide, propafenone, and quinidine

Anticonvulsants: Barbiturates may increase the metabolism of anticonvulsants; includes ethosuximide, felbamate (possibly), lamotrigine, phenytoin, tiagabine, topiramate, and zonisamide; does not appear to affect gabapentin or levetiracetam

Antineoplastics: Limited evidence suggests that enzyme-inducing anticonvulsant therapy may reduce the effectiveness of some chemotherapy regimens (specifically in ALL); teniposide and methotrexate may be cleared more rapidly in these patients

Antipsychotics: Barbiturates may enhance the metabolism (decrease the efficacy) of antipsychotics; monitor for altered response; dose adjustment may be needed

Beta-blockers: Metabolism of beta-blockers may be increased and clinical effect decreased; atenolol and nadolol are unlikely to interact given their renal elimination

Calcium channel blockers: Barbiturates may enhance the metabolism of calcium channel blockers, decreasing their clinical effect

Chloramphenicol: Barbiturates may increase the metabolism of chloramphenicol and chloramphenicol may inhibit barbiturate metabolism; monitor for altered response

Cimetidine: Barbiturates may enhance the metabolism of cimetidine, decreasing its clinical effect

CNS depressants: Sedative effects and/or respiratory depression with barbiturates may be additive with other CNS depressants; monitor for increased effect; includes ethanol, sedatives, antidepressants, narcotic analgesics, and benzodiazepines

Corticosteroids: Barbiturates may enhance the metabolism of corticosteroids, decreasing their clinical effect

Cyclosporine: Levels may be decreased by barbiturates; monitor

Immunosuppressants: Barbiturates may enhance the metabolism of immunosuppressants, decreasing its clinical effect; includes both cyclosporine and tacrolimus

Doxycycline: Barbiturates may enhance the metabolism of doxycycline, decreasing its clinical effect; higher dosages may be required

Estrogens: Barbiturates may increase the metabolism of estrogens and reduce their efficacy

Felbamate may inhibit the metabolism of barbiturates and barbiturates may increase the metabolism of felbamate

Griseofulvin: Barbiturates may impair the absorption of griseofulvin, and griseofulvin metabolism may be increased by barbiturates, decreasing clinical effect

Guanfacine: Effect may be decreased by barbiturates

Loop diuretics: Metabolism may be increased and clinical effects decreased; established for furosemide, effect with other loop diuretics not established

MAOIs: Metabolism of barbiturates may be inhibited, increasing clinical effect or toxicity of the barbiturates

Methadone: Barbiturates may enhance the metabolism of methadone resulting in methadone withdrawal

Methoxyflurane: Barbiturates may enhance the nephrotoxic effects of methoxyflurane

Oral contraceptives: Barbiturates may enhance the metabolism of oral contraceptives, decreasing their clinical effect; an alternative method of contraception should be considered

Theophylline: Barbiturates may increase metabolism of theophylline derivatives and decrease their clinical effect

Tricyclic antidepressants: Barbiturates may increase metabolism of tricyclic antidepressants and decrease their clinical effect; sedative effects may be additive

Valproic acid: Metabolism of barbiturates may be inhibited by valproic acid; monitor for excessive sedation; a dose reduction may be needed

Warfarin: Barbiturates inhibit the hypoprothrombinemic effects of oral anticoagulants via increased metabolism; this combination should generally be avoided

Mechanism of Action Interferes with transmission of impulses from the thalamus to the cortex of the brain resulting in an imbalance in central inhibitory and facilitatory mechanisms

Pharmacodynamics/Kinetics Duration of action: ~1 hour

Usual Dosage Oral:

Children 6 to 12 years: One-fourth ($\frac{1}{4}$) to one-half ($\frac{1}{2}$) tablet ~15 minutes before procedure

Children >12 years: One-half ($\frac{1}{2}$) to one tablet ~15 minutes before procedure

Adults: 1-2 tablets ~15 minutes before procedure

Additional Information This tranquilizer has a rapid 10-minute onset time and ultra-short duration of one hour. Developed exclusively for the dental industry to
(Continued)

Hexobarbital *(Continued)*

help reduce chair time. A comfortable patient will return and talk about the ease of his appointment.

Dosage Forms Tablet, scored: 260 mg

♦ **Histantil (Can)** *see* Promethazine *on page 337*

Hops

Synonyms *Humulus lupulus*

Pharmacologic Category Herb

Use In herbal medicine as a sleep aid (sometimes combined with valerian root)
Per Commission E: Mood disturbances such as restlessness and anxiety, sleep disturbances

Adverse Reactions None known relating to herb (as per Commission E); Dermatologic: Contact dermatitis (upon exposure to extracts)

Overdosage/Toxicology Decontamination:
Oral: **Do not** induce emesis; lavage (within 1 hour)/activated charcoal with cathartic
Dermal: Wash with soap and water

Drug Interactions CNS depressants: Sedative effects may be additive with CNS depressants; includes ethanol, barbiturates, narcotic analgesics, and other sedative agents; monitor for increased effect

Usual Dosage Per Commission E: Single dose: 0.5 g

Additional Information A perennial, climbing vine with heights up to 25 feet found in Germany and Pacific Northwest; loses most of its activity (85%) after 9 months of storage; not to be confused with Wild Hops (*Bryonia*)

♦ *Humulus lupulus* *see* Hops *on page 178*

♦ **Hydergine®** *see* Ergoloid Mesylates *on page 133*

♦ **Hydergine® LC** *see* Ergoloid Mesylates *on page 133*

♦ *Hydrastis canadensis* *see* Golden Seal *on page 169*

♦ **Hydrated Chloral** *see* Chloral Hydrate *on page 69*

Hydroxyzine *(hye DROKS i zeen)*

Related Information
Anxiolytic/Hypnotic Use in Long-Term Care Facilities *on page 562*
Federal OBRA Regulations Recommended Maximum Doses *on page 583*
Nonbenzodiazepine Anxiolytics and Hypnotics *on page 589*

U.S. Brand Names ANX®; Atarax®; Hyzine-50®; Restall®; Vistacot®; Vistaril®

Canadian Brand Names Apo®-Hydroxyzine; Multipax®; Novo-Hydroxyzine®; PMS-Hydroxyzine

Synonyms Hydroxyzine Hydrochloride; Hydroxyzine Pamoate

Pharmacologic Category Antianxiety Agent, Miscellaneous; Antiemetic; Antihistamine

Generic Available Yes

Use Treatment of anxiety; preoperative sedative; antipruritic

Unlabeled/Investigational Use Antiemetic; alcohol withdrawal symptoms

Pregnancy Risk Factor C

Contraindications Hypersensitivity to hydroxyzine or any component

Warnings/Precautions Causes sedation, caution must be used in performing tasks which require alertness (ie, operating machinery or driving). Sedative effects of CNS depressants or ethanol are potentiated. S.C., intra-arterial, and I.V. administration are not recommended since thrombosis and digital gangrene can occur; extravasation can result in sterile abscess and marked tissue induration; should be used with caution in patients with narrow-angle glaucoma, prostatic hypertrophy, and bladder neck obstruction; should also be used with caution in patients with asthma or COPD.

Anticholinergic effects are not well tolerated in the elderly. Hydroxyzine may be useful as a short-term antipruritic, but it is not recommended for use as a sedative or anxiolytic in the elderly.

Adverse Reactions

Central nervous system: Drowsiness, headache, fatigue, nervousness, dizziness

Gastrointestinal: Xerostomia

Neuromuscular & skeletal: Tremor, paresthesia, seizure

Ocular: Blurred vision

Respiratory: Thickening of bronchial secretions

Overdosage/Toxicology

Signs and symptoms: Seizures, sedation, hypotension; there is no specific treatment for an antihistamine overdose, however, most of its clinical toxicity is due to anticholinergic effects; anticholinesterase inhibitors may be useful by reducing acetylcholinesterase

Treatment: For anticholinergic overdose with severe life-threatening symptoms, physostigmine 1-2 mg (0.5 or 0.02 mg/kg for children) I.V., slowly may be given to reverse these effects.

Drug Interactions

Amantadine, rimantadine: Central and/or peripheral anticholinergic syndrome can occur when administered with amantadine or rimantadine

Anticholinergic agents: Central and/or peripheral anticholinergic syndrome can occur when administered with narcotic analgesics, phenothiazines and other antipsychotics (especially with high anticholinergic activity), tricyclic antidepressants, quinidine and some other antiarrhythmics, and antihistamines

Antipsychotics: Hydroxyzine may antagonize the therapeutic effects of antipsychotics

CNS depressants: Sedative effects of hydroxyzine may be additive with CNS depressants; includes ethanol, benzodiazepines, barbiturates, narcotic analgesics, and other sedative agents; monitor for increased effect

Ethanol/Nutrition/Herb Interactions

Ethanol: Avoid ethanol (may increase CNS depression).

Herb/Nutraceutical: Avoid valerian, St John's wort, kava kava, gotu kola (may increase CNS depression).

Stability Protect from light; store at 15°C to 30°C and protected from freezing; I.V. is **incompatible** when mixed with aminophylline, amobarbital, chloramphenicol, dimenhydrinate, heparin, penicillin G, pentobarbital, phenobarbital, phenytoin, ranitidine, sulfisoxazole, vitamin B complex with C

Mechanism of Action Competes with histamine for H_1-receptor sites on effector cells in the gastrointestinal tract, blood vessels, and respiratory tract. Possesses skeletal muscle relaxing, bronchodilator, antihistamine, antiemetic, and analgesic properties.

Pharmacodynamics/Kinetics

Onset of effect: Within 15-30 minutes

Duration: 4-6 hours

Absorption: Oral: Rapid

Metabolism: Exact fate is unknown

Half-life: 3-7 hours

Time to peak serum concentration: Within 2 hours

Usual Dosage

Children:

I.M.: 0.5-1.1 mg/kg/dose every 4-6 hours as needed

Oral: 0.6 mg/kg/dose every 6 hours

Adults:

Antiemetic: I.M.: 25-100 mg/dose every 4-6 hours as needed

Anxiety: Oral: 25-100 mg 4 times/day; maximum dose: 600 mg/day

Preoperative sedation:

Oral: 50-100 mg

I.M.: 25-100 mg

Management of pruritus: Oral: 25 mg 3-4 times/day

(Continued)

Hydroxyzine *(Continued)*

Dosing interval in hepatic impairment: Change dosing interval to every 24 hours in patients with primary biliary cirrhosis

Administration For I.M. administration in children, injections should be made into the midlateral muscles of the thigh; S.C., intra-arterial, and I.V. administration **not** recommended since thrombosis and digital gangrene can occur

Monitoring Parameters Relief of symptoms, mental status, blood pressure

Patient Information Will cause drowsiness, avoid alcohol and other CNS depressants, avoid driving and other hazardous tasks until the CNS effects are known

Nursing Implications Extravasation can result in sterile abscess and marked tissue induration; provide safety measures (ie, side rails, night light, and call button); remove smoking materials from area; supervise ambulation

Additional Information Although not recommended in the product labeling due to the possibility of arterial and venous spasms, intravascular hemolysis, and orthostatic hypotension, hydroxyzine can be administered as a short (15- to 30-minute) I.V. infusion.

Hydroxyzine hydrochloride: Anxanil®, Atarax®, Hydroxacen®, Quiess®, Vistaril® injection, Vistazine®
Hydroxyzine pamoate: Hy-Pam®, Vistaril® capsule and suspension

Dosage Forms
Capsule, as pamoate: 25 mg, 50 mg, 100 mg
Injection, as hydrochloride: 25 mg/mL (1 mL, 2 mL, 10 mL); 50 mg/mL (1 mL, 2 mL, 10 mL)
Suspension, oral, as pamoate: 25 mg/5 mL (120 mL, 480 mL)
Syrup, as hydrochloride: 10 mg/5 mL (120 mL, 480 mL, 4000 mL)
Tablet, as hydrochloride: 10 mg, 25 mg, 50 mg, 100 mg

Imipramine *(im IP ra meen)*

Related Information
Antidepressant Agents Comparison Chart *on page 553*
Discontinuation of Psychotropic Drugs - Withdrawal Symptoms and Recommendations *on page 582*
Federal OBRA Regulations Recommended Maximum Doses *on page 583*
Patient Information - Antidepressants (TCAs) *on page 454*
Teratogenic Risks of Psychotropic Medications *on page 594*

U.S. Brand Names Tofranil®; Tofranil-PM®

Canadian Brand Names Apo®-Imipramine; Novo-Pramine®; PMS-Imipramine

Synonyms Imipramine Hydrochloride; Imipramine Pamoate

Pharmacologic Category Antidepressant, Tricyclic (Tertiary Amine)

Generic Available Yes: Tablet

Use Treatment of various forms of depression

Unlabeled/Investigational Use Enuresis in children; analgesic for certain chronic and neuropathic pain; panic disorder

Pregnancy Risk Factor D

Contraindications Hypersensitivity to imipramine (cross-reactivity with other dibenzodiazepines may occur); concurrent use of monoamine oxidase inhibitors (within 14 days); acute recovery phase of MI; pregnancy

Warnings/Precautions May cause sedation, resulting in impaired performance of tasks requiring alertness (ie, operating machinery or driving). Sedative effects may be additive with other CNS depressants and/or ethanol. The degree of sedation is high relative to other antidepressants. May worsen psychosis in some patients or precipitate a shift to mania or hypomania in patients with bipolar disease. May increase the risks associated with electroconvulsive therapy. This agent should be discontinued, when possible, prior to elective surgery. Therapy should not be abruptly discontinued in patients receiving high doses for prolonged periods.

May cause orthostatic hypotension (risk is very high relative to other antidepressants) - use with caution in patients at risk of hypotension or in patients where transient hypotensive episodes would be poorly tolerated (cardiovascular disease or cerebrovascular disease). The degree of anticholinergic blockade produced by this agent is high relative to other cyclic antidepressants - use caution in patients with urinary retention, benign prostatic hypertrophy, narrow-angle glaucoma, xerostomia, visual problems, constipation, or history of bowel obstruction.

Use caution in patients with depression, particularly if suicidal risk may be present. Use with caution in patients with a history of cardiovascular disease (including previous MI, stroke, tachycardia, or conduction abnormalities). The risk of conduction abnormalities with this agent is high relative to other antidepressants. EKG monitoring is recommended if high dosages are used. Use caution in patients with a previous seizure disorder or condition predisposing to seizures such as brain damage, alcoholism, or concurrent therapy with other drugs which lower the seizure threshold. Use with caution in hyperthyroid patients or those receiving thyroid supplementation. Use with caution in patients with hepatic or renal dysfunction and in elderly patients. Has been associated with photosensitization.

Adverse Reactions

Cardiovascular: Orthostatic hypotension, arrhythmias, tachycardia, hypertension, palpitations, myocardial infarction, heart block, EKG changes, CHF, stroke

Central nervous system: Dizziness, drowsiness, headache, agitation, insomnia, nightmares, hypomania, psychosis, fatigue, confusion, hallucinations, disorientation, delusions, anxiety, restlessness, seizures

Endocrine & metabolic: Gynecomastia, breast enlargement, galactorrhea, increase or decrease in libido, increase or decrease in blood sugar, SIADH

Gastrointestinal: Nausea, unpleasant taste, weight gain, xerostomia, constipation, ileus, stomatitis, abdominal cramps, vomiting, anorexia, epigastric disorders, diarrhea, black tongue, weight loss

Genitourinary: Urinary retention, impotence

Neuromuscular & skeletal: Weakness, numbness, tingling, paresthesias, incoordination, ataxia, tremor, peripheral neuropathy, extrapyramidal symptoms

Ocular: Blurred vision, disturbances of accommodation, mydriasis

Otic: Tinnitus

Miscellaneous: Diaphoresis

<1%: Agranulocytosis, alopecia, cholestatic jaundice, eosinophilia, increased liver enzymes, itching, petechiae, photosensitivity, purpura, rash, thrombocytopenia, urticaria

Overdosage/Toxicology

Signs and symptoms: Confusion, hallucinations, constipation, cyanosis, tachycardia, urinary retention, ventricular tachycardia, seizures

Treatment: Following initiation of essential overdose management, toxic symptoms should be treated. Ventricular arrhythmias often respond to concurrent systemic alkalinization (sodium bicarbonate 0.5-2 mEq/kg I.V.). Arrhythmias unresponsive to this therapy may respond to lidocaine 1 mg/kg I.V. followed by a titrated infusion. Physostigmine (1-2 mg I.V. slowly for adults or 0.5 mg I.V. slowly for children) may be indicated in reversing cardiac arrhythmias that are life-threatening. Seizures usually respond to diazepam I.V. boluses (5-10 mg for adults up to 30 mg or 0.25-0.4 mg/kg/dose for children up to 10 mg/dose). If seizures are unresponsive or recur, phenytoin or phenobarbital may be required.

Drug Interactions CYP1A2, 2C9, 2C19, 2D6, and 3A3/4 enzyme substrate

Altretamine: Concurrent use may cause orthostatic hypertension

Amphetamines: TCAs may enhance the effect of amphetamines; monitor for adverse CV effects

Anticholinergics: Combined use with TCAs may produce additive anticholinergic effects

(Continued)

Imipramine *(Continued)*

Antihypertensives: TCAs may inhibit the antihypertensive response to bethanidine, clonidine, debrisoquin, guanadrel, guanethidine, guanabenz, guanfacine; monitor BP; consider alternate antihypertensive agent

Beta-agonists: When combined with TCAs may predispose patients to cardiac arrhythmias

Bupropion: May increase the levels of tricyclic antidepressants; based on limited information; monitor response

Carbamazepine: Tricyclic antidepressants may increase carbamazepine levels; monitor

Cholestyramine and colestipol: May bind TCAs and reduce their absorption; monitor for altered response

Clonidine: Abrupt discontinuation of clonidine may cause hypertensive crisis, amitriptyline may enhance the response

CNS depressants: Amitriptyline may be additive with or may potentiate sedation; sedative effects may be additive with TCAs; monitor for increased effect; includes benzodiazepines, barbiturates, antipsychotics, ethanol and other sedative medications

CYP2C8/9 inhibitors: Serum levels and/or toxicity of some tricyclic antidepressants may be increased; inhibitors include amiodarone, cimetidine, fluvoxamine, some NSAIDs, metronidazole, ritonavir, sulfonamides, troglitazone, valproic acid, and zafirlukast; monitor for increased effect/toxicity

CYP2D6 inhibitors: Serum levels and/or toxicity of some tricyclic antidepressants may be increased; inhibitors include amiodarone, cimetidine, delavirdine, fluoxetine, paroxetine, propafenone, quinidine, and ritonavir; monitor for increased effect/toxicity

CYP3A3/4 inhibitors: Serum level and/or toxicity of some tricyclic antidepressants may be increased; inhibitors include amiodarone, cimetidine, clarithromycin, erythromycin, delavirdine, diltiazem, dirithromycin, disulfiram, fluoxetine, fluvoxamine, grapefruit juice, indinavir, itraconazole, ketoconazole, nefazodone, nevirapine, propoxyphene, quinupristin-dalfopristin, ritonavir, saquinavir, verapamil, zafirlukast, zileuton; monitor for altered effects; a decrease in TCA dosage may be required

Enzyme inducers: May increase the metabolism of TCAs resulting in decreased effect; includes carbamazepine, phenobarbital, phenytoin, and rifampin; monitor for decreased response

Epinephrine (and other direct alpha-agonists): The pressor response to I.V. epinephrine, norepinephrine, and phenylephrine may be enhanced in patients receiving TCAs; this combination is best avoided

Fenfluramine: May increase tricyclic antidepressant levels/effects

Hypoglycemic agents (including insulin): TCAs may enhance the hypoglycemic effects of tolazamide, chlorpropamide, or insulin; monitor for changes in blood glucose levels; reported with chlorpropamide, tolazamide, and insulin

Levodopa: Tricyclic antidepressants may decrease the absorption (bioavailability) of levodopa; rare hypertensive episodes have also been attributed to this combination

Linezolid: Hyperpyrexia, hypertension, tachycardia, confusion, seizures, and **deaths have been reported** with agents which inhibit MAO (serotonin syndrome); this combination should be avoided

Lithium: Concurrent use with a TCA may increase the risk for neurotoxicity

MAO inhibitors: Hyperpyrexia, hypertension, tachycardia, confusion, seizures, and **deaths have been reported** (serotonin syndrome); this combination should be avoided

Methylphenidate: Metabolism of TCAs may be decreased

Phenothiazines: Serum concentrations of some TCAs may be increased; in addition, TCAs may increase concentration of phenothiazines; monitor for altered clinical response

QT_c-prolonging agents: Concurrent use of tricyclic agents with other drugs which may prolong QT_c interval may increase the risk of potentially fatal arrhythmias;

includes type Ia and type III antiarrhythmics agents, selected quinolones (sparfloxacin, gatifloxacin, moxifloxacin, grepafloxacin), cisapride, and other agents

Sucralfate: Absorption of tricyclic antidepressants may be reduced with coadministration

Sympathomimetics, indirect-acting: Tricyclic antidepressants may result in a decreased sensitivity to indirect-acting sympathomimetics; includes dopamine and ephedrine; also see interaction with epinephrine (and direct-acting sympathomimetics)

Tramadol: Tramadol's risk of seizures may be increased with TCAs

Valproic acid: May increase serum concentrations/adverse effects of some tricyclic antidepressants

Warfarin (and other oral anticoagulants): TCAs may increase the anticoagulant effect in patients stabilized on warfarin; monitor INR

Ethanol/Nutrition/Herb Interactions

Ethanol: Avoid ethanol (may decrease CNS depression).

Food: Grapefruit juice may inhibit the metabolism of some TCAs and clinical toxicity may result.

Herb/Nutraceutical: St John's wort may decrease imipramine levels. Avoid valerian, St John's wort, SAMe, kava kava (may increase risk of serotonin syndrome and/or excessive sedation).

Stability Solutions stable at a pH of 4-5; turns yellowish or reddish on exposure to light. Slight discoloration does not affect potency; marked discoloration is associated with loss of potency. Capsules stable for 3 years following date of manufacture.

Mechanism of Action Traditionally believed to increase the synaptic concentration of serotonin and/or norepinephrine in the central nervous system by inhibition of their reuptake by the presynaptic neuronal membrane. However, additional receptor effects have been found including desensitization of adenyl cyclase, down regulation of beta-adrenergic receptors, and down regulation of serotonin receptors.

Pharmacodynamics/Kinetics

Peak antidepressant effect: Usually ≥2 weeks

Absorption: Oral: Well absorbed

Distribution: Crosses the placenta

Metabolism: In the liver by microsomal enzymes to desipramine (active) and other metabolites; significant first-pass metabolism

Half-life: 6-18 hours

Elimination: Almost all compounds following metabolism are excreted in urine

Usual Dosage Oral:

Children:

Depression: 1.5 mg/kg/day with dosage increments of 1 mg/kg every 3-4 days to a maximum dose of 5 mg/kg/day in 1-4 divided doses; monitor carefully especially with doses ≥3.5 mg/kg/day

Enuresis: ≥6 years: Initial: 10-25 mg at bedtime, if inadequate response still seen after 1 week of therapy, increase by 25 mg/day; dose should not exceed 2.5 mg/kg/day or 50 mg at bedtime if 6-12 years of age or 75 mg at bedtime if ≥12 years of age

Adjunct in the treatment of cancer pain: Initial: 0.2-0.4 mg/kg at bedtime; dose may be increased by 50% every 2-3 days up to 1-3 mg/kg/dose at bedtime

Adolescents: Initial: 25-50 mg/day; increase gradually; maximum: 100 mg/day in single or divided doses

Adults: Initial: 25 mg 3-4 times/day, increase dose gradually, total dose may be given at bedtime; maximum: 300 mg/day

Elderly: Initial: 10-25 mg at bedtime; increase by 10-25 mg every 3 days for inpatients and weekly for outpatients if tolerated; average daily dose to achieve a therapeutic concentration: 100 mg/day; range: 50-150 mg/day

Monitoring Parameters Monitor blood pressure and pulse rate prior to and during initial therapy; EKG in older adults, CBC; evaluate mental status

(Continued)

Imipramine *(Continued)*

Reference Range Therapeutic: Imipramine and desipramine: 150-250 ng/mL (SI: 530-890 nmol/L); desipramine: 150-300 ng/mL (SI: 560-1125 nmol/L); Toxic: >500 ng/mL (SI: 446-893 nmol/L); utility of serum level monitoring controversial

Test Interactions ↑ glucose

Patient Information May require 4-6 weeks to achieve desired effect; avoid alcohol ingestion; do not discontinue medication abruptly; may cause urine to turn blue-green; may cause drowsiness, avoid alcohol and other CNS depressants; dry mouth may be helped by sips of water, sugarless gum, or hard candy; rise slowly to avoid dizziness

Nursing Implications Raise bed rails, institute safety measures

Dosage Forms

Capsule, as pamoate (Tofranil-PM®): 75 mg, 100 mg, 125 mg, 150 mg

Tablet, as hydrochloride (Tofranil®): 10 mg, 25 mg, 50 mg

♦ **Imipramine Hydrochloride** *see* Imipramine *on page 180*

♦ **Imipramine Pamoate** *see* Imipramine *on page 180*

♦ **Imitrex®** *see* Sumatriptan *on page 383*

♦ **Inapsine®** *see* Droperidol *on page 126*

♦ **Inderal®** *see* Propranolol *on page 340*

♦ **Inderal® LA** *see* Propranolol *on page 340*

♦ **Indian Eye: Orange Root** *see* Golden Seal *on page 169*

♦ **Indian Head** *see* Echinacea *on page 129*

♦ **Ionamin®** *see* Phentermine *on page 307*

Isocarboxazid *(eye soe kar BOKS a zid)*

Related Information

Patient Information - Antidepressants (MAOIs) *on page 462*

U.S. Brand Names Marplan®

Canadian Brand Names Marplan

Pharmacologic Category Antidepressant, Monoamine Oxidase Inhibitor

Generic Available No

Use Symptomatic treatment of atypical, nonendogenous or neurotic depression

Pregnancy Risk Factor C

Contraindications Hypersensitivity to isocarboxazid or any component of the formulation; uncontrolled hypertension; pheochromocytoma; hepatic or renal disease; cerebrovascular defect; cardiovascular disease (CHF); concurrent use of sympathomimetics (and related compounds), CNS depressants, ethanol, meperidine, bupropion, buspirone, guanethidine, and serotonergic drugs (including SSRIs) - do not use within 5 weeks of fluoxetine discontinuation or 2 weeks of other antidepressant discontinuation; general anesthesia, local vasoconstrictors; spinal anesthesia (hypotension may be exaggerated). Foods which are high in tyramine, tryptophan, or dopamine, chocolate, or caffeine.

Warnings/Precautions Safety in children <16 years of age has not been established; use with caution in patients who are hyperactive, hyperexcitable, or who have glaucoma, suicidal tendencies, hyperthyroidism, or diabetes; avoid use of meperidine within 2 weeks of isocarboxazid use. Toxic reactions have occurred with dextromethorphan. Hypertensive crisis may occur with tyramine, tryptophan, or dopamine-containing foods. Should not be used in combination with other antidepressants. Hypotensive effects of antihypertensives (beta-blockers, thiazides) may be exaggerated. Use with caution in depressed patients at risk of suicide. May cause orthostatic hypotension (especially at dosages >30 mg/day) - use with caution in patients with hypotension or patients who would not tolerate transient hypotensive episodes - effects may be additive when used with other agents known to cause orthostasis (phenothiazines). Has been associated with activation of hypomania and/or mania in bipolar patients. May worsen psychotic symptoms in some patients. Use with caution in patients at risk of seizures, or in patients receiving other drugs which may lower seizure threshold. Discontinue at least 48 hours prior to myelography. Use with caution in patients receiving disulfiram. Use with caution in patients with renal impairment.

The MAO inhibitors are effective and generally well tolerated by older patients. It is the potential interactions with tyramine- or tryptophan-containing foods and other drugs, and their effects on blood pressure that have limited their use.

Adverse Reactions

>10%:
Cardiovascular: Orthostatic hypotension
Central nervous system: Drowsiness
Endocrine & metabolic: Decreased sexual ability
Neuromuscular & skeletal: Weakness, trembling
Ocular: Blurred vision

1% to 10%:
Cardiovascular: Tachycardia, peripheral edema
Central nervous system: Nervousness, chills
Dermatologic: Xerostomia
Gastrointestinal: Diarrhea, anorexia, constipation

<1%: Hepatitis, leukopenia, parkinsonian syndrome

Drug Interactions

Amphetamines: MAO inhibitors in combination with amphetamines may result in severe hypertensive reaction; these combinations are best avoided

Anorexiants: Concurrent use of anorexiants may result in serotonin syndrome; these combinations are best avoided; includes dexfenfluramine, fenfluramine, or sibutramine

Barbiturates: MAO inhibitors may inhibit the metabolism of barbiturates and prolong their effect

CNS stimulants: MAO inhibitors in combination with stimulants (methylphenidate) may result in severe hypertensive reaction; these combinations are best avoided

Dextromethorphan: Concurrent use of MAO inhibitors may result in serotonin syndrome; these combinations are best avoided

Disulfiram: MAO inhibitors may produce delirium in patients receiving disulfiram; monitor

Guanadrel and guanethidine: MAO inhibitors inhibit the antihypertensive response to guanadrel or guanethidine; use an alternative antihypertensive agent

Hypoglycemic agents: MAO inhibitors may produce hypoglycemia in patients with diabetes; monitor

Levodopa: MAO inhibitors in combination with levodopa may result in hypertensive reactions; monitor

Lithium: MAO inhibitors in combination with lithium have resulted in malignant hyperpyrexia; this combination is best avoided

Meperidine: May cause serotonin syndrome when combined with an MAO inhibitor; avoid this combination

Nefazodone: Concurrent use of MAO inhibitors may result in serotonin syndrome; these combinations are best avoided

Norepinephrine: MAO inhibitors may increase the pressor response of norepinephrine (effect is generally small); monitor

Reserpine: MAO inhibitors in combination with reserpine may result in hypertensive reactions; monitor

Serotonin agonists: Theoretically, may increase the risk of serotonin syndrome; includes sumatriptan, naratriptan, rizatriptan, and zolmitriptan

SSRIs: May cause serotonin syndrome when combined with an MAO inhibitor; avoid this combination

Succinylcholine: MAO inhibitors may prolong the muscle relaxation produced by succinylcholine via decreased plasma pseudocholinesterase

Sympathomimetics (indirect-acting): MAO inhibitors in combination with sympathomimetics such as dopamine, metaraminol, phenylephrine, and decongestants (pseudoephedrine) may result in severe hypertensive reaction; these combinations are best avoided

(Continued)

Isocarboxazid *(Continued)*

Tramadol: May increase the risk of seizures and serotonin syndrome in patients receiving an MAO inhibitor

Trazodone: Concurrent use of MAO inhibitors may result in serotonin syndrome; these combinations are best avoided

Tricyclic antidepressants: May cause serotonin syndrome when combined with an MAO inhibitor; avoid this combination

Tyramine: Foods (eg, cheese) and beverages (eg, ethanol) containing tyramine, should be avoided in patients receiving an MAO inhibitor; hypertensive crisis may result

Venlafaxine: Concurrent use of MAO inhibitors may result in serotonin syndrome; these combinations are best avoided

Ethanol/Nutrition/Herb Interactions

Ethanol: Avoid ethanol (hypertensive crisis may result). May contain tyramine.

Food: Avoid tyramine-containing foods and beverages (hypertensive crisis may result).

Mechanism of Action Thought to act by increasing endogenous concentrations of epinephrine, norepinephrine, dopamine, and serotonin through inhibition of the enzyme (monoamine oxidase) responsible for the breakdown of these neurotransmitters

Usual Dosage Adults: Oral: 10 mg 3 times/day; reduce to 10-20 mg/day in divided doses when condition improves

Patient Information Avoid tyramine-containing foods and drinks

Dosage Forms Tablet: 10 mg

- **Isocom**® *see* Acetaminophen, Isometheptene, and Dichloralphenazone *on page 14*
- **Isollyl**® **Improved** *see* Butalbital Compound *on page 59*
- **Isometheptene, Acetaminophen, and Dichloralphenazone** *see* Acetaminophen, Isometheptene, and Dichloralphenazone *on page 14*
- **Isometheptene, Dichloralphenazone, and Acetaminophen** *see* Acetaminophen, Isometheptene, and Dichloralphenazone *on page 14*
- **Isopap**® *see* Acetaminophen, Isometheptene, and Dichloralphenazone *on page 14*
- **Jaundice Root** *see* Golden Seal *on page 169*
- **Jesuit's Tea** *see* Maté *on page 219*

Kava

Synonyms Awa; Kew; *Piper methysticum*; Tonga

Pharmacologic Category Herb

Use Conditions of nervous anxiety, stress, and restlessness per Commission E; used for sleep inducement and to reduce anxiety

Restrictions Not more than 3 months without medical advice per Commission E

Contraindications Per Commission E: Pregnancy, breast-feeding, endogenous depression. "Extended continuous intake can cause a temporary yellow discoloration of skin, hair and nails. In this case, further application must be discontinued. In rare cases, allergic skin reactions occur. Also, accommodative disturbances (eg, enlargement of the pupils and disturbances of the oculomotor equilibrium) have been described."

Adverse Reactions

Central nervous system: Euphoria, depression, somnolence

Dermatologic: Skin discoloration (prolonged use)

Neuromuscular & skeletal: Muscle weakness

Ocular: Eye disturbances

Overdosage/Toxicology

Signs and symptoms: Ataxia, deafness, yellow skin discoloration, sedation, extrapyramidal effects

Decontamination: Lavage (within 1 hour)/activated charcoal with cathartic

Treatment: Supportive therapy; can treat extrapyramidal reactions with benztropine and/or diphenhydramine

Drug Interactions

Alprazolam (and potentially all benzodiazepines): A case report of coma following concurrent alprazolam and kava has been reported. Combinations should be avoided

CNS depressants: Sedative effects may be additive with CNS depressants; includes ethanol, barbiturates, narcotic analgesics, and other sedative agents; monitor for increased effect

Levodopa: Effects may be antagonized by kava

Usual Dosage Per Commission E: Herb and preparations equivalent to 60-120 mg kavalactones

Additional Information Kava is used has a social and ceremonial drink in South Pacific Islands. It has medicinal use as a GU antiseptic, antipyretic, diuretic, local anesthetic, and muscle relaxant agent. The shrubs can grow 8-20 feet tall with green stems and rounded fruit. Patients may develop a characteristic yellow rash that resembles pellagra, but does not respond to nicotinamide.

♦ **Kemadrin®** *see* Procyclidine *on page 332*

♦ **Kew** *see* Kava *on page 186*

♦ **Klamath Weed** *see* St John's Wort *on page 382*

♦ **Klonopin™** *see* Clonazepam *on page 85*

♦ **L-3-Hydroxytyrosine** *see* Levodopa *on page 190*

♦ **Lamictal®** *see* Lamotrigine *on page 187*

Lamotrigine (la MOE tri jeen)

Related Information

Mood Stabilizers *on page 588*
Patient Information - Mood Stabilizers (Lamotrigine) *on page 479*

U.S. Brand Names Lamictal®

Canadian Brand Names Lamictal

Synonyms BW-430C; LTG

Pharmacologic Category Anticonvulsant, Miscellaneous

Generic Available No

Use Adjunctive therapy in the treatment of partial seizures in adults with epilepsy (safety and effectiveness in children <16 years of age have not been established); conversion to monotherapy in adults with partial seizures who are receiving treatment with a single enzyme-inducing antiepileptic drug

Orphan drug: Adjunctive therapy in the generalized seizures of Lennox-Gastaut syndrome in pediatrics and adults

Unlabeled/Investigational Use Bipolar disorder

Pregnancy Risk Factor C

Pregnancy/Breast-Feeding Implications Lamotrigine has been found to decrease folate concentrations in animal studies.

Contraindications Hypersensitivity to lamotrigine or any component of the formulation

Warnings/Precautions Use caution in patients with impaired renal, hepatic, or cardiac function. Avoid abrupt cessation, taper over at least 2 weeks if possible. Severe and potentially life-threatening skin rashes have been reported; this appears to occur most frequently in pediatric patients. Discontinue at first sign of rash unless rash is clearly not drug related. May cause CNS depression, which may impair physical or mental abilities. Patients must be cautioned about performing tasks which require mental alertness (ie, operating machinery or driving). Effects with other sedative drugs or ethanol may be potentiated. Binds to melanin and may accumulate in the eye and other melanin-rich tissues; the clinical significance of this is not known. Safety and efficacy has not been established for use as initial monotherapy, conversion to monotherapy from nonenzyme-inducing antiepileptic drugs (AED), or conversion to monotherapy from two or more AEDs. (Continued)

Lamotrigine *(Continued)*

Use caution in writing and/or interpreting prescriptions/orders. Confusion between Lamictal® (lamotrigine) and Lamisil® (terbinafine) has occurred.

Adverse Reactions

>10%:

Central nervous system: Headache (29%), dizziness (7% to 38%), ataxia (7% to 22%), somnolence

Gastrointestinal: Nausea (7% to 19%)

Ocular: Diplopia (28%), blurred vision (16%)

Respiratory: Rhinitis (7% to 14%)

1% to 10%:

Central nervous system: Depression (4%), anxiety (4%), irritability, emotional lability, confusion, speech disorder, difficulty concentrating, malaise, seizure (3% to 4%), incoordination, insomnia (5% to 6%)

Dermatologic: Hypersensitivity rash (10%), pruritus (3%)

Gastrointestinal: Abdominal pain, vomiting (9%), diarrhea (6%), dyspepsia (5% to 7%), constipation (4%), anorexia (2%)

Genitourinary: Vaginitis (4%), dysmenorrhea (7%)

Neuromuscular & skeletal: Tremor (6%), arthralgia, joint pain

Ocular: Nystagmus (2%)

Miscellaneous: Flu syndrome (7%), fever (2% to 6%)

<1%: Acute renal failure, allergic reactions, angina, atrial fibrillation, amnesia, angioedema, bronchospasm, depersonalization, dyspnea, dysarthria, dysphagia, eosinophilia, erythema multiforme, GI hemorrhage, gingival hyperplasia, hemorrhage, hepatitis, impotence, leukopenia, mania, movement disorder, paralysis, rash, stroke, suicidal ideation, urticaria

Postmarketing and/or case reports: Acne, agranulocytosis, alopecia, angioedema, aplastic anemia, apnea, disseminated intravascular coagulation (DIC), esophagitis, hemolytic anemia, hypersensitivity reactions (including rhabdomyolysis), immunosuppression (progressive), lupus-like reaction, multi-organ failure, neutropenia, pancreatitis, pancytopenia, Parkinson's disease exacerbation, red cell aplasia, Stevens-Johnson syndrome, tics, vasculitis

Overdosage/Toxicology Symptoms of overdose include QRS prolongation, AV block, dizziness, drowsiness, sedation, and ataxia. Enhancement of elimination: Multiple dosing of activated charcoal may be useful.

Drug Interactions

Acetaminophen: May reduce serum concentrations of lamotrigine; mechanism not defined; of clinical concern only with chronic acetaminophen dosing (not single doses)

Carbamazepine: Lamotrigine may increase the epoxide metabolite of carbamazepine resulting in toxicity

Enzyme inducers: Carbamazepine, phenytoin, phenobarbital may decrease concentrations of lamotrigine

SSRIs (sertraline): Toxicity has been reported following the addition of sertraline; limited documentation; monitor

Valproic acid: Inhibits the metabolism of lamotrigine; lamotrigine enhances the metabolism of valproic acid

Ethanol/Nutrition/Herb Interactions

Ethanol: Avoid ethanol (may increase CNS depression).

Food: Has no effect on absorption.

Herb/Nutraceutical: Avoid evening primrose (seizure threshold decreased).

Stability Store at 25°C (77°F); excursions are permitted to 15°C to 30°C (59°F to 86°F); protect from light

Mechanism of Action A triazine derivative which inhibits release of glutamate (an excitatory amino acid) and inhibits voltage-sensitive sodium channels, which stabilizes neuronal membranes. Lamotrigine has weak inhibitory effect on the 5-HT$_3$ receptor; *in vitro* inhibits dihydrofolate reductase.

Pharmacodynamics/Kinetics

Distribution: V_d: 1.1 L/kg

Protein binding: 55%

Metabolism: Hepatic and renal

Half-life: 24 hours; increases to 59 hours with concomitant valproic acid therapy; decreases with concomitant phenytoin or carbamazepine therapy to 15 hours

Peak levels: Within 1-4 hours

Elimination: In urine as the glucuronide conjugate

Usual Dosage Oral:

Children <6.7 kg: Not recommended

Children 2-12 years: Lennox-Gastaut (adjunctive): **Note:** Children 2-6 years will likely require maintenance doses at the higher end of recommended range; only whole tablets should be used for dosing, rounded down to the nearest whole tablet

Patients receiving AED regimens containing valproic acid:

Weeks 1 and 2: 0.15 mg/kg/day in 1-2 divided doses; round dose down to the nearest whole tablet. For patients >6.7 kg and <14 kg, dosing should be 2 mg every other day.

Weeks 3 and 4: 0.3 mg/kg/day in 1-2 divided doses; round dose down to the nearest whole tablet; may use combinations of 2 mg and 5 mg tablets. For patients >6.7 kg and <14 kg, dosing should be 2 mg/day.

Maintenance dose: Titrate dose to effect; after week 4, increase dose every 1-2 weeks by a calculated increment; calculate increment as 0.3 mg/kg/day rounded down to the nearest whole tablet; add this amount to the previously administered daily dose; usual maintenance: 1-5 mg/kg/day in 1-2 divided doses; maximum: 200 mg/day given in 1-2 divided doses

Patients receiving enzyme-inducing AED regimens without valproic acid:

Weeks 1 and 2: 0.6 mg/kg/day in 2 divided doses; round dose down to the nearest whole tablet

Weeks 3 and 4: 1.2 mg/kg/day in 2 divided doses; round dose down to the nearest whole tablet

Maintenance dose: Titrate dose to effect; after week 4, increase dose every 1-2 weeks by a calculated increment; calculate increment as 1.2 mg/kg/day rounded down to the nearest whole tablet; add this amount to the previously administered daily dose; usual maintenance: 5-15 mg/kg/day in 2 divided doses; maximum: 400 mg/day

Children >12 years: Lennox-Gastaut (adjunctive): See adult dosing

Children ≥16 years: Treatment of partial seizures (adjunctive) or conversion from single enzyme-inducing AED regimen to monotherapy: See adult dosing

Adults:

Lennox-Gastaut (adjunctive) or treatment of partial seizures (adjunctive):

Patients receiving AED regimens containing valproic acid:

Initial dose: 25 mg every other day for 2 weeks, then 25 mg every day for 2 weeks

Maintenance dose: 100-400 mg/day in 1-2 divided doses (usual range 100-200 mg/day). Dose may be increased by 25-50 mg every day for 1-2 weeks in order to achieve maintenance dose.

Patients receiving enzyme-inducing AED regimens without valproic acid:

Initial dose: 50 mg/day for 2 weeks, then 100 mg in 2 doses for 2 weeks; thereafter, daily dose can be increased by 100 mg every 1-2 weeks to be given in 2 divided doses

Usual maintenance dose: 300-500 mg/day in 2 divided doses; doses as high as 700 mg/day have been reported

Partial seizures (monotherapy) conversion from single enzyme-inducing AED regimen: Initial dose: 50 mg/day for 2 weeks, then 100 mg in 2 doses for 2 weeks; thereafter, daily dose should be increased by 100 mg every 1-2 weeks to be given in 2 divided doses until reaching a dose of 500 mg/day. Concomitant enzyme inducing AED should then be withdrawn by 20% decrements each week over a 4-week period. Patients should be monitored for rash.

Bipolar disorder (unlabeled use): 25 mg/day for 2 weeks, followed by 50 mg/day for 2 weeks, followed by 100 mg/day for 1 week; thereafter, daily dosage may

(Continued)

Lamotrigine *(Continued)*

be increased by 100 mg/week, up to a maximum of 500 mg/day as clinically indicated

Dosage adjustment in renal impairment: Decreased dosage may be effective in patients with significant renal impairment; use with caution

Dietary Considerations Take without regard to meals; drug may cause GI upset.

Administration Doses should be rounded down to the nearest whole tablet. Dispersible tablets may be chewed, dispersed in water or swallowed whole. To disperse tablets, add to a small amount of liquid (just enough to cover tablet); let sit ~1 minute until dispersed; swirl solution and consume immediately. Do not administer partial amounts of liquid. If tablets are chewed, a small amount of water or diluted fruit juice should be used to aid in swallowing.

Monitoring Parameters Seizure, frequency and duration, serum levels of concurrent anticonvulsants, hypersensitivity reactions, especially rash

Reference Range Therapeutic range: 2-4 µg/mL

Patient Information Notify physician immediately if skin rash develops or seizure control worsens; may cause dizziness or sedation; avoid activities needing good psychomotor activities until CNS effects are known; avoid abrupt discontinuation

Nursing Implications Doses should be rounded down to the nearest whole tablet. Chewable tablets may be swallowed whole, chewed, dispersed in water, or diluted in fruit juice. When tablets are chewed, follow with water or diluted fruit juice to aid in swallowing. To disperse chewable tablet, cover tablet with one teaspoonful of water and allow to dissolve for 1 minute; entire amount is then administered. Do not use partial amounts of dispersed tablets.

Dosage Forms
Tablet: 25 mg, 100 mg, 150 mg, 200 mg
Tablet, dispersible, chewable: 2 mg, 5 mg, 25 mg [black currant flavor]

♦ **Lanorinal**® *see* Butalbital Compound *on page 59*
♦ **Largactil**® **(Can)** *see* Chlorpromazine *on page 74*
♦ **Larodopa**® *see* Levodopa *on page 190*
♦ ***Larrea tridentata*** *see* Chaparral *on page 68*
♦ **L-Deprenyl** *see* Selegiline *on page 370*
♦ ***L-Dopa*** *see* Levodopa *on page 190*

Lemon Grass Oil

Pharmacologic Category Herb

Use Perfumes; flavoring agent; used also as a hypotensive and carminative in folk medicine

Overdosage/Toxicology
Signs and symptoms: Mucosal irritation, allergic contact dermatitis, skin irritation with citral concentrations >8%, CNS depression at high doses
Decontamination:
Oral: Dilute with milk or water
Dermal: Wash with cool water (warm water may increase severity of reactions)
Ocular: Irrigate copiously with saline

Usual Dosage Acceptable daily intake for food: 500 mcg of citral

Additional Information Not widely used in U.S. market as an herbal dietary supplement; plant is a perennial grass native to Ceylon and Southern India

♦ **Levate**® **(Can)** *see* Amitriptyline *on page 22*

Levodopa *(lee voe DOE pa)*

Related Information
Discontinuation of Psychotropic Drugs - Withdrawal Symptoms and Recommendations *on page 582*

U.S. Brand Names Dopar®; Larodopa®

Canadian Brand Names Larodopa

Synonyms *L*-3-Hydroxytyrosine; *L*-Dopa

Pharmacologic Category Anti-Parkinson's Agent (Dopamine Agonist)

Generic Available No

Use Treatment of Parkinson's disease

Unlabeled/Investigational Use Diagnostic agent for growth hormone deficiency

Pregnancy Risk Factor C

Contraindications Hypersensitivity to levodopa or any component of the formulation; narrow-angle glaucoma; use of MAO inhibitors within prior 14 days (however, may be administered concomitantly with the manufacturer's recommended dose of an MAO inhibitor with selectivity for MAO type B); history of melanoma or any undiagnosed skin lesions

Warnings/Precautions Use with caution in patients with history of cardiovascular disease (including myocardial infarction and arrhythmias); pulmonary diseases such as asthma, psychosis, wide-angle glaucoma, peptic ulcer disease; as well as in renal, hepatic, or endocrine disease. Sudden discontinuation of levodopa may cause a worsening of Parkinson's disease. Elderly may be more sensitive to CNS effects of levodopa. May cause or exacerbate dyskinesias. May cause orthostatic hypotension; Parkinson's disease patients appear to have an impaired capacity to respond to a postural challenge. Use with caution in patients at risk of hypotension (such as those receiving antihypertensive drugs) or where transient hypotensive episodes would be poorly tolerated (cardiovascular disease or cerebrovascular disease). Observe patients closely for development of depression with concomitant suicidal tendencies. Safety and effectiveness in pediatric patients have not been established. Some products may contain tartrazine. Dopaminergic agents have been associated with a syndrome resembling neuroleptic malignant syndrome on withdrawal or significant dosage reduction after long-term use. Pyridoxine may reverse effects of levodopa. Toxic reactions have occurred with dextromethorphan.

Adverse Reactions Frequency not defined.

Cardiovascular: Orthostatic hypotension, arrhythmias, chest pain, hypertension, syncope, palpitations, phlebitis

Central nervous system: Dizziness, anxiety, confusion, nightmares, headache, hallucinations, on-off phenomenon, decreased mental acuity, memory impairment, disorientation, delusions, euphoria, agitation, somnolence, insomnia, gait abnormalities, nervousness, ataxia, EPS, falling, psychosis

Gastrointestinal: Anorexia, nausea, vomiting, constipation, GI bleeding, duodenal ulcer, diarrhea, dyspepsia, taste alterations, sialorrhea, heartburn

Genitourinary: Discoloration of urine, urinary frequency

Hematologic: Hemolytic anemia, agranulocytosis, thrombocytopenia, leukopenia, decreased hemoglobin and hematocrit, abnormalities in AST and ALT, LDH, bilirubin, BUN, Coombs' test

Neuromuscular & skeletal: Choreiform and involuntary movements, paresthesia, bone pain, shoulder pain, muscle cramps, weakness

Ocular: Blepharospasm

Renal: Difficult urination

Respiratory: Dyspnea, cough

Miscellaneous: Hiccups, discoloration of sweat

Overdosage/Toxicology

Signs and symptoms: Palpitations, arrhythmias, spasms, hypertension or hypotension

Treatment: Use fluids judiciously to maintain pressures; may precipitate a variety of arrhythmias

Drug Interactions

Antacids: Levodopa absorption may be increased; monitor

Anticholinergics: May reduce the efficacy of levodopa, possibly due to reduced gastrointestinal absorption (also see tricyclic antidepressants); limited evidence of clinical significance; monitor

Antipsychotics: May inhibit the antiparkinsonian effects of levodopa via dopamine receptor blockade; use antipsychotics with low dopamine blockade (clozapine, olanzapine, quetiapine)

(Continued)

Levodopa (Continued)

Benzodiazepines: May inhibit the antiparkinsonian effects of levodopa; monitor for reduced effect

Clonidine: May reduce the efficacy of levodopa; monitor

Furazolidone: May increase the effect/toxicity of levodopa; hypertensive episodes have been reported; monitor

Iron salts: Binds levodopa and reduces its bioavailability; separate doses of iron and levodopa

Linezolid: Due to MAO inhibition (see note on MAO inhibitors), this agent is best avoided

MAO inhibitors: Concurrent use of levodopa with nonselective MAO inhibitors may result in hypertensive reactions via an increased storage and release of dopamine, norepinephrine, or both; use with carbidopa to minimize reactions if combination is necessary; otherwise avoid combination

L-methionine: May inhibit levodopa's antiparkinsonian effects; monitor for reduced effect

Metoclopramide: May increase the absorption/effect of levodopa; hypertensive episodes have been reported. Levodopa antagonizes metoclopramide's effects on lower esophageal sphincter pressure; avoid use of metoclopramide for reflux, monitor response to levodopa carefully if used.

Methyldopa: May potentiate the effects of levodopa; levodopa may increase the hypotensive response to methyldopa; monitor

Papaverine: May decrease the efficacy of levodopa; includes other similar agents (ethaverine); monitor

Penicillamine: May increase serum concentrations of levodopa; monitor for increased effect

Phenytoin: May inhibit levodopa's antiparkinsonian effects; monitor for reduced effect

Pyridoxine: May inhibit levodopa's antiparkinsonian effects; monitor for reduced effect (pyridoxine in doses >10-25 mg for levodopa alone, higher doses >200 mg/day may be a problem for levodopa/carbidopa)

Spiramycin: May inhibit levodopa's antiparkinsonian effects; monitor for reduced effect

Tacrine: May inhibit the effects of levodopa via enhanced cholinergic activity; monitor for reduced effect

Tricyclic antidepressants: May decrease the absorption (bioavailability) of levodopa; rare hypertensive episodes have also been attributed to this combination

Ethanol/Nutrition/Herb Interactions

Ethanol: Avoid ethanol (due to CNS depression).

Food: Avoid high protein diets and high intakes of vitamin B_6.

Herb/Nutraceutical: Pyridoxine in doses >10-25 mg (for levodopa alone) or higher doses >200 mg/day (for levodopa/carbidopa) may decrease efficacy.

Mechanism of Action Increases dopamine levels in the brain, then stimulates dopaminergic receptors in the basal ganglia to improve the balance between cholinergic and dopaminergic activity

Pharmacodynamics/Kinetics

Duration: Variable, usually 6-12 hours

Time to peak serum concentration: Oral: 1-2 hours

Metabolism: Majority of drug is peripherally decarboxylated to dopamine; small amounts of levodopa reach the brain where it is also decarboxylated to active dopamine

Half-life: 1.2-2.3 hours

Elimination: Primarily in urine (80%) as dopamine, norepinephrine, and homovanillic acid

Usual Dosage Oral:

Children (administer as a single dose to evaluate growth hormone deficiency):

0.5 g/m² **or**

<30 lb: 125 mg

30-70 lb: 250 mg

>70 lb: 500 mg

Adults: Parkinson's disease: 500-1000 mg/day in divided doses every 6-12 hours; increase by 100-750 mg/day every 3-7 days until response or total dose of 8000 mg is reached

A significant therapeutic response may not be obtained for 6 months

Dietary Considerations High-protein diets may decrease the efficacy of levodopa when used for parkinsonism via competition with amino acids in GI absorption .

Administration Administer with meals to decrease GI upset

Monitoring Parameters Serum growth hormone concentration

Test Interactions False-positive reaction for urinary glucose with Clinitest®; false-negative reaction using Clinistix®; false-positive urine ketones with Acetest®, Ketostix®, Labstix®

Patient Information Avoid vitamins with B₆ (pyridoxine); can take with food to prevent GI upset; do not stop taking this drug even if you do not think it is working; dizziness, lightheadedness, fainting may occur when you get up from a sitting or lying position.

Nursing Implications Sustained release product should not be crushed

Additional Information A single dose is not usually associated with the above adverse reactions.

Dosage Forms
Capsule: 100 mg, 250 mg, 500 mg
Tablet: 100 mg, 250 mg, 500 mg

Levodopa and Carbidopa (lee voe DOE pa & kar bi DOE pa)
Related Information
Patient Information - Miscellaneous Medications *on page 495*

U.S. Brand Names Sinemet®; Sinemet® CR

Canadian Brand Names Endo®-Levodopa/Carbidopa; Sinem t® CR

Synonyms Carbidopa and Levodopa

Pharmacologic Category Anti-Parkinson's Agent (Dopamine Agonist)

Generic Available Yes

Use Idiopathic Parkinson's disease; postencephalitic parkinsonism; symptomatic parkinsonism

Pregnancy Risk Factor C

Contraindications Hypersensitivity to levodopa, carbidopa, or any component of the formulation; narrow-angle glaucoma; use of MAO inhibitors within prior 14 days (however may be administered concomitantly with the manufacturer's recommended dose of an MAO inhibitor with selectivity for MAO type B); history of melanoma or undiagnosed skin lesions

Warnings/Precautions Use with caution in patients with history of cardiovascular disease (including myocardial infarction and arrhythmias); pulmonary diseases such as asthma, psychosis, wide-angle glaucoma, peptic ulcer disease; as well as in renal, hepatic, or endocrine disease. Sudden discontinuation of levodopa may cause a worsening of Parkinson's disease. Elderly may be more sensitive to CNS effects of levodopa. May cause or exacerbate dyskinesias. May cause orthostatic hypotension; Parkinson's disease patients appear to have an impaired capacity to respond to a postural challenge; use with caution in patients at risk of hypotension (such as those receiving antihypertensive drugs) or where transient hypotensive episodes would be poorly tolerated (cardiovascular disease or cerebrovascular disease). Observe patients closely for development of depression with concomitant suicidal tendencies. Some products may contain tartrazine. Has been associated with a syndrome resembling neuroleptic malignant syndrome on withdrawal or significant dosage reduction after long-term use. Toxic reactions have occurred with dextromethorphan. Protein in the diet should be distributed throughout the day to avoid fluctuations in levodopa absorption.

Adverse Reactions Frequency not defined.
Cardiovascular: Orthostatic hypotension, arrhythmias, chest pain, hypertension, syncope, palpitations, phlebitis
(Continued)

Levodopa and Carbidopa *(Continued)*

Central nervous system: Dizziness, anxiety, confusion, nightmares, headache, hallucinations, on-off phenomenon, decreased mental acuity, memory impairment, disorientation, delusions, euphoria, agitation, somnolence, insomnia, gait abnormalities, nervousness, ataxia, EPS, falling, psychosis, peripheral neuropathy, seizures (causal relationship not established)

Dermatologic: Rash, alopecia, malignant melanoma, hypersensitivity (angioedema, urticaria, pruritus, bullous lesions, Henoch-Schönlein purpura)

Endocrine & metabolic: Increased libido

Gastrointestinal: Anorexia, nausea, vomiting, constipation, GI bleeding, duodenal ulcer, diarrhea, dyspepsia, taste alterations, sialorrhea, heartburn

Genitourinary: Discoloration of urine, urinary frequency

Hematologic: Hemolytic anemia, agranulocytosis, thrombocytopenia, leukopenia; decreased hemoglobin and hematocrit; abnormalities in AST and ALT, LDH, bilirubin, BUN, Coombs' test

Neuromuscular & skeletal: Choreiform and involuntary movements, paresthesia, bone pain, shoulder pain, muscle cramps, weakness

Ocular: Blepharospasm, oculogyric crises

Renal: Difficult urination

Respiratory: Dyspnea, cough

Miscellaneous: Hiccups, discoloration of sweat, diaphoresis (increased)

Overdosage/Toxicology

Signs and symptoms: Palpitations, arrhythmias, spasms, hypotension; may cause hypertension or hypotension

Treatment: Use fluids judiciously to maintain pressures; may precipitate a variety of arrhythmias

Drug Interactions

Antacids: Levodopa absorption may be increased; monitor

Anticholinergics: May reduce the efficacy of levodopa, possibly due to reduced gastrointestinal absorption (also see tricyclic antidepressants); limited evidence of clinical significance; monitor

Antipsychotics: May inhibit the antiparkinsonian effects of levodopa via dopamine receptor blockade; use antipsychotics with low dopamine blockade (clozapine, olanzapine, quetiapine)

Benzodiazepines: May inhibit the antiparkinsonian effects of levodopa; monitor for reduced effect

Clonidine: May reduce the efficacy of levodopa; monitor

Dextromethorphan: Toxic reactions have occurred with dextromethorphan

Furazolidone: May increase the effect/toxicity of levodopa; hypertensive episodes have been reported; monitor

Iron salts: Binds levodopa and reduces its bioavailability; separate doses of iron and levodopa

Linezolid: Due to MAO inhibition (see note on MAO inhibitors), this agent is best avoided

MAO inhibitors: Concurrent use of levodopa with nonselective MAO inhibitors may result in hypertensive reactions via an increased storage and release of dopamine, norepinephrine, or both; use with carbidopa to minimize reactions if combination is necessary, otherwise avoid combination.

L-methionine: May inhibit levodopa's antiparkinsonian effects; monitor for reduced effect

Metoclopramide: May increase the absorption/effect of levodopa; hypertensive episodes have been reported. Levodopa antagonizes metoclopramide's effects on lower esophageal sphincter pressure. Avoid use of metoclopramide for reflux, monitor response to levodopa carefully if used.

Methyldopa: May potentiate the effects of levodopa; levodopa may increase the hypotensive response to methyldopa; monitor

Papaverine: May decrease the efficacy of levodopa; includes other similar agents (ethaverine); monitor

Penicillamine: May increase serum concentrations of levodopa; monitor for increased effect

Phenytoin: May inhibit levodopa's antiparkinsonian effects; monitor for reduced effect

Pyridoxine: May inhibit levodopa's antiparkinsonian effects; monitor for reduced effect (pyridoxine in doses >10-25 mg for levodopa alone, higher doses >200 mg/day may be a problem for levodopa/carbidopa)

Spiramycin: May inhibit levodopa's antiparkinsonian effects; monitor for reduced effect

Tacrine: May inhibit the effects of levodopa via enhanced cholinergic activity; monitor for reduced effect

Tricyclic antidepressants: May decrease the absorption (bioavailability) of levodopa; rare hypertensive episodes have also been attributed to this combination

Ethanol/Nutrition/Herb Interactions

Ethanol: Avoid ethanol (due to CNS depression).

Food: Avoid high protein diets and high intakes of vitamin B_6.

Herb/Nutraceutical: Avoid kava kava (may decrease effects). Pyridoxine in doses >10-25 mg (for levodopa alone) or higher doses >200 mg/day (for levodopa/carbidopa) may decrease efficacy.

Mechanism of Action Parkinson's symptoms are due to a lack of striatal dopamine; levodopa circulates in the plasma to the blood-brain-barrier (BBB), where it crosses, to be converted by striatal enzymes to dopamine; carbidopa inhibits the peripheral plasma breakdown of levodopa by inhibiting its decarboxylation, and thereby increases available levodopa at the BBB

Pharmacodynamics/Kinetics

Duration: Variable, 6-12 hours; longer with CR dosage forms

Carbidopa:

Absorption: Oral: 40% to 70%

Protein binding: 36%

Half-life: 1-2 hours

Elimination: Excreted unchanged

Levodopa:

Absorption: May be decreased if given with a high protein meal

Half-life: 1.2-2.3 hours

Elimination: Primarily in urine (80%) as dopamine, norepinephrine, and homovanillic acid

Usual Dosage Oral:

Adults: Initial: 25/100 2-4 times/day, increase as necessary to a maximum of 200/2000 mg/day

Elderly: Initial: 25/100 twice daily, increase as necessary

Conversion from Sinemet® to Sinemet® CR (50/200): (Sinemet® [total daily dose of levodopa] / Sinemet® CR)

300-400 mg / 1 tablet twice daily

500-600 mg / 1½ tablets twice daily or one 3 times/day

700-800 mg / 4 tablets in 3 or more divided doses

900-1000 mg / 5 tablets in 3 or more divided doses

Intervals between doses of Sinemet® CR should be 4-8 hours while awake

Dietary Considerations Levodopa peak serum concentrations may be decreased if taken with food. High protein diets (>2 g/kg) may decrease the efficacy of levodopa via competition with amino acids in crossing the blood-brain barrier.

Administration Administer with meals to decrease GI upset

Monitoring Parameters Blood pressure, standing and sitting/supine; symptoms of parkinsonism, dyskinesias, mental status

Test Interactions False-positive reaction for urinary glucose with Clinitest®; false-negative reaction using Clinistix®; false-positive urine ketones with Acetest®, Ketostix®, Labstix®

Patient Information Avoid vitamins with B_6 (pyridoxine); do not stop taking this drug even if you do not think it is working; take on an empty stomach if possible; if GI distress occurs, take with meals; sustained release product should not be

(Continued)

Levodopa and Carbidopa *(Continued)*

crushed; rise carefully from lying or sitting position as dizziness, lightheadedness, or fainting may occur

Nursing Implications Space doses evenly over the waking hours; sustained release product should not be crushed

Additional Information 50-100 mg/day of carbidopa is needed to block the peripheral conversion of levodopa to dopamine. "On-off" (a clinical syndrome characterized by sudden periods of drug activity/inactivity), can be managed by giving smaller, more frequent doses of Sinemet® or adding a dopamine agonist or selegiline; when adding a new agent, doses of Sinemet® can usually be decreased. Protein in the diet should be distributed throughout the day to avoid fluctuations in levodopa absorption. Levodopa is the drug of choice when rigidity is the predominant presenting symptom.

Dosage Forms

Tablet:

10/100: Carbidopa 10 mg and levodopa 100 mg

25/100: Carbidopa 25 mg and levodopa 100 mg

25/250: Carbidopa 25 mg and levodopa 250 mg

Tablet, sustained release:

Carbidopa 25 mg and levodopa 100 mg

Carbidopa 50 mg and levodopa 200 mg

Levomethadyl Acetate Hydrochloride

(lee voe METH a dil AS e tate hye droe KLOR ide)

Related Information

Addiction Treatments *on page 550*

Patient Information - Miscellaneous Medications *on page 495*

U.S. Brand Names ORLAAM®

Pharmacologic Category Analgesic, Narcotic

Generic Available No

Use Management of opiate dependence; should be reserved for use in treatment of opiate-addicted patients who fail to show an acceptable response to other adequate treatments for addiction

Restrictions C-II; must be dispensed in a designated clinic setting only

Pregnancy Risk Factor C

Contraindications Hypersensitivity to levomethadyl or any component of the formulation; known or suspected QT_c prolongation (male: 430 msec, female: 450 msec); bradycardia (<50 bpm); significant cardiac disease; concurrent treatment with drugs known to prolong QT interval, including class I and III antiarrhythmics; concurrent treatment with MAO inhibitors; hypokalemia or hypomagnesemia

Warnings/Precautions May cause QT prolongation. Use of levomethadyl has been associated with rare, but serious cardiac arrhythmias. Perform EKG prior to treatment, 12-14 days after initiation, and periodically thereafter. Not recommended for use outside of the treatment of opiate addiction; shall be dispensed only by treatment programs approved by FDA, DEA, and the designated state authority. Approved treatment programs shall dispense and use levomethadyl in oral form only and according to the treatment requirements stipulated in federal regulations. Failure to abide by these requirements may result in injunction precluding operation of the program, seizure of the drug supply, revocation of the program approval, and possible criminal prosecution.

Use only with **extreme caution** in patients with head injury or increased intracranial pressure (ICP). Use with caution in patients with respiratory disease or asthma. Has been studied only in 3 times/week or every-other-day dosing; daily administration may lead to accumulation/risk of overdose. Use caution in the elderly and in patients with hepatic or renal dysfunctions. Safety and efficacy in pediatric patients have not been established.

Adverse Reactions
>10%:
Central nervous system: Malaise
Miscellaneous: Flu syndrome
1% to 10%:
Central nervous system: CNS depression, sedation, chills, abnormal dreams, anxiety, euphoria, headache, insomnia, nervousness, hypesthesia
Endocrine & metabolic: Hot flashes (males 2:1)
Gastrointestinal: Abdominal pain, constipation, diarrhea, xerostomia, nausea, vomiting
Genitourinary: Urinary tract spasm, difficult ejaculation, impotence, decreased sex drive
Neuromuscular & skeletal: Arthralgia, back pain, weakness
Ocular: Miosis, blurred vision
<1%: Amenorrhea, amnesia, angina, confusion, hepatitis, incoordination, myalgia, postural hypotension, pyuria, seizures, S-T segment increased, tearing
Postmarketing and/or case reports: Apnea, breast enlargement, cardiac arrest, chest pain, dyspnea, hallucinations, migraine, myocardial infarction, QT_c prolongation, syncope, ventricular tachycardia; serious cardiac arrhythmias have been reported including torsade de pointes

Overdosage/Toxicology Consider possibility of multiple drug ingestion. Treatment should be symptom-directed and supportive. Naloxone may be used (as airway protection) and should be titrated to clinical effect. Due to duration of activity, repeated naloxone dosing may be needed.

Drug Interactions CYP3A3/4 enzyme substrate
Antiarrhythmics: Concurrent use is contraindicated.
CNS depressants: Sedative, tranquilizers, propoxyphene, antidepressants, benzodiazepines, alcohol used in combination with levomethadyl may result in serious overdose
Enzyme inducers: Carbamazepine, phenobarbital, rifampin, phenytoin may enhance the metabolism of levomethadyl leading to an increase in levomethadyl peak effect and shorten its duration of action
Enzyme inhibitors: Erythromycin, cimetidine, and ketoconazole may increase risk of arrhythmia, slow the onset, lower the activity, and/or increase the duration of action of levomethadyl
Linezolid: Due to MAO inhibition, use should be avoided.
MAO inhibitors: Concurrent use is contraindicated (per manufacturer).
Meperidine: May be ineffective in patients taking levomethadyl
Opiate antagonists and partial antagonists: Levomethadyl used in combination with naloxone, naltrexone, pentazocine, nalbuphine, butorphanol, and buprenorphine may result in withdrawal symptoms
QT_c-prolonging agents: Concurrent use is contraindicated. Includes antiarrhythmics, bepridil, cisapride, macrolides (erythromycin and clarithromycin), some fluoroquinolones (gatifloxacin, moxifloxacin, sparfloxacin), haloperidol, phenothiazines (particularly mesoridazine, thioridazine, or zonisamide), pimozide, terfenadine, and tricyclic antidepressants.
Selegiline: Concurrent use of nonselective MAO inhibitors is contraindicated. Safety of selective MAO type B inhibitors has not been established.

Ethanol/Nutrition/Herb Interactions Ethanol: Avoid ethanol (may increase CNS depression, may lead to overdose).

Stability Store at room temperature.

Mechanism of Action A synthetic opioid agonist with actions similar to morphine; principal actions are analgesia and sedation. Its clinical effects in the treatment of opiate abuse occur through two mechanisms: 1) cross-sensitivity for opiates of the morphine type, suppressing symptoms of withdrawal in opiate-dependent persons; 2) with chronic oral administration, can produce sufficient tolerance to block the subjective high of usual doses of parenterally administered opiates

Pharmacodynamics/Kinetics
Protein binding: 80%
(Continued)

Levomethadyl Acetate Hydrochloride *(Continued)*

Metabolism: Hepatic to L-alpha-noracetylmethadol and L-alpha-dinoracetylmethadol (active metabolites)

Half-life: 35-60 hours

Time to peak serum concentration: 1.5-6 hours

Elimination: Renal products as methadol and normethadol

Usual Dosage Adults: Oral: 20-40 mg at 48- or 72-hour intervals, with ranges of 10 mg to as high as 140 mg 3 times/week; adjust dose in increments of 5-10 mg (too rapid induction may lead to overdose); always dilute before administration and mix with diluent prior to dispensing

Monitoring Parameters Patient adherence with regimen and avoidance of illicit substances; random drug testing is recommended; EKG prior to treatment, 12-14 days after initiation, and periodically thereafter

Nursing Implications Drug administration and dispensing is to take place in an authorized clinic setting only; can potentially cause QT prolongation on EKG (not dose related)

Additional Information The product labeling for ORLAAM® (levomethadyl acetate hydrochloride) has been changed to reflect reports of 10 cases of serious arrhythmias submitted through MedWatch (as of March 30, 2001). On April 18, 2001, the manufacturer (Roxane Laboratories, Inc) mailed a Dear Healthcare Professional letter to physicians licensed to treat narcotic addiction. A black box warning has been added to highlight the seriousness of these reactions. In addition, the approved indication for levomethadyl has been revised, indicating levomethadyl should be reserved for use in treatment of opiate-addicted patients who fail to show an acceptable response to other adequate treatments for addiction.

Dosage Forms Solution, oral: 10 mg/mL (474 mL)

- ♦ **Levo-T**™ *see Levothyroxine on page 198*
- ♦ **Levotabs**® *see Levothyroxine on page 198*
- ♦ **Levothroid**® *see Levothyroxine on page 198*

Levothyroxine *(lee voe thye ROKS een)*

U.S. Brand Names Levo-T™; Levotabs®; Levothroid®; Levoxyl®; Synthroid®; Thyrox®; Unithroid™

Canadian Brand Names Eltroxin®; PMS-Levothyroxine Sodium

Synonyms Levothyroxine Sodium; *L*-Thyroxine Sodium; T_4

Pharmacologic Category Thyroid Product

Generic Available Yes

Use Replacement or supplemental therapy in hypothyroidism; some clinicians suggest levothyroxine is the drug of choice for replacement therapy

Pregnancy Risk Factor A

Contraindications Hypersensitivity to levothyroxine sodium or any component of the formulation; recent myocardial infarction or thyrotoxicosis; uncorrected adrenal insufficiency

Warnings/Precautions Ineffective for weight reduction; high doses may produce serious or even life-threatening toxic effects particularly when used with some anorectic drugs. Use with caution and reduce dosage in patients with angina pectoris or other cardiovascular disease; levothyroxine tablets contain tartrazine dye which may cause allergic reactions in susceptible individuals; use cautiously in elderly since they may be more likely to have compromised cardiovascular functions. Patients with adrenal insufficiency, myxedema, diabetes mellitus and insipidus may have symptoms exaggerated or aggravated; thyroid replacement requires periodic assessment of thyroid status. Chronic hypothyroidism predisposes patients to coronary artery disease.

Adverse Reactions Frequency not defined: Palpitations, cardiac arrhythmias, tachycardia, chest pain, nervousness, headache, insomnia, fever, ataxia, alopecia, changes in menstrual cycle, weight loss, increased appetite, diarrhea, abdominal cramps, constipation, myalgia, hand tremors, tremor, dyspnea, diaphoresis, vomiting, allergic skin reactions (rare)

Overdosage/Toxicology

Signs and symptoms: Chronic overdose may cause hyperthyroidism, weight loss, nervousness, sweating, tachycardia, insomnia, heat intolerance, menstrual irregularities, palpitations, psychosis, fever; acute overdose may cause fever, hypoglycemia, CHF, unrecognized adrenal insufficiency

Treatment: Chronic overdose is treated by withdrawal of the drug; massive overdose may require beta-blockers for increased sympathomimetic activity. Reduce dose or temporarily discontinue therapy; normal hypothalamic-pituitary-thyroid axis will return to normal in 6-8 weeks; serum T_4 levels do not correlate well with toxicity; in massive acute ingestion, reduce GI absorption, administer general supportive care; treat congestive heart failure with digitalis glycosides; excessive adrenergic activity (tachycardia) require propranolol 1-3 mg I.V. over 10 minutes or 80-160 mg orally/day; fever may be treated with acetaminophen.

Drug Interactions CYP enzyme substrate (T_3 and T_4); thyroid hormone may alter metabolic activity of cytochrome P450 enzymes

Aluminum- and magnesium-containing antacids, calcium carbonate, simethicone, or sucralfate: May decrease T_4 absorption; separate dose from levothyroxine by at least 4 hours.

Antidiabetic agents (biguanides, meglitinides, sulfonylureas, thiazolidinediones, insulin): Changes in thyroid function may alter requirements of antidiabetic agent. Monitor closely at initiation of therapy, or when dose is changed or discontinued.

Cholestyramine and colestipol: Decrease T_4 absorption; separate dose from levothyroxine by at least 4 hours.

CYP enzyme inducers: May increase the metabolism of T_3 and T_4. Inducers include barbiturates, carbamazepine, phenytoin, and rifampin/rifabutin.

Digoxin: Digoxin levels may be reduced in hyperthyroidism; therapeutic effect may be reduced. Impact of thyroid replacement should be monitored.

Iron: Decreases T_4 absorption; separate dose from levothyroxine by at least 4 hours.

Kayexalate®: Decreases T_4 absorption; separate dose from levothyroxine by at least 4 hours.

Ketamine: May cause marked hypertension and tachycardia; monitor.

Ritonavir: May alter response to levothyroxine (limited documentation/case report); monitor.

Somatrem, somatropin: Excessive thyroid hormone levels lead to accelerated epiphyseal closure; inadequate replacement interferes with growth response to growth hormone. Effect of thyroid replacement not specifically evaluated; use caution.

SSRI antidepressants: May need to increase dose of levothyroxine when SSRI is added to a previously stabilized patient.

Sympathomimetics: Effects of sympathomimetic agent or levothyroxine may be increased. Risk of coronary insufficiency is increased in patients with coronary artery disease when these agents are used together.

Theophylline, caffeine: Decreased theophylline clearance in hypothyroid patients; monitor during thyroid replacement.

Tricyclic and tetracyclic antidepressants: Therapeutic and toxic effects of levothyroxine and the antidepressant are increased.

Warfarin (and other oral anticoagulants): The hypoprothrombinemic response to warfarin may be altered by a change in thyroid function or replacement. Replacement may dramatically increase response to warfarin. However, initiation of warfarin in a patient stabilized on a dose of levothyroxine does not appear to require a significantly different approach.

Note: Several medications have effects on thyroid production or conversion. The impact in thyroid replacement has not been specifically evaluated, but patient response should be monitored:

Methimazole: Decreases thyroid hormone secretion, while propylthiouracil decrease thyroid hormone secretion and decreases conversion of T_4 to T_3.

(Continued)

Levothyroxine *(Continued)*

Beta-adrenergic antagonists: Decrease conversion of T_4 to T_3 (dose related, propranolol $\geq$160 mg/day); patients may be clinically euthyroid.

Iodide, iodine-containing radiographic contrast agents may decrease thyroid hormone secretion; may also increase thyroid hormone secretion, especially in patients with Graves' disease.

Other agents reported to impact on thyroid production/conversion include amino-glutethimide, amiodarone, chloral hydrate, diazepam, ethionamide, interferon-alpha, interleukin-2, lithium, lovastatin (case report), glucocorticoids (dose-related), 6-mercaptopurine, sulfonamides, thiazide diuretics, and tolbutamide.

In addition, a number of medications have been noted to cause transient depression in TSH secretion, which may complicate interpretation of monitoring tests for levothyroxine, including corticosteroids, octreotide, and dopamine. Metoclopramide may increase TSH secretion.

Ethanol/Nutrition/Herb Interactions Food: Taking levothyroxine with enteral nutrition may cause reduced bioavailability and may lower serum thyroxine levels leading to signs or symptoms of hypothyroidism. Limit intake of goitrogenic foods (eg, asparagus, cabbage, peas, turnip greens, broccoli, spinach, Brussels sprouts, lettuce, soybeans). Soybean flour (infant formula), walnuts, and dietary fiber may decrease absorption of levothyroxine from the GI tract.

Stability Protect tablets from light; do not mix I.V. solution with other I.V. infusion solutions; reconstituted solutions should be used immediately and any unused portions discarded

Mechanism of Action Exact mechanism of action is unknown; however, it is believed the thyroid hormone exerts its many metabolic effects through control of DNA transcription and protein synthesis; involved in normal metabolism, growth, and development; promotes gluconeogenesis, increases utilization and mobilization of glycogen stores, and stimulates protein synthesis, increases basal metabolic rate

Usual Dosage

Children: Congenital hypothyroidism:

Oral:

0-6 months: 8-10 mcg/kg/day **or** 25-50 mcg/day

6-12 months: 6-8 mcg/kg/day **or** 50-75 mcg/day

1-5 years: 5-6 mcg/kg/day **or** 75-100 mcg/day

6-12 years: 4-5 mcg/kg/day **or** 100-150 mcg/day

>12 years: 2-3 mcg/kg/day **or** $\geq$150 mcg/day

I.M., I.V.: 50% to 75% of the oral dose

Adults:

Oral: Initial: 0.05 mg/day, then increase by increments of 25 mcg/day at intervals of 2-3 weeks; average adult dose: 100-200 mcg/day; maximum dose: 200 mcg/day

I.M., I.V.: 50% of the oral dose

Myxedema coma or stupor: I.V.: 200-500 mcg one time, then 100-300 mcg the next day if necessary

Thyroid suppression therapy: Oral: 2-6 mcg/kg/day for 7-10 days

Dietary Considerations Should be administered on an empty stomach.

Administration

Oral: Administer on an empty stomach

Parenteral: Dilute vial with 5 mL normal saline; use immediately after reconstitution; administer by direct I.V. infusion over 2- to 3-minute period. I.V. form must be prepared immediately prior to administration; should not be admixed with other solutions

Monitoring Parameters Thyroid function test (serum thyroxine, thyrotropin concentrations), resin triiodothyronine uptake (RT_3U), free thyroxine index (FTI), T_4, TSH, heart rate, blood pressure, clinical signs of hypo- and hyperthyroidism; TSH is the most reliable guide for evaluating adequacy of thyroid replacement dosage. TSH may be elevated during the first few months of thyroid replacement despite patients being clinically euthyroid. In cases where T_4 remains low and TSH is within normal limits, an evaluation of "free" (unbound) T_4 is needed to evaluate further increase in dosage

Reference Range Pediatrics: Cord T_4 and values in the first few weeks are much higher, falling over the first months and years. ≥10 years: ~5.8-11 µg/dL (SI: 75-142 nmol/L). Borderline low: ≤4.5-5.7 µg/dL (SI: 58-73 nmol/L); low: ≤4.4 µg/dL (SI: 57 nmol/L); results <2.5 µg/dL (SI: <32 nmol/L) are strong evidence for hypothyroidism.

Approximate adult normal range: 4-12 µg/dL (SI: 51-154 nmol/L). Borderline high: 11.1-13 µg/dL (SI: 143-167 nmol/L); high: ≥13.1 µg/dL (SI: 169 nmol/L). Normal range is increased in women on birth control pills (5.5-12 µg/dL); normal range in pregnancy: ~5.5-16 µg/dL (SI: ~71-206 nmol/L). TSH: 0.4-10 (for those ≥80 years) mIU/L; T_4: 4-12 µg/dL (SI: 51-154 nmol/L); T_3 (RIA) (total T_3): 80-230 ng/dL (SI: 1.2-3.5 nmol/L); T_4 free (free T_4): 0.7-1.8 ng/dL (SI: 9-23 pmol/L).

Test Interactions Many drugs may have effects on thyroid function tests; para-aminosalicylic acid, aminoglutethimide, amiodarone, barbiturates, carbamazepine, chloral hydrate, clofibrate, colestipol, corticosteroids, danazol, diazepam, estrogens, ethionamide, fluorouracil, I.V. heparin, insulin, lithium, methadone, methimazole, mitotane, nitroprusside, oxyphenbutazone, phenylbutazone, PTU, perphenazine, phenytoin, propranolol, salicylates, sulfonylureas, and thiazides

Patient Information Thyroid replacement therapy is generally for life. Take as directed, in the morning before breakfast. Do not change brands and do not discontinue without consulting prescriber. Consult prescriber if drastically increasing or decreasing intake of goitrogenic food (eg, asparagus, cabbage, peas, turnip greens, broccoli, spinach, Brussels sprouts, lettuce, soybeans). Report chest pain, rapid heart rate, palpitations, heat intolerance, excessive sweating, increased nervousness, agitation, or lethargy.

Nursing Implications I.V. form must be prepared immediately prior to administration; should not be mixed with other solutions

Additional Information Levothroid® tablets contain lactose and tartrazine dye

Equivalent doses: Thyroid USP 60 mg ~ levothyroxine 0.05-0.06 mg ~ liothyronine 0.015-0.0375 mg

50-60 mg thyroid ~ 50-60 mcg levothyroxine and 12.5-15 mcg liothyronine Liotrix®

Dosage Forms

Powder for injection, lyophilized, as sodium: 200 mcg/vial (6 mL, 10 mL); 500 mcg/vial (6 mL, 10 mL)

Tablet, as sodium: 25 mcg, 50 mcg, 75 mcg, 88 mcg, 100 mcg, 112 mcg, 125 mcg, 137 mcg, 150 mcg, 175 mcg, 200 mcg, 300 mcg

♦ **Levothyroxine Sodium** *see* Levothyroxine *on page 198*

♦ **Levoxyl®** *see* Levothyroxine *on page 198*

♦ **Librium®** *see* Chlordiazepoxide *on page 71*

Licorice

Synonyms *Glycyrrhiza glabra*; *G. palidiflora*; *G. uralensis*; Sweet Root

Pharmacologic Category Herb

Use Foodstuff in chewing gum, chewing tobacco, cough preparations

Per Commission E: Catarrhs of the upper respiratory tract and gastric/duodenal ulcers

Restrictions Per Commission E: Not more than 4-6 weeks administration without medical advice; there is no objection of using licorice as a flavoring agent up to maximum daily dose: 100 mg glycyrrhizin

Pregnancy Risk Factor Contraindicated per Commission E

Contraindications Per Commission E: Cholestatic liver disorders, liver cirrhosis, hypertonia, hypokalemia, severe kidney insufficiency, pregnancy

Adverse Reactions

Cardiovascular: Hypertension

Central nervous system: Headache, seizures, tetany

(Continued)

Licorice *(Continued)*

Endocrine & metabolic: Amenorrhea, hyponatremia, hypokalemia, hypomagnesemia

Neuromuscular & skeletal: Myopathy, carpopedal spasms, rhabdomyolysis

Ocular: Bilateral ptosis

Renal: Myoglobinuria

Per Commission E: On prolonged use and with higher doses, mineral corticoid effects may occur in the form of sodium and water retention and potassium loss, accompanied by hypertension, edema, and hypokalemia, and in rare cases, myoglobinuria

Overdosage/Toxicology Treatment: Supportive therapy; fluid/electrolyte (especially potassium) replacement; spironolactone (1 g/day in divided doses) also may be useful in reversing electrolyte abnormalities; tetany can be treated with magnesium sulfate

Drug Interactions

Attenuated effect of strychnine, tetrodoxine, nicotine, cocaine, barbiturates, pilocarpine, urethane, epinephrine, and ephedrine through glucuronic-like conjugation action; traditional emmenagogue; increases progesterone and cortisol half-life; concomitant use of furosemide can exacerbate hypokalemia

Per Commission E: Potassium loss due to other drugs (eg, thiazide diuretics), can be increased; with potassium loss, sensitivity to digitalis glycosides increases

Usual Dosage

100 g (equivalent to 700 mg of glycyrrhizinic acid) of licorice found in 2-4 licorice twists; toxic effect can be seen if ingested daily (2-3 twists) for 2-4 weeks

Per Commission E: 5-15 g root/day, equivalent to 200-600 mg glycyrrhizin; succus liquiritiae (juice): 0.5-1 g for catarrhs of upper respiratory tract; 1.5-3 g for gastric/duodenal ulcers; equivalent preparations

Patient Information Considered unsafe

Additional Information Syndrome of pseudoprimary hyperaldosteronism is a complication of chronic licorice ingestion; serum potassium as low as 0.9 mmol/L has been noted

- ◆ **Limbitrol®** *see* Amitriptyline and Chlordiazepoxide *on page 25*
- ◆ **Limbitrol® DS** *see* Amitriptyline and Chlordiazepoxide *on page 25*

Liothyronine *(lye oh THYE roe neen)*

U.S. Brand Names Cytomel®; Triostat™

Canadian Brand Names Cytomel

Synonyms Liothyronine Sodium; Sodium *L*-Triiodothyronine; T_3 Sodium

Pharmacologic Category Thyroid Product

Generic Available Yes

Use Replacement or supplemental therapy in hypothyroidism; management of nontoxic goiter, chronic lymphocytic thyroiditis, as an adjunct in thyrotoxicosis and as a diagnostic aid; **levothyroxine is recommended for chronic therapy;** although previously thought to benefit cardiac patients with severely reduced fractions, liothyronine injection is no longer considered beneficial

Orphan drug: Triostat™: Treatment of myxedema coma/precoma

Pregnancy Risk Factor A

Contraindications Hypersensitivity to liothyronine sodium or any component of the formulation; undocumented or uncorrected adrenal insufficiency; recent myocardial infarction or thyrotoxicosis

Warnings/Precautions Ineffective for weight reduction; high doses may produce serious or even life-threatening toxic effects particularly when used with some anorectic drugs. Use with extreme caution in patients with angina pectoris or other cardiovascular disease (including hypertension) or coronary artery disease; use with caution in elderly patients since they may be more likely to have compromised cardiovascular function. Patients with adrenal insufficiency, myxedema, diabetes mellitus and insipidus may have symptoms exaggerated or aggravated; thyroid replacement requires periodic assessment of thyroid status. Chronic hypothyroidism predisposes patients to coronary artery disease.

Adverse Reactions Frequency not defined: Palpitations, cardiac arrhythmias, tachycardia, chest pain, nervousness, headache, insomnia, fever, ataxia, alopecia, changes in menstrual cycle, weight loss, increased appetite, diarrhea, abdominal cramps, constipation, myalgia, hand tremors, tremor, dyspnea, diaphoresis, vomiting, allergic skin reactions (rare)

Overdosage/Toxicology

Signs and symptoms: Chronic overdose may cause hyperthyroidism, weight loss, nervousness, sweating, tachycardia, insomnia, heat intolerance, menstrual irregularities, palpitations, psychosis, fever; acute overdose may cause fever, hypoglycemia, CHF, unrecognized adrenal insufficiency.

Treatment: Reduce dose or temporarily discontinue therapy; normal hypothalamic-pituitary-thyroid axis will return to normal in 6-8 weeks; serum T_4 levels do not correlate well with toxicity. In massive acute ingestion, reduce GI absorption, administer general supportive care; treat congestive heart failure with digitalis glycosides; excessive adrenergic activity (tachycardia) requires propranolol 1-3 mg I.V. over 10 minutes or 80-160 mg orally/day; fever may be treated with acetaminophen.

Drug Interactions

Aluminum- and magnesium-containing antacids, calcium carbonate, simethicone, or sucralfate: May decrease T_4 absorption; separate dose from thyroid hormones by at least 4 hours.

Antidiabetic agents (biguanides, meglitinides, sulfonylureas, thiazolidinediones, insulin): Changes in thyroid function may alter requirements of antidiabetic agent. Monitor closely at initiation of therapy, or when dose is changed or discontinued.

Cholestyramine and colestipol: Decrease T_4 absorption; separate dose from thyroid hormones by at least 4 hours.

CYP enzyme inducers: May increase the metabolism of T_3 and T_4. Inducers include barbiturates, carbamazepine, phenytoin, and rifampin/rifabutin.

Digoxin: Digoxin levels may be reduced in hyperthyroidism; therapeutic effect may be reduced. Impact of thyroid replacement should be monitored.

Iron: Decreases T_4 absorption; separate dose from thyroid hormones by at least 4 hours

Kayexalate®: Decreases T_4 absorption; separate dose from thyroid hormones by at least 4 hours

Ketamine: May cause marked hypertension and tachycardia; monitor

Ritonavir: May alter response to thyroid hormones (limited documentation/case report); monitor

Somatrem, somatropin: Excessive thyroid hormone levels lead to accelerated epiphyseal closure; inadequate replacement interferes with growth response to growth hormone. Effect of thyroid replacement not specifically evaluated; use caution.

SSRI antidepressants: May need to increase dose of thyroid hormones when SSRI is added to a previously stabilized patient.

Sympathomimetics: Effects of sympathomimetic agent or thyroid hormones may be increased. Risk of coronary insufficiency is increased in patients with coronary artery disease when these agents are used together.

Theophylline, caffeine: Decreased theophylline clearance in hypothyroid patients; monitor during thyroid replacement.

Tricyclic and tetracyclic antidepressants: Therapeutic and toxic effects of thyroid hormones and the antidepressant are increased.

Warfarin (and other oral anticoagulants): The hypoprothrombinemic response to warfarin may be altered by a change in thyroid function or replacement. Replacement may dramatically increase response to warfarin. However, initiation of warfarin in a patient stabilized on a dose of thyroid hormones does not appear to require a significantly different approach.

(Continued)

Liothyronine *(Continued)*

Note: Several medications have effects on thyroid production or conversion. The impact in thyroid replacement has not been specifically evaluated, but patient response should be monitored:

Methimazole: Decreases thyroid hormone secretion, while propylthiouracil decrease thyroid hormone secretion and decreases conversion of T_4 to T_3.

Beta-adrenergic antagonists: Decrease conversion of T_4 to T_3 (dose related, propranolol ≥160 mg/day); patients may be clinically euthyroid.

Iodide, iodine-containing radiographic contrast agents may decrease thyroid hormone secretion; may also increase thyroid hormone secretion, especially in patients with Graves' disease.

Other agents reported to impact on thyroid production/conversion include aminoglutethimide, amiodarone, chloral hydrate, diazepam, ethionamide, interferon-alpha, interleukin-2, lithium, lovastatin (case report), glucocorticoids (dose-related), 6-mercaptopurine, sulfonamides, thiazide diuretics, and tolbutamide.

In addition, a number of medications have been noted to cause transient depression in TSH secretion, which may complicate interpretation of monitoring tests for thyroid hormones, including corticosteroids, octreotide, and dopamine. Metoclopramide may increase TSH secretion.

Ethanol/Nutrition/Herb Interactions Food: Limit intake of goitrogenic foods (asparagus, cabbage, peas, turnip greens, broccoli, spinach, Brussels sprouts, lettuce, soybeans)

Stability Vials must be stored under refrigeration at 2°C to 8°C (36°F to 46°F)

Mechanism of Action Primary active compound is T_3 (triiodothyronine), which may be converted from T_4 (thyroxine) and then circulates throughout the body to influence growth and maturation of various tissues; exact mechanism of action is unknown; however, it is believed the thyroid hormone exerts its many metabolic effects through control of DNA transcription and protein synthesis; involved in normal metabolism, growth, and development; promotes gluconeogenesis, increases utilization and mobilization of glycogen stores, and stimulates protein synthesis, increases basal metabolic rate

Usual Dosage

Congenital hypothyroidism: Children: Oral: 5 mcg/day increase by 5 mcg every 3-4 days until the desired response is achieved. Usual maintenance dose: 20 mcg/day for infants, 50 mcg/day for children 1-3 years of age, and adult dose for children >3 years.

Hypothyroidism: Oral:

Adults: 25 mcg/day increase by increments of 12.5-25 mcg/day every 1-2 weeks to a maximum of 100 mcg/day; usual maintenance dose: 25-75 mcg/day

Elderly: Initial: 5 mcg/day, increase by 5 mcg/day every 1-2 weeks; usual maintenance dose: 25-75 mcg/day

T_3 suppression test: Oral: 75-100 mcg/day for 7 days; use lowest dose for elderly

Myxedema: Oral: Initial: 5 mcg/day; increase in increments of 5-10 mcg/day every 1-2 weeks. When 25 mcg/day is reached, dosage may be increased at intervals of 12.5-25 mcg/day every 1-2 weeks. Usual maintenance dose: 50-100 mcg/day.

Myxedema coma: I.V.: 25-50 mcg

Patients with known or suspected cardiovascular disease: 10-20 mcg

Note: Normally, at least 4 hours should be allowed between doses to adequately assess therapeutic response and no more than 12 hours should elapse between doses to avoid fluctuations in hormone levels. Oral therapy should be resumed as soon as the clinical situation has been stabilized and the patient is able to take oral medication. If levothyroxine rather than liothyronine sodium is used in initiating oral therapy, the physician should bear in mind that there is a delay of several days in the onset of levothyroxine activity and that I.V. therapy should be discontinued gradually.

Administration For I.V. use only - **do not administer I.M. or S.C.**

Administer doses at least 4 hours, and no more than 12 hours, apart

Resume oral therapy as soon as the clinical situation has been stabilized and the patient is able to take oral medication

When switching to tablets, discontinue the injectable, initiate oral therapy at a low dosage and increase gradually according to response

If **levothyroxine** is used for oral therapy, there is a delay of several days in the onset of activity; therefore, discontinue I.V. therapy gradually

Monitoring Parameters T_4, TSH, heart rate, blood pressure, clinical signs of hypo- and hyperthyroidism; TSH is the most reliable guide for evaluating adequacy of thyroid replacement dosage. TSH may be elevated during the first few months of thyroid replacement despite patients being clinically euthyroid. In cases where T_4 remains low and TSH is within normal limits, an evaluation of "free" (unbound) T_4 is needed to evaluate further increase in dosage.

Reference Range Free T_3, serum: 250-390 pg/dL; TSH: 0.4 and up to 10 (≥80 years) mIU/L; remains normal in pregnancy

Test Interactions Many drugs may have effects on thyroid function tests; para-aminosalicylic acid, aminoglutethimide, amiodarone, barbiturates, carbamazepine, chloral hydrate, clofibrate, colestipol, corticosteroids, danazol, diazepam, estrogens, ethionamide, fluorouracil, I.V. heparin, insulin, lithium, methadone, methimazole, mitotane, nitroprusside, oxyphenbutazone, phenylbutazone, PTU, perphenazine, phenytoin, propranolol, salicylates, sulfonylureas, and thiazides

Patient Information Take as directed; do not change brands of medication or discontinue without consulting prescriber. Do not change diet without consulting prescriber. Report chest pain, increased heartbeat, palpitations, excessive weight gain or loss, change in level of energy (increased or decreased), excessive sweating, or intolerance to heat.

Nursing Implications I.V. form must be prepared immediately prior to administration; dilute 200 mcg/mL vial with 2 mL of 0.9% sodium chloride injection and shake well until a clear solution is obtained; should not be admixed with other solutions

Additional Information

Equivalent doses: Thyroid USP 60 mg ~ levothyroxine 0.05-0.06 mg ~ liothyronine 0.015-0.0375 mg

50-60 mg thyroid ~ 50-60 mcg levothyroxine and 12.5-15 mcg liothyronine

Dosage Forms

Injection, as sodium: 10 mcg/mL (1 mL)

Tablet, as sodium: 5 mcg, 25 mcg, 50 mcg

♦ **Liothyronine Sodium** *see* Liothyronine *on page 202*

♦ **Liquid Compatibility With Antipsychotics and Mood Stabilizers** *see page 587*

Lithium (LITH ee um)

Related Information

Liquid Compatibility With Antipsychotics and Mood Stabilizers *on page 587*
Mood Stabilizers *on page 588*
Patient Information - Mood Stabilizers (Lithium) *on page 471*
Teratogenic Risks of Psychotropic Medications *on page 594*

U.S. Brand Names Eskalith®; Eskalith CR®; Lithobid®; Lithostat®

Canadian Brand Names Carbolith™; Duralith®; Lithizine

Synonyms Lithium Carbonate; Lithium Citrate

Pharmacologic Category Lithium

Generic Available Yes

Use Management of bipolar disorders

Unlabeled/Investigational Use Potential augmenting agent for antidepressants; aggression, post-traumatic stress disorder, conduct disorder in children

Pregnancy Risk Factor D

Contraindications Hypersensitivity to lithium or any component of the formulation; severe cardiovascular or renal disease; severe debilitation, dehydration, or sodium depletion; pregnancy

(Continued)

Lithium (Continued)

Warnings/Precautions Lithium toxicity is closely related to serum levels and can occur at therapeutic doses; serum lithium determinations are required to monitor therapy. Use with caution in patients with cardiovascular or thyroid disease, or in patients receiving medications which alter sodium excretion (eg, diuretics, ACE inhibitors, NSAIDs). Some elderly patients may be extremely sensitive to the effects of lithium, see Usual Dosage and Reference Range. Chronic therapy results in diminished renal concentrating ability (nephrogenic DI). Changes in renal function should be monitored, and re-evaluation of treatment may be necessary.

Use with caution in patients receiving neuroleptic medications - a syndrome resembling NMS has been associated with concurrent therapy. Lithium may impair the patient's alertness, affecting the ability to operate machinery or driving a vehicle. Neuromuscular blocking agents should be administered with caution - the response may be prolonged.

Higher serum concentrations may be required and tolerated during an acute manic phase; however, the tolerance decreases when symptoms subside. Normal fluid and salt intake must be maintained during therapy.

Adverse Reactions

Cardiovascular: Cardiac arrhythmias, hypotension, sinus node dysfunction, flattened or inverted T waves (reversible), edema

Central nervous system: Dizziness, vertigo, slurred speech, blackout spells, seizures, sedation, restlessness, confusion, psychomotor retardation, stupor, coma, dystonia, fatigue, lethargy, headache, pseudotumor cerebri

Dermatologic: Dry or thinning of hair, folliculitis, alopecia, exacerbation of psoriasis, rash

Endocrine & metabolic: Euthyroid goiter and/or hypothyroidism, hyperthyroidism, hyperglycemia, diabetes insipidus

Gastrointestinal: Polydipsia, anorexia, nausea, vomiting, diarrhea, xerostomia, metallic taste, weight gain

Genitourinary: Incontinence, polyuria, glycosuria, oliguria, albuminuria

Hematologic: Leukocytosis

Neuromuscular & skeletal: Tremor, muscle hyperirritability, ataxia, choreoathetoid movements, hyperactive deep tendon reflexes

Ocular: Nystagmus, blurred vision

Miscellaneous: Discoloration of fingers and toes

Overdosage/Toxicology

Signs and symptoms: Sedation, confusion, tremors, joint pain, visual changes, seizures, coma

Treatment: There is no specific antidote for lithium poisoning. In the acute ingestion following initiation of essential overdose management, correction of fluid and electrolyte imbalances should be commenced.

Hemodialysis is the treatment of choice for severe intoxications

Charcoal is ineffective

Drug Interactions

ACE inhibitors: May increase the risk of lithium toxicity via sodium depletion; monitor

Angiotensin receptor antagonists (losartan): May reduce the renal clearance of lithium; monitor

Carbamazepine: Concurrent use of lithium with carbamazepine, diltiazem may increase the risk for neurotoxicity; monitor

Carbonic anhydrase inhibitors: May decrease lithium levels; includes acetazolamide; monitor

Calcium channel blockers (diltiazem and verapamil): May increase the risk for neurotoxicity; monitor; does not appear to involve dihydropyridine class

Chlorpromazine: May lower serum concentrations of both drugs; monitor

Haloperidol: May increase the risk for neurotoxicity; monitor

Iodine salts: May enhance the hypothyroid effects of lithium; monitor

Loop diuretics: May decrease the renal excretion of lithium, leading to toxicity; monitor

MAO inhibitors: Should generally be avoided due to use reports of fatal malignant hyperpyrexia when combined with lithium

Methyldopa: May increase the risk for neurotoxicity; monitor

Metronidazole: May increase lithium toxicity (rare); monitor

Neuromuscular blocking agents: Lithium may potentiate the response to neuro-muscular blockade, resulting in prolonged blockade and possible delayed recovery

NSAIDs: Renal lithium excretion may be decreased leading to increased serum lithium concentrations; sulindac and aspirin may be the exceptions; monitor

Phenothiazines: May increase the risk for neurotoxicity; monitor

Phenytoin: May enhance lithium toxicity; monitor

Selegiline: Risk of severe reactions when combined with MAO inhibitors may be decreased when administered with selective MAO type-B inhibitor, particularly at selegiline doses <10 mg/day; however, theoretical risk is still present

SSRIs: May increase the risk for neurotoxicity; monitor; effect noted with fluoxe-tine, fluvoxamine

Sibutramine: Combined use of lithium with sibutramine may increase the risk of serotonin syndrome; this combination is best avoided

Sodium-containing products: Bicarbonate and/or high sodium intake may reduce serum lithium concentrations via enhanced excretion; monitor

Sympathomimetics: Lithium may blunt the pressor response to sympathomimetics (epinephrine, phenylephrine, norepinephrine)

Tetracyclines: May increase lithium levels; monitor

Theophylline: May increase real clearance of lithium, resulting in a decrease in serum lithium concentrations; monitor

Thiazide diuretics: May increase serum lithium concentration via sodium depletion and decreased lithium clearance; a lithium dose reduction of 50% is commonly recommended

Tricyclic antidepressants: May increase the risk for neurotoxicity; monitor

Ethanol/Nutrition/Herb Interactions Food: Lithium serum concentrations may be increased if taken with food. Limit caffeine.

Mechanism of Action Alters cation transport across cell membrane in nerve and muscle cells and influences reuptake of serotonin and/or norepinephrine; second messenger systems involving the phosphatidylinositol cycle are inhibited; postsyn-aptic D2 receptor supersensitivity is inhibited

Pharmacodynamics/Kinetics

Distribution: V_d: Initial: 0.3-0.4 L/kg; V_{dss}: 0.7-1 L/kg; crosses the placenta; appears in breast milk at 35% to 50% the concentrations in serum

Half-life: 18-24 hours; can increase to more than 36 hours in elderly or patients with renal impairment

Time to peak serum concentration (nonsustained release product): Within 0.5-2 hours following oral absorption

Elimination: 90% to 98% of dose excreted in urine as unchanged drug; other excretory routes include feces (1%) and sweat (4% to 5%)

Usual Dosage Oral: Monitor serum concentrations and clinical response (efficacy and toxicity) to determine proper dose

Children 6-12 years:

Bipolar disorder: 15-60 mg/kg/day in 3-4 divided doses; dose not to exceed usual adult dosage

Conduct disorder (unlabeled use): 15-30 mg/kg/day in 3-4 divided doses; dose not to exceed usual adult dosage

Adults: Bipolar disorder: 900-2400 mg/day in 3-4 divided doses or 900-1800 mg/day (sustained release) in 2 divided doses

Elderly: Bipolar disorder: Initial dose: 300 mg once or twice daily; increase weekly in increments of 300 mg/day, monitoring levels; rarely need >900-1200 mg/day

Dosing adjustment in renal impairment:

Cl_{cr} 10-50 mL/minute: Administer 50% to 75% of normal dose

(Continued)

Lithium *(Continued)*

Cl$_{cr}$ <10 mL/minute: Administer 25% to 50% of normal dose

Hemodialysis: Dialyzable (50% to 100%)

Dietary Considerations May be administered with meals to avoid GI upset; have patient drink 2-3 L of water daily.

Administration Administer with meals to decrease GI upset

Monitoring Parameters Serum lithium every 4-5 days during initial therapy; draw lithium serum concentrations 12 hours postdose; renal, thyroid, and cardiovascular function; fluid status; serum electrolytes; CBC with differential, urinalysis; monitor for signs of toxicity; b-HCG pregnancy test for all females not known to be sterile

Reference Range Levels should be obtained twice weekly until both patient's clinical status and levels are stable then levels may be obtained every 1-2 months

Timing of serum samples: Draw trough just before next dose

Therapeutic levels:

Acute mania: 0.6-1.2 mEq/L (SI: 0.6-1.2 mmol/L)

Protection against future episodes in most patients with bipolar disorder: 0.8-1 mEq/L (SI: 0.8-1.0 mmol/L); a higher rate of relapse is described in subjects who are maintained at <0.4 mEq/L (SI: 0.4 mmol/L)

Elderly patients can usually be maintained at lower end of therapeutic range (0.6-0.8 mEq/L)

Toxic concentration: >2 mEq/L (SI: >2 mmol/L)

Adverse effect levels:

GI complaints/tremor: 1.5-2 mEq/L

Confusion/somnolence: 2-2.5 mEq/L

Seizures/death: >2.5 mEq/L

Test Interactions ↑ calcium (S), glucose, magnesium, potassium (S); ↓ thyroxine (S)

Patient Information Avoid tasks requiring psychomotor coordination until the CNS effects are known; blood level monitoring is required to determine the proper dose; maintain a steady salt and fluid intake especially during the summer months; do not crush or chew slow or extended release dosage form, swallow whole

Nursing Implications Avoid dehydration

Dosage Forms

Capsule, as carbonate: 150 mg, 300 mg, 600 mg

Syrup, as citrate: 300 mg/5 mL (5 mL, 10 mL, 480 mL)

Tablet, as carbonate: 300 mg

Tablet, controlled release, as carbonate: 450 mg

Tablet, extended release, as carbonate: 300 mg

♦ **Lithium Carbonate** *see Lithium on page 205*

♦ **Lithium Citrate** *see Lithium on page 205*

♦ **Lithizine (Can)** *see Lithium on page 205*

♦ **Lithobid®** *see Lithium on page 205*

♦ **Lithostat®** *see Lithium on page 205*

♦ *Lobela inflata* *see Lobelia on page 208*

Lobelia

Synonyms *Lobela inflata*

Pharmacologic Category Herb

Use Primary use is in homeopathic products; in herbal medicine used as an expectorant; relief of muscle spasms; also incorporated (in doses of 2-4 mg) in tablets/lozenges or chewing gum to aid in smoking cessation

Overdosage/Toxicology

Signs and symptoms: Hypothermia, hypertension, respiratory depression, coma, paralysis, seizures, euphoria, nausea, vomiting, abdominal pain, salivation, dermal irritation, tachycardia, diaphoresis

Decontamination:

Oral: **Do not** induce emesis; lavage (within 1 hour)/ingestions >8 mg of lobeline, 50 mg of dried herb or 1 mL of tincture of lobelia; activated charcoal with cathartic can then be used

Occular: Irrigate with saline copiously

Dermal: Wash with soap and water

Treatment: Supportive therapy; seizures can be treated with benzodiazepines; phenobarbital or phenytoin can be used for refractory seizures; hypotension can be treated with intravenous fluid bolus (10-20 mL/kg) and placement in Trendelenburg position; dopamine or norepinephrine can be used for refractory cases

Usual Dosage

Toxic dose:

Dried herb: 50 mg

Lobelia, tincture: 1 mL

Lobeline: 8 mg

Toxic daily dose: >20 mg

Therapeutic dose:

Lobeline hydrochloride:

S.C.: 10 mg (up to 20 mg/day)

I.V.: 3 mg (maximum daily dose: 20 mg)

Lobeline sulfate: 2-4 mg

Patient Information Considered unsafe; nicotine-like effect; use only for short-term and <50 mg

Additional Information Not reviewed by Commission E; found in eastern North America with small, pale blue flowers; acrid/bitter taste; can cause euphoria; an annual weed which grows by roadsides and in open woods; irritating odor; contains 6% piperidine alkaloids

Lorazepam (lor A ze pam)

Related Information

Anxiolytic/Hypnotic Use in Long-Term Care Facilities *on page 562*

Benzodiazepines Comparison Chart *on page 566*

Federal OBRA Regulations Recommended Maximum Doses *on page 583*

Patient Information - Anxiolytics & Sedative Hypnotics (Benzodiazepines) *on page 483*

U.S. Brand Names Ativan®

Canadian Brand Names Apo®-Lorazepam; Novo-Lorazepam®; Nu-Loraz®; PMS-Lorazepam; Pro-Lorazepam®

Pharmacologic Category Benzodiazepine

Generic Available Yes

Use

Oral: Management of anxiety disorders or short-term relief of the symptoms of anxiety or anxiety associated with depressive symptoms

I.V.: Status epilepticus, preanesthesia for desired amnesia, antiemetic adjunct

Unlabeled/Investigational Use Alcohol detoxification; insomnia; psychogenic catatonia; partial complex seizures

Restrictions C-IV

Pregnancy Risk Factor D

Pregnancy/Breast-Feeding Implications

Clinical effects on the fetus: Crosses the placenta. Respiratory depression or hypotonia if administered near time of delivery.

Breast-feeding/lactation: Crosses into breast milk and no data on clinical effects on the infant. AAP states MAY BE OF CONCERN.

Contraindications Hypersensitivity to lorazepam or any component of the formulation (cross-sensitivity with other benzodiazepines may exist); acute narrow-angle glaucoma; sleep apnea (parenteral); intra-arterial injection of parenteral formulation; severe respiratory insufficiency (except during mechanical ventilation); pregnancy

(Continued)

Lorazepam *(Continued)*

Warnings/Precautions Use with caution in elderly or debilitated patients, patients with hepatic disease (including alcoholics) or renal impairment. Use with caution in patients with respiratory disease or impaired gag reflex. Initial doses in elderly or debilitated patients should not exceed 2 mg. Prolonged lorazepam use may have a possible relationship to GI disease, including esophageal dilation.

The parenteral formulation of lorazepam contains polyethylene glycol and propylene glycol. Each agent has been associated with specific toxicities when administered in prolonged infusions at high dosages. Also contains benzyl alcohol - avoid rapid injection in neonates or prolonged infusions. Intra-arterial injection or extravasation should be avoided. Concurrent administration with scopolamine results in an increased risk of hallucinations, sedation, and irrational behavior.

Causes CNS depression (dose-related) resulting in sedation, dizziness, confusion, or ataxia which may impair physical and mental capabilities. Patients must be cautioned about performing tasks which require mental alertness (ie, operating machinery or driving). Use with caution in patients receiving other CNS depressants or psychoactive agents. Effects with other sedative drugs or ethanol may be potentiated. Benzodiazepines have been associated with falls and traumatic injury and should be used with extreme caution in patients who are at risk of these events (especially the elderly).

Lorazepam may cause anterograde amnesia. Paradoxical reactions, including hyperactive or aggressive behavior have been reported with benzodiazepines, particularly in adolescent/pediatric or psychiatric patients. Does not have analgesic, antidepressant, or antipsychotic properties.

Use caution in patients with depression, particularly if suicidal risk may be present. Use with caution in patients with a history of drug dependence. Benzodiazepines have been associated with dependence and acute withdrawal symptoms on discontinuation or reduction in dose. Acute withdrawal, including seizures, may be precipitated after administration of flumazenil to patients receiving long-term benzodiazepine therapy.

As a hypnotic agent, should be used only after evaluation of potential causes of sleep disturbance. Failure of sleep disturbance to resolve after 7-10 days may indicate psychiatric or medical illness. A worsening of insomnia or the emergence of new abnormalities of thought or behavior may represent unrecognized psychiatric or medical illness and requires immediate and careful evaluation.

Adverse Reactions

>10%:
  Central nervous system: Sedation
  Respiratory: Respiratory depression

1% to 10%:
  Cardiovascular: Hypotension
  Central nervous system: Confusion, dizziness, akathisia, unsteadiness, headache, depression, disorientation, amnesia
  Dermatologic: Dermatitis, rash
  Gastrointestinal: Weight gain/loss, nausea, changes in appetite
  Neuromuscular & skeletal: Weakness
  Respiratory: Nasal congestion, hyperventilation, apnea

<1%: Blood dyscrasias, increased salivation, menstrual irregularities, physical and psychological dependence with prolonged use, reflex slowing

Overdosage/Toxicology

Signs and symptoms: Confusion, coma, hypoactive reflexes, dyspnea, labored breathing

Treatment for benzodiazepine overdose is supportive. Rarely is mechanical ventilation required.

Flumazenil has been shown to selectively block the binding of benzodiazepines to CNS receptors, resulting in a reversal of benzodiazepine-induced CNS depression but not respiratory depression

Drug Interactions CYP3A3/4 enzyme substrate

CNS depressants: Sedative effects and/or respiratory depression may be additive with CNS depressants; includes ethanol, barbiturates, narcotic analgesics, and other sedative agents; monitor for increased effect

CYP3A3/4 inhibitors: Serum level and/or toxicity of some benzodiazepines may be increased; inhibitors include amiodarone, cimetidine, clarithromycin, erythromycin, delavirdine, diltiazem, dirithromycin, disulfiram, fluoxetine, fluvoxamine, grapefruit juice, indinavir, itraconazole, ketoconazole, metronidazole, nefazodone, nevirapine, propoxyphene, quinupristin-dalfopristin, ritonavir, saquinavir, verapamil, zafirlukast, zileuton; monitor for altered benzodiazepine response

Enzyme inducers: Metabolism of some benzodiazepines may be increased, decreasing their therapeutic effect; consider using an alternative sedative/hypnotic agent; potential inducers include phenobarbital, phenytoin, carbamazepine, rifampin, and rifabutin

Levodopa: Lorazepam may decrease the antiparkinsonian efficacy of levodopa (limited documentation); monitor

Loxapine: There are rare reports of significant respiratory depression, stupor, and/or hypotension with concomitant use of loxapine and lorazepam; use caution if concomitant administration of loxapine and CNS drugs is required

Oral contraceptives: May decrease the clearance of some benzodiazepines (those which undergo oxidative metabolism); monitor for increased benzodiazepine effect

Scopolamine: May increase the incidence of sedation, hallucinations, and irrational behavior; reported only with parenteral lorazepam

Theophylline: May partially antagonize some of the effects of benzodiazepines; monitor for decreased response; may require higher doses for sedation

Ethanol/Nutrition/Herb Interactions

Ethanol: Avoid or limit ethanol (may increase CNS depression).

Herb/Nutraceutical: Avoid valerian, St John's wort, kava kava, gotu kola (may increase CNS depression).

Stability

Intact vials should be refrigerated, protected from light; do not use discolored or precipitate containing solutions

May be stored at room temperature for up to 60 days

Stability of parenteral admixture at room temperature (25°C): 24 hours

Standard diluent: 1 mg/100 mL D_5W

I.V. is **incompatible** when administered in the same line with foscarnet, ondansetron, sargramostim

Mechanism of Action Binds to stereospecific benzodiazepine receptors on the postsynaptic GABA neuron at several sites within the central nervous system, including the limbic system, reticular formation. Enhancement of the inhibitory effect of GABA on neuronal excitability results by increased neuronal membrane permeability to chloride ions. This shift in chloride ions results in hyperpolarization (a less excitable state) and stabilization.

Pharmacodynamics/Kinetics

Onset of hypnosis: I.M.: 20-30 minutes

Onset of sedation, anticonvulsant: I.V.: 5 minutes; oral: 30 minutes to 1 hour

Duration: 6-8 hours

Absorption: Oral, I.M.: Prompt following administration

Distribution: Crosses the placenta; appears in breast milk

V_d:
Neonates: 0.76 L/kg
Adults: 1.3 L/kg

Protein binding: 85%, free fraction may be significantly higher in elderly

Metabolism: In the liver to inactive compounds

Half-life:
Neonates: 40.2 hours
Older Children: 10.5 hours
Adults: 12.9 hours

(Continued)

Lorazepam *(Continued)*

Elderly: 15.9 hours

End-stage renal disease: 32-70 hours

Elimination: Urinary excretion and minimal fecal clearance

Usual Dosage

Antiemetic:

Children 2-15 years: I.V.: 0.05 mg/kg (up to 2 mg/dose) prior to chemotherapy

Adults: Oral, I.V.: 0.5-2 mg every 4-6 hours as needed

Anxiety and sedation:

Infants and Children: Oral, I.V.: Usual: 0.05 mg/kg/dose (range: 0.02-0.09 mg/kg) every 4-8 hours

Adults: Oral: 1-10 mg/day in 2-3 divided doses; usual dose: 2-6 mg/day in divided doses

Elderly: 0.5-4 mg/day

Insomnia: Adults: Oral: 2-4 mg at bedtime

Preoperative: Adults:

I.M.: 0.05 mg/kg administered 2 hours before surgery (maximum: 4 mg/dose)

I.V.: 0.044 mg/kg 15-20 minutes before surgery (usual maximum: 2 mg/dose)

Operative amnesia: Adults: I.V.: Up to 0.05 mg/kg (maximum: 4 mg/dose)

Sedation (preprocedure): Infants and Children:

Oral, I.M., I.V.: Usual: 0.05 mg/kg (range: 0.02-0.09 mg/kg)

I.V.: May use smaller doses (eg, 0.01-0.03 mg/kg) and repeat every 20 minutes, as needed to titrate to effect

Status epilepticus: I.V.:

Infants and Children: 0.1 mg/kg slow I.V. over 2-5 minutes; do not exceed 4 mg/single dose; may repeat second dose of 0.05 mg/kg slow I.V. in 10-15 minutes if needed

Adolescents: 0.07 mg/kg slow I.V. over 2-5 minutes; maximum: 4 mg/dose; may repeat in 10-15 minutes

Adults: 4 mg/dose slow I.V. over 2-5 minutes; may repeat in 10-15 minutes; usual maximum dose: 8 mg

Rapid tranquilization of agitated patient (administer every 30-60 minutes):

Oral: 1-2 mg

I.M.: 0.5-1 mg

Average total dose for tranquilization: Oral, I.M.: 4-8 mg

Administration

Lorazepam may be administered by I.M. or I.V.

I.M.: Should be administered deep into the muscle mass

I.V.: Do not exceed 2 mg/minute or 0.05 mg/kg over 2-5 minutes

Dilute I.V. dose with equal volume of compatible diluent (D_5W, NS, SWI)

Injection must be made slowly with repeated aspiration to make sure the injection is not intra-arterial and that perivascular extravasation has not occurred

Monitoring Parameters Respiratory and cardiovascular status, blood pressure, heart rate, symptoms of anxiety

Reference Range Therapeutic: 50-240 ng/mL (SI: 156-746 nmol/L)

Test Interactions May increase the results of liver function tests

Patient Information Advise patient of potential for physical and psychological dependence with chronic use; do not use alcohol; advise patient of possible retrograde amnesia after I.V. or I.M. use; will cause drowsiness, impairment of judgment or coordination

Nursing Implications Keep injectable form in the refrigerator; **inadvertent intra-arterial injection may produce arteriospasm resulting in gangrene which may require amputation;** emergency resuscitative equipment should be available when administering by I.V.; prior to I.V. use, lorazepam injection must be diluted with an equal amount of compatible diluent; injection must be made slowly with repeated aspiration to make sure the injection is not intra-arterial and that perivascular extravasation has not occurred; provide safety measures (ie, side rails, night light, and call button); supervise ambulation

Additional Information Oral doses >0.09 mg/kg produced ↑ ataxia without ↑ sedative benefit vs lower doses; preferred anxiolytic when I.M. route needed. Abrupt discontinuation after sustained use (generally >10 days) may cause withdrawal symptoms.

Dosage Forms
Injection: 2 mg/mL (1 mL, 10 mL); 4 mg/mL (1 mL, 10 mL)
Solution, oral concentrate: 2 mg/mL (30 mL) [alcohol free, dye free]
Tablet: 0.5 mg, 1 mg, 2 mg

♦ **Loxapac® (Can)** *see* Loxapine *on page 213*

Loxapine (LOKS a peen)

Related Information
Antipsychotic Agents Comparison Chart *on page 557*
Antipsychotic Medication Guidelines *on page 559*
Discontinuation of Psychotropic Drugs - Withdrawal Symptoms and Recommendations *on page 582*
Federal OBRA Regulations Recommended Maximum Doses *on page 583*
Liquid Compatibility With Antipsychotics and Mood Stabilizers *on page 587*
Patient Information - Antipsychotics (General) *on page 466*

U.S. Brand Names Loxitane®; Loxitane® C; Loxitane® I.M.
Canadian Brand Names Loxapac®
Synonyms Loxapine Hydrochloride; Loxapine Succinate; Oxilapine Succinate
Pharmacologic Category Antipsychotic Agent, Dibenzoxazepine
Generic Available Yes
Use Management of psychotic disorders
Pregnancy Risk Factor C
Contraindications Hypersensitivity to loxapine or any component of the formulation; severe CNS depression; coma
Warnings/Precautions May cause hypotension, particularly with I.M. administration. Moderately sedating, use with caution in disorders where CNS depression is a feature. Use with caution in Parkinson's disease. Caution in patients with hemodynamic instability; bone marrow suppression; predisposition to seizures; subcortical brain damage; severe cardiac, hepatic, renal or respiratory disease. Esophageal dysmotility and aspiration have been associated with antipsychotic use - use with caution in patients at risk of pneumonia (ie, Alzheimer's disease). Caution in breast cancer or other prolactin-dependent tumors (may elevate prolactin levels). May alter temperature regulation or mask toxicity of other drugs due to antiemetic effects. May alter cardiac conduction; life-threatening arrhythmias have occurred with therapeutic doses of phenothiazines. May cause orthostatic hypotension - use with caution in patients at risk of this effect or those who would tolerate transient hypotensive episodes (cerebrovascular disease, cardiovascular disease, or other medications which may predispose). Safety and effectiveness of loxapine in pediatric patients have not been established.

Phenothiazines may cause anticholinergic effects (confusion, agitation, constipation, dry mouth, blurred vision, urinary retention); therefore, they should be used with caution in patients with decreased gastrointestinal motility, urinary retention, BPH, xerostomia, or visual problems. Conditions which also may be exacerbated by cholinergic blockade include narrow-angle glaucoma (screening is recommended) and worsening of myasthenia gravis. Relative to other antipsychotics, loxapine has a low potency of cholinergic blockade.

May cause extrapyramidal reactions, including pseudoparkinsonism, acute dystonic reactions, akathisia, and tardive dyskinesia (risk of these reactions is moderate-high relative to other neuroleptics). May be associated with neuroleptic malignant syndrome (NMS) or pigmentary retinopathy.

Adverse Reactions Frequency not defined.
Cardiovascular: Orthostatic hypotension, tachycardia, arrhythmias, abnormal T-waves with prolonged ventricular repolarization, hypertension, hypotension, lightheadedness, syncope
(Continued)

Loxapine *(Continued)*

Central nervous system: Drowsiness, extrapyramidal reactions (dystonia, akathisia, pseudoparkinsonism, tardive dyskinesia, akinesia), dizziness, faintness, ataxia, insomnia, agitation, tension, seizures, slurred speech, confusion, headache, neuroleptic malignant syndrome (NMS), altered central temperature regulation

Dermatologic: Rash, pruritus, photosensitivity, dermatitis, alopecia, seborrhea

Endocrine & metabolic: Enlargement of breasts, galactorrhea, amenorrhea, gynecomastia, menstrual irregularity

Gastrointestinal: Xerostomia, constipation, nausea, vomiting, nasal congestion, weight gain/loss, adynamic ileus, polydipsia

Genitourinary: Urinary retention, sexual dysfunction

Hematologic: Agranulocytosis, leukopenia, thrombocytopenia

Neuromuscular & skeletal: Weakness

Ocular: Blurred vision

Overdosage/Toxicology

Signs and symptoms: Deep sleep, dystonia, agitation, dysrhythmias, extrapyramidal symptoms, hypotension, seizures

Treatment:

Following initiation of essential overdose management, toxic symptom treatment and supportive treatment should be initiated

Hypotension usually responds to I.V. fluids or Trendelenburg positioning. If unresponsive to these measures, the use of a parenteral inotrope may be required (eg, norepinephrine 0.1-0.2 mcg/kg/minute titrated to response).

Seizures commonly respond to diazepam (I.V. 5-10 mg bolus in adults every 15 minutes if needed up to a total of 30 mg; I.V. 0.25-0.4 mg/kg/dose up to a total of 10 mg in children) or to phenytoin or phenobarbital.

Critical cardiac arrhythmias often respond to I.V. phenytoin (15 mg/kg up to 1 gram), while other antiarrhythmics can be used

Neuroleptics often cause extrapyramidal symptoms (eg, dystonic reactions) requiring management with diphenhydramine 1-2 mg/kg (adults) up to a maximum of 50 mg I.M. or I.V. slow push followed by a maintenance dose for 48-72 hours. Alternatively, benztropine mesylate I.V. 1-2 mg (adults) may be effective. These agents are generally effective within 2-5 minutes.

Drug Interactions

Aluminum salts: May decrease the absorption of antipsychotics; monitor

Amphetamines: Efficacy may be diminished by antipsychotics; in addition, amphetamines may increase psychotic symptoms; avoid concurrent use

Anticholinergics: May inhibit the therapeutic response to antipsychotics and excess anticholinergic effects may occur; includes benztropine, trihexyphenidyl, biperiden, and drugs with significant anticholinergic activity (TCAs, antihistamines, disopyramide)

Antihypertensives: Concurrent use of antipsychotics with an antihypertensive may produce additive hypotensive effects (particularly orthostasis)

Bromocriptine: Antipsychotics inhibit the ability of bromocriptine to lower serum prolactin concentrations

CNS depressants: Sedative effects may be additive with antipsychotics; monitor for increased effect; includes barbiturates, benzodiazepines, narcotic analgesics, ethanol, and other sedative agents

Enzyme inducers: May enhance the hepatic metabolism of antipsychotics. Larger doses may be required; includes rifampin, rifabutin, barbiturates, phenytoin, and cigarette smoking

Epinephrine: Chlorpromazine (and possibly other low potency antipsychotics) may diminish the pressor effects of epinephrine

Guanethidine and guanadrel: Antihypertensive effects may be inhibited by antipsychotics

Levodopa: Antipsychotics may inhibit the antiparkinsonian effect of levodopa; avoid this combination

Lithium: Antipsychotics may produce neurotoxicity with lithium; this is a rare effect

Phenytoin: May reduce serum levels of antipsychotics; antipsychotics may increase phenytoin serum levels

Propranolol: Serum concentrations of antipsychotics may be increased; propranolol also increases antipsychotic concentrations

QT_c-prolonging agents: Effects on QT_c interval may be additive with antipsychotics, increasing the risk of malignant arrhythmias. Includes type Ia antiarrhythmics, TCAs, and some quinolone antibiotics (sparfloxacin, moxifloxacin and gatifloxacin)

Sulfadoxine-pyrimethamine: May increase antipsychotic concentrations

Tricyclic antidepressants: Concurrent use may produce increased toxicity or altered therapeutic response

Trazodone: Antipsychotics and trazodone may produce additive hypotensive effects

Valproic acid: Serum levels may be increased by antipsychotics

Ethanol/Nutrition/Herb Interactions
Ethanol: Avoid ethanol (may increase CNS depression).
Herb/Nutraceutical: Avoid kava kava, gotu kola, valerian, St John's wort (may increase CNS depression).

Stability Protect from light; dispense in amber or opaque vials

Mechanism of Action Blocks postsynaptic mesolimbic D_1 and D_2 receptors in the brain, and also possesses serotonin 5-HT_2 blocking activity

Pharmacodynamics/Kinetics
Onset of neuroleptic effect: Oral: Within 20-30 minutes
Peak effect: 1.5-3 hours
Duration: ~12 hours
Metabolism: Hepatic to glucuronide conjugates
Half-life, biphasic:
  Initial: 5 hours
  Terminal: 12-19 hours
Elimination: In urine, and to a smaller degree, feces

Usual Dosage Adults:
Oral: 10 mg twice daily, increase dose until psychotic symptoms are controlled; usual dose range: 20-100 mg/day in divided doses 2-4 times/day; dosages >250 mg/day are not recommended
  Elderly: 20-60 mg/day
I.M.: 12.5-50 mg every 4-6 hours or longer as needed and change to oral therapy as soon as possible

Administration Injectable is for I.M. use only

Monitoring Parameters EKG, CBC, blood pressure, electrolytes, pH

Test Interactions False-positives for phenylketonuria, amylase, uroporphyrins, urobilinogen; elevated liver function tests

Patient Information May cause drowsiness; avoid alcoholic beverages; may impair judgment or coordination; may cause photosensitivity; avoid excessive sunlight; do not stop taking without consulting physician

Nursing Implications
Injectable is for I.M. use only; dilute the oral concentrate with water or juice before administration; avoid skin contact with oral suspension or solution; may cause contact dermatitis
Monitor orthostatic blood pressures 3-5 days after initiation of therapy or a dose increase; observe for tremor and abnormal movement or posturing (extrapyramidal symptoms)

Dosage Forms
Capsule, as succinate (Loxitane®): 5 mg, 10 mg, 25 mg, 50 mg
Injection, as hydrochloride (Loxitane® IM): 50 mg/mL (1 mL)
Solution, oral concentrate, as hydrochloride (Loxitane® C): 25 mg/mL (120 mL dropper bottle)

♦ **Loxapine Hydrochloride** *see* Loxapine *on page 213*

♦ **Loxapine Succinate** *see* Loxapine *on page 213*

- **Loxitane**® *see* Loxapine *on page 213*
- **Loxitane**® **C** *see* Loxapine *on page 213*
- **Loxitane**® **I.M.** *see* Loxapine *on page 213*
- **LTG** *see* Lamotrigine *on page 187*
- ***L*-Thyroxine Sodium** *see* Levothyroxine *on page 198*
- **Ludiomil**® *see* Maprotiline *on page 216*
- **Luminal**® **Sodium** *see* Phenobarbital *on page 302*
- **Luvox**® *see* Fluvoxamine *on page 157*
- **LY170053** *see* Olanzapine *on page 272*
- **Ma-Huang** *see* Ephedra *on page 131*

Maprotiline (ma PROE ti leen)

Related Information

Antidepressant Agents Comparison Chart *on page 553*
Discontinuation of Psychotropic Drugs - Withdrawal Symptoms and Recommendations *on page 582*
Federal OBRA Regulations Recommended Maximum Doses *on page 583*
Patient Information - Antidepressants (TCAs) *on page 454*
Teratogenic Risks of Psychotropic Medications *on page 594*

U.S. Brand Names Ludiomil®

Canadian Brand Names Ludiomil

Synonyms Maprotiline Hydrochloride

Pharmacologic Category Antidepressant, Tetracyclic

Generic Available Yes

Use Treatment of depression and anxiety associated with depression

Unlabeled/Investigational Use Bulimia; duodenal ulcers; enuresis; urinary symptoms of multiple sclerosis; pain; panic attacks; tension headache; cocaine withdrawal

Pregnancy Risk Factor B

Contraindications Hypersensitivity to maprotiline or any component of the formulation; use of monoamine oxidase inhibitors within 14 days; use in a patient during the acute recovery phase of MI

Warnings/Precautions May cause sedation, resulting in impaired performance of tasks requiring alertness (ie, operating machinery or driving). Sedative effects may be additive with other CNS depressants and/or ethanol. The degree of sedation is high relative to other antidepressants. May worsen psychosis in some patients or precipitate a shift to mania or hypomania in patients with bipolar disease. May increase the risks associated with electroconvulsive therapy. This agent should be discontinued, when possible, prior to elective surgery. Therapy should not be abruptly discontinued in patients receiving high doses for prolonged periods.

May cause orthostatic hypotension (risk is moderate relative to other antidepressants) - use with caution in patients at risk of hypotension or in patients where transient hypotensive episodes would be poorly tolerated (cardiovascular disease or cerebrovascular disease). The degree of anticholinergic blockade produced by this agent is moderate relative to other cyclic antidepressants, however, caution should still be used in patients with urinary retention, benign prostatic hypertrophy, narrow-angle glaucoma, xerostomia, visual problems, constipation, or history of bowel obstruction.

Use caution in patients with depression, particularly if suicidal risk may be present. Use with caution in patients with a history of cardiovascular disease (including previous MI, stroke, tachycardia, or conduction abnormalities). The risk conduction abnormalities with this agent is moderate relative to other antidepressants. Use caution in patients with a previous seizure disorder or condition predisposing to seizures such as brain damage, alcoholism, or concurrent therapy with other drugs which lower the seizure threshold. Use with caution in hyperthyroid patients or those receiving thyroid supplementation. Use with caution in patients with hepatic or renal dysfunction and in elderly patients.

Adverse Reactions

>10%:

Central nervous system: Drowsiness

Gastrointestinal: Xerostomia

1% to 10%:

Central nervous system: Insomnia, nervousness, anxiety, agitation, dizziness, fatigue, headache

Gastrointestinal: Constipation, nausea

Neuromuscular & skeletal: Tremor, weakness

Ocular: Blurred vision

<1%: Abdominal cramps, accommodation disturbances, akathisia, arrhythmias, ataxia, bitter taste, breast enlargement, confusion, decreased libido, delusions, diaphoresis (excessive), diarrhea, disorientation, dysarthria, dysphagia, edema of testicles, epigastric distress, EPS, exacerbation of psychosis, hallucinations, heart block, hyperglycemia, hypertension, hypomania, hypotension, impotence, mania, motor hyperactivity, mydriasis, nightmares, numbness, palpitations, petechiae, photosensitivity, rash, restlessness, seizures, syncope, tachycardia, tingling, tinnitus, urinary retention, vomiting, weight gain/loss

Overdosage/Toxicology

Signs and symptoms: Agitation, confusion, hallucinations, urinary retention, hypothermia, hypotension, seizures, ventricular tachycardia

Treatment:

Following initiation of essential overdose management, toxic symptoms should be treated

Ventricular arrhythmias often respond to systemic alkalinization (sodium bicarbonate 0.5-2 mEq/kg I.V.). Arrhythmias unresponsive to this therapy may respond to lidocaine 1 mg/kg I.V. followed by a titrated infusion. Physostigmine (1-2 mg I.V. slowly for adults or 0.5 mg I.V. slowly for children) may be indicated in reversing cardiac arrhythmias that are life-threatening.

Seizures usually respond to diazepam I.V. boluses (5-10 mg for adults up to 30 mg or 0.25-0.4 mg/kg/dose for children up to 10 mg/dose). If seizures are unresponsive or recur, phenytoin or phenobarbital may be required.

Drug Interactions CYP1A2 and 2D6 enzyme substrate

Altretamine: Concurrent use may cause orthostatic hypertension

Amphetamines: Cyclic antidepressants may enhance the effect of amphetamines; monitor for adverse CV effects

Anticholinergics: Combined use with cyclic antidepressants may produce additive anticholinergic effects

Antihypertensives: Cyclic antidepressants may inhibit the antihypertensive response to bethanidine, clonidine, debrisoquin, guanadrel, guanethidine, guanabenz, guanfacine; monitor BP; consider alternate antihypertensive agent

Beta-agonists: When combined with cyclic antidepressants may predispose patients to cardiac arrhythmias

Bupropion: May increase the levels of cyclic antidepressants; based on limited information; monitor response

Carbamazepine: Cyclic antidepressants may increase carbamazepine levels; monitor

Cholestyramine and colestipol: May bind cyclic antidepressants and reduce their absorption; monitor for altered response

Clonidine: Abrupt discontinuation of clonidine may cause hypertensive crisis, cyclic antidepressants may enhance the response

CNS depressants: Sedative effects may be additive with cyclic antidepressants; monitor for increased effect; includes benzodiazepines, barbiturates, antipsychotics, ethanol and other sedative medications

CYP1A2 inhibitors: Serum levels and/or toxicity of some cyclic antidepressants may be increased; inhibitors include cimetidine, ciprofloxacin, fluvoxamine, isoniazid, ritonavir, and zileuton

(Continued)

Maprotiline (Continued)

CYP2D6 inhibitors: Serum levels and/or toxicity of some cyclic antidepressants may be increased; inhibitors include amiodarone, cimetidine, delavirdine, fluoxetine, paroxetine, propafenone, quinidine, and ritonavir; monitor for increased effect/toxicity

Enzyme inducers: May increase the metabolism of cyclic antidepressants resulting in decreased effect; includes carbamazepine, phenobarbital, phenytoin, and rifampin; monitor for decreased response

Epinephrine (and other direct alpha-agonists): The pressor response to I.V. epinephrine, norepinephrine, and phenylephrine may be enhanced in patients receiving cyclic antidepressants; this combination is best avoided

Fenfluramine: May increase cyclic antidepressant levels/effects

Hypoglycemic agents (including insulin): Hypoglycemic effects may be enhanced, profound hypoglycemia has been reported; monitor for changes in blood glucose levels; reported with chlorpropamide, tolazamide, and insulin

Levodopa: Cyclic antidepressants may decrease the absorption (bioavailability) of levodopa; rare hypertensive episodes have also been attributed to this combination

Linezolid: Hyperpyrexia, hypertension, tachycardia, confusion, seizures, and **deaths have been reported** with agents which inhibit MAO (serotonin syndrome); this combination should be avoided

Lithium: Concurrent use with a cyclic antidepressant may increase the risk for neurotoxicity

MAO inhibitors: Hyperpyrexia, hypertension, tachycardia, confusion, seizures, and **deaths have been reported** (serotonin syndrome); this combination should be avoided

Methylphenidate: Metabolism of maprotiline may be decreased

Phenothiazines: Serum concentrations of some TCAs may be increased; in addition, TCAs may increase concentration of phenothiazines; monitor for altered clinical response

QT_c-prolonging agents: Concurrent use of cyclic agents with other drugs which may prolong QT_c interval may increase the risk of potentially fatal arrhythmias; includes type Ia and type III antiarrhythmics agents, selected quinolones (sparfloxacin, gatifloxacin, moxifloxacin, grepafloxacin), cisapride, and other agents

Sucralfate: Absorption of cyclic antidepressants may be reduced with coadministration.

Sympathomimetics, indirect-acting: Cyclic antidepressants may result in a decreased sensitivity to indirect-acting sympathomimetics; includes dopamine and ephedrine; also see interaction with epinephrine (and direct-acting sympathomimetics)

Tramadol: Tramadol's risk of seizures may be increased with TCAs

Valproic acid: May increase serum concentrations/adverse effects of some cyclic antidepressants

Warfarin (and other oral anticoagulants): Cyclic antidepressants may increase the anticoagulant effect in patients stabilized on warfarin; monitor INR

Ethanol/Nutrition/Herb Interactions Ethanol: Avoid ethanol (may increase CNS depression).

Mechanism of Action Traditionally believed to increase the synaptic concentration of norepinephrine in the central nervous system by inhibition of their reuptake by the presynaptic neuronal membrane. However, additional receptor effects have been found including desensitization of adenyl cyclase, down regulation of beta-adrenergic receptors, and down regulation of serotonin receptors.

Pharmacodynamics/Kinetics

Absorption: Slow

Protein binding: 88%

Metabolism: In the liver to active and inactive compounds

Half-life: 27-58 hours (mean, 43 hours)

Time to peak serum concentration: Within 12 hours

Elimination: In urine (70%) and feces (30%)

Usual Dosage Oral:

Children 6-14 years: Depression: 10 mg/day; increase to a maximum daily dose of 75 mg

Adults: Depression: 75 mg/day to start, increase by 25 mg every 2 weeks up to 150-225 mg/day; given in 3 divided doses or in a single daily dose

Elderly: Depression: Initial: 25 mg at bedtime, increase by 25 mg every 3 days for inpatients and weekly for outpatients if tolerated; usual maintenance dose: 50-75 mg/day, higher doses may be necessary in nonresponders

Monitoring Parameters Monitor blood pressure and pulse rate prior to and during initial therapy; evaluate mood and somatic complaints; monitor appetite and weight; EKG in older adults

Patient Information Avoid alcohol ingestion; do not discontinue medication abruptly; may cause drowsiness; full effect may not occur for 4-6 weeks; dry mouth may be helped by sips of water, sugarless gum, or hard candy; rise slowly to avoid dizziness

Nursing Implications

Offer patient sugarless hard candy for dry mouth

Monitor blood pressure and pulse rate prior to and during initial therapy; evaluate mental status; monitor weight and appetite

Additional Information Odorless, bitter tasting; seizures are rarely seen 5-30 hours postdrug ingestion.

Dosage Forms Tablet, as hydrochloride: 25 mg, 50 mg, 75 mg

♦ **Maprotiline Hydrochloride** *see Maprotiline on page 216*

♦ **Margesic**® *see Butalbital Compound on page 59*

Margosa Oil

Pharmacologic Category Herb

Use A folk remedy in India, Japan, and Southeast Asia; antihelminthic, insecticidal, or analgesic agent; an extract from the dried stem bark and tree leaves of *Azadirachta indica* (Neem tree)

Adverse Reactions

Cardiovascular: Reye's-like syndrome, cerebral edema

Central nervous system: Lethargy, seizures, coma

Endocrine & metabolic: Metabolic acidosis

Gastrointestinal: Vomiting (15 minutes to 4 hours)

Hematology: Leukocytosis

Hepatic: Steatosis of the liver

Neuromuscular & skeletal: Tremor

Respiratory: Tachypnea, dyspnea

Overdosage/Toxicology

Decontamination: Do **not** induce emesis; lavage within 1 hour (if spontaneous emesis has not already occurred), activated charcoal with cathartic

Treatment: Supportive therapy; benzodiazepines have been used to treat seizures; paraldehyde has also been used to terminate seizures; mannitol and/or dexamethasone should be used to treat cerebral edema

Additional Information Not generally available in U.S. market; not listed with Commission E; some Neem extracts are used as ingredients in imported (from India) toothpastes and in natural cosmetics, but **not** as a dietary supplement for oral consumption

♦ **Marnal**® **Medigesic**® *see Butalbital Compound on page 59*

♦ **Marplan**® *see Isocarboxazid on page 184*

Maté

Synonyms *Ilex paraguariensis*; Jesuit's Tea; Paraguay Tea; St Bartholomew's Tea

Pharmacologic Category Herb

Use Herbal medicine as a depurative, stimulant, diuretic, urinary tract infection, kidney and bladder stones, CHF

Per Commission E: Physical fatigue

(Continued)

Maté *(Continued)*

Adverse Reactions
Cardiovascular: Tachycardia

Central nervous system: Fever, disorientation

Dermatologic: Flushed skin

Gastrointestinal: Xerostomia

Genitourinary: Urinary retention

Ocular: Mydriasis

Miscellaneous: Incidence of esophageal cancer and bladder cancer increased when used with tobacco (in chronic users)

Overdosage/Toxicology
Decontamination: Lavage (within 1 hour)/activated charcoal with cathartic

Treatment: Supportive therapy; physostigmine (0.5 mg in children, up to 4 mg in adult as a total dose) has been used to treat severe anticholinergic toxicity due to ingestion of Paraguay tea contaminated with anticholinergic agents. This modality should not be used for treating effects of caffeine exposure.

Drug Interactions
CYP1A2, 2E1, and 3A3/4 enzyme substrate

Note: Contains significant amounts of caffeine; interactions noted are for caffeine content

Adenosine: Caffeine may antagonize the cardiovascular effects of adenosine

Beta-agonists: Therapeutic effect of beta-agonists (bronchodilation) and toxicity (tachycardia, tremor) may be additive; use caution

CYP1A2 inhibitors: Metabolism of caffeine may be decreased, increasing clinical effect or toxicity; inhibitors include cimetidine, ciprofloxacin, fluvoxamine, isoniazid, ritonavir, and zileuton

CNS stimulants: Effects on CNS stimulation are additive with caffeine; cardiovascular side effects may also be additive; includes phenylpropanolamine, amphetamines, methylphenidate and others

Disulfiram: May increase the effects of caffeine

Theophylline: Therapeutic effect of theophylline (respiratory stimulation, bronchodilation) and toxicity (tachycardia, tremor, possible seizures) may be additive; avoid combinations

Usual Dosage
One cup of maté (6 ounces) is equivalent to 25-50 mg of caffeine

Per Commission E: Daily dose: 3 g of drug (dried herb); equivalent preparations

Additional Information
A climbing evergreen shrub which can grow to 20 feet; native to South American countries; greenish white flowers with small deep red berries; leaves contain as much as 2% caffeine along with theophylline (0.05%); apnea has occurred in an infant after breast-feeding from a mother ingesting maté; teas should be used with caution in patients with elevated blood pressure, diabetes or ulcer disease

- *Matricaria chamomilla* see Chamomile on page 68
- *Matricarta recutita* see Chamomile on page 68
- *Maxalt®* see Rizatriptan on page 360
- *Maxalt-MLT™* see Rizatriptan on page 360
- *Maximum Strength Nytol® [OTC]* see Diphenhydramine on page 116
- *Maybush* see Hawthorn on page 175
- *Mazanor®* see Mazindol on page 220
- *Mazepine® (Can)* see Carbamazepine on page 61

Mazindol *(MAY zin dole)*

U.S. Brand Names Mazanor®; Sanorex®

Canadian Brand Names Sanorex

Pharmacologic Category Anorexiant

Generic Available No

Use Short-term adjunct in exogenous obesity

Restrictions C-IV

Pregnancy Risk Factor C

Contraindications Hypersensitivity to mazindol or any component of the formulation; agitated states; history of drug abuse; MAO inhibitors

Warnings/Precautions Tolerance may develop within a few weeks. If this occurs, discontinue drug. Do not increase dose. Not recommended for severe hypertensive patients or patients with symptomatic cardiovascular disease including arrhythmias. Stimulants may unmask tics in individuals with coexisting Tourette's syndrome.

Adverse Reactions

Cardiovascular: Palpitation, tachycardia, edema

Central nervous system: Insomnia, overstimulation, dizziness, dysphoria, drowsiness, depression, headache, restlessness

Dermatologic: Rash, clamminess

Endocrine & metabolic: Changes in libido

Gastrointestinal: Nausea, constipation, vomiting, xerostomia, unpleasant taste, diarrhea, abdominal cramps

Genitourinary: Dysuria, polyuria, impotence

Neuromuscular & skeletal: Tremor, weakness

Ocular: Blurred vision, corneal opacities

Miscellaneous: Diaphoresis (excessive)

Overdosage/Toxicology Symptoms of overdose include hypertension, tachycardia, and hyperthermia. Treatment is supportive.

Drug Interactions

Antipsychotics: Efficacy of CNS stimulants may be decreased by antipsychotics; in addition, amphetamines may induce an increase in psychotic symptoms in some patients

Furazolidone: Amphetamine-like compounds may induce hypertensive episodes in patients receiving furazolidone

Guanethidine: Amphetamine-like compounds inhibit the antihypertensive response to guanethidine; probably also may occur with guanadrel

MAO inhibitors: Severe hypertensive episodes have occurred with amphetamines when used in patients receiving MAO inhibitors; likely to occur with related compounds; concurrent use or use within 14 days is contraindicated

Norepinephrine: Amphetamine-like compounds may enhance the pressor response to norepinephrine

Sibutramine: Concurrent use of sibutramine and amphetamine-like compounds may cause severe hypertension and tachycardia; use is contraindicated (benzphetamine)

SSRIs: Amphetamine-like compounds may increase the potential for serotonin syndrome when used concurrently with selective serotonin reuptake inhibitors (including fluoxetine, fluvoxamine, paroxetine, and sertraline)

Ethanol/Nutrition/Herb Interactions Ethanol: Avoid ethanol (may increase CNS depression).

Mechanism of Action An isoindole with pharmacologic activity similar to amphetamine; produces CNS stimulation in humans and animals and appears to work primarily in the limbic system

Pharmacodynamics/Kinetics

Half-life: 33-55 hours

Elimination: Renal

Usual Dosage Oral: Adults:

Initial: 1 mg once daily; adjust to patient response

Usual maintenance range: 2-3 mg/day in 1-3 divided doses

Note: Take 1 hour before meals to avoid GI discomfort

Dosage Forms

Tablet:

Mazanor®: 1 mg

Sanorex®: 1 mg, 2 mg

♦ **Medilium**® **(Can)** *see* Chlordiazepoxide *on page 71*

♦ **Meditran**® **(Can)** *see* Meprobamate *on page 223*

Melaleuca Oil

Pharmacologic Category Herb

Use Marketed as having fungicidal, bactericidal properties; also used as a topical dermal agent for burns

Overdosage/Toxicology
Signs and symptoms: CNS depression, ataxia, aspiration pneumonitis, lethargy
Decontamination: Activated charcoal with cathartic

Usual Dosage Minimal toxic dose: Infant: <10 mL

Additional Information Found in New South Wales (Australia) on the north coast in swampy lowlands, this paper-bark tree can grow up to 20 ft high; the tree may also be found in southern U.S. (Florida), Spain, or Portugal; nutmeg odor; has been used to treat acne vulgaris, athlete's foot, and vaginitis

Oral: Mildly toxic
Dermal: Very mild irritant; no dermal sensitization; no phototoxicity

Melatonin (mel ah TOE nin)

Synonyms N-Acetyl-5-methoxytryptamine

Pharmacologic Category Hormone; Hypnotic, Miscellaneous

Use Sleep disorders (insomnia), circadian rhythm disturbances (ie, jet lag); only FDA approval (as an orphan drug) is for treatment of circadian rhythm sleep disorders in blind people with no light perception

Adverse Reactions Percentage unknown:
Central nervous system: Drowsiness, dysphoria (especially in depressed patients), giddiness, headache
Dermatologic: Pruritus
Gastrointestinal: Nausea
Miscellaneous: Increase in alkaline phosphatase

Drug Interactions
CNS depressants: Sedative effects may be additive with other sedative agents; monitor for increased effect; includes benzodiazepines, barbiturates, antipsychotics, antihistamines, ethanol, and other sedative medications
Fluvoxamine: The bioavailability of melatonin has been reported to be increased by fluvoxamine
Nifedipine: Melatonin has been reported to decrease the antihypertensive efficacy of nifedipine

Mechanism of Action A hormone produced and secreted in the pineal gland causes an increase in hypothalamus aminobutyric acid and serotonin. Increased secretion occurs during dark hours; decreases neopterin release; counteracts apoptosis; increases thymus activity

Pharmacodynamics/Kinetics
Absorption: Rapid
Peak plasma level: 1 hour

Usual Dosage Oral:
Jet lag: 5 mg/day (at 6 PM) for 1 week starting 3 days before the flight
Hypnotic effects: Oral: 0.1-0.3 mg (daytime); 1-10 mg (nighttime)
Insomnia: 5-75 mg at night have been used

Reference Range Mean baseline melatonin serum levels 80 pg/mL (range: 0-200) between 2-4 AM. Elevated endogenous levels seen after 9 AM; after a 2.5 mg oral dose, plasma melatonin level may be as high as 8.50 pg/mL.

Dosage Forms
Tablet: 3 mg
Tablet, sublingual: 2.5 mg

◆ **Melfiat®: Obezine®** *see* Phendimetrazine *on page 298*

◆ **Mellaril®** *see* Thioridazine *on page 393*

◆ **Mentha pulegium** *see* Pennyroyal Oil *on page 289*

Meprobamate (me proe BA mate)

Related Information
Anxiolytic/Hypnotic Use in Long-Term Care Facilities *on page 562*
Federal OBRA Regulations Recommended Maximum Doses *on page 583*

U.S. Brand Names Equanil®; Miltown®

Canadian Brand Names Apo®-Meprobamate; Meditran®; Novo-Mepro®

Pharmacologic Category Antianxiety Agent, Miscellaneous

Generic Available Yes

Use Management of anxiety disorders

Unlabeled/Investigational Use Demonstrated value for muscle contraction, headache, premenstrual tension, external sphincter spasticity, muscle rigidity, opisthotonos-associated with tetanus

Restrictions C-IV

Pregnancy Risk Factor D

Contraindications Hypersensitivity to meprobamate, related compounds (including carisoprodol), or any component of the formulation; acute intermittent porphyria; pre-existing CNS depression; narrow-angle glaucoma; severe uncontrolled pain; pregnancy

Warnings/Precautions Physical and psychological dependence and abuse may occur; abrupt cessation may precipitate withdrawal. Use with caution in patients with depression or suicidal tendencies, or in patients with a history of drug abuse. May cause CNS depression, which may impair physical or mental abilities. Patients must be cautioned about performing tasks which require mental alertness (ie, operating machinery or driving). Effects with other sedative drugs or ethanol may be potentiated. Not recommended in children <6 years of age; allergic reaction may occur in patients with history of dermatological condition (usually by fourth dose). Use with caution in patients with renal or hepatic impairment, or with a history of seizures. Use caution in the elderly as it may cause confusion, cognitive impairment, or excessive sedation.

Adverse Reactions Frequency not defined.
Cardiovascular: Syncope, peripheral edema, palpitations, tachycardia, arrhythmia
Central nervous system: Drowsiness, ataxia, dizziness, paradoxical excitement, confusion, slurred speech, headache, euphoria, chills, vertigo, paresthesia, overstimulation
Dermatologic: Rashes, purpura, dermatitis, Stevens-Johnson syndrome, petechiae, ecchymosis
Gastrointestinal: Diarrhea, vomiting, nausea
Hematologic: Leukopenia, eosinophilia, agranulocytosis, aplastic anemia
Neuromuscular & skeletal: Weakness
Ocular: Blurred vision, impairment of accommodation
Renal: Renal failure
Respiratory: Wheezing, dyspnea, bronchospasm, angioneurotic edema

Overdosage/Toxicology Symptoms of overdose include drowsiness, lethargy, ataxia, coma, hypotension, shock, and death. Treatment is supportive following attempts to enhance drug elimination.

Drug Interactions CNS depressants: Sedative effects may be additive with other CNS depressants; monitor for increased effect; includes barbiturates, benzodiazepines, narcotic analgesics, ethanol, and other sedative agents

Ethanol/Nutrition/Herb Interactions
Ethanol: Avoid ethanol (may increase CNS depression).
Herb/Nutraceutical: Avoid valerian, St John's wort, kava kava, gotu kola (may increase CNS depression).

Mechanism of Action Affects the thalamus and limbic system; also appears to inhibit multineuronal spinal reflexes

Pharmacodynamics/Kinetics
Onset of sedation: Oral: Within 1 hour
Distribution: Crosses the placenta; appears in breast milk
Metabolism: Promptly in the liver
(Continued)

Meprobamate *(Continued)*

Half-life: 10 hours

Elimination: In urine (8% to 20% as unchanged drug) and feces (10% as metabolites)

Usual Dosage Oral:

Children 6-12 years: Anxiety: 100-200 mg 2-3 times/day

Adults: Anxiety: 400 mg 3-4 times/day, up to 2400 mg/day

Dosing interval in renal impairment:

Cl_{cr} 10-50 mL/minute: Administer every 9-12 hours

Cl_{cr} <10 mL/minute: Administer every 12-18 hours

Hemodialysis: Moderately dialyzable (20% to 50%)

Dosing adjustment in hepatic impairment: Probably necessary in patients with liver disease

Monitoring Parameters Mental status

Reference Range Therapeutic: 6-12 µg/mL (SI: 28-55 µmol/L); Toxic: >60 µg/mL (SI: >275 µmol/L)

Patient Information May cause drowsiness and dependence; avoid alcoholic beverages

Nursing Implications Assist with ambulation; monitor mental status

Additional Information Withdrawal should be gradual over 1-2 weeks. Benzodiazepine and buspirone are better choices for treatment of anxiety disorders.

Dosage Forms Tablet: 200 mg, 400 mg

♦ **Meridia**® *see* Sibutramine *on page 378*

Mesoridazine *(mez oh RID a zeen)*

Related Information

Antipsychotic Agents Comparison Chart *on page 557*

Antipsychotic Medication Guidelines *on page 559*

Discontinuation of Psychotropic Drugs - Withdrawal Symptoms and Recommendations *on page 582*

Federal OBRA Regulations Recommended Maximum Doses *on page 583*

Liquid Compatibility With Antipsychotics and Mood Stabilizers *on page 587*

Patient Information - Antipsychotics (General) *on page 466*

U.S. Brand Names Serentil®

Canadian Brand Names Serentil

Synonyms Mesoridazine Besylate

Pharmacologic Category Antipsychotic Agent, Phenothiazine, Piperidine

Generic Available No

Use Management of schizophrenic patients who fail to respond adequately to treatment with other antipsychotic drugs, either because of insufficient effectiveness or the inability to achieve an effective dose due to intolerable adverse effects from these drugs

Unlabeled/Investigational Use Psychosis

Pregnancy Risk Factor C

Contraindications Hypersensitivity to mesoridazine or any component of the formulation (cross-reactivity between phenothiazines may occur); severe CNS depression and coma; prolonged QT interval (>450 msec), including prolongation due to congenital causes; history of arrhythmias; concurrent use of medications which prolong QT_c (including type Ia and type III antiarrhythmics, cyclic antidepressants, some fluoroquinolones, cisapride); concurrent use of mesoridazine with fluvoxamine, fluoxetine, paroxetine, pindolol, or propranolol

Warnings/Precautions Has been shown to prolong QT_c interval in a dose-dependent manner (associated with an increased risk of torsade de pointes). Patients should have a baseline EKG prior to initiation, and should not receive mesoridazine if baseline QT_c >450 msec. Mesoridazine should be discontinued in patients with a QT_c interval >500 msec. Potassium levels must be evaluated and normalized prior to and throughout treatment.

May cause hypotension, particularly with I.M. administration. Highly sedating, use with caution in disorders where CNS depression is a feature. Use with caution in Parkinson's disease. Caution in patients with hemodynamic instability; bone marrow suppression; predisposition to seizures; subcortical brain damage; severe cardiac, hepatic, renal, or respiratory disease. Esophageal dysmotility and aspiration have been associated with antipsychotic use; use with caution in patients at risk of pneumonia (ie, Alzheimer's disease). Caution in breast cancer or other prolactin-dependent tumors (may elevate prolactin levels). May alter temperature regulation or mask toxicity of other drugs due to antiemetic effects. May cause orthostatic hypotension - use with caution in patients at risk of this effect or those who would tolerate transient hypotensive episodes (cerebrovascular disease, cardiovascular disease, or other medications which may predispose).

Phenothiazines may cause anticholinergic effects (confusion, agitation, constipation, dry mouth, blurred vision, urinary retention). Therefore, they should be used with caution in patients with decreased gastrointestinal motility, urinary retention, BPH, xerostomia, or visual problems. Conditions which also may be exacerbated by cholinergic blockade include narrow-angle glaucoma (screening is recommended) and worsening of myasthenia gravis. Relative to other antipsychotics, mesoridazine has a high potency of cholinergic blockade.

May cause extrapyramidal reactions, including pseudoparkinsonism, acute dystonic reactions, akathisia, and tardive dyskinesia (risk of these reactions is low relative to other neuroleptics). May be associated with neuroleptic malignant syndrome (NMS) or pigmentary retinopathy (particularly at doses >1 g/day).

Adverse Reactions Frequency not defined.

Cardiovascular: Hypotension, orthostatic hypotension, tachycardia, QT prolongation (dose dependent, up to 100% of patients at higher dosages), syncope, edema

Central nervous system: Pseudoparkinsonism, akathisia, dystonias, tardive dyskinesia, dizziness, drowsiness, restlessness, ataxia, slurred speech, neuroleptic malignant syndrome (NMS), impairment of temperature regulation, lowering of seizure threshold

Dermatologic: Increased sensitivity to sun, rash, itching, angioneurotic edema, dermatitis, discoloration of skin (blue-gray)

Endocrine & metabolic: Changes in menstrual cycle, changes in libido, gynecomastia, lactation, galactorrhea

Gastrointestinal: Constipation, xerostomia, weight gain, nausea, vomiting, stomach pain

Genitourinary: Difficulty in urination, ejaculatory disturbances, impotence, enuresis, incontinence, priapism, urinary retention

Hematologic: Agranulocytosis, leukopenia, eosinophilia, thrombocytopenia, anemia, aplastic anemia

Hepatic: Cholestatic jaundice, hepatotoxicity

Neuromuscular & skeletal: Weakness, tremor, rigidity

Ocular: Pigmentary retinopathy, photophobia, blurred vision, cornea and lens changes

Respiratory: Nasal congestion

Miscellaneous: Diaphoresis (decreased), lupus-like syndrome

Overdosage/Toxicology

Signs and symptoms: Deep sleep, coma, extrapyramidal symptoms, abnormal involuntary muscle movements, hypotension

Treatment:

Following initiation of essential overdose management, toxic symptom treatment and supportive treatment should be initiated

Hypotension usually responds to I.V. fluids or Trendelenburg positioning. If unresponsive to these measures, the use of a parenteral inotrope may be required.

Seizures commonly respond to diazepam (I.V. 5-10 mg bolus in adults every 15 minutes if needed up to a total of 30 mg; I.V. 0.25-0.4 mg/kg/dose up to a total of 10 mg in children) or to phenytoin or phenobarbital.

(Continued)

Mesoridazine *(Continued)*

Critical cardiac arrhythmias often respond to I.V. phenytoin (15 mg/kg up to 1 g), while other antiarrhythmics can be used.

Extrapyramidal symptoms (eg, dystonic reactions) can be managed with benztropine mesylate I.V. 1-2 mg (adults)

Drug Interactions CYP1A2, 2D6, and 3A3/4 enzyme substrate; CYP2D6 enzyme inhibitor

Aluminum salts: May decrease the absorption of phenothiazines; monitor

Amphetamines: Efficacy may be diminished by antipsychotics; in addition, amphetamines may increase psychotic symptoms; avoid concurrent use

Anticholinergics: May inhibit the therapeutic response to phenothiazines and excess anticholinergic effects may occur; includes benztropine, trihyexyphenidyl, biperiden, and drugs with significant anticholinergic activity (TCAs, antihistamines, disopyramide)

Antihypertensives: Concurrent use of phenothiazines with an antihypertensive may produce additive hypotensive effects (particularly orthostasis)

Bromocriptine: Phenothiazines inhibit the ability of bromocriptine to lower serum prolactin concentrations

Chloroquine: Serum concentrations of chlorpromazine may be increased by chloroquine

CNS depressants: Sedative effects may be additive with phenothiazines; monitor for increased effect; includes barbiturates, benzodiazepines, narcotic analgesics, ethanol, and other sedative agents

CYP1A2 inhibitors: Metabolism of phenothiazines may be decreased; increasing clinical effect or toxicity. Inhibitors include cimetidine, ciprofloxacin, fluvoxamine, isoniazid, ritonavir, and zileuton. **Concurrent use with fluvoxamine is contraindicated.**

CYP2D6 inhibitors: Metabolism of phenothiazines may be decreased; increasing clinical effect or toxicity. Inhibitors include amiodarone, cimetidine, delavirdine, fluoxetine, paroxetine, propafenone, quinidine, and ritonavir; monitor for increased effect/toxicity. **Concurrent use with fluoxetine and paroxetine is contraindicated.**

CYP3A3/4 inhibitors: Metabolism of phenothiazines may be decreased; increasing clinical effect or toxicity; inhibitors include amiodarone, cimetidine, clarithromycin, erythromycin, delavirdine, diltiazem, dirithromycin, disulfiram, fluoxetine, fluvoxamine, grapefruit juice, indinavir, itraconazole, ketoconazole, nefazodone, nevirapine, propoxyphene, quinupristin-dalfopristin, ritonavir, saquinavir, verapamil, zafirlukast, zileuton

Enzyme inducers: May enhance the hepatic metabolism of phenothiazines; larger doses may be required. Includes rifampin, rifabutin, barbiturates, phenytoin, and cigarette smoking

Epinephrine: Chlorpromazine (and possibly other low potency antipsychotics) may diminish the pressor effects of epinephrine

Guanethidine and guanadrel: Antihypertensive effects may be inhibited by chlorpromazine

Levodopa: Chlorpromazine may inhibit the antiparkinsonian effect of levodopa; avoid this combination

Lithium: Chlorpromazine may produce neurotoxicity with lithium; this is a rare effect

Phenytoin: May reduce serum levels of phenothiazines; phenothiazines may increase phenytoin serum levels

Propranolol: Serum concentrations of phenothiazines may be increased; propranolol also increases phenothiazine concentrations; may also occur with pindolol. **These agents are contraindicated with mesoridazine.**

Polypeptide antibiotics: Rare cases of respiratory paralysis have been reported with concurrent use of phenothiazines

QT$_c$-prolonging agents: Effects on QT$_c$ interval may be additive with phenothiazines, increasing the risk of malignant arrhythmias; includes type Ia antiarrhythmics, TCAs, and some quinolone antibiotics (sparfloxacin, moxifloxacin and gatifloxacin). **Concurrent use is contraindicated.**

Sulfadoxine-pyrimethamine: May increase phenothiazine concentrations

Tricyclic antidepressants: Concurrent use may produce increased toxicity or altered therapeutic response

Trazodone: Phenothiazines and trazodone may produce additive hypotensive effects

Valproic acid: Serum levels may be increased by phenothiazines

Ethanol/Nutrition/Herb Interactions

Ethanol: Avoid ethanol (may increase CNS depression).

Herb/Nutraceutical: Avoid valerian, St John's wort, kava kava, gotu kola (may increase CNS depression).

Stability Protect all dosage forms from light; clear or slightly yellow solutions may be used; should be dispensed in amber or opaque vials/bottles. Solutions may be diluted or mixed with fruit juices or other liquids but must be administered immediately after mixing; do not prepare bulk dilutions or store bulk dilutions.

Mechanism of Action Blockade of postsynaptic CNS dopamine$_2$ receptors in the mesolimbic and mesocortical areas

Pharmacodynamics/Kinetics

Duration of action: 4-6 hours

Absorption: Very erratic with oral tablet; oral liquids much more dependable

Protein binding: 91% to 99%

Half-life: 24-48 hours

Time to peak serum concentration: 2-4 hours

Time to steady-state serum: 4-7 days

Elimination: In urine

Usual Dosage Concentrate may be diluted just prior to administration with distilled water, acidified tap water, orange or grape juice; do not prepare and store bulk dilutions

Adults: Schizophrenia/psychoses:

Oral: 25-50 mg 3 times/day; maximum: 100-400 mg/day

I.M.: Initial: 25 mg, repeat in 30-60 minutes as needed; optimal dosage range: 25-200 mg/day

Elderly: Behavioral symptoms associated with dementia:

Oral: Initial: 10 mg 1-2 times/day; if <10 mg/day is desired, consider administering 10 mg every other day (qod). Increase dose at 4- to 7-day intervals by 10-25 mg/day; increase dose intervals (bid, tid, etc) as necessary to control response or side effects. Maximum daily dose: 250 mg. Gradual increases (titration) may prevent some side effects or decrease their severity.

I.M.: Initial: 25 mg; repeat doses in 30-60 minutes if necessary. Dose range: 25-200 mg/day. Elderly usually require less than maximal daily dose.

Hemodialysis: Not dialyzable (0% to 5%)

Administration When administering I.M. or I.V., watch for hypotension. Dilute oral concentrate just prior to administration with distilled water, acidified tap water, orange or grape juice. Do not prepare and store bulk dilutions. Do not mix oral solutions of mesoridazine and lithium, these oral liquids are incompatible when mixed. **Note:** Avoid skin contact with oral medication; may cause contact dermatitis.

Monitoring Parameters Orthostatic blood pressures; tremors, gait changes, abnormal movement in trunk, neck, buccal area or extremities; monitor target behaviors for which the agent is given; monitor hepatic function (especially if fever with flu-like symptoms); baseline EKG, baseline (and periodic) serum potassium; do not initiate if QT$_c$ >450 msec (discontinue in any patient with a QT$_c$ >500 msec)

Test Interactions ↑ cholesterol (S), ↑ glucose; ↓ uric acid (S)

Patient Information May cause drowsiness or restlessness, avoid alcohol and other CNS depressants; do not alter dosage or discontinue without consulting (Continued)

Mesoridazine *(Continued)*

physician; avoid excessive/intense sunlight, yearly ophthalmic examinations are necessary

Nursing Implications

Dilute oral concentrate with water or juice before administration; avoid skin contact with oral suspension or solution; may cause contact dermatitis; monitor orthostatic blood pressures 3-5 days after initiation of therapy or a dose increase

Monitor orthostatic blood pressures; tremors, gait changes, abnormal movement in trunk, neck, buccal area or extremities; monitor target behaviors for which the agent is administered; monitor hepatic function (especially if fever with flu-like symptoms); watch for hypotension when administering I.M. or I.V.

Additional Information Coadministration of two or more antipsychotics does not improve clinical response and may increase the potential for adverse effects.

Dosage Forms

Injection, as besylate: 25 mg/mL (1 mL)

Liquid, oral, as besylate: 25 mg/mL (118 mL)

Tablet, as besylate: 10 mg, 25 mg, 50 mg, 100 mg

♦ **Mesoridazine Besylate** *see* Mesoridazine *on page 224*

♦ **Metadate® CD** *see* Methylphenidate *on page 236*

♦ **Metadate™ ER** *see* Methylphenidate *on page 236*

Methadone *(METH a done)*

Related Information

Addiction Treatments *on page 550*

Patient Information - Miscellaneous Medications *on page 495*

U.S. Brand Names Dolophine®; Methadose®

Canadian Brand Names Methadose®

Synonyms Methadone Hydrochloride

Pharmacologic Category Analgesic, Narcotic

Generic Available Yes

Use Management of severe pain; detoxification and maintenance treatment of narcotic addiction (if used for detoxification and maintenance treatment of narcotic addiction, it must be part of an FDA-approved program)

Restrictions C-II

Pregnancy Risk Factor B/D (prolonged use or high doses at term)

Contraindications Hypersensitivity to methadone or any component of the formulation; pregnancy (prolonged use or high doses near term)

Warnings/Precautions Because methadone's effects on respiration last much longer than its analgesic effects, the dose must be titrated slowly; because of its long half-life and risk of accumulation, it is not considered a drug of first choice in the elderly, who may be particularly susceptible to its CNS depressant and constipating effects. May cause respiratory depression - use caution in patients with respiratory disease or pre-existing respiratory depression. Potential for drug dependency exists, abrupt cessation may precipitate withdrawal. Use caution in elderly, debilitated, or pediatric patients. Use with caution in patients with depression or suicidal tendencies, or in patients with a history of drug abuse. Tolerance or psychological and physical dependence may occur with prolonged use.

Use with caution in patients with hepatic, pulmonary, or renal function impairment. May cause CNS depression, which may impair physical or mental abilities. Patients must be cautioned about performing tasks which require mental alertness (ie, operating machinery or driving). Effects with other sedative drugs or ethanol may be potentiated. Elderly may be more sensitive to CNS depressant and constipating effects. Use with caution in patients with head injury or increased ICP, biliary tract dysfunction or pancreatitis; history of ileus or bowel obstruction, glaucoma, hyperthyroidism, adrenal insufficiency, prostatic hypertrophy or urinary stricture, CNS depression, toxic psychosis, alcoholism, delirium tremens, or kyphoscoliosis. Tablets are to be used only for oral administration and must not be used for injection.

Adverse Reactions Frequency not defined.

Cardiovascular: Bradycardia, peripheral vasodilation, cardiac arrest, syncope, faintness

Central nervous system: Euphoria, dysphoria, headache, insomnia, agitation, disorientation, drowsiness, dizziness, lightheadedness, sedation

Dermatologic: Pruritus, urticaria, rash

Endocrine & metabolic: Decreased libido

Gastrointestinal: Nausea, vomiting, constipation, anorexia, stomach cramps, xerostomia, biliary tract spasm

Genitourinary: Urinary retention or hesitancy, antidiuretic effect, impotence

Neuromuscular & skeletal: Weakness

Ocular: Miosis, visual disturbances

Respiratory: Respiratory depression, respiratory arrest

Miscellaneous: Physical and psychological dependence

Overdosage/Toxicology

Signs and symptoms: Respiratory depression, CNS depression, miosis, hypothermia, circulatory collapse, convulsions

Treatment: Naloxone 2 mg I.V. (0.01 mg/kg for children) with repeat administration as necessary up to a total of 10 mg

Drug Interactions CYP1A2, 2D6, and 3A3/4 enzyme substrate; CYP2D6 enzyme inhibitor

CYP1A2 inhibitors: Serum level and/or toxicity of methadone may be increased, increasing clinical effect or toxicity; inhibitors include cimetidine, ciprofloxacin, fluvoxamine, isoniazid, ritonavir, and zileuton.

CYP2D6 inhibitors: Serum level and/or toxicity of methadone may be increased, increasing clinical effect or toxicity; inhibitors include amiodarone, cimetidine, delavirdine, fluoxetine, paroxetine, propafenone, quinidine, and ritonavir; monitor for increased effect/toxicity

CYP3A3/4 inhibitors: Serum level and/or toxicity of methadone may be increased; inhibitors include amiodarone, cimetidine, clarithromycin, erythromycin, delavirdine, diltiazem, dirithromycin, disulfiram, fluoxetine, fluvoxamine, grapefruit juice, indinavir, itraconazole, ketoconazole, metronidazole, nefazodone, nevirapine, propoxyphene, quinupristin-dalfopristin, ritonavir, saquinavir, verapamil, zafirlukast, zileuton; monitor for altered response

Enzyme inducers: Barbiturates, carbamazepine, phenytoin, primidone, and rifampin may decrease serum methadone concentrations via enhanced hepatic metabolism; monitor for methadone withdrawal; larger doses of methadone may be required

Somatostatin: Therapeutic effect of methadone may be decreased; limited documentation; monitor

Zidovudine: serum concentrations may be increased by methadone; monitor

Ethanol/Nutrition/Herb Interactions

Ethanol: Avoid ethanol (may increase CNS effects). Watch for sedation.

Herb/Nutraceutical: Avoid St John's wort (may decrease methadone levels; may increase CNS depression). Avoid valerian, kava kava, gotu kola (may increase CNS depression). Methadone is metabolized by CYP3A4 in the intestines; avoid concurrent use of grapefruit juice.

Stability Highly **incompatible** with all other I.V. agents when mixed together

Mechanism of Action Binds to opiate receptors in the CNS, causing inhibition of ascending pain pathways, altering the perception of and response to pain; produces generalized CNS depression

Pharmacodynamics/Kinetics

Oral:

Onset of analgesia: Within 0.5-1 hour

Duration: 6-8 hours, increases to 22-48 hours with repeated doses

Parenteral:

Onset of effect: Within 10-20 minutes

(Continued)

Methadone (Continued)

Peak effect: Within 1-2 hours

Distribution: Crosses the placenta; appears in breast milk

Protein binding: 80% to 85%

Metabolism: In the liver (N-demethylation)

Half-life: 15-29 hours, may be prolonged with alkaline pH

Elimination: In urine (<10% as unchanged drug); increased renal excretion with urine pH <6

Usual Dosage Doses should be titrated to appropriate effects

Children:

Analgesia:

Oral, I.M., S.C.: 0.7 mg/kg/24 hours divided every 4-6 hours as needed or 0.1-0.2 mg/kg every 4-12 hours as needed; maximum: 10 mg/dose

I.V.: 0.1 mg/kg every 4 hours initially for 2-3 doses, then every 6-12 hours as needed; maximum: 10 mg/dose

Iatrogenic narcotic dependency: Oral: General guidelines: Initial: 0.05-0.1 mg/kg/dose every 6 hours; increase by 0.05 mg/kg/dose until withdrawal symptoms are controlled; after 24-48 hours, the dosing interval can be lengthened to every 12-24 hours; to taper dose, wean by 0.05 mg/kg/day; if withdrawal symptoms recur, taper at a slower rate

Adults:

Analgesia: Oral, I.M., S.C.: 2.5-10 mg every 3-8 hours as needed, up to 5-20 mg every 6-8 hours

Detoxification: Oral: 15-40 mg/day

Maintenance treatment of opiate dependence: Oral: 20-120 mg/day

Dosing adjustment in renal impairment: Cl_{cr} <10 mL/minute: Administer at 50% to 75% of normal dose

Dosing adjustment/comments in hepatic disease: Avoid in severe liver disease

Important note: Methadone accumulates with repeated doses and dosage may need to be adjusted downward after 3-5 days to prevent toxic effects. Some patients may benefit from every 8- to 12-hour dosing interval (pain control).

Monitoring Parameters Pain relief, respiratory and mental status, blood pressure

Reference Range Therapeutic: 100-400 ng/mL (SI: 0.32-1.29 µmol/L); Toxic: >2 µg/mL (SI: >6.46 µmol/L)

Patient Information May cause drowsiness, avoid alcohol and other CNS depressants

Nursing Implications Observe patient for excessive sedation, respiratory depression, implement safety measures, assist with ambulation

Additional Information Methadone accumulates with repeated doses and dosage may need to be adjusted downward after 3-5 days to prevent toxic effects. Some patients may benefit from every 8- to 12-hour dosing interval (pain control). Oral dose for detoxification and maintenance may be administered in Tang®, Kool-Aid®, apple juice, grape Crystal Light®.

Dosage Forms

Injection, as hydrochloride: 10 mg/mL (20 mL)

Solution, oral, as hydrochloride: 5 mg/5 mL (5 mL, 500 mL); 10 mg/5 mL (500 mL)

Solution, oral concentrate, as hydrochloride: 10 mg/mL (30 mL)

Tablet, as hydrochloride: 5 mg, 10 mg

Tablet, dispersible, as hydrochloride: 40 mg

♦ **Methadone Hydrochloride** *see* Methadone *on page 228*

♦ **Methadose®** *see* Methadone *on page 228*

♦ **Methaminodiazepoxide Hydrochloride** *see* Chlordiazepoxide *on page 71*

Methamphetamine (meth am FET a meen)

Related Information

Patient Information - Stimulants *on page 481*

Stimulant Agents Used for ADHD *on page 593*

U.S. Brand Names Desoxyn®; Desoxyn® Gradumet®

Synonyms Desoxyephedrine Hydrochloride; Methamphetamine Hydrochloride

Pharmacologic Category Stimulant

Generic Available Yes

Use Treatment of attention-deficit/hyperactivity disorder (ADHD); exogenous obesity (short-term adjunct)

Unlabeled/Investigational Use Narcolepsy

Restrictions C-II

Pregnancy Risk Factor C

Contraindications Hypersensitivity or idiosyncrasy to sympathomimetic amines; patients with advanced arteriosclerosis, symptomatic cardiovascular disease, moderate to severe hypertension (stage II or III), hyperthyroidism, glaucoma, agitated states; patients with a history of drug abuse; use during or within 14 days following MAO inhibitor therapy; stimulant medications are contraindicated for use in children with attention-deficit/hyperactivity disorders and concomitant Tourette's syndrome or tics

Warnings/Precautions Use with caution in patients with bipolar disorder, diabetes mellitus, cardiovascular disease, seizure disorders, insomnia, porphyria, or mild hypertension (stage I). May exacerbate symptoms of behavior and thought disorder in psychotic patients. Potential for drug dependency exists - avoid abrupt discontinuation in patients who have received for prolonged periods. Use in weight reduction programs only when alternative therapy has been ineffective. Products may contain tartrazine - use with caution in potentially sensitive individuals. Stimulant use in children has been associated with growth suppression. Stimulants may unmask tics in individuals with coexisting Tourette's syndrome.

Adverse Reactions Frequency not defined.

Cardiovascular: Hypertension, tachycardia, palpitations

Central nervous system: Restlessness, headache, exacerbation of motor and phonic tics and Tourette's syndrome, dizziness, psychosis, dysphoria, overstimulation, euphoria, insomnia

Dermatologic: Rash, urticaria

Endocrine & metabolic: Change in libido

Gastrointestinal: Diarrhea, nausea, vomiting, stomach cramps, constipation, anorexia, weight loss, xerostomia, unpleasant taste

Genitourinary: Impotence

Neuromuscular & skeletal: Tremor

Miscellaneous: Suppression of growth in children, tolerance and withdrawal with prolonged use

Overdosage/Toxicology

Signs and symptoms: Seizures, hyperactivity, coma, hypertension

Treatment: There is no specific antidote for amphetamine intoxication and the bulk of the treatment is supportive. Hyperactivity and agitation usually respond to reduced sensory input, however with extreme agitation haloperidol (2-5 mg I.M. for adults) may be required. Hyperthermia is best treated with external cooling measures, or when severe or unresponsive, muscle paralysis with pancuronium may be needed. Hypertension is usually transient and generally does not require treatment unless severe. For diastolic blood pressures >110 mm Hg, a nitroprusside infusion should be initiated. Seizures usually respond to diazepam IVP and/or phenytoin maintenance regimens.

Drug Interactions CYP2D6 enzyme substrate

Acidifiers: Very large doses of potassium acid phosphate or ammonium chloride may increase the renal elimination of amphetamines due to urinary acidification

Alkalinizers: Large doses of sodium bicarbonate or other alkalinizers may increase renal tubular reabsorption (decreased elimination) and diminish the effect of amphetamine; includes potassium or sodium citrate and acetate

Antipsychotics: Efficacy of amphetamines may be decreased by antipsychotics; in addition, amphetamines may induce an increase in psychotic symptoms in some patients

(Continued)

Methamphetamine *(Continued)*

CYP2D6 inhibitors: Serum levels and/or toxicity of methamphetamine may be increased; inhibitors include amiodarone, cimetidine, delavirdine, fluoxetine, paroxetine, propafenone, quinidine, and ritonavir; monitor for increased effect/toxicity

Enzyme inducers: Metabolism of amphetamine may be increased; decreasing clinical effect; inducers include barbiturates, carbamazepine, phenytoin, and rifampin

Furazolidone: Amphetamines may induce hypertensive episodes in patients receiving furazolidone

Guanethidine: Amphetamines inhibit the antihypertensive response to guanethidine; probably also may occur with guanadrel

MAO inhibitors: Severe hypertensive episodes have occurred with amphetamine when used in patients receiving MAO inhibitors; concurrent use or use within 14 days is contraindicated

Norepinephrine: Amphetamines enhance the pressor response to norepinephrine

Sibutramine: Concurrent use of sibutramine and amphetamines may cause severe hypertension and tachycardia; use is contraindicated (benzphetamine)

SSRIs: Amphetamines may increase the potential for serotonin syndrome when used concurrently with selective serotonin reuptake inhibitors (including fluoxetine, fluvoxamine, paroxetine, and sertraline)

Tricyclic antidepressants: Concurrent of amphetamines with TCAs may result in hypertension and CNS stimulation; avoid this combination

Ethanol/Nutrition/Herb Interactions

Ethanol: Avoid ethanol (may cause CNS depression).

Food: Amphetamine serum levels may be altered if taken with acidic food, juices, or vitamin C. Avoid caffeine.

Herb/Nutraceutical: Avoid ephedra (may cause hypertension or arrhythmias).

Mechanism of Action A sympathomimetic amine related to ephedrine and amphetamine with CNS stimulant activity; peripheral actions include elevation of systolic and diastolic blood pressure and weak bronchodilator and respiratory stimulant action

Pharmacodynamics/Kinetics

Absorption: Rapid from GI tract

Metabolism: In the liver

Half-Life: 4-5 hours

Elimination: Primarily in urine; dependent on urine pH

Usual Dosage

Children >6 years: ADHD: 2.5-5 mg 1-2 times/day; may increase by 5 mg increments at weekly intervals until optimum response is achieved, usually 20-25 mg/day

Children >12 years and Adults: Exogenous obesity: 5 mg 30 minutes before each meal; long-acting formulation: 10-15 mg in morning; treatment duration should not exceed a few weeks

Dietary Considerations Should be administered 30 minutes before meals.

Monitoring Parameters Heart rate, respiratory rate, blood pressure, and CNS activity

Patient Information Take during day to avoid insomnia; do not discontinue abruptly, may cause physical and psychological dependence with prolonged use; do not crush or chew extended release tablet

Nursing Implications Dose should not be given in evening or at bedtime; do not crush extended release tablet

Additional Information Illicit methamphetamine may contain lead; alkalinizing urine can result in longer methamphetamine half-life and elevated blood level; ephedrine is a precursor in the illicit manufacture of methamphetamine; ephedrine is extracted by dissolving ephedrine tablets in water or alcohol (50,000 tablets can result in 1 kg of ephedrine); conversion to methamphetamine occurs at a rate of 50% to 70% of the weight of ephedrine. 3,4-methylene dioxymethamphetamine (slang: XTC, Ecstasy, Adam) affects the serotonergic, dopaminergic, and noradrenergic pathways. As such, it can cause the serotonin syndrome associated with malignant hyperthermia and rhabdomyolysis.

Dosage Forms

Tablet, as hydrochloride: 5 mg

Tablet, extended release, as hydrochloride (Desoxyn® Gradumet®): 5 mg, 10 mg, 15 mg

♦ **Methamphetamine Hydrochloride** *see* Methamphetamine *on page 230*

Methohexital (meth oh HEKS i tal)

U.S. Brand Names Brevital® Sodium

Canadian Brand Names Brietal Sodium®

Synonyms Methohexital Sodium

Pharmacologic Category Barbiturate

Generic Available No

Use Induction and maintenance of general anesthesia for short procedures

Can be used in pediatric patients >1 month of age as follows: For rectal or intramuscular induction of anesthesia prior to the use of other general anesthetic agents, as an adjunct to subpotent inhalational anesthetic agents for short surgical procedures, or for short surgical, diagnostic, or therapeutic procedures associated with minimal painful stimuli

Restrictions C-IV

Pregnancy Risk Factor C

Contraindications Porphyria, hypersensitivity to methohexital or any component

Warnings/Precautions Use with extreme caution in patients with liver impairment, asthma, cardiovascular instability

Adverse Reactions Frequency not defined.

Cardiovascular: Hypotension, peripheral vascular collapse,

Central nervous system: Seizures, headache

Gastrointestinal: Cramping, diarrhea, rectal bleeding, nausea, vomiting

Hematologic: Hemolytic anemia, thrombophlebitis

Local: Pain on I.M. injection

Neuromuscular & skeletal: Tremor, twitching, rigidity, involuntary muscle movement, radial nerve palsy

Respiratory: Apnea, respiratory depression, laryngospasm, coughing, hiccups

Overdosage/Toxicology

Signs and symptoms: Apnea, tachycardia, hypotension

Treatment: Primarily supportive with mechanical ventilation if needed

Drug Interactions CYP1A2, 2C, 3A3/4, and 3A5-7 inducer

Note: Barbiturates are enzyme inducers; patients should be monitored when these drugs are started or stopped for a decreased or increased therapeutic effect respectively

Acetaminophen: Barbiturates may enhance the hepatotoxic potential of acetaminophen overdoses

Antiarrhythmics: Barbiturates may increase the metabolism of antiarrhythmics, decreasing their clinical effect; includes disopyramide, propafenone, and quinidine

Anticonvulsants: Barbiturates may increase the metabolism of anticonvulsants; includes ethosuximide, felbamate (possibly), lamotrigine, phenytoin, tiagabine, topiramate, and zonisamide; does not appear to affect gabapentin or levetiracetam

Antineoplastics: Limited evidence suggests that enzyme-inducing anticonvulsant therapy may reduce the effectiveness of some chemotherapy regimens (specifically in ALL); teniposide and methotrexate may be cleared more rapidly in these patients

Antipsychotics: Barbiturates may enhance the metabolism (decrease the efficacy) of antipsychotics; monitor for altered response; dose adjustment may be needed

(Continued)

Methohexital *(Continued)*

Beta-blockers: Metabolism of beta-blockers may be increased and clinical effect decreased; atenolol and nadolol are unlikely to interact given their renal elimination

Calcium channel blockers: Barbiturates may enhance the metabolism of calcium channel blockers, decreasing their clinical effect

Chloramphenicol: Barbiturates may increase the metabolism of chloramphenicol and chloramphenicol may inhibit barbiturate metabolism; monitor for altered response

Cimetidine: Barbiturates may enhance the metabolism of cimetidine, decreasing its clinical effect

CNS depressants: Sedative effects and/or respiratory depression with barbiturates may be additive with other CNS depressants; monitor for increased effect; includes ethanol, sedatives, antidepressants, narcotic analgesics, and benzodiazepines

Corticosteroids: Barbiturates may enhance the metabolism of corticosteroids, decreasing their clinical effect

Cyclosporine: Levels may be decreased by barbiturates; monitor

Doxycycline: Barbiturates may enhance the metabolism of doxycycline, decreasing its clinical effect; higher dosages may be required

Estrogens: Barbiturates may increase the metabolism of estrogens and reduce their efficacy

Felbamate may inhibit the metabolism of barbiturates and barbiturates may increase the metabolism of felbamate

Griseofulvin: Barbiturates may impair the absorption of griseofulvin, and griseofulvin metabolism may be increased by barbiturates, decreasing clinical effect

Guanfacine: Effect may be decreased by barbiturates

Immunosuppressants: Barbiturates may enhance the metabolism of immunosuppressants, decreasing its clinical effect; includes both cyclosporine and tacrolimus

Loop diuretics: Metabolism may be increased and clinical effects decreased; established for furosemide, effect with other loop diuretics not established

MAO inhibitors: Metabolism of barbiturates may be inhibited, increasing clinical effect or toxicity of the barbiturates

Methadone: Barbiturates may enhance the metabolism of methadone resulting in methadone withdrawal

Methoxyflurane: Barbiturates may enhance the nephrotoxic effects of methoxyflurane

Oral contraceptives: Barbiturates may enhance the metabolism of oral contraceptives, decreasing their clinical effect; an alternative method of contraception should be considered

Theophylline: Barbiturates may increase metabolism of theophylline derivatives and decrease their clinical effect

Tricyclic antidepressants: Barbiturates may increase metabolism of tricyclic antidepressants and decrease their clinical effect; sedative effects may be additive

Valproic acid: Metabolism of barbiturates may be inhibited by valproic acid; monitor for excessive sedation; a dose reduction may be needed

Warfarin: Barbiturates inhibit the hypoprothrombinemic effects of oral anticoagulants via increased metabolism; this combination should generally be avoided

Stability Do not dilute with solutions containing bacteriostatic agents; solutions are alkaline (pH 9.5-11) and **incompatible** with acids (eg, atropine sulfate, succinylcholine, silicone), also **incompatible** with phenol-containing solutions and silicone

Mechanism of Action Ultra short-acting I.V. barbiturate anesthetic

Usual Dosage Doses must be titrated to effect

Children 3-12 years:

I.M.: Preop: 5-10 mg/kg/dose

I.V.: Induction: 1-2 mg/kg/dose

Rectal: Preop/induction: 20-35 mg/kg/dose; usual 25 mg/kg/dose; administer as 10% aqueous solution

Adults: I.V.: Induction: 50-120 mg to start; 20-40 mg every 4-7 minutes

Dosing adjustment/comments in hepatic impairment: Lower dosage and monitor closely

Dietary Considerations Should not be given to patients with food in stomach because of danger of vomiting during anesthesia.

Administration Dilute to a maximum concentration of 1% for I.V. use

Patient Information May cause drowsiness

Nursing Implications Avoid extravasation or intra-arterial administration

Dosage Forms Injection, as sodium: 500 mg, 2.5 g, 5 g

♦ **Methohexital Sodium** *see* Methohexital *on page 233*

Methsuximide (meth SUKS i mide)

U.S. Brand Names Celontin®

Canadian Brand Names Celontin

Pharmacologic Category Anticonvulsant, Succinimide

Generic Available No

Use Control of absence (petit mal) seizures that are refractory to other drugs

Unlabeled/Investigational Use Partial complex (psychomotor) seizures

Pregnancy Risk Factor C

Contraindications Hypersensitivity to succinimides or any component of the formulation

Warnings/Precautions Use with caution in patients with hepatic or renal disease; abrupt withdrawal of the drug may precipitate absence status; methsuximide may increase tonic-clonic seizures in patients with mixed seizure disorders; methsuximide must be used in combination with other anticonvulsants in patients with both absence and tonic-clonic seizures. Succinimides have been associated with severe blood dyscrasias and cases of systemic lupus erythematosus.

Adverse Reactions Frequency not defined.

Cardiovascular: Hyperemia

Central nervous system: Ataxia, dizziness, drowsiness, headache, aggressiveness, mental depression, irritability, nervousness, insomnia, confusion, psychosis, suicidal behavior, auditory hallucinations

Dermatologic: Stevens-Johnson syndrome, rash, urticaria, pruritus

Gastrointestinal: Anorexia, nausea, vomiting, weight loss, diarrhea, epigastric and abdominal pain, constipation

Genitourinary: Proteinuria, hematuria (microscopic); cases of blood dyscrasias have been reported with succinimides

Hematologic: Leukopenia, pancytopenia, eosinophilia, monocytosis

Neuromuscular & skeletal: Cases of systemic lupus erythematosus have been reported

Ocular: Blurred vision, photophobia, peripheral edema

Overdosage/Toxicology

Signs and symptoms: Acute overdosage can cause CNS depression, ataxia, stupor, coma, hypotension; chronic overdose can cause skin rash, confusion, ataxia, proteinuria, hepatic dysfunction, hematuria

Treatment: Supportive; hemoperfusion and hemodialysis may be useful

Drug Interactions CYP3A3/4 enzyme substrate

CNS depressants: Sedative effects and/or respiratory depression may be additive with CNS depressants; includes ethanol, benzodiazepines, barbiturates, narcotic analgesics, and other sedative agents; monitor for increased effect

CYP3A3/4 inhibitors: Serum level and/or toxicity of succimides may be increased; inhibitors include amiodarone, cimetidine, clarithromycin, erythromycin, delavirdine, diltiazem, dirithromycin, disulfiram, fluoxetine, fluvoxamine, grapefruit juice, indinavir, itraconazole, ketoconazole, nefazodone, nevirapine, propoxyphene, quinupristin-dalfopristin, ritonavir, saquinavir, verapamil, zafirlukast, zileuton

(Continued)

Methsuximide *(Continued)*

Enzyme inducers: Metabolism of succimides may be increased, decreasing their therapeutic effect; consider using an alternative sedative/hypnotic agent; potential inducers include phenobarbital, phenytoin, carbamazepine, rifampin, and rifabutin

Phenobarbital: Methsuximide may increase phenobarbital concentration.

Phenytoin: Methsuximide may increase phenytoin concentration.

Stability Protect from high temperature.

Mechanism of Action Increases the seizure threshold and suppresses paroxysmal spike-and-wave pattern in absence seizures; depresses nerve transmission in the motor cortex

Pharmacodynamics/Kinetics

Metabolism: Rapidly demethylated in the liver to N-desmethylmethsuximide (active metabolite)

Half-life: 2-4 hours

Time to peak serum concentration: Oral: Within 1-3 hours

Elimination: <1% excreted in urine as unchanged drug

Usual Dosage Oral:

Children: Anticonvulsant: Initial: 10-15 mg/kg/day in 3-4 divided doses; increase weekly up to maximum of 30 mg/kg/day

Adults: Anticonvulsant: 300 mg/day for the first week; may increase by 300 mg/day at weekly intervals up to 1.2 g/day in 2-4 divided doses/day

Monitoring Parameters CBC, hepatic function tests, urinalysis

Patient Information Take with food; do not discontinue abruptly; may cause drowsiness and impair judgment

Nursing Implications Monitor CBC, hepatic function tests, urinalysis

Dosage Forms Capsule: 150 mg, 300 mg

♦ **Methylin**™ *see Methylphenidate on page 236*
♦ **Methylin**™ **ER** *see Methylphenidate on page 236*

Methylphenidate *(meth il FEN i date)*

Related Information

Clozapine-Induced Side Effects *on page 568*
Patient Information - Stimulants *on page 481*
Stimulant Agents Used for ADHD *on page 593*

U.S. Brand Names Concerta™; Metadate® CD; Metadate™ ER; Methylin™; Methylin™ ER; Ritalin®; Ritalin-SR®

Canadian Brand Names PMS-Methylphenidate

Synonyms Methylphenidate Hydrochloride

Pharmacologic Category Stimulant

Generic Available Yes

Use Treatment of attention-deficit/hyperactivity disorder (ADHD); symptomatic management of narcolepsy

Unlabeled/Investigational Use Depression (especially elderly or medically ill)

Restrictions C-II

Pregnancy Risk Factor C

Pregnancy/Breast-Feeding Implications There are no well-controlled studies establishing safety in pregnant women. Animal studies have shown teratogenic effects to the fetus. Do not use in women of childbearing age unless the potential benefit outweighs the possible risk. It is unknown if methylphenidate is excreted in human milk. Use caution if administering to a nursing woman.

Contraindications Hypersensitivity to methylphenidate, any component of the formulation, or idiosyncrasy to sympathomimetic amines; marked anxiety, tension, and agitation; patients with advanced arteriosclerosis, symptomatic cardiovascular disease, moderate to severe hypertension (stage II or III), hyperthyroidism, glaucoma; patients with a history of drug abuse; use during or within 14 days following

MAO inhibitor therapy; stimulant medications are contraindicated for use in children with attention-deficit/hyperactivity disorders and concomitant Tourette's syndrome or tics

Warnings/Precautions Safety and efficacy in children <6 years of age not established. Use with caution in patients with bipolar disorder, diabetes mellitus, cardiovascular disease, seizure disorders, insomnia, porphyria, or mild hypertension (stage I). May exacerbate symptoms of behavior and thought disorder in psychotic patients. Do not use to treat severe depression or fatigue states. Potential for drug dependency exists - avoid abrupt discontinuation in patients who have received for prolonged periods. Visual disturbances have been reported (rare). Stimulant use has been associated with growth suppression. Stimulants may unmask tics in individuals with coexisting Tourette's syndrome. Concerta™ should not be used in patients with pre-existing severe gastrointestinal narrowing (small bowel disease, short gut syndrome, history of peritonitis, cystic fibrosis, chronic intestinal pseudo-obstruction, Meckel's diverticulum)

Adverse Reactions Frequency not defined.

Cardiovascular: Tachycardia, bradycardia, angina, hypertension, hypotension, palpitations, cardiac arrhythmias

Central nervous system: Nervousness, insomnia, headache, dyskinesia, toxic psychosis, Tourette's syndrome, NMS, dizziness, drowsiness

Dermatologic: Rash, exfoliative dermatitis, erythema multiforme,

Endocrine & metabolic: Growth retardation

Gastrointestinal: Nausea, vomiting, anorexia, nausea, abdominal pain, weight loss

Hematologic: Thrombocytopenia, anemia, leukopenia, thrombocytopenic purpura

Ocular: Blurred vision

Renal: Necrotizing vasculitis

Respiratory: Upper respiratory tract infection, increased cough, pharyngitis, sinusitis

Miscellaneous: Hypersensitivity reactions

Overdosage/Toxicology

Symptoms of overdose include vomiting, agitation, tremors, hyperpyrexia, muscle twitching, hallucinations, tachycardia, mydriasis, sweating, palpitations

There is no specific antidote for methylphenidate intoxication and the bulk of the treatment is supportive. Hyperactivity and agitation usually respond to reduced sensory input or benzodiazepines, however, with extreme agitation haloperidol (2-5 mg I.M. for adults) may be required. Hyperthermia is best treated with external cooling measures, or when severe or unresponsive, muscle paralysis with pancuronium may be needed. Hypertension is usually transient and generally does not require treatment unless severe. For diastolic blood pressures >110 mm Hg, a nitroprusside infusion should be initiated. Seizures usually respond to diazepam I.V. and/or phenytoin maintenance regimens.

Drug Interactions

Clonidine: Severe toxic reactions have been reported in combined use with methylphenidate.

Guanethidine: Methylphenidate inhibits the antihypertensive response to guanethidine; probably also may occur with guanadrel

Linezolid: Due to MAO inhibition (see note on MAO inhibitors), concurrent use with methylphenidate should generally be avoided

MAO inhibitors: Severe hypertensive episodes have occurred with amphetamine when used in patients receiving nonselective MAO inhibitors; methylphenidate may be less likely to interact, or reactions may be less severe; use with caution only when warranted; wait 14 days following discontinuation of MAO inhibitor

Phenobarbital: Serum levels may be increased by methylphenidate (in some patients); monitor

Phenytoin: Serum levels may be increased by methylphenidate (in some patients); monitor

Selegiline: When selegiline is used at low dosages (<10 mg/day), an interaction with methylphenidate is less likely than with nonselective MAO inhibitors (see MAO inhibitor information), but theoretically possible; monitor

(Continued)

Methylphenidate *(Continued)*

Sibutramine: Potential for reactions noted with amphetamines (severe hypertension and tachycardia) appears to be low; use with caution

SSRIs: Methylphenidate may increase the serum concentration of some SSRIs; clinical reports are limited.

Tricyclic antidepressants: Methylphenidate may increase serum concentrations of some tricyclic agents; clinical reports of toxicity are limited; dosage reduction of tricyclic antidepressants may be required; monitor

Venlafaxine: NMS has been reported in a patient receiving methylphenidate and venlafaxine

Warfarin: Methylphenidate may decrease metabolism of coumarin anticoagulants; effect has not been confirmed in all studies; monitor INR

Ethanol/Nutrition/Herb Interactions

Ethanol: Avoid ethanol (may cause CNS depression).

Food: Food may increase oral absorption; Concerta™ formulation is not affected. Food delays early peak and high-fat meals increase C_{max} and AUC of Metadate® CD formulation.

Herb/Nutraceutical: Avoid ephedra (may cause hypertension or arrhythmias)

Stability

Tablet: Do not store above 30°C (86°F); protect from light

Extended release capsule: Store in dose pack provided at 25°C (77°F)

Sustained release tablet: Do not store above 30°C (86°F); protect from moisture

Osmotic controlled release tablet (Concerta™): Store at 25°C (77°F); protect from humidity

Mechanism of Action
Mild CNS stimulant; blocks the reuptake mechanism of dopaminergic neurons; appears to stimulate the cerebral cortex and subcortical structures similar to amphetamines

Pharmacodynamics/Kinetics

Immediate release tablet:
  Peak cerebral stimulation effect: Within 2 hours
  Duration: 3-6 hours

Extended release capsule (Metadate® CD): Biphasic; initial peak similar to immediate release product, followed by second rising portion (corresponding to extended release portion)

Sustained release tablet:
  Peak effect: Within 4-7 hours
  Duration: 8 hours

Osmotic release tablet (Concerta™):
  Peak effect: Initial: 1-2 hours; C_{max}: 6-8 hours

Absorption: Readily absorbed from GI tract

Metabolism: In liver via de-esterification to an active metabolite

Half-life: 2-4 hours

Elimination: 90% in urine as metabolites and unchanged drug

Usual Dosage
Oral (discontinue periodically to re-evaluate or if no improvement occurs within 1 month):

Children ≥6 years: ADHD: Initial: 0.3 mg/kg/dose or 2.5-5 mg/dose given before breakfast and lunch; increase by 0.1 mg/kg/dose or by 5-10 mg/day at weekly intervals; usual dose: 0.5-1 mg/kg/day; maximum dose: 2 mg/kg/day or 90 mg/day

Extended release products:

Metadate™ ER, Methylin™ ER, Ritalin® SR: Duration of action is 8 hours. May be given in place of regular tablets, once the daily dose is titrated using the regular tablets and the titrated 8-hour dosage corresponds to sustained release tablet size.

Metadate® CD: Initial: 20 mg once daily; may be adjusted in 20 mg increments at weekly intervals; maximum: 60 mg/day

Concerta™: Duration of action is 12 hours:
  Children not currently taking methylphenidate:
    Initial: 18 mg once daily in the morning
    Adjustment: May increase to 54 mg/day; dose may be adjusted at weekly intervals
  Children currently taking methylphenidate: **Note:** Dosing based on current regimen and clinical judgment; suggested dosing listed below:
    Patients taking methylphenidate 5 mg 2-3 times/day or 20 mg/day sustained release formulation: Initial dose: 18 mg once every morning (maximum: 54 mg/day)
    Patients taking methylphenidate 10 mg 2-3 times/day or 40 mg/day sustained release formulation: Initial dose: 36 mg once every morning (maximum: 54 mg/day)
    Patients taking methylphenidate 15 mg 2-3 times/day or 60 mg/day sustained release formulation: Initial dose: 54 mg once every morning (maximum: 54 mg/day)

Adults:
  Narcolepsy: 10 mg 2-3 times/day, up to 60 mg/day
  Depression (unlabeled use): Initial: 2.5 mg every morning before 9 AM; dosage may be increased by 2.5-5 mg every 2-3 days as tolerated to a maximum of 20 mg/day; may be divided (ie, 7 AM and 12 noon), but should not be given after noon; do not use sustained release product

Dietary Considerations Should be taken 30-45 minutes before meals. Concerta™ is not affected by food and may be taken with or without meals. Metadate® CD should be taken before breakfast. Metadate™ ER should be taken before breakfast and lunch.

Administration Do not crush or allow patient to chew sustained release dosage form. To effectively avoid insomnia, dosing should be completed by noon.
  Concerta™: Administer dose once daily in the morning. May be taken with or without food, but must be taken with water, milk, or juice.

Monitoring Parameters Blood pressure, heart rate, signs and symptoms of depression

Patient Information Take exactly as directed; do not change dosage or discontinue without consulting prescriber. Response may take some time. Do not crush or chew sustained release dosage forms. Tablets and sustained release tablets should be taken 30-45 minutes before meals. Concerta™ may be taken with or without food, but must be taken with water, milk, or juice. Avoid alcohol, caffeine, or other stimulants. Maintain adequate fluid intake (2-3 L/day of fluids unless instructed to restrict fluid intake). You may experience decreased appetite or weight loss (small frequent meals may help maintain adequate nutrition); restlessness, impaired judgment, or dizziness, especially during early therapy (use caution when driving or engaging in tasks requiring alertness until response to drug is known); Report unresolved rapid heartbeat; excessive agitation, nervousness, insomnia, tremors, or dizziness; blackened stool; skin rash or irritation; or altered gait or movement. Concerta™ tablet shell may appear intact in stool; this is normal.

Nursing Implications Do not crush or allow patient to chew sustained release dosage forms; to effectively avoid insomnia, dosing should be completed by noon. Concerta™ tablet shell may appear intact in stool; this is normal. Must be taken with water, milk, or juice.

Additional Information Treatment with methylphenidate should include "drug holidays" or periodic discontinuation in order to assess the patient's requirements and to decrease tolerance and limit suppression of linear growth and weight. Specific patients may require 3 doses/day for treatment of ADHD (ie, additional dose at 4 PM).

Concerta™ is an osmotic controlled release formulation (OROS®) of methylphenidate. The tablet has an immediate-release overcoat that provides an initial dose of methylphenidate within 1 hour. The overcoat covers a trilayer core. The trilayer core is composed of two layers containing the drug and excipients, and one layer (Continued)

Methylphenidate *(Continued)*

of osmotic components. As water from the gastrointestinal tract enters the core, the osmotic components expand and methylphenidate is released.

Metadate® CD capsules contain a mixture of immediate release and extended release beads, designed to release 30% of the dose (6 mg) immediately and 70% (14 mg) over an extended period.

Dosage Forms

Capsule, extended release, as hydrochloride (Metadate® CD): 20 mg
Tablet, as hydrochloride: 5 mg, 10 mg, 20 mg
  Methylin™, Ritalin®: 5 mg, 10 mg, 20 mg
Tablet, extended release, as hydrochloride (Metadate™ ER): 10 mg, 20 mg
Tablet, osmotic controlled release, as hydrochloride (Concerta™): 18 mg, 36 mg, 54 mg
Tablet, sustained release, as hydrochloride: 20 mg
  Methylin™ ER: 10 mg, 20 mg
  Ritalin-SR®: 20 mg

♦ **Methylphenidate Hydrochloride** *see Methylphenidate on page 236*

♦ **Meval® (Can)** *see Diazepam on page 110*

Midazolam *(MID aye zoe lam)*

Related Information

Benzodiazepines Comparison Chart *on page 566*
Patient Information - Anxiolytics & Sedative Hypnotics (Benzodiazepines) *on page 483*

U.S. Brand Names Versed®
Canadian Brand Names Versed
Synonyms Midazolam Hydrochloride
Pharmacologic Category Benzodiazepine
Generic Available No
Use Preoperative sedation and provides conscious sedation prior to diagnostic or radiographic procedures; ICU sedation (continuous infusion); intravenous anesthesia (induction); intravenous anesthesia (maintenance)
Unlabeled/Investigational Use Anxiety, status epilepticus
Restrictions C-IV
Pregnancy Risk Factor D
Pregnancy/Breast-Feeding Implications Midazolam has been found to cross the placenta; not recommended for use during pregnancy
Contraindications Hypersensitivity to midazolam or any component of the formulation, including benzyl alcohol (cross-sensitivity with other benzodiazepines may exist); parenteral form is not for intrathecal or epidural injection; narrow-angle glaucoma; pregnancy
Warnings/Precautions May cause severe respiratory depression, respiratory arrest, or apnea. Use with extreme caution, particularly in noncritical care settings. Appropriate resuscitative equipment and qualified personnel must be available for administration and monitoring. Initial dosing must be cautiously titrated and individualized, particularly in elderly or debilitated patients, patients with hepatic impairment (including alcoholics), or in renal impairment, particularly if other CNS depressants (including opiates) are used concurrently. Initial doses in elderly or debilitated patients should not exceed 2.5 mg. Use with caution in patients with respiratory disease or impaired gag reflex. Use during upper airway procedures may increase risk of hypoventilation. Prolonged responses have been noted following extended administration by continuous infusion (possibly due to metabolite accumulation) or in the presence of drugs which inhibit midazolam metabolism.

May cause hypotension - hemodynamic events are more common in pediatric patients or patients with hemodynamic instability. Hypotension and/or respiratory depression may occur more frequently in patients who have received narcotic analgesics. Use with caution in obese patients, chronic renal failure, and CHF.

Parenteral form contains benzyl alcohol - avoid rapid injection in neonates or prolonged infusions. Does not protect against increases in heart rate or blood pressure during intubation. Should not be used in shock, coma, or acute alcohol intoxication. Avoid intra-arterial administration or extravasation of parenteral formulation.

Causes CNS depression (dose-related) resulting in sedation, dizziness, confusion, or ataxia which may impair physical and mental capabilities. Patients must be cautioned about performing tasks which require mental alertness (ie, operating machinery or driving). A minimum of 1 day should elapse after midazolam administration before attempting these tasks. Use with caution in patients receiving other CNS depressants or psychoactive agents. Effects with other sedative drugs or ethanol may be potentiated. Benzodiazepines have been associated with falls and traumatic injury and should be used with extreme caution in patients who are at risk of these events (especially the elderly).

Midazolam causes anterograde amnesia. Paradoxical reactions, including hyperactive or aggressive behavior have been reported with benzodiazepines, particularly in adolescent/pediatric or psychiatric patients. Does not have analgesic, antidepressant, or antipsychotic properties.

Benzodiazepines have been associated with dependence and acute withdrawal symptoms on discontinuation or reduction in dose. Acute withdrawal, including seizures, may be precipitated after administration of flumazenil to patients receiving long-term benzodiazepine therapy.

Adverse Reactions As reported in adults unless otherwise noted:
>10%: Respiratory: Decreased tidal volume and/or respiratory rate decrease, apnea (3% children)
1% to 10%:
  Cardiovascular: Hypotension (3% children)
  Central nervous system: Drowsiness (1%), oversedation, headache (1%), seizure-like activity (1% children)
  Gastrointestinal: Nausea (3%), vomiting (3%)
  Local: Pain and local reactions at injection site (4% I.M., 5% I.V.; severity less than diazepam)
  Ocular: Nystagmus (1% children)
  Respiratory: Cough (1%)
  Miscellaneous: Physical and psychological dependence with prolonged use, hiccups (4%, 1% children), paradoxical reaction (2% children)
<1%: Acid taste, agitation, amnesia, bigeminy, bradycardia, bronchospasm, confusion, dyspnea, emergence delirium, euphoria, excessive salivation, hallucinations, hyperventilation, laryngospasm, PVC, rash, tachycardia, wheezing

Overdosage/Toxicology
Signs and symptoms: Respiratory depression, hypotension, coma, stupor, confusion, apnea
Treatment: Treatment for benzodiazepine overdose is supportive. Rarely is mechanical ventilation required. Flumazenil has been shown to selectively block the binding of benzodiazepines to CNS receptors, resulting in a reversal of benzodiazepine-induced CNS depression; respiratory reaction to hypoxia may not be restored

Drug Interactions CYP3A3/4 enzyme substrate
CNS depressants: Sedative effects and/or respiratory depression may be additive with CNS depressants; includes ethanol, barbiturates, narcotic analgesics, and other sedative agents; monitor for increased effect. **If narcotics or other CNS depressants are administered concomitantly, the midazolam dose should be reduced by 30% if <65 years of age, or by at least 50% if >65 years of age.**
Enzyme inducers: Metabolism of some benzodiazepines may be increased, decreasing their therapeutic effect; consider using an alternative sedative/hypnotic agent; potential inducers include phenobarbital, phenytoin, carbamazepine, rifampin, and rifabutin
(Continued)

Midazolam *(Continued)*

CYP3A3/4 inhibitors: Serum level and/or toxicity of some benzodiazepines may be increased; inhibitors include amiodarone, cimetidine, clarithromycin, erythromycin, delavirdine, diltiazem, dirithromycin, disulfiram, fluoxetine, fluvoxamine, grapefruit juice, indinavir, itraconazole, ketoconazole, nefazodone, nevirapine, propoxyphene, quinupristin-dalfopristin, ritonavir, saquinavir, verapamil, zafirlukast, zileuton; monitor for altered benzodiazepine response. **Use is contraindicated with amprenavir and ritonavir.**

Levodopa: Therapeutic effects may be diminished in some patients following the addition of a benzodiazepine; limited/inconsistent data

Oral contraceptives: May decrease the clearance of some benzodiazepines (those which undergo oxidative metabolism); monitor for increased benzodiazepine effect

Theophylline: May partially antagonize some of the effects of benzodiazepines; monitor for decreased response; may require higher doses for sedation

Ethanol/Nutrition/Herb Interactions

Ethanol: Avoid ethanol (may increase CNS depression).

Food: Grapefruit juice may increase serum concentrations of midazolam; avoid concurrent use with oral form.

Herb/Nutraceutical: Avoid concurrent use with St John's wort (may decrease midazolam levels, may increase CNS depression). Avoid concurrent use with valerian, kava kava, gotu kola (may increase CNS depression).

Stability Stable for 24 hours at room temperature/refrigeration; at a final concentration of 0.5 mg/mL, stable for up to 24 hours when diluted with D_5W or NS, or for up to 4 hours when diluted with lactated Ringer's; admixtures do not require protection from light for short-term storage

Mechanism of Action Binds to stereospecific benzodiazepine receptors on the postsynaptic GABA neuron at several sites within the central nervous system, including the limbic system, reticular formation. Enhancement of the inhibitory effect of GABA on neuronal excitability results by increased neuronal membrane permeability to chloride ions. This shift in chloride ions results in hyperpolarization (a less excitable state) and stabilization.

Pharmacodynamics/Kinetics

I.M.:

Onset of sedation: Within 15 minutes

Peak effect: 0.5-1 hour

Duration: 2 hours mean, up to 6 hours

I.V.: Onset of action: Within 1-5 minutes

Absorption: Oral: Rapid

Distribution: V_d: 0.8-2.5 L/kg; increased with congestive heart failure (CHF) and chronic renal failure

Protein binding: 95%

Metabolism: Extensively in the liver (microsomally)

Bioavailability: 45% mean

Half-life, elimination: 1-4 hours, increased with cirrhosis, CHF, obesity, elderly

Elimination: As glucuronide conjugated metabolites in urine, ~2% to 10% excreted in feces

Usual Dosage The dose of midazolam needs to be individualized based on the patient's age, underlying diseases, and concurrent medications. Decrease dose (by ~30%) if narcotics or other CNS depressants are administered concomitantly. **Personnel and equipment needed for standard respiratory resuscitation should be immediately available during midazolam administration.**

Children <6 years may require higher doses and closer monitoring than older children; calculate dose on ideal body weight

Conscious sedation for procedures or preoperative sedation:
Oral: 0.25-0.5 mg/kg as a single dose preprocedure, up to a maximum of 20 mg; administer 30-45 minutes prior to procedure. Children <6 years or less cooperative patients may require as much as 1 mg/kg as a single dose; 0.25 mg/kg may suffice for children 6-16 years of age.
Intranasal (not an approved route): 0.2 mg/kg (up to 0.4 mg/kg in some studies), to a maximum of 15 mg; may be administered 30-45 minutes prior to procedure
I.M.: 0.1-0.15 mg/kg 30-60 minutes before surgery or procedure; range 0.05-0.15 mg/kg; doses up to 0.5 mg/kg have been used in more anxious patients; maximum total dose: 10 mg
I.V.:
Infants <6 months: Limited information is available in nonintubated infants; dosing recommendations not clear; infants <6 months are at higher risk for airway obstruction and hypoventilation; titrate dose in small increments to desired effect; monitor carefully
Infants 6 months to Children 5 years: Initial: 0.05-0.1 mg/kg; titrate dose carefully; total dose of 0.6 mg/kg may be required; usual maximum total dose: 6 mg
Children 6-12 years: Initial: 0.025-0.05 mg/kg; titrate dose carefully; total doses of 0.4 mg/kg may be required; usual maximum total dose: 10 mg
Children 12-16 years: Dose as adults; usual maximum total dose: 10 mg
Conscious sedation during mechanical ventilation: Children: Loading dose: 0.05-0.2 mg/kg, followed by initial continuous infusion: 0.06-0.12 mg/kg/hour (1-2 mcg/kg/minute); titrate to the desired effect; usual range: 0.4-6 mcg/kg/minute
Status epilepticus refractory to standard therapy (unlabeled use): Infants >2 months and Children: Loading dose: 0.15 mg/kg followed by a continuous infusion of 1 mcg/kg/minute; titrate dose upward very 5 minutes until clinical seizure activity is controlled; mean infusion rate required in 24 children was 2.3 mcg/kg/minute with a range of 1-18 mcg/kg/minute
Adults:
Preoperative sedation:
I.M.: 0.07-0.08 mg/kg 30-60 minutes prior to surgery/procedure; usual dose: 5 mg; **Note:** Reduce dose in patients with COPD, high-risk patients, patients ≥60 years of age, and patients receiving other narcotics or CNS depressants
I.V.: 0.02-0.04 mg/kg; repeat every 5 minutes as needed to desired effect or up to 0.1-0.2 mg/kg
Intranasal (not an approved route): 0.2 mg/kg (up to 0.4 mg/kg in some studies); administer 30-45 minutes prior to surgery/procedure
Conscious sedation: I.V.: Initial: 0.5-2 mg slow I.V. over at least 2 minutes; slowly titrate to effect by repeating doses every 2-3 minutes if needed; usual total dose: 2.5-5 mg; use decreased doses in elderly
Healthy Adults <60 years: Some patients respond to doses as low as 1 mg; no more than 2.5 mg should be administered over a period of 2 minutes. Additional doses of midazolam may be administered after a 2-minute waiting period and evaluation of sedation after each dose increment. A total dose >5 mg is generally not needed. If narcotics or other CNS depressants are administered concomitantly, the midazolam dose should be reduced by 30%.
Anesthesia: I.V.:
Induction:
Unpremedicated patients: 0.3-0.35 mg/kg (up to 0.6 mg/kg in resistant cases)
Premedicated patients: 0.15-0.35 mg/kg
Maintenance: 0.05-0.3 mg/kg as needed, or continuous infusion 0.25-1.5 mcg/kg/minute
Sedation in mechanically-ventilated patients: I.V. continuous infusion: 100 mg in 250 mL D_5W or NS (if patient is fluid-restricted, may concentrate up to a maximum of 0.5 mg/mL); initial dose: 0.01-0.05 mg/kg (~0.5-4 mg for a typical adult) initially and either repeated at 10-15 minute intervals until adequate
(Continued)

Midazolam *(Continued)*

sedation is achieved or continuous infusion rates of 0.02-0.1 mg/kg/hour (1-7 mg/hour) and titrate to reach desired level of sedation

Elderly: I.V.: Conscious sedation: Initial: 0.5 mg slow I.V.; give no more than 1.5 mg in a 2-minute period; if additional titration is needed, give no more than 1 mg over 2 minutes, waiting another 2 or more minutes to evaluate sedative effect; a total dose of >3.5 mg is rarely necessary

Dosage adjustment in renal impairment:
Hemodialysis: Supplemental dose is not necessary
Peritoneal dialysis: Significant drug removal is unlikely based on physiochemical characteristics

Dietary Considerations Sodium content of 1 mL: 0.14 mEq

Administration

Intranasal: Administer using a 1 mL needleless syringe into the nares over 15 seconds; use the 5 mg/mL injection; $1/2$ of the dose may be administered to each nare

Oral: Do not mix with any liquid (such as grapefruit juice) prior to administration
Parenteral:
I.M.: Administer deep I.M. into large muscle.
I.V.: Administer by slow I.V. injection over at least 2-5 minutes at a concentration of 1-5 mg/mL or by I.V. infusion. Continuous infusions should be administered via an infusion pump.

Monitoring Parameters Respiratory and cardiovascular status, blood pressure, blood pressure monitor required during I.V. administration

Patient Information May cause drowsiness; do not drive or operate hazardous machinery until the effects of the drug are gone or until the day after administration

Nursing Implications Midazolam is a short-acting benzodiazepine; recovery occurs within 2 hours in most patients, however, may require up to 6 hours in some cases

Additional Information Abrupt discontinuation after sustained use (generally >10 days) may cause withdrawal symptoms. For neonates, since both concentrations of the injection contain 1% benzyl alcohol, use the 5 mg/mL injection and dilute to 0.5 mg/mL with SWI without preservatives to decrease the amount of benzyl alcohol delivered to the neonate; with continuous infusion, midazolam may accumulate in peripheral tissues; use lowest effective infusion rate to reduce accumulation effects; midazolam is 3-4 times as potent as diazepam; paradoxical reactions associated with midazolam use in children (eg, agitation, restlessness, combativeness) have been successfully treated with flumazenil (see Massanari, 1997).

Dosage Forms
Injection, as hydrochloride: 1 mg/mL (2 mL, 5 mL, 10 mL); 5 mg/mL (1 mL, 2 mL, 5 mL, 10 mL)
Syrup, as hydrochloride: 2 mg/mL (118 mL)

Mirtazapine *(mir TAZ a peen)*

Related Information
Antidepressant Agents Comparison Chart *on page 553*

Patient Information - Antidepressants (Mirtazapine) *on page 464*
Teratogenic Risks of Psychotropic Medications *on page 594*

U.S. Brand Names Remeron®; Remeron® SolTab™

Pharmacologic Category Antidepressant, Alpha-2 Antagonist

Generic Available No

Use Treatment of depression

Pregnancy Risk Factor C

Pregnancy/Breast-Feeding Implications Animal studies did not show teratogenic effects, however there was an increase in fetal loss and decrease in birth weight; use during pregnancy only if clearly needed. Excretion in human breast milk unknown; breast-feeding is not recommended

Contraindications Hypersensitivity to mirtazapine or any component of the formulation; use of MAO inhibitors within 14 days

Warnings/Precautions Discontinue immediately if signs and symptoms of neutropenia/agranulocytosis occur. May cause sedation, resulting in impaired performance of tasks requiring alertness (ie, operating machinery or driving). Sedative effects may be additive with other CNS depressants and/or ethanol. The degree of sedation is moderate-high relative to other antidepressants. May worsen psychosis in some patients or precipitate a shift to mania or hypomania in patients with bipolar disease. The risks of orthostatic hypotension or anticholinergic effects are low relative to other antidepressants. The incidence of sexual dysfunction with mirtazapine is generally lower than with SSRIs.

May increase appetite and stimulate weight gain, may increase serum cholesterol and triglyceride levels. Use caution in patients with depression, particularly if suicidal risk may be present. Use caution in patients with a previous seizure disorder or condition predisposing to seizures such as brain damage, alcoholism, or concurrent therapy with other drugs which lower the seizure threshold. Use with caution in patients with hepatic or renal dysfunction and in elderly patients.

SolTab™ formulation contains phenylalanine

Adverse Reactions

>10%:

Central nervous system: Somnolence (54%)

Endocrine & metabolic: Increased cholesterol

Gastrointestinal: Constipation (13%), xerostomia (25%), increased appetite (17%), weight gain (12%)

1% to 10%:

Cardiovascular: Hypertension, vasodilatation, peripheral edema (2%), edema (1%)

Central nervous system: Dizziness (7%), abnormal dreams (4%), abnormal thoughts (3%), confusion (2%), malaise

Endocrine & metabolic: Increased triglycerides

Gastrointestinal: Vomiting, anorexia, abdominal pain

Genitourinary: Urinary frequency (2%)

Neuromuscular & skeletal: Myalgia (2%), back pain (2%), arthralgias, tremor (2%), weakness (8%)

Respiratory: Dyspnea (1%)

Miscellaneous: Flu-like symptoms (5%), thirst

<1%: Abdomen enlarged, abnormal ejaculation, accommodation abnormality, acne, agitation, agranulocytosis, akathisia, alopecia, amenorrhea, amnesia, anemia, angina pectoris, anxiety, apathy, aphasia, aphthous stomatitis, arthrosis, arthritis, asphyxia, asthma, ataxia, atrial arrhythmia, bigeminy, blepharitis, bone pain, bradycardia, breast engorgement, breast enlargement, breast pain, bronchitis, bursitis, cardiomegaly, cellulitis, cerebral ischemia, chest pain, chills, cholecystitis, cirrhosis, colitis, conjunctivitis, coordination abnormal, cough, cystitis, deafness, dehydration, delirium, delusions, dementia, depersonalization, depression, diabetes mellitus, diplopia, drug dependence, dry skin, dysarthria, dyskinesia, dysmenorrhea, dystonia, dysuria, ear pain, emotional lability, epistaxis, eructation, euphoria, exfoliative dermatitis, extrapyramidal

(Continued)

245

Mirtazapine *(Continued)*

syndrome, eye pain, facial edema, fever, fracture, gastritis, gastroenteritis, glaucoma, glossitis, goiter, gout, grand mal seizure, gum hemorrhage, hallucinations, hematuria, herpes simplex, herpes zoster, hiccup, hostility, hypokinesia, hyperacusis, hyperkinesias, hypesthesia, hypotension, hypothyroidism, hypotonia, impotence, increased salivation, intestinal obstruction, keratoconjunctivitis, kidney calculus, lacrimation disorder, laryngitis, left heart failure, leukopenia, leukorrhea, libido increased, liver function tests abnormal, lymphadenopathy, lymphocytosis, manic reaction, menorrhagia, metrorrhagia, migraine, myocardial infarction, myoclonus, myositis, nausea, neck pain, neck rigidity, neurosis, nystagmus, oral moniliasis, osteoporosis, otitis media, pancreatitis, pancytopenia, paralysis, paranoid reaction, paresthesia, parosmia, petechia, phlebitis, photosensitivity reaction, pneumonia, pneumothorax, polyuria, pruritus, psychotic depression, pulmonary embolus, rash, reflexes increased, salivary gland enlargement, seborrhea, sinusitis, skin hypertrophy, skin ulcer, stomatitis, stupor, syncope, taste loss, tendon rupture, tenosynovitis, thrombocytopenia, tongue discoloration, tongue edema, twitching, ulcer, ulcerative stomatitis, urethritis, urinary incontinence, urinary retention, urinary tract infection, urinary urgency, urticaria, vaginitis, vascular headache, ventricular extrasystoles, vertigo, weight loss, withdrawal syndrome

Postmarketing and/or case reports: Torsade de pointes (1 case reported)

Overdosage/Toxicology

Signs and symptoms of overdose include disorientation, drowsiness, impaired memory, and tachycardia

Treatment: No specific antidotes; establish and maintain an airway to ensure adequate oxygenation and ventilation; activated charcoal should be considered in treatment; monitor cardiac and vital signs along with general symptomatic and supportive measures; consider possibility of multiple-drug involvement

Drug Interactions CYP1A2, 2C9, 2D6, and 3A3/4 enzyme substrate

Clonidine: Antihypertensive effects of clonidine may be antagonized by mirtazapine (hypertensive urgency has been reported following addition of mirtazapine to clonidine); in addition, mirtazapine may potentially enhance the hypertensive response associated with abrupt clonidine withdrawal. Avoid this combination; consider an alternative agent.

CNS depressants: Sedative effects may be additive with other CNS depressants; monitor for increased effect; includes barbiturates, benzodiazepines, narcotic analgesics, ethanol and other sedative agents

CYP inhibitors: May increase serum concentrations of mirtazapine; monitor

Enzyme inducers: Metabolism of mirtazapine may be increased; decreasing clinical effect; inducers include barbiturates, carbamazepine, phenytoin, and rifampin

Linezolid: Due to MAO inhibition (see note on MAO inhibitors), this combination should be avoided

MAO inhibitors: Possibly serious or fatal reactions can occur when given with or when given within 14 days of an MAO inhibitor

Selegiline: Interaction is less likely than with nonselective MAO inhibitors (see MAO inhibitor information), but theoretically possible; monitor

Sibutramine: Potential for serotonin syndrome when used in combination

Ethanol/Nutrition/Herb Interactions

Ethanol: Avoid ethanol (may increase CNS depression).

Herb/Nutraceutical: Avoid St John's wort (may decrease mirtazapine levels). Avoid valerian, St John's wort, SAMe, kava kava (may increase CNS depression).

Stability Store at controlled room temperature

SolTab™: Protect from light and moisture; use immediately upon opening tablet blister

Mechanism of Action Mirtazapine is a tetracyclic antidepressant that works by its central presynaptic alpha$_2$-adrenergic antagonist effects, which results in increased release of norepinephrine and serotonin. It is also a potent antagonist of 5-HT$_2$ and 5-HT$_3$ serotonin receptors and H1 histamine receptors and a moderate

---

peripheral alpha₁-adrenergic and muscarinic antagonist; it does not inhibit the reuptake of norepinephrine or serotonin.

Pharmacodynamics/Kinetics
Protein binding: 85%
Metabolism: Extensive by cytochrome P450 enzymes in the liver
Bioavailability: 50%
Half-life: 20-40 hours
Time to peak serum concentration: 2 hours
Elimination: Extensive hepatic metabolism via demethylation and hydroxylation, metabolites eliminated primarily renally (75%) and some via the feces (15%); elimination is hampered with renal dysfunction or hepatic dysfunction.

Usual Dosage
Children: Safety and efficacy in children have not been established
Treatment of depression: Adults: Oral: Initial: 15 mg nightly, titrate up to 15-45 mg/day with dose increases made no more frequently than every 1-2 weeks; there is an inverse relationship between dose and sedation
Elderly: Decreased clearance seen (40% males, 10% females); no specific dosage adjustment recommended by manufacturer

Dosage adjustment in renal impairment:
Cl_cr 11-39 mL/minute: 30% decreased clearance
Cl_cr <10 mL/minute: 50% decreased clearance
Dosage adjustment in hepatic impairment: Clearance decreased by 30%
Dietary Considerations Remeron® SolTab™ contains phenylalanine: 2.6 mg per 15 mg tablet; 5.2 mg per 30 mg tablet; 7.8 mg per 45 mg tablet
Administration SolTab™: Open blister pack and place tablet on the tongue. Do not split tablet. Tablet is formulated to dissolve on the tongue without water.
Monitoring Parameters Patients should be monitored for signs of agranulocytosis or severe neutropenia such as sore throat, stomatitis or other signs of infection or a low WBC; monitor for improvement in clinical signs and symptoms of depression, improvement may be observed within 1-4 weeks after initiating therapy
Patient Information Be aware of the risk of developing agranulocytosis; contact physician if any indication of infection (ie, fever, chills, sore throat, mucous membrane ulceration, and especially flu-like symptoms) occur; may impair judgment, thinking, and particularly motor skills; may impair ability to drive, use machines, or perform tasks requiring alertness; avoid engaging in hazardous activities until certain that therapy does not affect ability to engage in these activities; avoid alcohol consumption
Additional Information Note: At least 14 days should elapse between discontinuation of an MAO inhibitor and initiation of therapy with mirtazapine; at least 14 days should be allowed after discontinuing mirtazapine before starting an MAO inhibitor.

Dosage Forms
Tablet: 15 mg, 30 mg, 45 mg
Tablet, orally disintegrating:
15 mg [phenylalanine 2.6 mg/tablet] [orange flavor]
30 mg [phenylalanine 5.2 mg/tablet] [orange flavor]
45 mg [phenylalanine 7.8 mg/tablet] [orange flavor]

♦ **MK462** see Rizatriptan on page 360
♦ **Moban**® see Molindone on page 250

Modafinil (moe DAF i nil)
Related Information
Patient Information - Stimulants on page 481
U.S. Brand Names Provigil®
Canadian Brand Names Alertec®
Pharmacologic Category Stimulant
Generic Available No
Use Improve wakefulness in patients with excessive daytime sleepiness associated with narcolepsy
(Continued)

Modafinil *(Continued)*

Unlabeled/Investigational Use Attention-deficit/hyperactivity disorder (ADHD); treatment of fatigue in MS and other disorders

Restrictions C-IV

Pregnancy Risk Factor C

Pregnancy/Breast-Feeding Implications Currently, there are no studies in humans evaluating its teratogenicity. Embryotoxicity of modafinil has been observed in animal models at dosages above those employed therapeutically. As a result, it should be used cautiously during pregnancy and should be used only when the potential risk of drug therapy is outweighed by the drug's benefits. It remains unknown if modafinil is secreted into human milk and, therefore, should be used cautiously in nursing women.

Contraindications Hypersensitivity to modafinil or any component of the formulation

Warnings/Precautions History of angina, ischemic EKG changes, left ventricular hypertrophy, or clinically significant mitral valve prolapse in association with CNS stimulant use; caution should be exercised when modafinil is given to patients with a history of psychosis, recent history of myocardial infarction, and because it has not yet been adequately studied in patients with hypertension, periodic monitoring of hypertensive patients receiving modafinil may be appropriate; caution is warranted when operating machinery or driving, although functional impairment has not been demonstrated with modafinil, all CNS-active agents may alter judgment, thinking and/or motor skills. Efficacy of oral contraceptives may be reduced, therefore, use of alternative contraception should be considered. Stimulants may unmask tics in individuals with coexisting Tourette's syndrome.

Adverse Reactions Limited to reports equal to or greater than placebo-related events.

<10%:

    Cardiovascular: Chest pain (2%), hypertension (2%), hypotension (2%), vasodilation (1%), arrhythmia (1%), syncope (1%)

    Central nervous system: Headache (50%, compared to 40% with placebo), nervousness (8%), dizziness (5%), depression (4%), anxiety (4%), cataplexy (3%), insomnia (3%), chills (2%), fever (1%), confusion (1%), amnesia (1%), emotional lability (1%), ataxia (1%)

    Dermatologic: Dry skin (1%)

    Endocrine & metabolic: Hyperglycemia (1%), albuminuria (1%)

    Gastrointestinal: Diarrhea (8%), nausea (13%, compared to 4% with placebo), xerostomia (5%), anorexia (5%), vomiting (1%), mouth ulceration (1%), gingivitis (1%)

    Genitourinary: Abnormal urine (1%), urinary retention (1%), ejaculatory disturbance (1%)

    Hematologic: Eosinophilia (1%)

    Hepatic: Abnormal LFTs (3%)

    Neuromuscular & skeletal: Paresthesias (3%), dyskinesia (2%), neck pain (2%), hypertonia (2%), neck rigidity (1%), joint disorder (1%), tremor (1%)

    Ocular: Amblyopia (2%), abnormal vision (2%)

    Respiratory: Pharyngitis (6%), rhinitis (11%, compared to 8% with placebo), lung disorder (4%), dyspnea (2%), asthma (1%), epistaxis (1%)

Overdosage/Toxicology Symptoms of overdose include agitation, irritability, aggressiveness, confusion, nervousness, tremor, insomnia, palpitations, and elevations in hemodynamic parameters. Treatment is symptomatic and supportive. Cardiac monitoring is warranted.

Drug Interactions CYP3A3/4 substrate; CYP2C19 inhibitor; weak inducer of CYP1A2, 2B6, and 3A3/4

    CYP2C19 substrates: Serum concentrations of drugs metabolized by this enzyme can be increased, these agents include diazepam, mephenytoin, phenytoin, and propranolol

    CYP3A3/4 substrates: May decrease serum concentrations of CYP3A3/4 metabolized drugs such as oral contraceptives, benzodiazepines, and cyclosporine

Enzyme inducers (including phenobarbital, carbamazepine, and rifampin): May result in decreased modafinil levels; there is evidence to suggest that modafinil may induce its own metabolism

Oral contraceptives; serum concentrations may be reduced (enzyme induction); contraceptive failure may result; consider alternative contraceptive measures

Phenytoin: Serum concentrations may be increased by modafinil (enzyme inhibition); modafinil concentrations may be reduced by phenytoin (enzyme induction)

SSRIs: In populations genetically deficient in the CYP2D6 isoenzyme, where CYP2C19 acts as a secondary metabolic pathway, concentrations of selective serotonin reuptake inhibitors may be increased during coadministration

Tricyclic antidepressants: In populations genetically deficient in the CYP2D6 isoenzyme, where CYP2C19 acts as a secondary metabolic pathway, concentrations of tricyclic antidepressants may be increased during coadministration

Warfarin: Serum concentrations/effect may be increased by modafinil

Mechanism of Action The exact mechanism of action is unclear, it does not appear to alter the release of dopamine or norepinephrine, it may exert its stimulant effects by decreasing GABA-mediated neurotransmission, although this theory has not yet been fully evaluated; several studies also suggest that an intact central alpha-adrenergic system is required for modafinil's activity; the drug increases high-frequency alpha waves while decreasing both delta and theta wave activity, and these effects are consistent with generalized increases in mental alertness

Pharmacodynamics/Kinetics Modafinil is a racemic compound (10% *d*-isomer and 90% *l*-isomer at steady state), whose enantiomers have different pharmacokinetics

Distribution: V_d: 0.9 L/kg

Protein binding: 60%, mostly to albumin

Metabolism: In the liver; multiple pathways including the cytochrome P450 system

Half-life: Effective half-life: 15 hours; time to steady-state: 2-4 days

Time to peak serum concentration: 2-4 hours

Elimination: Renal, as metabolites (<10% excreted unchanged)

Usual Dosage

Children: ADHD (unlabeled use): 50-100 mg once daily

Adults:

ADHD (unlabeled use): 100-300 mg once daily

Narcolepsy: Initial: 200 mg as a single daily dose in the morning

Doses of 400 mg/day, given as a single dose, have been well tolerated, but there is no consistent evidence that this dose confers additional benefit

Elderly: Elimination of modafinil and its metabolites may be reduced as a consequence of aging and as a result, lower doses should be considered.

Dosing adjustment in renal impairment: Inadequate data to determine safety and efficacy in severe renal impairment

Dosing adjustment in hepatic impairment: Dose should be reduced to one-half of that recommended for patients with normal liver function

Child/Adolescent Considerations Eleven children with attention-deficit/hyperactivity disorder (ADHD) 5-15 years of age received modafinil for an average of 4.6 weeks (Rugino, 2001).

Patient Information Take during the day to avoid insomnia; may cause dependence with prolonged use; patients should be reminded to notify their physician if they become pregnant, intend to become pregnant, or are breast-feeding an infant; patients should be advised that combined use with alcohol has not been studied and that it is prudent to avoid this combination. Patients should notify their physician and/or pharmacist of any concomitant medications they are taking, due to the drug interaction potential this might represent.

Dosage Forms Tablet: 100 mg, 200 mg

♦ **Modecate® [Fluphenazine Decanoate] (Can)** *see* Fluphenazine *on page 151*

♦ **Modecate Enanthate [Fluphenazine Enanthate] (Can)** *see* Fluphenazine *on page 151*

♦ **Moditen Hydrochloride (Can)** *see* Fluphenazine *on page 151*

Molindone (moe LIN done)

Related Information

Antipsychotic Agents Comparison Chart *on page 557*

Antipsychotic Medication Guidelines *on page 559*

Discontinuation of Psychotropic Drugs - Withdrawal Symptoms and Recommendations *on page 582*

Federal OBRA Regulations Recommended Maximum Doses *on page 583*

Patient Information - Antipsychotics (General) *on page 466*

U.S. Brand Names Moban®

Synonyms Molindone Hydrochloride

Pharmacologic Category Antipsychotic Agent, Dihydoindoline

Generic Available No

Use Management of schizophrenia

Unlabeled/Investigational Use Management of psychotic disorders

Pregnancy Risk Factor C

Contraindications Hypersensitivity to molindone or any component of the formulation (cross-reactivity between phenothiazines may occur); severe CNS depression; coma

Warnings/Precautions May be sedating, use with caution in disorders where CNS depression is a feature. Use with caution in Parkinson's disease. Caution in patients with hemodynamic instability; bone marrow suppression; predisposition to seizures; subcortical brain damage; severe cardiac, hepatic, renal, or respiratory disease. Esophageal dysmotility and aspiration have been associated with antipsychotic use - use with caution in patients at risk of pneumonia (ie, Alzheimer's disease). Caution in breast cancer or other prolactin-dependent tumors (may elevate prolactin levels). May alter temperature regulation or mask toxicity of other drugs due to antiemetic effects. May alter cardiac conduction; life-threatening arrhythmias have occurred with therapeutic doses of neuroleptics. May cause orthostatic hypotension - use with caution in patients at risk of this effect or those who would tolerate transient hypotensive episodes (cerebrovascular disease, cardiovascular disease, or other medications which may predispose).

May cause anticholinergic effects (confusion, agitation, constipation, dry mouth, blurred vision, urinary retention); therefore, they should be used with caution in patients with decreased gastrointestinal motility, urinary retention, BPH, xerostomia, or visual problems. Conditions which also may be exacerbated by cholinergic blockade include narrow-angle glaucoma (screening is recommended) and worsening of myasthenia gravis. Relative to other neuroleptics, molindone has a low potency of cholinergic blockade.

May cause extrapyramidal reactions, including pseudoparkinsonism, acute dystonic reactions, akathisia, and tardive dyskinesia (risk of these reactions is moderate-high relative to other antipsychotics). May be associated with neuroleptic malignant syndrome (NMS) or pigmentary retinopathy.

Adverse Reactions Frequency not defined.

Cardiovascular: Orthostatic hypotension, tachycardia, arrhythmias

Central nervous system: Extrapyramidal reactions (akathisia, pseudoparkinsonism, dystonia, tardive dyskinesia), mental depression, altered central temperature regulation, sedation, drowsiness, restlessness, anxiety, hyperactivity, euphoria, seizures, neuroleptic malignant syndrome (NMS)

Dermatologic: Pruritus, rash, photosensitivity

Endocrine & metabolic: Change in menstrual periods, edema of breasts, amenorrhea, galactorrhea, gynecomastia

Gastrointestinal: Constipation, xerostomia, nausea, salivation, weight gain (minimal compared to other antipsychotics), weight loss

Genitourinary: Urinary retention, priapism

Hematologic: Leukopenia, leukocytosis

Ocular: Blurred vision, retinal pigmentation

Miscellaneous: Diaphoresis (decreased)

Overdosage/Toxicology

Signs and symptoms: Deep sleep, extrapyramidal symptoms, cardiac arrhythmias, seizures, hypotension

Treatment: Following initiation of essential overdose management, toxic symptom treatment and supportive treatment should be initiated. Hypotension usually responds to I.V. fluids or Trendelenburg positioning. If unresponsive to these measures, the use of a parenteral inotrope may be required (eg, norepinephrine 0.1-0.2 mcg/kg/minute titrated to response). Seizures commonly respond to diazepam (I.V. 5-10 mg bolus in adults every 15 minutes if needed up to a total of 30 mg; I.V. 0.25-0.4 mg/kg/dose up to a total of 10 mg in children) or to phenytoin or phenobarbital. Also critical cardiac arrhythmias often respond to I.V. phenytoin (15 mg/kg up to 1 gram), while other antiarrhythmics can be used. Neuroleptics often cause extrapyramidal symptoms (eg, dystonic reactions) requiring management with diphenhydramine 1-2 mg/kg (adults) up to a maximum of 50 mg I.M. or I.V. slow push followed by a maintenance dose for 48-72 hours. Alternatively, benztropine mesylate I.V. 1-2 mg (adults) may be effective. These agents are generally effective within 2-5 minutes.

Drug Interactions CYP2D6 enzyme substrate

Aluminum salts: May decrease the absorption of antipsychotics; monitor

Amphetamines: Efficacy may be diminished by antipsychotics; in addition, amphetamines may increase psychotic symptoms; avoid concurrent use

Anticholinergics: May inhibit the therapeutic response to antipsychotics and excess anticholinergic effects may occur; includes benztropine, trihexyphenidyl, biperiden, and drugs with significant anticholinergic activity (TCAs, antihistamines, disopyramide)

Antihypertensives: Concurrent use of antipsychotics with an antihypertensive may produce additive hypotensive effects (particularly orthostasis)

Bromocriptine: Antipsychotics inhibit the ability of bromocriptine to lower serum prolactin concentrations

CNS depressants: Sedative effects may be additive with antipsychotics; monitor for increased effect; includes barbiturates, benzodiazepines, narcotic analgesics, ethanol and other sedative agents

CYP2D6 inhibitors: Metabolism of antipsychotics may be decreased; increasing clinical effect or toxicity; inhibitors include amiodarone, cimetidine, delavirdine, fluoxetine, paroxetine, propafenone, quinidine, and ritonavir; monitor for increased effect/toxicity

Enzyme inducers: May enhance the hepatic metabolism of antipsychotics; larger doses may be required; includes rifampin, rifabutin, barbiturates, phenytoin, and cigarette smoking

Epinephrine: Chlorpromazine (and possibly other low potency antipsychotics) may diminish the pressor effects of epinephrine

Guanethidine and guanadrel: Antihypertensive effects may be inhibited by antipsychotics Levodopa: Antipsychotics may inhibit the antiparkinsonian effect of levodopa; avoid this combination

Lithium: Antipsychotics may produce neurotoxicity with lithium; this is a rare effect

Phenytoin: May reduce serum levels of antipsychotics; antipsychotics may increase phenytoin serum levels

Propranolol: Serum concentrations of antipsychotics may be increased; propranolol also increases antipsychotic concentrations

QT_c-prolonging agents: Effects on QT_c interval may be additive with antipsychotics, increasing the risk of malignant arrhythmias; includes type Ia antiarrhythmics, TCAs, and some quinolone antibiotics (sparfloxacin, moxifloxacin, and gatifloxacin)

Sulfadoxine-pyrimethamine: May increase antipsychotics concentrations

Tricyclic antidepressants: Concurrent use may produce increased toxicity or altered therapeutic response

Trazodone: Antipsychotics and trazodone may produce additive hypotensive effects

Valproic acid: Serum levels may be increased by antipsychotics
(Continued)

Molindone *(Continued)*

Ethanol/Nutrition/Herb Interactions

Ethanol: Avoid ethanol (may increase CNS depression).

Herb/Nutraceutical: Avoid kava kava, gotu kola, valerian, St John's wort (may increase CNS depression).

Stability Protect from light; dispense in amber or opaque vials

Mechanism of Action Mechanism of action mimics that of chlorpromazine; however, it produces more extrapyramidal effects and less sedation than chlorpromazine

Pharmacodynamics/Kinetics

Metabolism: In the liver

Half-life: 1.5 hours

Time to peak serum concentration: Oral: Within 1.5 hours

Elimination: Principally in urine and feces (90% within 24 hours)

Usual Dosage Oral:

Children: Schizophrenia/psychoses:

3-5 years: 1-2.5 mg/day in 4 divided doses

5-12 years: 0.5-1 mg/kg/day in 4 divided doses

Adults: Schizophrenia/psychoses: 50-75 mg/day increase at 3- to 4-day intervals up to 225 mg/day

Elderly: Behavioral symptoms associated with dementia: Initial: 5-10 mg 1-2 times/day; increase at 4- to 7-day intervals by 5-10 mg/day; increase dosing intervals (bid, tid, etc) as necessary to control response or side effects.

Monitoring Parameters Monitor blood pressure and pulse rate prior to and during initial therapy; evaluate mental status

Patient Information Dry mouth may be helped by sips of water, sugarless gum or hard candy; avoid alcohol; very important to maintain established dosage regimen; photosensitivity to sunlight can occur, do not discontinue abruptly; full effect may not occur for 3-4 weeks; full dosage may be taken at bedtime to avoid daytime sedation; report to physician any involuntary movements or feelings of restlessness

Nursing Implications May increase appetite and possibly a craving for sweets; recognize signs of neuroleptic malignant syndrome and tardive dyskinesia

Additional Information Coadministration of two or more antipsychotics does not improve clinical response and may increase the potential for adverse effects.

Dosage Forms

Solution, oral concentrate, as hydrochloride: 20 mg/mL (120 mL)

Tablet, as hydrochloride: 5 mg, 10 mg, 25 mg, 50 mg, 100 mg

- ♦ **Molindone Hydrochloride** *see* Molindone *on page 250*
- ♦ **Mood Stabilizers** *see page 588*
- ♦ **Mormon Tea** *see* Ephedra *on page 131*
- ♦ **Multipax® (Can)** *see* Hydroxyzine *on page 178*
- ♦ **Mysoline®** *see* Primidone *on page 325*
- ♦ **N-Acetyl-5-methoxytryptamine** *see* Melatonin *on page 222*
- ♦ **N-allylnoroxymorphine Hydrochloride** *see* Naloxone *on page 254*

Nalmefene *(NAL me feen)*

U.S. Brand Names Revex®

Synonyms Nalmefene Hydrochloride

Pharmacologic Category Antidote

Generic Available No

Use Complete or partial reversal of opioid drug effects, including respiratory depression induced by natural or synthetic opioids; reversal of postoperative opioid depression; management of known or suspected opioid overdose

Pregnancy Risk Factor B

Pregnancy/Breast-Feeding Implications Limited information available; do not use in pregnant or lactating women if possible

Contraindications Hypersensitivity to nalmefene, naltrexone, or any component of the formulation

Warnings/Precautions May induce symptoms of acute withdrawal in opioid-dependent patients; recurrence of respiratory depression is possible if the opioid involved is long-acting; observe patients until there is no reasonable risk of recurrent respiratory depression. Safety and efficacy have not been established in children. Avoid abrupt reversal of opioid effects in patients of high cardiovascular risk or who have received potentially cardiotoxic drugs. Pulmonary edema and cardiovascular instability have been reported in association with abrupt reversal with other narcotic antagonists. Animal studies indicate nalmefene may not completely reverse buprenorphine-induced respiratory depression.

Adverse Reactions

>10%: Gastrointestinal: Nausea

1% to 10%:
   Cardiovascular: Tachycardia, hypertension, hypotension, vasodilation
   Central nervous system: Fever, dizziness, headache, chills
   Gastrointestinal: Vomiting
   Miscellaneous: Postoperative pain

<1%: Agitation, arrhythmia, bradycardia, confusion, depression, diarrhea, myoclonus, nervousness, pharyngitis, pruritus, somnolence, tremor, urinary retention, xerostomia

Overdosage/Toxicology Signs and symptoms: No known symptoms in significant overdose; large doses of opioids administered to overcome a full blockade of opioid antagonists, however, has resulted in adverse respiratory and circulatory reactions

Drug Interactions

   Flumazenil: May increase the risk of toxicity with flumazenil. An increased risk of seizures has been associated with flumazenil and nalmefene coadministration
   Narcotic analgesics: Decreased effect of narcotic analgesics; may precipitate acute withdrawal reaction in physically dependent patients

Mechanism of Action As a 6-methylene analog of naltrexone, nalmefene acts as a competitive antagonist at opioid receptor sites, preventing or reversing the respiratory depression, sedation, and hypotension induced by opiates; no pharmacologic activity of its own (eg, opioid agonist activity) has been demonstrated

Pharmacodynamics/Kinetics

   Onset of action: I.M., S.C.: 5-15 minutes
   Distribution: V_d: 8.6 L/kg; rapid
   Protein binding: 45%
   Metabolism: Hepatic by glucuronide conjugation to metabolites with little or no activity
   Bioavailability: I.M., I.V., S.C.: 100%
   T_{max}: I.M.: 2.3 hours; I.V.: <2 minutes; S.C.: 1.5 hours
   Half-life: 10.8 hours
   Time to peak serum concentration: 2.3 hours
   Elimination: <5% excreted unchanged in urine, 17% in feces; clearance: 0.8 L/hour/kg

Usual Dosage

   Reversal of postoperative opioid depression: Blue labeled product (100 mcg/mL): Titrate to reverse the undesired effects of opioids; initial dose for nonopioid dependent patients: 0.25 mcg/kg followed by 0.25 mcg/kg incremental doses at 2- to 5-minute intervals; after a total dose >1 mcg/kg, further therapeutic response is unlikely

   Management of known/suspected opioid overdose: Green labeled product (1000 mcg/mL): Initial dose: 0.5 mg/70 kg; may repeat with 1 mg/70 kg in 2-5 minutes; further increase beyond a total dose of 1.5 mg/70 kg will not likely result in improved response and may result in cardiovascular stress and precipitated withdrawal syndrome. (If opioid dependency is suspected, administer a challenge dose of 0.1 mg/70 kg; if no withdrawal symptoms are observed in 2 minutes, the recommended doses can be administered.)

(Continued)

Nalmefene *(Continued)*

Note: If recurrence of respiratory depression is noted, dose may again be titrated to clinical effect using incremental doses.

Note: If I.V. access is lost or not readily obtainable, a single S.C. or I.M. dose of 1 mg may be effective in 5-15 minutes.

Dosing adjustment in renal or hepatic impairment: Not necessary with single uses, however, slow administration (over 60 seconds) of incremental doses is recommended to minimize hypertension and dizziness

Administration Dilute drug (1:1) with diluent and use smaller doses in patients known to be at increased cardiovascular risk; may be administered via I.M. or S.C. routes if I.V. access is not feasible

Nursing Implications Check dosage strength carefully before use to avoid error (labeling is color-coded; postoperative reversal - blue, overdose management - green); monitor patients for signs of withdrawal, especially those physically dependent who are in pain or at high cardiovascular risk

Additional Information Proper steps should be used to prevent use of the incorrect dosage strength. The goal of treatment in the postoperative setting is to achieve reversal of excessive opioid effects without inducing a complete reversal and acute pain.

If opioid dependence is suspected, nalmefene should only be used in opioid overdose if the likelihood of overdose is high based on history or the clinical presentation of respiratory depression with concurrent pupillary constriction is present.

Dosage Forms Injection, as hydrochloride: 100 mcg/mL [blue label] (1 mL); 1000 mcg/mL [green label] (2 mL)

♦ **Nalmefene Hydrochloride** *see* Nalmefene on page 252

Naloxone *(nal OKS one)*

U.S. Brand Names Narcan®

Canadian Brand Names Narcan

Synonyms *N*-allylnoroxymorphine Hydrochloride; Naloxone Hydrochloride

Pharmacologic Category Antidote

Generic Available Yes

Use

Complete or partial reversal of opioid depression, including respiratory depression, induced by natural and synthetic opioids, including propoxyphene, methadone, and certain mixed agonist-antagonist analgesics: nalbuphine, pentazocine, and butorphanol

Diagnosis of suspected opioid tolerance or acute opioid overdose

Adjunctive agent to increase blood pressure in the management of septic shock

Unlabeled/Investigational Use PCP and ethanol ingestion

Pregnancy Risk Factor B

Contraindications Hypersensitivity to naloxone or any component

Warnings/Precautions Due to an association between naloxone and acute pulmonary edema, use with caution in patients with cardiovascular disease or in patients receiving medications with potential adverse cardiovascular effects (eg, hypotension, pulmonary edema or arrhythmias). Excessive dosages should be avoided after use of opiates in surgery, because naloxone may cause an increase in blood pressure and reversal of anesthesia; may precipitate withdrawal symptoms in patients addicted to opiates, including pain, hypertension, sweating, agitation, irritability; in neonates: shrill cry, failure to feed. Recurrence of respiratory depression is possible if the opioid involved is long-acting; observe patients until there is no reasonable risk of recurrent respiratory depression.

Adverse Reactions Frequency not defined.

Cardiovascular: Hypertension, hypotension, tachycardia, ventricular arrhythmias, cardiac arrest

Central nervous system: Irritability, anxiety, narcotic withdrawal, restlessness, seizures

Gastrointestinal: Nausea, vomiting, diarrhea

Neuromuscular & skeletal: Tremulousness

Respiratory: Dyspnea, pulmonary edema, runny nose, sneezing

Miscellaneous: Diaphoresis

Overdosage/Toxicology Treatment: Naloxone is the drug of choice for respiratory depression that is known or suspected to be caused by an overdose of an opiate or opioid

Caution: Naloxone's effects are due to its action on narcotic reversal, not due to any direct effect upon opiate receptors. Therefore, adverse events occur secondarily to reversal (withdrawal) of narcotic analgesia and sedation, which can cause severe reactions.

Drug Interactions Narcotic analgesics: Decreased effect of narcotic analgesics; may precipitate acute withdrawal reaction in physically dependent patients

Stability Protect from light; stable in 0.9% sodium chloride and D_5W at 4 mcg/mL for 24 hours; do not mix with alkaline solutions

Mechanism of Action Pure opioid antagonist that competes and displaces narcotics at opioid receptor sites

Pharmacodynamics/Kinetics

Onset of effect:

Endotracheal, I.M., S.C.: Within 2-5 minutes

I.V.: Within 2 minutes

Duration: 20-60 minutes; since shorter than that of most opioids, repeated doses are usually needed

Distribution: Crosses the placenta

Metabolism: Primarily by glucuronidation in the liver

Half-life:

Neonates: 1.2-3 hours

Adults: 1-1.5 hours

Elimination: In urine as metabolites

Usual Dosage I.M., I.V. (preferred), intratracheal, S.C.:

Postanesthesia narcotic reversal: Infants and Children: 0.01 mg/kg; may repeat every 2-3 minutes, as needed based on response

Opiate intoxication:

Children:

Birth (including premature infants) to 5 years or <20 kg: 0.1 mg/kg; repeat every 2-3 minutes if needed; may need to repeat doses every 20-60 minutes

>5 years or ≥20 kg: 2 mg/dose; if no response, repeat every 2-3 minutes; may need to repeat doses every 20-60 minutes

Children and Adults: Continuous infusion: I.V.: If continuous infusion is required, calculate dosage/hour based on effective intermittent dose used and duration of adequate response seen, titrate dose 0.04-0.16 mg/kg/hour for 2-5 days in children, adult dose typically 0.25-6.25 mg/hour (short-term infusions as high as 2.4 mg/kg/hour have been tolerated in adults during treatment for septic shock); alternatively, continuous infusion utilizes $2/3$ of the initial naloxone bolus on an hourly basis; add 10 times this dose to each liter of D_5W and infuse at a rate of 100 mL/hour; $1/2$ of the initial bolus dose should be readministered 15 minutes after initiation of the continuous infusion to prevent a drop in naloxone levels; increase infusion rate as needed to assure adequate ventilation

Narcotic overdose: Adults: I.V.: 0.4-2 mg every 2-3 minutes as needed; may need to repeat doses every 20-60 minutes, if no response is observed after 10 mg, question the diagnosis. **Note:** Use 0.1-0.2 mg increments in patients who are opioid dependent and in postoperative patients to avoid large cardiovascular changes.

Administration

Endotracheal: Dilute to 1-2 mL with normal saline

I.V. push: Administer over 30 seconds as undiluted preparation

(Continued)

Naloxone *(Continued)*

I.V. continuous infusion: Dilute to 4 mcg/mL in D_5W or normal saline

Monitoring Parameters Respiratory rate, heart rate, blood pressure

Nursing Implications The use of neonatal naloxone (0.02 mg/mL) is no longer recommended because unacceptable fluid volumes will result, especially to small neonates; the 0.4 mg/mL preparation is available and can be accurately dosed with appropriately sized syringes (1 mL)

Additional Information May contain methyl and propylparabens

Dosage Forms

Injection, as hydrochloride: 0.4 mg/mL (1 mL, 2 mL, 10 mL); 1 mg/mL (2 mL, 10 mL)

Injection, neonatal, as hydrochloride: 0.02 mg/mL (2 mL)

♦ **Naloxone Hydrochloride** *see Naloxone on page 254*

Naltrexone *(nal TREKS one)*

Related Information

Addiction Treatments *on page 550*
Patient Information - Miscellaneous Medications *on page 495*

U.S. Brand Names ReVia®

Canadian Brand Names Revia

Synonyms Naltrexone Hydrochloride

Pharmacologic Category Antidote

Generic Available Yes

Use Treatment of alcohol dependence; blockade of the effects of exogenously administered opioids

Pregnancy Risk Factor C

Contraindications Hypersensitivity to naltrexone or any component of the formulation; narcotic dependence or current use of opioid analgesics; acute opioid withdrawal; failure to pass Narcan® challenge or positive urine screen for opioids; acute hepatitis; liver failure

Warnings/Precautions Dose-related hepatocellular injury is possible; the margin of separation between the apparent safe and hepatotoxic doses appear to be only fivefold or less. May precipitate withdrawal symptoms in patients addicted to opiates, including pain, hypertension, sweating, agitation, irritability; in neonates: shrill cry, failure to feed. Use with caution in patients with hepatic or renal impairment.

Patients who had been treated with naltrexone may respond to lower opioid doses than previously used. This could result in potentially life-threatening opioid intoxication. Patients should be aware that they may be more sensitive to lower doses of opioids after naltrexone treatment is discontinued. Use of naltrexone does not eliminate or diminish withdrawal symptoms.

Adverse Reactions

>10%:
Central nervous system: Insomnia, nervousness, headache, low energy
Gastrointestinal: Abdominal cramping, nausea, vomiting
Neuromuscular & skeletal: Arthralgia

1% to 10%:
Central nervous system: Increased energy, feeling down, irritability, dizziness, anxiety, somnolence
Dermatologic: Rash
Endocrine & metabolic: Polydipsia
Gastrointestinal: Diarrhea, constipation
Genitourinary: Delayed ejaculation, impotency

<1%: Bad dreams, blurred vision, confusion, depression, disorientation, edema, fatigue, hallucinations, increased blood pressure, itching, rhinorrhea, narcotic withdrawal, nasal congestion, nightmares, palpitations, paranoia, restlessness, sneezing, suicide attempts, tachycardia

Overdosage/Toxicology Signs and symptoms: Clonic-tonic convulsions, respiratory failure; patients receiving up to 800 mg/day for 1 week have shown no toxicity; seizures and respiratory failure have been seen in animals

Drug Interactions

Narcotic analgesics: Decreased effect of narcotic analgesics; may precipitate acute withdrawal reaction in physically dependent patients; concurrent use is contraindicated

Thioridazine: Lethargy and somnolence have been reported with the combination of naltrexone and thioridazine

Mechanism of Action Naltrexone (a pure opioid antagonist) is a cyclopropyl derivative of oxymorphone similar in structure to naloxone and nalorphine (a morphine derivative); it acts as a competitive antagonist at opioid receptor sites

Pharmacodynamics/Kinetics

Duration of action:
  50 mg: 24 hours
  100 mg: 48 hours
  150 mg: 72 hours

Absorption: Oral: Almost completely

Distribution: V_d: 19 L/kg; distributed widely throughout the body but considerable interindividual variation exists

Protein binding: 21%

Metabolism: Undergoes extensive first-pass metabolism to 6-β-naltrexol

Half-life: 4 hours; 6-β-naltrexol: 13 hours

Time to peak serum concentration: Within 60 minutes

Elimination: Principally in urine as metabolites and unchanged drug

Usual Dosage Do not give until patient is opioid-free for 7-10 days as determined by urine analysis

Adults: Oral: 25 mg; if no withdrawal signs within 1 hour give another 25 mg; maintenance regimen is flexible, variable and individualized (50 mg/day to 100-150 mg 3 times/week for 12 weeks); up to 800 mg/day has been tolerated in adults without an adverse effect

Dosing cautions in renal/hepatic impairment: Caution in patients with renal and hepatic impairment. An increase in naltrexone AUC of approximately five- and tenfold in patients with compensated or decompensated liver cirrhosis respectively, compared with normal liver function has been reported.

Administration If there is any question of occult opioid dependence, perform a naloxone challenge test; do not attempt treatment until naloxone challenge is negative

Naltrexone is administered orally; to minimize adverse gastrointestinal effects, give with food or antacids or after meals; advise patient not to self-administer opiates while receiving naltrexone therapy

Monitoring Parameters For narcotic withdrawal; liver function tests

Patient Information Will cause narcotic withdrawal; serious overdose can occur after attempts to overcome the blocking effect of naltrexone

Nursing Implications Monitor for narcotic withdrawal

Dosage Forms Tablet, as hydrochloride: 50 mg

♦ **Naltrexone Hydrochloride** *see* Naltrexone *on page 256*

Naratriptan (NAR a trip tan)

Related Information

Patient Information - Miscellaneous Medications - Antimigraine Medications *on page 521*

U.S. Brand Names Amerge®

Canadian Brand Names Amerge

Synonyms Naratriptan Hydrochloride

Pharmacologic Category Serotonin 5-HT$_{1D}$ Receptor Agonist

Generic Available No

Use Treatment of acute migraine headache with or without aura

(Continued)

Naratriptan *(Continued)*

Pregnancy Risk Factor C

Contraindications Hypersensitivity to naratriptan or any component of the formulation; cerebrovascular, peripheral vascular disease (ischemic bowel disease), ischemic heart disease (angina pectoris, history of myocardial infarction, or proven silent ischemia); or in patients with symptoms consistent with ischemic heart disease, coronary artery vasospasm, or Prinzmetal's angina; uncontrolled hypertension or patients who have received within 24 hours another 5-HT agonist (sumatriptan, zolmitriptan) or ergotamine-containing product; patients with known risk factors associated with coronary artery disease; patients with severe hepatic or renal disease (Cl$_{cr}$ <15 mL/minute); do not administer naratriptan to patients with hemiplegic or basilar migraine

Warnings/Precautions Use only if there is a clear diagnosis of migraine. Patients who are at risk of CAD but have had a satisfactory cardiovascular evaluation may receive naratriptan but with extreme caution (ie, in a physician's office where there are adequate precautions in place to protect the patient). Blood pressure may increase with the administration of naratriptan. Monitor closely, especially with the first administration of the drug. If the patient does not respond to the first dose, re-evaluate the diagnosis of migraine before trying a second dose.

Adverse Reactions

1% to 10%:
Central nervous system: Dizziness, drowsiness, malaise/fatigue
Gastrointestinal: Nausea, vomiting
Neuromuscular & skeletal: Paresthesias
Miscellaneous: Pain or pressure in throat or neck

<1% (Limited to important or life-threatening symptoms): Coronary artery vasospasm, transient myocardial ischemia, myocardial infarction, ventricular tachycardia, ventricular fibrillation, palpitations, hypertension, EKG changes (PR prolongation, QT$_c$ prolongation, premature ventricular contractions, atrial flutter, or atrial fibrillation) hypotension, heart murmurs, bradycardia, hyperlipidemia, hypercholesterolemia, hypothyroidism, hyperglycemia, glycosuria, ketonuria, eye hemorrhage, abnormal liver function tests, abnormal bilirubin tests, convulsions, allergic reaction, panic, hallucinations

Drug Interactions

Decreased effect: Smoking increases the clearance of naratriptan

Increased effect/toxicity: Ergot-containing drugs (dihydroergotamine or methysergide) may cause vasospastic reactions when taken with naratriptan. Avoid concomitant use with ergots; separate dose of naratriptan and ergots by at least 24 hours. Oral contraceptives taken with naratriptan reduced the clearance of naratriptan ~30% which may contribute to adverse effects. Selective serotonin reuptake inhibitors (SSRIs) (eg, fluoxetine, fluvoxamine, paroxetine, sertraline) may cause lack of coordination, hyper-reflexia, or weakness and should be avoided when taking naratriptan.

Mechanism of Action The therapeutic effect for migraine is due to serotonin agonist activity

Usual Dosage

Adults: Oral: 1-2.5 mg at the onset of headache; it is recommended to use the lowest possible dose to minimize adverse effects. If headache returns or does not fully resolve, the dose may be repeated after 4 hours; do not exceed 5 mg in 24 hours.

Elderly: Not recommended for use in the elderly

Dosing in renal impairment:
Cl$_{cr}$: 18-39 mL/minute: Initial: 1 mg; do not exceed 2.5 mg in 24 hours
Cl$_{cr}$: <15 mL/minute: Do not use

Dosing in hepatic impairment: Contraindicated in patients with severe liver failure; maximum dose: 2.5 mg in 24 hours for patients with mild or moderate liver failure; recommended starting dose: 1 mg

Patient Information This drug is to be used to reduce your migraine, not to prevent or reduce the number of attacks. If headache returns or is not fully resolved, the dose may be repeated after 4 hours. If you have no relief with first dose, do not take a second dose without consulting prescriber. **Do not exceed 5 mg in 24 hours. Do not take within 24 hours of any other migraine medication without first consulting prescriber.** You may experience some dizziness, fatigue, or drowsiness; use caution when driving or engaging in tasks that require alertness until response to drug is known. Frequent mouth care and sucking on lozenges may relieve dry mouth. Report immediately any chest pain, heart throbbing, tightness in throat, skin rash or hives, hallucinations, anxiety, or panic.

Dosage Forms Tablet: 1 mg, 2.5 mg

- ◆ **Naratriptan Hydrochloride** *see Naratriptan on page 257*
- ◆ **Narcan**® *see Naloxone on page 254*
- ◆ **Nardil**® *see Phenelzine on page 300*
- ◆ **Navane**® *see Thiothixene on page 396*
- ◆ **Nectar of the Gods** *see Garlic on page 166*

Nefazodone (nef AY zoe done)

Related Information

Antidepressant Agents Comparison Chart *on page 553*
Patient Information - Antidepressants (Serotonin Blocker) *on page 460*

U.S. Brand Names Serzone®

Canadian Brand Names Serzone

Synonyms Nefazodone Hydrochloride

Pharmacologic Category Antidepressant, Serotonin Reuptake Inhibitor/Antagonist

Generic Available No

Use Treatment of depression

Unlabeled/Investigational Use Post-traumatic stress disorder

Pregnancy Risk Factor C

Contraindications Hypersensitivity to nefazodone, related compounds (phenylpiperazines), or any component of the formulation; concurrent use or use of MAO inhibitors within previous 14 days; use in a patient during the acute recovery phase of MI; concurrent use with astemizole, carbamazepine, cisapride, pimozide, or terfenadine; concurrent therapy with triazolam or alprazolam is generally contraindicated (dosage must be reduced by 75%, which often may not be possible with available dosage forms).

Warnings/Precautions May cause sedation, resulting in impaired performance of tasks requiring alertness (ie, operating machinery or driving). Sedative effects may be additive with other CNS depressants. Does not potentiate ethanol but use is not advised. The degree of sedation is low relative to other antidepressants. May worsen psychosis in some patients or precipitate a shift to mania or hypomania in patients with bipolar disease. May increase the risks associated with electroconvulsive therapy. This agent should be discontinued, when possible, prior to elective surgery. Therapy should not be abruptly discontinued in patients receiving high doses for prolonged periods. Rare reports of priapism have occurred. The incidence of sexual dysfunction with nefazodone is generally lower than with SSRIs.

Use with caution in patients at risk of hypotension or in patients where transient hypotensive episodes would be poorly tolerated (cardiovascular disease or cerebrovascular disease). The risk of postural hypotension is low relative to other antidepressants. Use with caution in patients with urinary retention, benign prostatic hypertrophy, narrow-angle glaucoma, xerostomia, visual problems, constipation, or history of bowel obstruction (due to anticholinergic effects). The degree of anticholinergic blockade produced by this agent is very low relative to other cyclic antidepressants.

Use caution in patients with depression, particularly if suicidal risk may be present. Use caution in patients with a previous seizure disorder or condition predisposing to seizures such as brain damage, alcoholism, or concurrent therapy with other drugs which lower the seizure threshold. Use with caution in patients with hepatic (Continued)

Nefazodone *(Continued)*

or renal dysfunction and in elderly patients. Use with caution in patients with a history of cardiovascular disease (including previous MI, stroke, tachycardia, or conduction abnormalities). However, the risk of conduction abnormalities with this agent is very low relative to other antidepressants.

Adverse Reactions

>10%:

Central nervous system: Headache, drowsiness, insomnia, agitation, dizziness

Gastrointestinal: Xerostomia, nausea, constipation

Neuromuscular & skeletal: Weakness

1% to 10%:

Cardiovascular: Postural hypotension

Central nervous system: Lightheadedness, confusion, memory impairment, abnormal dreams, decreased concentration, ataxia

Dermatologic: Pruritus, rash

Gastrointestinal: Vomiting, dyspepsia, diarrhea, increased appetite, thirst, taste perversion

Neuromuscular & skeletal: Arthralgia, paresthesia, tremor

Ocular: Blurred vision (9%), abnormal vision (7%), visual field defect

Otic: Tinnitus

Respiratory: Cough

Miscellaneous: Flu syndrome

<1%, postmarketing and/or case reports: Allergic reaction, angioedema, AV block, bronchitis, dyspnea, eye pain, galactorrhea, gynecomastia, hallucinations, hepatic failure, hepatic necrosis, hyponatremia, impotence, increased prolactin, leukopenia, photosensitivity, priapism, rhabdomyolysis (with lovastatin/simvastatin), seizures, serotonin syndrome, Stevens-Johnson syndrome, thrombocytopenia

Overdosage/Toxicology

Signs and symptoms: Drowsiness, vomiting, hypotension, tachycardia, incontinence, coma, priapism

Treatment: Following initiation of essential overdose management, toxic symptoms should be treated. Ventricular arrhythmias often respond to lidocaine 1.5 mg/kg bolus followed by 2 mg/minute infusion with concurrent systemic alkalinization (sodium bicarbonate 0.5-2 mEq/kg I.V.). Seizures usually respond to diazepam I.V. boluses (5-10 mg for adults up to 30 mg or 0.25-0.4 mg/kg/dose for children up to 10 mg/dose). If seizures are unresponsive or recur, phenytoin or phenobarbital may be required. Hypotension is best treated by I.V. fluids and by placing the patient in the Trendelenburg position.

Drug Interactions CYP3A3/4 enzyme substrate; CYP3A3/4 enzyme inhibitor

Antiarrhythmics: Serum concentrations may be increased due to enzyme inhibition; monitor; includes amiodarone, lidocaine, propafenone, quinidine

Antipsychotics: Serum concentrations of some antipsychotics may be increased by nefazodone due to enzyme inhibition; includes clozapine, haloperidol, mesoridazine, pimozide, quetiapine, and risperidone

Benzodiazepines: Nefazodone inhibits the metabolism of triazolam (decrease dose by 75%) and alprazolam (decrease dose by 50%); triazolam is contraindicated per manufacturer

Buspirone: Concurrent use may result in serotonin syndrome; serum concentrations may be increased due to enzyme inhibition; these combinations are best avoided or limit buspirone to 2.5 mg/day

Calcium channel blockers: Serum concentrations may be increased due to enzyme inhibition; monitor for increased effect (hypotension)

Carbamazepine: Significantly reduces serum concentrations of nefazodone; coadministration is contraindicated

Cisapride: Nefazodone likely increases cisapride serum concentrations via CYP3A3/4 inhibition; this combination may lead to cardiac arrhythmias and should be avoided

Cyclosporine and tacrolimus: Serum levels and toxicity may be increased by nefazodone; monitor

CYP3A3/4 inhibitors: Serum level and/or toxicity of nefazodone may be increased; inhibitors include amiodarone, cimetidine, clarithromycin, erythromycin, delavirdine, diltiazem, dirithromycin, disulfiram, fluoxetine, fluvoxamine, grapefruit juice, indinavir, itraconazole, ketoconazole, metronidazole, nevirapine, propoxyphene, quinupristin-dalfopristin, ritonavir, saquinavir, verapamil, zafirlukast, zileuton

CYP3A3/4 substrates: Serum concentrations of drugs metabolized by CYP3A3/4 may be elevated by nefazodone; cisapride, pimozide, and triazolam are contraindicated; also see notes on individual drug classes

Digoxin: Serum levels may be increased by nefazodone (modest increases); monitor for digoxin toxicity or increased serum levels

Donepezil: Serum concentrations may be increased due to enzyme inhibition; monitor

HMG-CoA reductase inhibitors (statins) have been associated with myositis and rhabdomyolysis when used in combination with nefazodone; this has been associated most strongly with lovastatin and simvastatin

Linezolid: Due to MAO inhibition (see note on MAO inhibitors), this combination should be avoided

MAO inhibitors: Concurrent use may lead to serotonin syndrome; avoid concurrent use or use within 14 days

Meperidine: Combined use theoretically may increase the risk of serotonin syndrome

Methadone: Serum concentrations may be increased due to enzyme inhibition; monitor

Oral contraceptives: Serum concentrations may be increased due to enzyme inhibition; monitor

Pimozide: Serum concentrations may be increased due to enzyme inhibition; may result in life-threatening arrhythmias (also see note on antipsychotics); avoid use

Protease inhibitors: Indinavir, ritonavir saquinavir; serum concentrations may be increased due to enzyme inhibition; monitor

Quinidine: Metabolism is likely to be inhibited by nefazodone; avoid concurrent use

Selegiline: Concurrent use with nefazodone may be associated with a risk of serotonin syndrome, particularly at higher dosages (>10 mg/day)

Serotonin agonists: Theoretically may increase the risk of serotonin syndrome; includes sumatriptan, naratriptan, rizatriptan, and zolmitriptan

Sibutramine: Serum concentrations may be increased by nefazodone; monitor

Sildenafil: Serum concentrations may be increased due to enzyme inhibition; monitor

SSRIs: Combined use of nefazodone with an SSRI may produce serotonin syndrome; in addition, nefazodone may increase serum concentrations of some SSRIs due to enzyme inhibition (fluoxetine and citalopram)

Tricyclic antidepressants: Serum concentrations of some tricyclic antidepressants (amitriptyline, clomipramine) may be increased; monitor for increased effect or toxicity

Venlafaxine: Combined use with nefazodone may increase the risk of serotonin syndrome

Vinca alkaloids (vincristine, and vinblastine): Serum concentrations may be increased due to enzyme inhibition; may result in increased toxicity

Zolpidem: Serum concentrations may be increased due to enzyme inhibition; monitor

Ethanol/Nutrition/Herb Interactions

Ethanol: Avoid ethanol (may increase CNS depression).

Food: Nefazodone absorption may be delayed and bioavailability may be decreased if taken with food.

Herb/Nutraceutical: Avoid valerian, St John's wort, SAMe, kava kava (may increase risk of serotonin syndrome and/or excessive sedation).

(Continued)

Nefazodone *(Continued)*

Mechanism of Action Inhibits neuronal reuptake of serotonin and norepinephrine; also blocks 5-HT$_2$ and alpha$_1$ receptors; has no significant affinity for alpha$_2$, beta-adrenergic, 5-HT$_{1A}$, cholinergic, dopaminergic, or benzodiazepine receptors

Pharmacodynamics/Kinetics

Onset of effect: Full therapeutic effects may take up to 6 weeks to appear

Metabolism: In the liver to 3 active metabolites; triazoledione, hydroxynefazodone and m-chlorophenylpiperazine (mCPP)

Bioavailability: 20% (variable)

Half-life: 2-4 hours (parent compound), active metabolites persist longer

Time to peak serum concentration: 1 hour, prolonged in presence of food

Elimination: Primarily as metabolites in urine and secondarily in feces

Usual Dosage Oral:

Children and Adolescents: Depression: Target dose: 300-400 mg/day (mean: 3.4 mg/kg)

Adults: Depression: 200 mg/day, administered in 2 divided doses initially, with a range of 300-600 mg/day in 2 divided doses thereafter

Child/Adolescent Considerations Seven treatment-refractory and very comorbid children and adolescents (mean age: 12.4 years) with a juvenile mood disorder were treated with a mean daily dose of 357 mg (3.4 mg/kg) for 13 weeks (Wilens, 1997).

Administration Dosing after meals may decrease lightheadedness and postural hypotension, but may also decrease absorption and therefore effectiveness.

Reference Range Therapeutic plasma levels have not yet been defined

Patient Information Take shortly after a meal or light snack; can be given at bedtime dose if drowsiness occurs; optimum effect may take 2-4 weeks to be achieved; avoid alcohol; avoid sudden changes in position

Nursing Implications Dosing after meals may decrease lightheadedness and postural hypotension, but may also decrease absorption and therefore effectiveness; use side rails on bed if administered to the elderly; observe patient's activity and compare with admission level; assist with ambulation; sitting and standing blood pressure and pulse

Additional Information May cause less sexual dysfunction than other antidepressants. Women and elderly receiving single doses attain significant higher peak concentrations than male volunteers.

Dosage Forms Tablet, as hydrochloride: 50 mg, 100 mg, 150 mg, 200 mg, 250 mg

♦ **Nefazodone Hydrochloride** *see* Nefazodone *on page 259*

♦ **Nembutal**® *see* Pentobarbital *on page 289*

Neostigmine *(nee oh STIG meen)*

U.S. Brand Names Prostigmin®

Canadian Brand Names Prostigmin

Synonyms Neostigmine Bromide; Neostigmine Methylsulfate

Pharmacologic Category Acetylcholinesterase Inhibitor (Central)

Generic Available Yes

Use Diagnosis and treatment of myasthenia gravis; prevention and treatment of postoperative bladder distention and urinary retention; reversal of the effects of nondepolarizing neuromuscular-blocking agents after surgery

Pregnancy Risk Factor C

Contraindications Hypersensitivity to neostigmine, bromides, or any component of the formulation; GI or GU obstruction

Warnings/Precautions Does **not** antagonize and may prolong the phase I block of depolarizing muscle relaxants (eg, succinylcholine); use with caution in patients with epilepsy, asthma, bradycardia, hyperthyroidism, cardiac arrhythmias, or peptic ulcer; adequate facilities should be available for cardiopulmonary resuscitation when testing and adjusting dose for myasthenia gravis; have atropine and epinephrine ready to treat hypersensitivity reactions; overdosage may result in cholinergic crisis, this must be distinguished from myasthenic crisis; anticholinesterase insensitivity can develop for brief or prolonged periods

Adverse Reactions Frequency not defined.

Cardiovascular: Arrhythmias (especially bradycardia), hypotension, decreased carbon monoxide, tachycardia, AV block, nodal rhythm, nonspecific EKG changes, cardiac arrest, syncope, flushing

Central nervous system: Convulsions, dysarthria, dysphonia, dizziness, loss of consciousness, drowsiness, headache

Dermatologic: Skin rash, thrombophlebitis (I.V.), urticaria

Gastrointestinal: Hyperperistalsis, nausea, vomiting, salivation, diarrhea, stomach cramps, dysphagia, flatulence

Genitourinary: Urinary urgency

Neuromuscular & skeletal: Weakness, fasciculations, muscle cramps, spasms, arthralgias

Ocular: Small pupils, lacrimation

Respiratory: Increased bronchial secretions, laryngospasm, bronchiolar constriction, respiratory muscle paralysis, dyspnea, respiratory depression, respiratory arrest, bronchospasm

Miscellaneous: Diaphoresis (increased), anaphylaxis, allergic reactions

Overdosage/Toxicology Symptoms of overdose include muscle weakness, blurred vision, excessive sweating, tearing and salivation, nausea, vomiting, diarrhea, hypertension, bradycardia, muscle weakness, and paralysis. Atropine sulfate injection should be readily available as an antagonist for the effects of neostigmine.

Drug Interactions

Anticholinergics: Effects may be reduced with cholinesterase inhibitors; atropine antagonizes the muscarinic effects of cholinesterase inhibitors

Beta-blockers without ISA: Activity may increase risk of bradycardia

Calcium channel blockers (diltiazem or verapamil): May increase risk of bradycardia

Cholinergic agonists: Effects may be increased with cholinesterase inhibitors

Corticosteroids: May see increased muscle weakness and decreased response to anticholinesterases shortly after onset of corticosteroid therapy in the treatment of myasthenia gravis. Deterioration in muscle strength, including severe muscular depression, has been documented in patients with myasthenia gravis while receiving corticosteroids and anticholinesterases.

Digoxin: Increased risk of bradycardia with concurrent use

Neuromuscular blockers: Depolarizing neuromuscular blocking agents effects may be increased with cholinesterase inhibitors; nondepolarizing agents are antagonized by cholinesterase inhibitors

Mechanism of Action Inhibits destruction of acetylcholine by acetylcholinesterase which facilitates transmission of impulses across myoneural junction

Pharmacodynamics/Kinetics

Onset of effect: I.M.: Within 20-30 minutes; I.V.: Within 1-20 minutes

Duration: I.M.: 2.5-4 hours; I.V.: 1-2 hours

Absorption: Oral: Poor, <2%

Metabolism: In the liver

Half-life: Normal renal function: 0.5-2.1 hours; End-stage renal disease: Prolonged

Elimination: 50% excreted renally as unchanged drug

Usual Dosage

Myasthenia gravis: Diagnosis: I.M.:

Children: 0.04 mg/kg as a single dose

Adults: 0.02 mg/kg as a single dose

Myasthenia gravis: Treatment:

Children:

Oral: 2 mg/kg/day divided every 3-4 hours

I.M., I.V., S.C.: 0.01-0.04 mg/kg every 2-4 hours

Adults:

Oral: 15 mg/dose every 3-4 hours up to 375 mg/day maximum

I.M., I.V., S.C.: 0.5-2.5 mg every 1-3 hours up to 10 mg/24 hours maximum

(Continued)

Neostigmine *(Continued)*

Reversal of nondepolarizing neuromuscular blockade after surgery in conjunction with atropine: I.V.:
Infants: 0.025-0.1 mg/kg/dose
Children: 0.025-0.08 mg/kg/dose
Adults: 0.5-2.5 mg; total dose not to exceed 5 mg
Bladder atony: Adults: I.M., S.C.:
Prevention: 0.25 mg every 4-6 hours for 2-3 days
Treatment: 0.5-1 mg every 3 hours for 5 doses after bladder has emptied
Dosing adjustment in renal impairment:
Cl_{cr} 10-50 mL/minute: Administer 50% of normal dose
Cl_{cr} <10 mL/minute: Administer 25% of normal dose

Administration May be given undiluted by slow I.V. injection over several minutes

Test Interactions ↑ aminotransferase [ALT (SGPT)/AST (SGOT)] (S), ↑ amylase (S)

Nursing Implications In the diagnosis of myasthenia gravis, all anticholinesterase medications should be discontinued for at least 8 hours before administering neostigmine

Dosage Forms
Injection, as methylsulfate: 0.5 mg/mL (1 mL, 10 mL); 1 mg/mL (10 mL)
Tablet, as bromide: 15 mg

♦ **Neostigmine Bromide** *see* Neostigmine *on page 262*
♦ **Neostigmine Methylsulfate** *see* Neostigmine *on page 262*
♦ **Neurontin®** *see* Gabapentin *on page 161*
♦ **NicoDerm® CQ® Patch** *see* Nicotine *on page 264*
♦ **Nicorette® DS Gum** *see* Nicotine *on page 264*
♦ **Nicorette® Gum** *see* Nicotine *on page 264*
♦ **Nicorette™ Plus (Can)** *see* Nicotine *on page 264*

Nicotine *(nik oh TEEN)*

Related Information
Addiction Treatments *on page 550*
Patient Information - Miscellaneous Medications *on page 495*

U.S. Brand Names Habitrol™ Patch; NicoDerm® CQ® Patch; Nicorette® DS Gum; Nicorette® Gum; Nicotrol® NS; Nicotrol® Patch [OTC]; ProStep® Patch

Canadian Brand Names Nicorette™ Plus

Pharmacologic Category Smoking Cessation Aid

Generic Available Yes: Transdermal patch and gum

Use Treatment to aid smoking cessation for the relief of nicotine withdrawal symptoms

Unlabeled/Investigational Use Management of ulcerative colitis (transdermal)

Pregnancy Risk Factor D (transdermal); X (chewing gum)

Contraindications Hypersensitivity to nicotine or any component of the formulation; patients who are smoking during the postmyocardial infarction period; patients with life-threatening arrhythmias, or severe or worsening angina pectoris; active temporomandibular joint disease (gum); pregnancy; not for use in nonsmokers

Warnings/Precautions The risk versus the benefits must be weighed for each of these groups: patients with CAD, serious cardiac arrhythmias, vasospastic disease. Use caution in patients with hyperthyroidism, pheochromocytoma, or insulin-dependent diabetes. Use with caution in oropharyngeal inflammation and in patients with history of esophagitis, peptic ulcer, coronary artery disease, vasospastic disease, angina, hypertension, hyperthyroidism, pheochromocytoma, diabetes, severe renal dysfunction, and hepatic dysfunction. The inhaler should be used with caution in patients with bronchospastic disease (other forms of nicotine replacement may be preferred). Safety and efficacy have not been established in pediatric patients. Cautious use of topical nicotine in patients with certain skin diseases. Hypersensitivity to the topical products can occur. Dental problems may be worsened by chewing the gum. Urge patients to stop smoking completely when initiating therapy.

Adverse Reactions
Chewing gum:
>10%:

Cardiovascular: Tachycardia

Central nervous system: Headache (mild)

Gastrointestinal: Nausea, vomiting, indigestion, excessive salivation, belching, increased appetite

Miscellaneous: Mouth or throat soreness, jaw muscle ache, hiccups

1% to 10%:

Central nervous system: Insomnia, dizziness, nervousness

Endocrine & metabolic: Dysmenorrhea

Gastrointestinal: GI distress, eructation

Neuromuscular & skeletal: Muscle pain

Respiratory: Hoarseness

Miscellaneous: Hiccups

<1%: Atrial fibrillation, erythema, hypersensitivity reactions, itching

Transdermal systems:
>10%:

Central nervous system: Insomnia, abnormal dreams

Dermatologic: Pruritus, erythema

Local: Application site reaction

Respiratory: Rhinitis, cough, pharyngitis, sinusitis

1% to 10%:

Cardiovascular: Chest pain

Central nervous system: Dysphoria, anxiety, difficulty concentrating, dizziness, somnolence

Dermatologic: Rash

Gastrointestinal: Diarrhea, dyspepsia, nausea, xerostomia, constipation, anorexia, abdominal pain

Neuromuscular & skeletal: Arthralgia, myalgia

<1%: Atrial fibrillation, hypersensitivity reactions, itching, nervousness, taste perversion, thirst, tremor

Overdosage/Toxicology
Signs and symptoms: Nausea, vomiting, abdominal pain, mental confusion, diarrhea, salivation, tachycardia, respiratory and cardiovascular collapse

Treatment: After decontamination is symptomatic and supportive; remove patch, rinse area with water and dry, do not use soap as this may increase absorption

Drug Interactions
CYP2B6 and 2A6 enzyme substrate; CYP1A2 enzyme inducer

Adenosine: Nicotine increases the hemodynamic and AV blocking effects of adenosine; monitor

Bupropion: Monitor for treatment-emergent hypertension in patients treated with the combination of nicotine patch and bupropion

Cimetidine; May increases nicotine concentrations; therefore, may decrease amount of gum or patches needed

CYP1A2 substrates: May decrease serum concentrations of drugs metabolized by this isoenzyme, including theophylline and tacrine

Stability
Store inhaler cartridge at room temperature not to exceed 30°C (86°F); protect cartridges from light

Mechanism of Action
Nicotine is one of two naturally-occurring alkaloids which exhibit their primary effects via autonomic ganglia stimulation. The other alkaloid is lobeline which has many actions similar to those of nicotine but is less potent. Nicotine is a potent ganglionic and central nervous system stimulant, the actions of which are mediated via nicotine-specific receptors. Biphasic actions are observed depending upon the dose administered. The main effect of nicotine in small doses is stimulation of all autonomic ganglia; with larger doses, initial stimulation is followed by blockade of transmission. Biphasic effects are also evident in the adrenal medulla; discharge of catecholamines occurs with small doses, whereas prevention of catecholamines release is seen with higher doses as a response to
(Continued)

Nicotine *(Continued)*

splanchnic nerve stimulation. Stimulation of the central nervous system (CNS) is characterized by tremors and respiratory excitation. However, convulsions may occur with higher doses, along with respiratory failure secondary to both central paralysis and peripheral blockade to respiratory muscles.

Pharmacodynamics/Kinetics Intranasal nicotine may more closely approximate the time course of plasma nicotine levels observed after cigarette smoking than other dosage forms

Duration of action: Transdermal: 24 hours

Absorption: Transdermal: Slow

Metabolism: In the liver, primarily to cotinine, which is $1/5$ as active.

Half-life, elimination: 4 hours

Time to peak serum concentration: Transdermal: 8-9 hours

Elimination: Via the kidneys; renal clearance is pH-dependent

Usual Dosage

Gum: Chew 1 piece of gum when urge to smoke, up to 30 pieces/day; most patients require 10-12 pieces of gum/day

Transdermal patch

Smoking deterrent: Patients should be advised to completely stop smoking upon initiation of therapy: Apply new patch every 24 hours to nonhairy, clean, dry skin on the upper body or upper outer arm; each patch should be applied to a different site

Initial starting dose: 21 mg/day for 4-8 weeks for most patients

First weaning dose: 14 mg/day for 2-4 weeks

Second weaning dose: 7 mg/day for 2-4 weeks

Initial starting dose for patients <100 pounds, smoke <10 cigarettes/day, have a history of cardiovascular disease: 14 mg/day for 4-8 weeks followed by 7 mg/day for 2-4 weeks

In patients who are receiving >600 mg/day of cimetidine: Decrease to the next lower patch size

Benefits of use of nicotine transdermal patches beyond 3 months have not been demonstrated

Ulcerative colitis: Titrated to 22-25 mg/day

Spray: 1-2 sprays/hour; do not exceed more than 5 doses (10 sprays) per hour; each dose (2 sprays) contains 1 mg of nicotine. **Warning:** A dose of 40 mg can cause fatalities.

Monitoring Parameters Heart rate and blood pressure periodically during therapy; discontinue therapy if signs of nicotine toxicity occur (eg, severe headache, dizziness, mental confusion, disturbed hearing and vision, abdominal pain; rapid, weak and irregular pulse; salivation, nausea, vomiting, diarrhea, cold sweat, weakness); therapy should be discontinued if rash develops; discontinuation may be considered if other adverse effects of patch occur such as myalgia, arthralgia, abnormal dreams, insomnia, nervousness, dry mouth, sweating

Patient Information Instructions for the proper use of the patch should be given to the patient; notify physician if persistent rash, itching, or burning may occur with the patch; do not smoke while wearing patches chew slowly to avoid jaw ache and to maximize benefit

Nursing Implications

Chew gum formulation: Patient should be instructed to chew slowly to avoid jaw ache and to maximize benefit

Transdermal patch: Patches cannot be cut; use of an aerosol corticosteroid may diminish local irritation under patches

Additional Information A cigarette has 10-25 mg nicotine. Use of an aerosol corticosteroid may diminish local irritation under patches.

Dosage Forms

Gum, chewing pieces, as polacrilex: 2 mg/square [OTC] (96 pieces/box); 4 mg/square (96 pieces/box)

Liquid for oral inhalation (Nicotrol® Inhaler): 10 mg cartridge [delivering 4 mg] (42s); each unit consists of one mouthpiece, 7 storage trays each containing 6 cartridges and one storage case

Patch, transdermal:
Habitrol™: 21 mg/day; 14 mg/day; 7 mg/day (30 systems/box)
NicoDerm® CQ® [OTC]: 21 mg/day; 14 mg/day; 7 mg/day (14 systems/box)
Nicotrol® [OTC]: 15 mg/day (gradually released over 16 hours)
ProStep®: 22 mg/day; 11 mg/day (7 systems/box)
Solution, intranasal [spray] (Nicotrol® NS): 0.5 mg/actuation [10 mg/mL - 200 actuations] (10 mL)

Nortriptyline (nor TRIP ti leen)

Related Information
Antidepressant Agents Comparison Chart *on page 553*
Discontinuation of Psychotropic Drugs - Withdrawal Symptoms and Recommendations *on page 582*
Federal OBRA Regulations Recommended Maximum Doses *on page 583*
Patient Information - Antidepressants (TCAs) *on page 454*

U.S. Brand Names Aventyl®; Pamelor®

Canadian Brand Names Apo®-Nortriptyline

Synonyms Nortriptyline Hydrochloride

Pharmacologic Category Antidepressant, Tricyclic (Secondary Amine)

Generic Available Yes

Use Treatment of symptoms of depression

Unlabeled/Investigational Use Chronic pain, anxiety disorders, enuresis, attention-deficit/hyperactivity disorder (ADHD)

Pregnancy Risk Factor D

Contraindications Hypersensitivity to nortriptyline and similar chemical class, or any component of the formulation; use of MAO inhibitors within 14 days; use in a patient during the acute recovery phase of MI; pregnancy

Warnings/Precautions May cause sedation, resulting in impaired performance of tasks requiring alertness (ie, operating machinery or driving). Sedative effects may be additive with other CNS depressants and/or ethanol. The degree of sedation is low-moderate relative to other antidepressants. May worsen psychosis in some patients or precipitate a shift to mania or hypomania in patients with bipolar disease. May increase the risks associated with electroconvulsive therapy. This agent should be discontinued, when possible, prior to elective surgery. Therapy should not be abruptly discontinued in patients receiving high doses for prolonged periods. May alter glucose regulation - use caution in patients with diabetes.

May cause orthostatic hypotension (risk is low relative to other antidepressants) - use with caution in patients at risk of hypotension or in patients where transient hypotensive episodes would be poorly tolerated (cardiovascular disease or cerebrovascular disease). The degree of anticholinergic blockade produced by this agent is moderate relative to other cyclic antidepressants, however, caution should still be used in patients with urinary retention, benign prostatic hypertrophy, narrow-angle glaucoma, xerostomia, visual problems, constipation, or history of bowel obstruction.

Use caution in patients with depression, particularly if suicidal risk may be present. Use with caution in patients with a history of cardiovascular disease (including previous MI, stroke, tachycardia, or conduction abnormalities). The risk conduction (Continued)

Nortriptyline *(Continued)*

abnormalities with this agent is moderate relative to other antidepressants. Use caution in patients with a previous seizure disorder or condition predisposing to seizures such as brain damage, alcoholism, or concurrent therapy with other drugs which lower the seizure threshold. Use with caution in hyperthyroid patients or those receiving thyroid supplementation. Use with caution in patients with hepatic or renal dysfunction and in elderly patients.

Adverse Reactions Frequency not defined.

Cardiovascular: Postural hypotension, arrhythmias, hypertension, heart block, tachycardia, palpitations, myocardial infarction

Central nervous system: Confusion, delirium, hallucinations, restlessness, insomnia, disorientation, delusions, anxiety, agitation, panic, nightmares, hypomania, exacerbation of psychosis, incoordination, ataxia, extrapyramidal symptoms, seizures

Dermatologic: Alopecia, photosensitivity, rash, petechiae, urticaria, itching

Endocrine & metabolic: Sexual dysfunction, gynecomastia, breast enlargement, galactorrhea, increase or decrease in libido, increase in blood sugar, SIADH

Gastrointestinal: Xerostomia, constipation, vomiting, anorexia, diarrhea, abdominal cramps, black tongue, nausea, unpleasant taste, weight gain/loss

Genitourinary: Urinary retention, delayed micturition, impotence, testicular edema

Hematologic: Rarely agranulocytosis, eosinophilia, purpura, thrombocytopenia

Hepatic: Increased liver enzymes, cholestatic jaundice

Neuromuscular & skeletal: Tremor, numbness, tingling, paresthesias, peripheral neuropathy

Ocular: Blurred vision, eye pain, disturbances in accommodation, mydriasis

Otic: Tinnitus

Miscellaneous: Diaphoresis (excessive), allergic reactions

Overdosage/Toxicology

Signs and symptoms: Agitation, confusion, hallucinations, urinary retention, hypothermia, hypotension, seizures, ventricular tachycardia

Treatment: Following initiation of essential overdose management, toxic symptoms should be treated. Ventricular arrhythmias often respond to phenytoin 15-20 mg/kg (adults) with concurrent systemic alkalinization (sodium bicarbonate 0.5-2 mEq/kg I.V.). Arrhythmias unresponsive to this therapy may respond to lidocaine 1 mg/kg I.V. followed by a titrated infusion. Physostigmine (1-2 mg I.V. slowly for adults or 0.5 mg I.V. slowly for children) may be indicated in reversing cardiac arrhythmias that are life-threatening. Seizures usually respond to diazepam I.V. boluses (5-10 mg for adults up to 30 mg or 0.25-0.4 mg/kg/dose for children up to 10 mg/dose). If seizures are unresponsive or recur, phenytoin or phenobarbital may be required.

Drug Interactions CYP1A2 and 2D6 enzyme substrate

Altretamine: Concurrent use may cause orthostatic hypertension

Amphetamines: TCAs may enhance the effect of amphetamines; monitor for adverse CV effects

Anticholinergics: Combined use with TCAs may produce additive anticholinergic effects

Antihypertensives: TCAs may inhibit the antihypertensive response to bethanidine, clonidine, debrisoquin, guanadrel, guanethidine, guanabenz, guanfacine; monitor BP; consider alternate antihypertensive agent

Beta-agonists: When combined with TCAs may predispose patients to cardiac arrhythmias

Bupropion: May increase the levels of tricyclic antidepressants; based on limited information; monitor response

Carbamazepine: Tricyclic antidepressants may increase carbamazepine levels; monitor

Cholestyramine and colestipol: May bind TCAs and reduce their absorption; monitor for altered response

Clonidine: Abrupt discontinuation of clonidine may cause hypertensive crisis, amitriptyline may enhance the response

CNS depressants: Sedative effects may be additive with TCAs; monitor for increased effect; includes benzodiazepines, barbiturates, antipsychotics, ethanol and other sedative medications

CYP1A2 inhibitors: Serum levels and/or toxicity of some tricyclic antidepressants may be increased; inhibitors include cimetidine, ciprofloxacin, fluvoxamine, isoniazid, ritonavir, and zileuton

CYP2D6 inhibitors: Serum levels and/or toxicity of some tricyclic antidepressants may be increased; inhibitors include amiodarone, cimetidine, delavirdine, fluoxetine, paroxetine, propafenone, quinidine, and ritonavir; monitor for increased effect/toxicity

Enzyme inducers: May increase the metabolism of TCAs resulting in decreased effect; includes carbamazepine, phenobarbital, phenytoin, and rifampin; monitor for decreased response

Epinephrine (and other direct alpha-agonists): Pressor response to I.V. epinephrine, norepinephrine, and phenylephrine may be enhanced in patients receiving TCAs (**Note:** Effect is unlikely with epinephrine or levonordefrin dosages typically administered as infiltration in combination with local anesthetics)

Fenfluramine: May increase tricyclic antidepressant levels/effects

Hypoglycemic agents (including insulin): TCAs may enhance the hypoglycemic effects of tolazamide, chlorpropamide, or insulin; monitor for changes in blood glucose levels; reported with chlorpropamide, tolazamide, and insulin

Levodopa: Tricyclic antidepressants may decrease the absorption (bioavailability) of levodopa; rare hypertensive episodes have also been attributed to this combination

Linezolid: Hyperpyrexia, hypertension, tachycardia, confusion, seizures, and **deaths have been reported** with agents which inhibit MAO (serotonin syndrome); this combination should be avoided

Lithium: Concurrent use with a TCA may increase the risk for neurotoxicity

MAO inhibitors: Hyperpyrexia, hypertension, tachycardia, confusion, seizures, and **deaths have been reported** (serotonin syndrome); this combination should be avoided

Methylphenidate: Metabolism of TCAs may be decreased

Phenothiazines: Serum concentrations of some TCAs may be increased; in addition, TCAs may increase concentration of phenothiazines; monitor for altered clinical response

QT_c-prolonging agents: Concurrent use of tricyclic agents with other drugs which may prolong QT_c interval may increase the risk of potentially fatal arrhythmias; includes type Ia and type III antiarrhythmics agents, selected quinolones (sparfloxacin, gatifloxacin, moxifloxacin, grepafloxacin), cisapride, and other agents

Sucralfate: Absorption of tricyclic antidepressants may be reduced with coadministration

Sympathomimetics, indirect-acting: Tricyclic antidepressants may result in a decreased sensitivity to indirect-acting sympathomimetics; includes dopamine and ephedrine; also see interaction with epinephrine (and direct-acting sympathomimetics)

Tramadol: Tramadol's risk of seizures may be increased with TCAs

Valproic acid: May increase serum concentrations/adverse effects of some tricyclic antidepressants

Warfarin (and other oral anticoagulants): TCAs may increase the anticoagulant effect in patients stabilized on warfarin; monitor INR

Ethanol/Nutrition/Herb Interactions

Ethanol: Avoid ethanol (may increase CNS depression).

Food: Grapefruit juice may inhibit the metabolism of some TCAs and clinical toxicity may result.

Herb/Nutraceutical: Avoid valerian, St John's wort, SAMe, kava kava (may increase risk of serotonin syndrome and/or excessive sedation).

Stability Protect from light

Mechanism of Action Traditionally believed to increase the synaptic concentration of serotonin and/or norepinephrine in the central nervous system by inhibition of their reuptake by the presynaptic neuronal membrane. However, additional (Continued)

Nortriptyline *(Continued)*

receptor effects have been found including desensitization of adenyl cyclase, down regulation of beta-adrenergic receptors, and down regulation of serotonin receptors.

Pharmacodynamics/Kinetics

Onset of action: 1-3 weeks

Distribution: V_d: 21 L/kg

Protein binding: 93% to 95%

Metabolism: Undergoes significant first-pass metabolism; primarily detoxified in the liver

Half-life: 28-31 hours

Time to peak serum concentration: Oral: Within 7-8.5 hours

Elimination: As metabolites and small amounts of unchanged drug in urine; small amounts of biliary elimination occur

Usual Dosage Oral:

Nocturnal enuresis:

Children:

6-7 years (20-25 kg): 10 mg/day

8-11 years (25-35 kg): 10-20 mg/day

>11 years (35-54 kg): 25-35 mg/day

Depression or ADHD (unlabeled use):

Children 6-12 years: 1-3 mg/kg/day or 10-20 mg/day in 3-4 divided doses

Adolescents: 30-100 mg/day in divided doses

Depression:

Adults: 25 mg 3-4 times/day up to 150 mg/day

Elderly (**Note:** Nortriptyline is one of the best tolerated TCAs in the elderly)

Initial: 10-25 mg at bedtime

Dosage can be increased by 25 mg every 3 days for inpatients and weekly for outpatients if tolerated

Usual maintenance dose: 75 mg as a single bedtime dose or 2 divided doses; however, lower or higher doses may be required to stay within the therapeutic window

Dosing adjustment in hepatic impairment: Lower doses and slower titration dependent on individualization of dosage is recommended

Monitoring Parameters Blood pressure and pulse rate (EKG, cardiac monitoring) prior to and during initial therapy in older adults; weight

Reference Range

Plasma levels do not always correlate with clinical effectiveness

Therapeutic: 50-150 ng/mL (SI: 190-570 nmol/L)

Toxic: >500 ng/mL (SI: >1900 nmol/L)

Test Interactions ↑ glucose

Patient Information Avoid alcohol ingestion; do not discontinue medication abruptly; may cause urine to turn blue-green; may cause drowsiness; full effect may not occur for 4-6 weeks; dry mouth may be helped by sips of water, sugarless gum, or hard candy

Nursing Implications May increase appetite and possibly a craving for sweets

Dosage Forms

Capsule, as hydrochloride: 10 mg, 25 mg, 50 mg, 75 mg

Solution, as hydrochloride: 10 mg/5 mL (473 mL)

Nutmeg

Pharmacologic Category Herb

Use In folk medicine for delayed menses; stomach complains

Adverse Reactions

Cardiovascular: Sinus tachycardia

Dermatologic: Contact dermatitis

Overdosage/Toxicology Signs and symptoms: The most prominent effects of significant ingestions appear to be hallucinations, nausea, and profound vomiting; miosis, tachycardia, mydriasis, hypothermia, dry skin, hypotension, and a feeling of impending doom may also be seen; symptoms may be delayed up to 8 hours after ingestion

Drug Interactions

Decreased effect of antihypertensives

Increased toxicity with disulfiram (possible seizures, delirium), fluoxetine (and other serotonin active agents), TCAs (cardiovascular instability), meperidine (cardiovascular instability), phenothiazine (hyperpyretic crisis), levodopa, sympathomimetics (hyperpyretic crisis), barbiturates, Rauwolfia alkaloids (eg, reserpine), dextroamphetamine (psychoses), foods containing tyramine (hypertension, headache, seizures); theophylline/caffeine (hyperthermia), cyclobenzaprine (fever/seizures)

Potentiation of hypoglycemia with oral hypoglycemic agents

Serotonin syndrome (shivering, muscle rigidity, salivation, agitation, and hyperthermia) can occur with concomitant administration of venlafaxine and tranylcypromine

Usual Dosage It is estimated that 2 tablespoons of ground nutmeg will produce toxicity; however, amounts may vary depending on the content of volatile oil

Toxic dose: 1-3 nutmegs can cause toxic symptoms

(Continued)

Nutmeg *(Continued)*

Additional Information Nutmeg is the seed of *Myristica fragrans*; the spice mace is from the seed coat of *Myristica fragrans*

Family: Myristicaceae

Toxin: Myristicin, elemicin, geraniol

Range: Grows in India, Ceylon, and Grenada

Toxic parts: Volatile oil in seed and seed coat appears to be responsible for pharmacologic effects

- ♦ **Nu-Triazo® (Can)** *see* Triazolam *on page 410*
- ♦ **Nu-Trimipramine® (Can)** *see* Trimipramine *on page 421*
- ♦ **Nutrol E (Can)** *see* Vitamin E *on page 433*
- ♦ **Nytol® [OTC]** *see* Diphenhydramine *on page 116*

Olanzapine *(oh LAN za peen)*

Related Information

Antipsychotic Agents Comparison Chart *on page 557*

Antipsychotic Medication Guidelines *on page 559*

Atypical Antipsychotics *on page 565*

Discontinuation of Psychotropic Drugs - Withdrawal Symptoms and Recommendations *on page 582*

Patient Information - Antipsychotics (General) *on page 466*

U.S. Brand Names Zyprexa®; Zyprexa® Zydis®

Canadian Brand Names Zyprexa

Synonyms LY170053

Pharmacologic Category Antipsychotic Agent, Thienobenzodiaepine

Generic Available No

Use Treatment of the manifestations of schizophrenia; short-term treatment of acute mania episodes associated with bipolar mania

Unlabeled/Investigational Use Treatment of psychotic symptoms

Pregnancy Risk Factor C

Contraindications Hypersensitivity to olanzapine or any component of the formulation

Warnings/Precautions Moderate to highly sedating, use with caution in disorders where CNS depression is a feature. Use with caution in Parkinson's disease. Caution in patients with hemodynamic instability; bone marrow suppression; predisposition to seizures; subcortical brain damage; severe cardiac, hepatic, renal, or respiratory disease. Esophageal dysmotility and aspiration have been associated with antipsychotic use - use with caution in patients at risk of pneumonia (ie, Alzheimer's disease). Caution in breast cancer or other prolactin-dependent tumors (may elevate prolactin levels). May alter temperature regulation or mask toxicity of other drugs due to antiemetic effects. Life-threatening arrhythmias have occurred with therapeutic doses of some neuroleptics. Significant weight gain may occur.

May cause anticholinergic effects (constipation, dry mouth, blurred vision, urinary retention); therefore, they should be used with caution in patients with decreased gastrointestinal motility, urinary retention, BPH, xerostomia, or visual problems. Conditions which also may be exacerbated by cholinergic blockade include narrow-angle glaucoma (screening is recommended) and worsening of myasthenia gravis. Relative to other neuroleptics, olanzapine has a moderate potency of cholinergic blockade.

May cause extrapyramidal reactions, including pseudoparkinsonism, acute dystonic reactions, akathisia, and tardive dyskinesia (risk of these reactions is very low relative to other neuroleptics). May be associated with neuroleptic malignant syndrome (NMS).

Adverse Reactions

>10%: Central nervous system: Headache, somnolence, insomnia, agitation, nervousness, hostility, dizziness

1% to 10%:

Cardiovascular: Postural hypotension, tachycardia, hypotension, peripheral edema

Central nervous system: Dystonic reactions, parkinsonian events, amnesia, euphoria, stuttering, akathisia, anxiety, personality changes, fever

Dermatologic: Rash

Gastrointestinal: Xerostomia, constipation, abdominal pain, weight gain, increased appetite

Genitourinary: Premenstrual syndrome

Neuromuscular & skeletal: Arthralgia, neck rigidity, twitching, hypertonia, tremor

Ocular: Amblyopia

Respiratory: Rhinitis, cough, pharyngitis

<1%: Neuroleptic malignant syndrome, priapism, seizures, tardive dyskinesia, neutropenia, agranulocytosis

Overdosage/Toxicology

Signs and symptoms: Drowsiness and slurred developed in one patient taking 300 mg of olanzapine

Treatment: Supportive; activated charcoal 1 g reduced the C_{max} and AUC by ~60

Drug Interactions CYP1A2 enzyme substrate, CYP2C19 enzyme substrate (minor), and CYP2D6 enzyme substrate (minor)

Activated charcoal: Decreases the C_{max} and AUC of olanzapine by 60%

Antihypertensives: Increased risk of hypotension and orthostatic hypotension with antihypertensives

Clomipramine: When used in combination, clomipramine and olanzapine have been reported to be associated with the development of seizures; limited documentation (case report)

CNS depressants: Sedative effects and may be additive with CNS depressants; includes ethanol, barbiturates, narcotic analgesics, and other sedative agents; monitor for increased effect

CYP1A2 inhibitors: Serum levels may be increased and effect/toxicity increased by CYP1A2 inhibitors; examples include cimetidine, ciprofloxacin, fluvoxamine, isoniazid, and ritonavir

Enzyme inducers: May increase the metabolism of olanzapine resulting in decreased effect; includes carbamazepine, phenobarbital, phenytoin, rifampin, and cigarette smoking; monitor for decreased response

Haloperidol: A case of severe Parkinsonism following the addition of olanzapine to haloperidol therapy has been reported

Levodopa: Antipsychotics may inhibit the antiparkinsonian effect of levodopa; avoid this combination

Ethanol/Nutrition/Herb Interactions

Ethanol: Avoid ethanol (may increase CNS depression).

Herb/Nutraceutical: Avoid dong quai, St John's wort (may also cause photosensitization). Avoid kava kava, gotu kola, valerian, St John's wort (may increase CNS depression).

Stability Store at room temperature (20°C to 25°C); protect from light

Mechanism of Action Olanzapine is a thienobenzodiazepine neuroleptic; thought to work by antagonizing dopamine and serotonin activities. It is a selective monoaminergic antagonist with high affinity binding to serotonin $5-HT_{2a}$ and $5-HT_{2c}$, dopamine D_{1-4}, muscarinic M_{1-5}, histamine H_1- and alpha$_1$-adrenergic receptor sites. Olanzapine binds weakly to GABA-A, BZD, and beta-adrenergic receptors.

Pharmacodynamics/Kinetics

Absorption: Well absorbed; not affected by food; tablets and orally-disintegrating tablets are bioequivalent

Distribution: V_d: Extensive, 1000 L

Protein binding, plasma: 93% bound to albumin and alpha$_1$-glycoprotein

Metabolism: Highly metabolized via direct glucuronidation and cytochrome P450 mediated oxidation (CYP1A2, CYP2D6)

Time to peak serum concentrations: ~6 hours

Half-life: 21-54 hours; approximately 1.5 times greater in elderly

(Continued)

Olanzapine *(Continued)*

Elimination: 40% removed via first pass metabolism; 57% in urine, 30% feces, 7% excreted unchanged; 40% increase in olanzapine clearance in smokers

Not removed by dialysis

Usual Dosage Oral:

Children: Schizophrenia/bipolar disorder: Initial: 2.5 mg/day; titrate as necessary to 20 mg/day (0.12-0.29 mg/kg/day)

Adults:

Schizophrenia: Usual starting dose: 5-10 mg once daily; increase to 10 mg once daily within 5-7 days, thereafter adjust by 5-10 mg/day at 1-week intervals, up to a maximum of 20 mg/day; doses of 30-50 mg/day have been used; typical dosage range: 10-30 mg/day

Bipolar mania: Usual starting dose: 10-15 mg once daily; increase by 5 mg/day at intervals of not less than 24 hours; maximum dose: 20 mg/day

Elderly: Schizophrenia: Usual starting dose: 2.5 mg/day, increase as clinically indicated and monitor blood pressure; typical dosage range: 2.5-10 mg/day

Child/Adolescent Considerations Five hospitalized children 6-11 years of age with varying diagnoses were treated with a mean daily dose of 7.5 mg/day (2.5-10 mg/day) or 0.22 mg/kg/day (0.12-0.29 mg/kg/day) for a mean of 32 days (Krishnamoorthy, 1998). Seven adolescents 12-17 years of age with DSM-IV bipolar disorder, manic episode were treated with a mean dose of 11 mg/day or 0.146 ± 0.086 mg/kg/day (Soutullo, 1999).

Administration Orally-disintegrating tablets: Remove from foil blister by peeling back (do not push tablet through the foil); place tablet in mouth immediately upon removal; tablet dissolves rapidly in saliva and may be swallowed with or without liquid

Patient Information Use exactly as directed (do not increase dose or frequency); may cause physical and/or psychological dependence. It may take 2-3 weeks to achieve desired results; do not discontinue without consulting prescriber. Avoid excess alcohol or caffeine and other prescription or OTC medications not approved by prescriber. Maintain adequate hydration (2-3 L/day of fluids unless instructed to restrict fluid intake). You may experience excess drowsiness, restlessness, dizziness, or blurred vision (use caution driving or when engaging in tasks requiring alertness until response to drug is known); or constipation (increased exercise, fluids, or dietary fruit and fiber may help). Report persistent CNS effects (eg, trembling fingers, altered gait or balance, excessive sedation, seizures, unusual movements, anxiety, abnormal thoughts, confusion, personality changes); unresolved constipation or gastrointestinal effects; vision changes; difficulty breathing; unusual cough or flu-like symptoms; or worsening of condition.

Orally-disintegrating tablets: Remove from foil blister by peeling back (do not push tablet through the foil); place tablet in mouth immediately upon removal; tablet dissolves rapidly in saliva and may be swallowed with or without liquid

Dosage Forms

Tablet (Zyprexa®): 2.5 mg, 5 mg, 7.5 mg, 10 mg, 15 mg, 20 mg

Tablet, orally-disintegrating (Zyprexa® Zydis®): 5 mg, 10 mg, 15 mg, 20 mg

♦ **Orap**™ *see* Pimozide *on page 316*

♦ **Organex (Can)** *see* Vitamin E *on page 433*

♦ **ORLAAM**® *see* Levomethadyl Acetate Hydrochloride *on page 196*

Orlistat *(OR li stat)*

Related Information

Patient Information - Miscellaneous Medications *on page 495*

U.S. Brand Names Xenical®

Canadian Brand Names Xenical

Pharmacologic Category Lipase Inhibitor

Generic Available No

Use Management of obesity, including weight loss and weight management when used in conjunction with a reduced-calorie diet; reduce the risk of weight regain after prior weight loss; indicated for obese patients with an initial body mass index (BMI) ≥30 kg/m^2 or ≥27 kg/m^2 in the presence of other risk factors; see Body Mass Index *on page 569* in the Appendix)

Pregnancy Risk Factor B

Pregnancy/Breast-Feeding Implications There are no adequate and well-controlled studies of orlistat in pregnant women. Because animal reproductive studies are not always predictive of human response, orlistat is not recommended for use during pregnancy. Teratogenicity studies were conducted in rats and rabbits at doses up to 800 mg/kg/day. Neither study showed embryotoxicity or teratogenicity. This dose is 23 and 47 times the daily human dose calculated on a body surface area basis for rats and rabbits, respectively. It is not know if orlistat is secreted in human milk. Therefore, it should not be taken by nursing women.

Contraindications Hypersensitivity to orlistat or any component of the formulation; chronic malabsorption syndrome or cholestasis

Warnings/Precautions Patients should be advised to adhere to dietary guidelines; gastrointestinal adverse events may increase if taken with a diet high in fat (>30% total daily calories from fat). The daily intake of fat should be distributed over three main meals. If taken with any one meal very high in fat, the possibility of gastrointestinal effects increases. Patients should be counseled to take a multivitamin supplement that contains fat-soluble vitamins to ensure adequate nutrition because orlistat has been shown to reduce the absorption of some fat-soluble vitamins and beta-carotene. The supplement should be taken once daily at least 2 hours before or after the administration of orlistat (ie, bedtime). Some patients may develop increased levels of urinary oxalate following treatment; caution should be exercised when prescribing it to patients with a history of hyperoxaluria or calcium oxalate nephrolithiasis. As with any weight-loss agent, the potential exists for misuse in appropriate patient populations (eg, patients with anorexia nervosa or bulimia). Write/fill prescription carefully. Dispensing errors have been made between Xenical® (orlistat) and Xeloda® (capecitabine).

Adverse Reactions

>10%

Central nervous system: Headache (31%)

Gastrointestinal: Oily spotting (27%), abdominal pain/discomfort (26%), flatus with discharge (24%), fatty/oily stool (20%), fecal urgency (22%), oily evacuation (12%), increased defecation (11%)

Neuromuscular and skeletal: Back pain (14%)

Respiratory: Upper respiratory infection (38%)

1% to 10%

Central nervous system: Fatigue (7%), anxiety (5%), sleep disorder (4%)

Dermatologic: Dry skin (2%)

Endocrine and metabolic: Menstrual irregularities (10%)

Gastrointestinal: Fecal incontinence (8%), nausea (8%), infectious diarrhea (5%), rectal pain/discomfort (5%), vomiting (4%)

Neuromuscular and skeletal: Arthritis (5%), myalgia (4%)

Otic: Otitis (4%)

<1%: Allergic reactions, anaphylaxis, angioedema, pruritus, rash, urticaria

Overdosage/Toxicology Single doses of 800 mg and multiple doses of up to 400 mg 3 times daily for 15 days have been studied in normal weight and obese patients without significant adverse findings; in case of significant overdose, it is recommended that the patient be observed for 24 hours

Drug Interactions

Fat-soluble vitamins: Absorption of vitamins A,D,E, and K may be decreased by orlistat (also see note on warfarin)

Nifedipine: Serum levels may be slightly reduced during coadministration of orlistat; monitor

(Continued)

Orlistat *(Continued)*

Warfarin: Vitamin K absorption may be decreased when taken with orlistat; because of a potential alteration in vitamin K absorption, patients stabilized on warfarin must be closely monitored; dosage adjustment may be required

Usual Dosage Oral: Adults: 120 mg 3 times/day with each main meal containing fat (during or up to 1 hour after the meal); omit dose if meal is occasionally missed or contains no fat

Monitoring Parameters Changes in coagulation parameters

Patient Information Patient should be on a nutritionally balanced, reduced-calorie diet that contains approximately 30% of calories from fat; daily intake of fat, carbohydrate, and protein should be distributed over the three main meals

Dosage Forms Capsule: 120 mg

Oxazepam *(oks A ze pam)*

Related Information

Anxiolytic/Hypnotic Use in Long-Term Care Facilities *on page 562*
Benzodiazepines Comparison Chart *on page 566*
Federal OBRA Regulations Recommended Maximum Doses *on page 583*
Patient Information - Anxiolytics & Sedative Hypnotics (Benzodiazepines) *on page 483*

U.S. Brand Names Serax®

Canadian Brand Names Apo®-Oxazepam; Novo-Oxazepam®; Oxpam®; PMS-Oxazepam; Zapex®

Pharmacologic Category Benzodiazepine

Generic Available Yes

Use Treatment of anxiety; management of alcohol withdrawal

Unlabeled/Investigational Use Anticonvulsant in management of simple partial seizures; hypnotic

Restrictions C-IV

Pregnancy Risk Factor D

Contraindications Hypersensitivity to oxazepam or any component of the formulation (cross-sensitivity with other benzodiazepines may exist); narrow-angle glaucoma (not in product labeling, however, benzodiazepines are contraindicated); not indicated for use in the treatment of psychosis; pregnancy

Warnings/Precautions May cause hypotension (rare) - use with caution in patients with cardiovascular or cerebrovascular disease, or in patients who would not tolerate transient decreases in blood pressure. Serax® 15 mg tablet contains tartrazine; use is not recommended in pediatric patients <6 years of age; dose has not been established between 6-12 years of age.

Use with caution in elderly or debilitated patients, patients with hepatic disease (including alcoholics), or renal impairment. Use with caution in patients with respiratory disease or impaired gag reflex. Avoid use in patients with sleep apnea.

Causes CNS depression (dose-related) resulting in sedation, dizziness, confusion, or ataxia which may impair physical and mental capabilities. Patients must be cautioned about performing tasks which require mental alertness (ie, operating machinery or driving). Use with caution in patients receiving other CNS depressants or psychoactive agents. Effects with other sedative drugs or ethanol may be potentiated. Benzodiazepines have been associated with falls and traumatic injury and should be used with extreme caution in patients who are at risk of these events (especially the elderly).

Use caution in patients with depression, particularly if suicidal risk may be present. Use with caution in patients with a history of drug dependence. Benzodiazepines have been associated with dependence and acute withdrawal symptoms on discontinuation or reduction in dose. Acute withdrawal, including seizures, may be precipitated after administration of flumazenil to patients receiving long-term benzodiazepine therapy.

Benzodiazepines have been associated with anterograde amnesia. Paradoxical reactions, including hyperactive or aggressive behavior have been reported with benzodiazepines, particularly in adolescent/pediatric or psychiatric patients. Does not have analgesic, antidepressant, or antipsychotic properties.

Adverse Reactions Frequency not defined.

Cardiovascular: Syncope (rare), edema

Central nervous system: Drowsiness, ataxia, dizziness, vertigo, memory impairment, headache, paradoxical reactions (excitement, stimulation of effect), lethargy, amnesia, euphoria

Dermatologic: Rash

Endocrine & metabolic: Decreased libido, menstrual irregularities

Genitourinary: Incontinence

Hematologic: Leukopenia, blood dyscrasias

Hepatic: Jaundice

Neuromuscular & skeletal: Dysarthria, tremor, reflex slowing

Ocular: Blurred vision, diplopia

Miscellaneous: Drug dependence

Overdosage/Toxicology

Signs and symptoms: Somnolence, confusion, coma, hypoactive reflexes, dyspnea, hypotension, slurred speech, impaired coordination

Treatment: Treatment for benzodiazepine overdose is supportive. Rarely is mechanical ventilation required. Flumazenil has been shown to selectively block the binding of benzodiazepines to CNS receptors, resulting in a reversal of benzodiazepine-induced CNS depression but not the respiratory depression due to toxicity.

Drug Interactions

Alcohol and other CNS depressants may increase the CNS effects of oxazepam

Levodopa: Therapeutic effects may be diminished in some patients following the addition of a benzodiazepine; limited/inconsistent data

Theophylline and other CNS stimulants may antagonize the sedative effects of oxazepam

Zidovudine: Increased incidence of headache with concurrent use.

Ethanol/Nutrition/Herb Interactions

Ethanol: Avoid ethanol (may increase CNS depression).

Herb/Nutraceutical: Avoid valerian, St John's wort, kava kava, gotu kola (may increase CNS depression).

Mechanism of Action Binds to stereospecific benzodiazepine receptors on the postsynaptic GABA neuron at several sites within the central nervous system, including the limbic system, reticular formation. Enhancement of the inhibitory effect of GABA on neuronal excitability results by increased neuronal membrane permeability to chloride ions. This shift in chloride ions results in hyperpolarization (a less excitable state) and stabilization.

Pharmacodynamics/Kinetics

Absorption: Oral: Almost completely

Protein binding: 86% to 99%

Metabolism: In the liver to inactive compounds (primarily as glucuronides)

Half-life: 2.8-5.7 hours

Time to peak serum concentration: Within 2-4 hours

Elimination: Excretion of unchanged drug (50%) and metabolites; excreted without need for liver metabolism

Usual Dosage Oral:

Children: Anxiety: 1 mg/kg/day has been administered

Adults:

Anxiety: 10-30 mg 3-4 times/day

Alcohol withdrawal: 15-30 mg 3-4 times/day

Hypnotic: 15-30 mg

Hemodialysis: Not dialyzable (0% to 5%)

Administration Give orally in divided doses

Monitoring Parameters Respiratory and cardiovascular status

(Continued)

Oxazepam *(Continued)*

Reference Range Therapeutic: 0.2-1.4 µg/mL (SI: 0.7-4.9 µmol/L)

Patient Information Avoid alcohol and other CNS depressants; avoid activities needing good psychomotor coordination until CNS effects are known; drug may cause physical or psychological dependence; avoid abrupt discontinuation after prolonged use

Nursing Implications Provide safety measures (ie, side rails, night light, and call button); remove smoking materials from area; supervise ambulation

Additional Information Not intended for management of anxieties and minor distresses associated with everyday life. Treatment longer than 4 months should be re-evaluated to determine the patient's need for the drug. Abrupt discontinuation after sustained use (generally >10 days) may cause withdrawal symptoms.

Dosage Forms
Capsule: 10 mg, 15 mg, 30 mg
Tablet: 15 mg

Oxcarbazepine *(ox car BAZ e peen)*

U.S. Brand Names Trileptal®

Synonyms GP 47680

Pharmacologic Category Anticonvulsant, Miscellaneous

Generic Available No

Use Monotherapy or adjunctive therapy in the treatment of partial seizures in adults with epilepsy; adjunctive therapy in the treatment of partial seizures in children (4-16 years of age) with epilepsy

Unlabeled/Investigational Use Antimanic

Pregnancy Risk Factor C

Pregnancy/Breast-Feeding Implications Although many epidemiological studies of congenital anomalies in infants born to women treated with various anticonvulsants during pregnancy have been reported, none of these investigations includes enough women treated with oxcarbazepine to assess possible teratogenic effects of this drug. Given that teratogenic effects have been observed in animal studies, and that oxcarbazepine is structurally related to carbamazepine (teratogenic in humans), use during pregnancy only if the benefit to the mother outweighs the potential risk to the fetus. Nonhormonal forms of contraception should be used during therapy.

Contraindications Hypersensitivity to oxcarbazepine or any component of the formulation

Warnings/Precautions Clinically significant hyponatremia (sodium <125 mmol/L) can develop during oxcarbazepine use. As with all antiepileptic drugs, oxcarbazepine should be withdrawn gradually to minimize the potential of increased seizure frequency. Use of oxcarbazepine has been associated with CNS related adverse events, most significant of these were cognitive symptoms including psychomotor slowing, difficulty with concentration, and speech or language problems, somnolence or fatigue, and coordination abnormalities, including ataxia and gait disturbances. Use caution in patients with previous hypersensitivity to carbamazepine (cross-sensitivity occurs in 25% to 30%). May reduce the efficacy of oral contraceptives (nonhormonal contraceptive measures are recommended).

Adverse Reactions As reported in adults with doses of up to 2400 mg/day (includes patients on monotherapy, adjunctive therapy, and those not previously on AEDs); incidence in children was similar.

>10%:
  Central nervous system: Dizziness (22% to 49%), somnolence (20% to 36%), headache (13% to 32%, placebo 23%), ataxia (5% to 31%), fatigue (12% to 15%), vertigo (6% to 15%)
  Gastrointestinal: Vomiting (7% to 36%), nausea (15% to 29%), abdominal pain (10% to 13%)
  Neuromuscular & skeletal: Abnormal gait (5% to 17%), tremor (3% to 16%)

Ocular: Diplopia (14% to 40%), nystagmus (7% to 26%), abnormal vision (4% to 14%)

1% to 10%:

Cardiovascular: Hypotension (1% to 2%), leg edema (1% to 2%, placebo 1%)

Central nervous system: Nervousness (2% to 5%, placebo 1% to 2%), amnesia (4%), abnormal thinking (2% to 4%), insomnia (2% to 4%), speech disorder (1% to 3%), EEG abnormalities (2%), abnormal feelings (1% to 2%), agitation (1% to 2%, placebo 1%), confusion (1% to 2%, placebo 1%)

Dermatologic: Rash (4%), acne (1% to 2%)

Endocrine & metabolic: Hyponatremia (1% to 3%, placebo 1%)

Gastrointestinal: Diarrhea (5% to 7%), dyspepsia (5% to 6%), constipation (2% to 6%, placebo 0% to 4%), gastritis (1% to 2%, placebo 1%), weight gain (1% to 2%, placebo 1%)

Neuromuscular & skeletal: Weakness (3% to 6%, placebo 5%), back pain (4%), falling down (4%), abnormal coordination (1% to 4%, placebo 1% to 2%), dysmetria (1% to 3%), sprains/strains (2%), muscle weakness (1% to 2%)

Ocular: Abnormal accommodation (2%)

Respiratory: Upper respiratory tract infection (7%), rhinitis (2% to 5%, placebo 4%), chest infection (4%), epistaxis (4%), sinusitis (4%)

Postmarketing and/or case reports: Aggressive reaction, alopecia, amnesia, angioedema, anguish, anxiety, apathy, aphasia, appetite increased, asthma, arthralgia, aura, biliary pain, blood in stool, bradycardia, bruising, cardiac failure, cataract, cerebral hemorrhage, chest pain, cholelithiasis, colitis, conjunctival hemorrhage, consciousness decreased, contact dermatitis, convulsions aggravated, delirium, delusion, dry mouth, duodenal ulcer, dysphagia, dysphonia, dyspnea, dystonia, dysuria, eczema, emotional lability, enteritis, eructation, erythema multiforme, erythematosus rash, esophagitis, eosinophilia, euphoria, eye edema, extrapyramidal disorder, facial rash, feeling drunk, fever, flatulence, flushing, folliculitis, gastric ulcer, genital pruritus, GGT increased, gingival bleeding, gum hyperplasia, heat rash, hematuria, hemianopia, hemiplegia, hematemesis, hemorrhoids, hiccups, hot flushes, hyperglycemia, hyperkinesia, hyper-reflexia, hypersensitivity reaction, hypertonia, hypertension, hypocalcemia, hypochondrium pain, hypoesthesia, hypoglycemia, hypokalemia, hypokinesia, hyporeflexia, hypotonia, hysteria, intermenstrual bleeding, laryngismus, leukopenia, leukorrhea, libido decreased/increased, liver enzymes elevated, lymphadenopathy, maculopapular rash, malaise, manic reaction, migraine, menorrhagia, micturition frequency, muscle contractions (involuntary), mydriasis, neuralgia, oculogyric crisis, otitis externa, palpitation, panic disorder, paralysis, paroniria, personality disorder, photophobia, photosensitivity reaction, pleurisy, postural hypotension, priapism, psoriasis, purpura, psychosis, ptosis, rectal hemorrhage, renal calculus, renal pain, retching, rigors, scotoma, sialoadenitis, serum transaminase increased, Stevens-Johnson syndrome, stupor, syncope, systemic lupus erythematosus, tachycardia, taste perversion, tetany, thrombocytopenia, tinnitus, toxic epidermal necrolysis, ulcerative stomatitis, urinary tract pain, vitiligo, weight loss, xerophthalmia

Overdosage/Toxicology Symptoms may include CNS depression (somnolence, ataxia). Treatment is symptomatic and supportive.

Drug Interactions CYP2C19 enzyme inhibitor; CYP3A4/5 enzyme inducer

Carbamazepine: Oxcarbazepine serum concentrations may be reduced by a mean 40%

Felodipine: Metabolism is increased due to enzyme induction; similar effects may be anticipated with other dihydropyridine calcium channel blockers

Oral contraceptives: Metabolism may be increased due to enzyme induction; use alternative contraceptive measures; oxcarbazepine with oral contraceptives has been shown to decrease plasma concentrations of the two hormonal components, ethinyl estradiol (48% and 52%) and levonorgestrel (32% and 52%).

Phenobarbital: Phenobarbital levels are increased (average of 14%); oxcarbazepine levels decreases (average of 25%)

(Continued)

Oxcarbazepine *(Continued)*

Phenytoin: Phenytoin levels may be increased (high dosages) by an average of 40%; oxcarbazepine levels may be decreased (by an average of 30%) during concurrent therapy; monitor phenytoin levels

Valproic acid decreases oxcarbazepine levels by an average of 18%

Verapamil's metabolism may be increased due to enzyme induction; verapamil may reduce blood levels of oxcarbazepine's active metabolite (MHD)

Note: No evidence of an interaction was noted with erythromycin, cimetidine, dextropropoxyphene, or warfarin

Ethanol/Nutrition/Herb Interactions

Ethanol: Avoid ethanol (may increase CNS depression).

Herb/Nutraceutical: St John's wort may decrease oxcarbazepine levels. Avoid evening primrose (seizure threshold decreased). Avoid valerian, St John's wort, kava kava, gotu kola

Stability Store tablets and suspension at 25°C (77°F). Use suspension within 7 weeks of first opening container.

Mechanism of Action Pharmacological activity results from both oxcarbazepine and its monohydroxy metabolite (MHD). Precise mechanism of anticonvulsant effect has not been defined. Oxcarbazepine and MHD block voltage sensitive sodium channels, stabilizing hyperexcited neuronal membranes, inhibiting repetitive firing, and decreasing the propagation of synaptic impulses. These actions are believed to prevent the spread of seizures. Oxcarbazepine and MHD also increase potassium conductance and modulate the activity of high-voltage activated calcium channels.

Pharmacodynamics/Kinetics

Absorption: Completely absorbed and extensively metabolized to its pharmacologically active 10-monohydroxy metabolite (MHD)

Distribution: MHD: V_d: 49 L

Protein binding: 40% of MHD is bound to serum proteins

Metabolism: Hepatic, further by conjugation with glucuronic acid.

Half-life: 2 hours (parent), 9 hours (MHD)

Time to peak serum concentration: 4.5 hours (3-13 hours)

Elimination: 95% of the dose appears in the urine, <1% as unchanged oxcarbazepine; fecal (4%)

Dialyzable: Half-life of MHD is prolonged to 19 hours when 300 mg of oxcarbazepine is administered to renally-impaired patients (Cl_{cr} <30 mL/min)

Usual Dosage Oral:

Children:

Adjunctive therapy: 8-10 mg/kg/day, not to exceed 600 mg/day, given in 2 divided daily doses. Maintenance dose should be achieved over 2 weeks, and is dependent upon patient weight, according to the following:

20-29 kg: 900 mg/day in 2 divided doses

29.1-39 kg: 1200 mg/day in 2 divided doses

>39 kg: 1800 mg/day in 2 divided doses

Adults:

Adjunctive therapy: Initial: 300 mg twice daily; dose may be increased by as much as 600 mg/day at weekly intervals; recommended daily dose: 1200 mg/day in 2 divided doses. Although daily doses >1200 mg/day demonstrated greater efficacy, most patients were unable to tolerate 2400 mg/day (due to CNS effects).

Conversion to monotherapy: Oxcarbazepine 600 mg/day in twice daily divided doses while simultaneously initiating the reduction of the dose of the concomitant antiepileptic drug. The concomitant dosage should be withdrawn over 3-6 weeks, while the maximum dose of oxcarbazepine should be reached in about 2-4 weeks. Recommended daily dose: 2400 mg/day.

Initiation of monotherapy: Oxcarbazepine should be initiated at a dose of 600 mg/day in twice daily divided doses; doses may be titrated upward by 300 mg/day every third day to a final dose of 1200 mg/day given in 2 daily divided doses

Dosing adjustment in renal impairment: Therapy should be initiated at one-half the usual starting dose (300 mg/day) and increased slowly to achieve the desired clinical response

Dietary Considerations May be taken with or without food.

Administration Suspension: Prior to using for the first time, firmly insert the plastic adapter provided with the bottle. Cover adapter with child-resistant cap when not in use. Shake bottle for at least 10 seconds, remove child-resistant cap and insert the oral dosing syringe provided to withdraw appropriate dose. Dose may be taken directly from oral syringe or may be mixed in a small glass of water immediately prior to swallowing. Rinse syringe with warm water after use and allow to dry thoroughly. Discard any unused portion after 7 weeks of first opening bottle.

Monitoring Parameters Serum sodium

Test Interactions Thyroid function tests may depress serum T_4 without affecting T_3 levels or TSH.

Patient Information Hormonal contraceptives may be less effective when used with oxcarbazepine; caution should be exercised if alcohol is taken with oxcarbazepine, due to the possible additive sedative effects and that it may cause dizziness and somnolence; therefore, early in therapy are advised not to drive or operate machinery

Nursing Implications Inform those patients who have exhibited hypersensitivity reactions to carbamazepine that there is the possibility of cross-sensitivity reactions with oxcarbazepine. Inform patients of childbearing age that hormonal contraceptives may be less effective when used with oxcarbazepine. Caution should be exercised if alcohol is taken with oxcarbazepine, due to the possible additive sedative effects. Advise patients that oxcarbazepine may cause dizziness and somnolence and that early in therapy they are advised not to drive or operate machinery.

Dosage Forms
Suspension, oral: 300 mg/5 mL (250 mL)
Tablet: 150 mg, 300 mg, 600 mg

♦ **Oxilapine Succinate** *see* Loxapine *on page 213*
♦ **Oxpam®** **(Can)** *see* Oxazepam *on page 276*
♦ **Palmetto Scrub** *see* Saw Palmetto *on page 367*
♦ **Pamelor®** *see* Nortriptyline *on page 267*
♦ **Paracetaldehyde** *see* Paraldehyde *on page 281*
♦ **Paraguay Tea** *see* Maté *on page 219*
♦ **Paral®** *see* Paraldehyde *on page 281*

Paraldehyde (par AL de hyde)
Related Information
Anxiolytic/Hypnotic Use in Long-Term Care Facilities *on page 562*
U.S. Brand Names Paral®
Synonyms Paracetaldehyde
Pharmacologic Category Anticonvulsant
Generic Available Yes
Use Treatment of seizures associated with status epilepticus, tetanus, eclampsia, and convulsant drug toxicity
Unlabeled/Investigational Use Delirium tremors, sedative/hypnotic
Restrictions C-IV
Pregnancy Risk Factor C
Contraindications Hypersensitivity to paraldehyde or any component of the formulation; severe hepatic insufficiency; respiratory disease; GI inflammation or ulceration; concurrent disulfiram
Warnings/Precautions Use with caution in patients with asthma or other bronchopulmonary disease; do not abruptly discontinue in patients receiving chronic therapy
Adverse Reactions Frequency not defined.
(Continued)

Paraldehyde *(Continued)*

Cardiovascular: Cardiovascular collapse

Central nervous system: Drowsiness, clumsiness, dizziness, "hangover effect"

Dermatologic: Skin rash

Endocrine & metabolic: Metabolic acidosis

Gastrointestinal: Strong, unpleasant breath odor; nausea, vomiting, stomach pain, irritation of mucous membrane

Hepatic: Hepatitis

Local: Thrombophlebitis

Respiratory: Coughing, respiratory depression, pulmonary edema

Miscellaneous: Psychological and physical dependence with prolonged use

Overdosage/Toxicology

Signs and symptoms: Hypotension, respiratory depression, metabolic acidosis, pulmonary edema, pulmonary hemorrhage, hemorrhagic gastritis, renal failure; death has occurred with as little as 12-25 mL

Treatment: Metabolic acidosis should be treated with sodium bicarbonate; hemodialysis may be required to treat acidosis and to support renal function

Drug Interactions

CNS depressants: Sedative effects and/or respiratory depression may be additive with CNS depressants; includes ethanol, barbiturates, narcotic analgesics, and other sedative agents; monitor for increased effect

Disulfiram: Concurrent use of paraldehyde and disulfiram produces a "disulfiram reaction," this combination is contraindicated

Ethanol/Nutrition/Herb Interactions Ethanol: Avoid ethanol (may increase CNS depression).

Stability Decomposes with exposure to air and light to acetaldehyde which then oxidizes to acetic acid. Store in tightly closed containers. Protect from light. Discard unused contents of any container which has been opened for >24 hours.

Mechanism of Action Unknown mechanism of action; causes depression of CNS, including the ascending reticular activating system to provide sedation/hypnosis and anticonvulsant activity. Hypnotic activity is rapid, with sleep induction in 10-15 minutes. It has no analgesic properties and may reduce excitement or delirium in the presence of pain.

Pharmacodynamics/Kinetics

Onset of hypnosis:

Oral: Within 10-15 minutes

I.M.: Within 2-3 minutes

Duration: 6-8 hours

Distribution: Crosses the placenta

Metabolism: ~70% to 80% of a dose metabolized in the liver

Half-life: Adults: 3.5-10 hours

Elimination: Up to 30% excreted as unchanged drug in expired air via the lungs; trace amounts excreted in urine unchanged

Usual Dosage Oral, rectal:

Note: Oral: Dilute in milk or iced fruit juice to mask taste and odor

Note: Rectal: Mix paraldehyde 2:1 with oil (cottonseed or olive)

Children:

Sedative: 0.15 mL/kg

Hypnotic: 0.3 mL/kg

Seizure: 0.3 mL/kg every 2-4 hours per rectum; maximum dose: 5 mL

Adults:

Sedative: 5-10 mL

Hypnotic dose: 10-30 mL

Dosing adjustment in hepatic impairment: Dosage may need to be reduced

Patient Information Do not attempt tasks requiring psychomotor coordination until the CNS effects by the drug are known; do not drink alcohol; may cause physical and psychological dependence; do not use if solution has a brownish color

Nursing Implications Discard unused contents of any container which has been opened for more than 24 hours; do **not** use discolored solution or solutions with

strong smell of acetic acid (vinegar); do **not** use any plastic equipment for administration, use glass syringes and rubber tubing; outdated preparations can be toxic
Oral: Dilute oral formulation in milk or iced fruit juice
Rectal: Mix paraldehyde 2:1 with oil (cottonseed or olive)
Dosage Forms Liquid, oral or rectal: 1 g/mL (30 mL)

♦ **Parlodel**® see Bromocriptine on page 49
♦ **Parnate**® see Tranylcypromine on page 405

Paroxetine (pa ROKS e teen)
Related Information
Antidepressant Agents Comparison Chart on page 553
Discontinuation of Psychotropic Drugs - Withdrawal Symptoms and Recommendations on page 582
Patient Information - Antidepressants (SSRIs) on page 452
Pharmacokinetics of Selective Serotonin-Reuptake Inhibitors (SSRIs) on page 590
U.S. Brand Names Paxil™; Paxil® CR™
Canadian Brand Names Paxil
Pharmacologic Category Antidepressant, Selective Serotonin Reuptake Inhibitor
Generic Available No
Use Treatment of depression in adults; treatment of panic disorder with or without agoraphobia; obsessive-compulsive disorder (OCD) in adults; social anxiety disorder (social phobia); generalized anxiety disorder (GAD)
Unlabeled/Investigational Use May be useful in eating disorders, impulse control disorders, self-injurious behavior, post-traumatic stress disorder; premenstrual disorders, vasomotor symptoms of menopause; treatment of depression and obsessive-compulsive disorder (OCD) in children
Pregnancy Risk Factor C
Pregnancy/Breast-Feeding Implications Enters breast milk; use caution in breast-feeding
Contraindications Hypersensitivity to paroxetine or any component of the formulation; use of MAO inhibitors or within 14 days; concurrent use with thioridazine or mesoridazine
Warnings/Precautions Potential for severe reaction when used with MAO inhibitors - serotonin syndrome (hyperthermia, muscular rigidity, mental status changes/agitation, autonomic instability) may occur. May precipitate a shift to mania or hypomania in patients with bipolar disease. Has a low potential to impair cognitive or motor performance - caution operating hazardous machinery or driving. Low potential for sedation or anticholinergic effects relative to cyclic antidepressants. Use caution in patients with depression, particularly if suicidal risk may be present. Use caution in patients with a previous seizure disorder or condition predisposing to seizures such as brain damage, alcoholism, or concurrent therapy with other drugs which lower the seizure threshold. Use with caution in patients with hepatic or dysfunction and in elderly patients. May cause hyponatremia/SIADH. Use with caution in patients at risk of bleeding or receiving anticoagulant therapy - may cause impairment in platelet aggregation. Use with caution in patients with renal insufficiency or other concurrent illness (due to limited experience). May cause or exacerbate sexual dysfunction.
Adverse Reactions
>10%:
Central nervous system: Headache, somnolence, dizziness, insomnia
Gastrointestinal: Nausea, xerostomia, constipation, diarrhea
Genitourinary: Ejaculatory disturbances
Neuromuscular & skeletal: Weakness
Miscellaneous: Diaphoresis
1% to 10%:
Cardiovascular: Palpitations, vasodilation, postural hypotension
Central nervous system: Nervousness, anxiety, yawning, abnormal dreams
Dermatologic: Rash
(Continued)

Paroxetine *(Continued)*

Endocrine & metabolic: Decreased libido, delayed ejaculation

Gastrointestinal: Anorexia, flatulence, vomiting, dyspepsia, taste perversion

Genitourinary: Urinary frequency, impotence

Neuromuscular & skeletal: Tremor, paresthesia, myopathy, myalgia

<1%: Acne, akinesia, alopecia, amenorrhea, anemia, arthritis, asthma, brady-cardia, bruxism, colitis, ear pain, eye pain, EPS, hypotension, leukopenia, mania, migraine, thirst

Postmarketing and/or case reports: Acute renal failure, allergic alveolitis, anaphyl-axis, aplastic anemia, agranulocytosis, bone marrow aplasia, eclampsia, Guillain-Barré syndrome, hemolytic anemia, hepatic necrosis, laryngismus, neuroleptic malignant syndrome, optic neuritis, pancreatitis, pancytopenia, porphyria, priapism, pulmonary hypertension, seizures (including status epilep-ticus), serotonin syndrome, SIADH, thrombocytopenia, torsade de pointes, toxic epidermal necrolysis, ventricular fibrillation, ventricular tachycardia, withdrawal reactions (dizziness, agitation, anxiety, nausea, diaphoresis - particularly following abrupt withdrawal)

Overdosage/Toxicology

Signs and symptoms: Nausea, vomiting, drowsiness, sinus tachycardia, and dilated pupils

Treatment: There are no specific antidotes, following attempts at decontamination, treatment is supportive and symptomatic; forced diuresis, dialysis, and hemoper-fusion are unlikely to be beneficial

Drug Interactions CYP2D6 enzyme substrate (minor); CYP2D6 and 1A2 enzyme inhibitor (weak), and CYP3A3/4 enzyme inhibitor (weak)

Amphetamines: SSRIs may increase the sensitivity to amphetamines, and amphetamines may increase the risk of serotonin syndrome

Buspirone: Combined use with SSRIs may cause serotonin syndrome

Carvedilol: Serum concentrations may be increased; monitor carefully for increased carvedilol effect (hypotension and bradycardia)

Cimetidine: Cimetidine may reduce the first-pass metabolism of paroxetine resulting in elevated paroxetine serum concentrations; consider an alternative H_2 antagonist

Clozapine: May increase serum levels of clozapine; monitor for increased effect/toxicity

Cyproheptadine: May inhibit the effects of serotonin reuptake inhibitors; monitor for altered antidepressant response; cyproheptadine acts as a serotonin agonist

Dextromethorphan: Metabolism of dextromethorphan may be inhibited; visual hallucinations occurred; monitor

Haloperidol: Metabolism may be inhibited and cause extrapyramidal symptoms (EPS); monitor patients for EPS if combination is utilized

HMG-CoA reductase inhibitors: Metabolism may be inhibited by SSRIs; particularly lovastatin and simvastatin resulting in myositis and rhabdomyolysis; paroxetine appears to have weak interaction with CYP3A3/4, and therefore, appears to have a low risk of this interaction

Lithium: Patients receiving SSRIs and lithium have developed neurotoxicity; if combination is used; monitor for neurotoxicity

Loop diuretics: SSRIs may cause hyponatremia; additive hyponatremic effects may be seen with combined use of a loop diuretic (bumetanide, furosemide, torsemide); monitor for hyponatremia

MAO inhibitors: SSRIs should not be used with nonselective MAO inhibitors (isocarboxazid, phenelzine); fatal reactions have been reported; this combination should be avoided

Meperidine: Combined use may cause serotonin syndrome; monitor

Mesoridazine: Paroxetine may inhibit the metabolism of mesoridazine, resulting in increased plasma levels and increasing the risk of QT_c interval prolongation. Concurrent use is contraindicated.

Nefazodone and trazodone: May increase the risk of serotonin syndrome with SSRIs; monitor

Phenytoin: Metabolism of phenytoin may be inhibited, resulting in phenytoin toxicity; monitor for toxicity (ataxia, confusion, dizziness, nystagmus, involuntary muscle movement)

Selegiline: SSRIs have been reported to cause mania or hypertension when combined with selegiline; this combination is best avoided; concurrent use with SSRIs has also been reported to cause serotonin syndrome; as an MAO type-B inhibitor, the risk of serotonin syndrome may be less than with nonselective MAO inhibitors

Serotonergic uptake inhibitors: Combined use with other drugs which inhibit the reuptake may cause serotonin syndrome

Sibutramine: May increase the risk of serotonin syndrome with SSRIs; avoid coadministration

Sumatriptan (and other serotonin agonists): Concurrent use may result in toxicity; weakness, hyper-reflexia, and incoordination have been observed with suma-triptan and SSRIs. In addition, concurrent use may theoretically increase the risk of serotonin syndrome; includes sumatriptan, naratriptan, rizatriptan, and zolmi-triptan.

Sympathomimetics: May increase the risk of serotonin syndrome with SSRIs

Thioridazine: Paroxetine may inhibit the metabolism of thioridazine, resulting in increased plasma levels and increasing the risk of QT_c interval prolongation. Concurrent use is contraindicated.

Tramadol: Combined use may cause serotonin syndrome; monitor

Tricyclic antidepressants: The metabolism of tricyclic antidepressants (amitripty-line, desipramine, imipramine, nortriptyline) may be inhibited by SSRIs resulting is elevated serum levels; if combination is warranted, a low dose of TCA (10-25 mg/day) should be utilized

Tryptophan: Combination with tryptophan, a serotonin precursor, may cause agita-tion and restlessness; this combination is best avoided

Venlafaxine: Combined use with paroxetine may increase the risk of serotonin syndrome

Warfarin: May alter the hypoprothrombinemic response to warfarin; monitor INR

Zolpidem: At least one case of acute delirium in association with combined therapy has been reported

Ethanol/Nutrition/Herb Interactions

Ethanol: Avoid ethanol.

Food: Peak concentration is increased, but bioavailability is not significantly altered by food.

Herb/Nutraceutical: Avoid valerian, St John's wort, SAMe, kava kava.

Stability

Suspension: Store at ≤25°C (≤77°F)

Tablet: Store at 15°C to 30°C (59°F to 86°F)

Mechanism of Action Paroxetine is a selective serotonin reuptake inhibitor, chemically unrelated to tricyclic, tetracyclic, or other antidepressants; presumably, the inhibition of serotonin reuptake from brain synapse stimulated serotonin activity in the brain

Pharmacodynamics/Kinetics

Protein binding: 93% to 95%

Metabolism: Extensive following absorption by cytochrome P450 enzymes (CYP2D6)

Half-life: 21 hours

Time to peak serum concentration: 5.2 hours

Elimination: Metabolites are excreted in bile and urine

Usual Dosage Oral:

Children:

Depression (unlabeled use): Initial: 10 mg/day and adjusted upward on an indi-vidual basis to 20 mg/day

OCD (unlabeled use): Initial: 10 mg/day and titrate up as necessary to 60 mg/day

Self-Injurious behavior (unlabeled use): 20 mg/day

(Continued)

Paroxetine (Continued)

Adults:
  Depression: Initial: 20 mg/day given once daily preferably in the morning; increase if needed by 10 mg/day increments at intervals of at least 1 week; maximum dose: 50 mg/day

  Paxil® CR™: Initial: 25 mg once daily; may be increased in 12.5 mg increments at intervals of at least 1 week (range: 25-62.5 mg)

  OCD: Initial: 20 mg/day given once daily preferably in the morning; increase by 10 mg/day increments at intervals of at least 1 week; recommended dose: 40 mg/day; range: 20-60 mg/day; maximum dose: 60 mg/day

  Panic disorder: Initial: 10 mg/day given once daily preferably in the morning; increase by 10 mg/day increments at intervals of at least 1 week; recommended dose: 40 mg/day; range: 10-60 mg/day; maximum dose: 60 mg/day

  Social anxiety disorder: Initial: 20 mg/day given once daily preferably in the morning; recommended dose: 20 mg/day; range: 20-60 mg/day; doses >20 mg may not have additional benefit

  GAD: Initial: 20 mg once daily preferably administered in the morning; doses of 20-50 mg/day were used in clinical trials, however, no greater benefit was seen with doses >20 mg. If dose is increased, adjust in increments of 10 mg/day at 1-week intervals.

  Elderly: Initial: 10 mg/day; increase (if needed) in increments of 10 mg/day at intervals of at least 1 week; maximum dose: 40 mg/day

Dosage adjustment in severe renal/hepatic impairment: Adults: Initial: 10 mg/day; increase (if needed) in increments of 10 mg/day at intervals of at least 1 week; maximum dose: 40 mg/day

Child/Adolescent Considerations

  Depression: Paroxetine was shown to be effective and well tolerated in an open label clinical trial in 45 children <14 years of age (mean: 10.7 ± 2 years) with major depression (Rey-Sanchoz, 1997). Doses were initiated at 10 mg/day and adjusted upward on an individual basis with a mean dose of 16.2 mg/day used for an average of 8.4 months. Further studies are needed.

  Obsessive-compulsive disorder (OCD): Twenty OCD outpatients 8-17 years of age were treated with daily doses ranging from 10-60 mg/day for 12 weeks (Rosenberg, 1999).

  Self-injurious behavior: A 15-year old autistic male with self-injurious behavior was successfully treated with 20 mg/day (Snead, 1994). Further studies are needed.

Dietary Considerations May be administered with or without food.

Monitoring Parameters Hepatic and renal function tests, blood pressure, heart rate

Test Interactions Increased LFTs

Patient Information Caution should be used in activities that require alertness like driving or operating machinery; avoid alcoholic beverage intake; notify physician if pregnant or breast feeding

Nursing Implications Monitor hepatic and renal function tests, blood pressure, heart rate

Additional Information Has properties similar to fluvoxamine maleate; buspirone (15-60 mg/day) may be useful in treatment of sexual dysfunction during treatment with a selective serotonin reuptake inhibitor.

Dosage Forms

  Suspension, oral: 10 mg/5 mL (250 mL) [orange flavor]
  Tablet: 10 mg, 20 mg, 30 mg, 40 mg
  Tablet, controlled release (Paxil® CR™): 12.5 mg, 25 mg

♦ **Patient Information - Agents for the Treatment of Alzheimer's Disease** see page 491
♦ **Patient Information - Agents for Treatment of Extrapyramidal Symptoms** see page 493
♦ **Patient Information - Antidepressants (Bupropion)** see page 456
♦ **Patient Information - Antidepressants (MAOIs)** see page 462

Pemoline (PEM oh leen)

Related Information

Patient Information - Stimulants *on page 481*
Stimulant Agents Used for ADHD *on page 593*

U.S. Brand Names Cylert®; PemADD®; PemADD® CT

Canadian Brand Names Cylert

Synonyms Phenylisohydantoin; PIO

Pharmacologic Category Stimulant

Generic Available Yes

Use Treatment of attention-deficit/hyperactivity disorder (ADHD) (not first-line)

Unlabeled/Investigational Use Narcolepsy

Restrictions C-IV

Pregnancy Risk Factor B

Contraindications Hypersensitivity to pemoline or any component of the formulation; hepatic impairment (including abnormalities on baseline liver function tests); children <6 years of age; Tourette's syndrome; psychosis

Warnings/Precautions Not considered first-line therapy for ADHD due to association with hepatic failure. The manufacturer has recommended that signed informed consent following a discussion of risks and benefits must or should be obtained prior to the initiation of therapy. Therapy should be discontinued if a response is not evident after 3 weeks of therapy. Pemoline should not be started in patients with abnormalities in baseline liver function tests, and should be discontinued if clinically significant liver function test abnormalities are revealed at any time during therapy. Use with caution in patients with renal dysfunction or psychosis. In general, stimulant medications should be used with caution in patients with bipolar disorder, diabetes mellitus, cardiovascular disease, seizure disorders, insomnia, (Continued)

Pemoline (Continued)

porphyria, or hypertension (although pemoline has been demonstrated to have a low potential to elevate blood pressure relative to other stimulants). May exacerbate symptoms of behavior and thought disorder in psychotic patients. Potential for drug dependency exists - avoid abrupt discontinuation in patients who have received for prolonged periods. Stimulant use has been associated with growth suppression, and careful monitoring is recommended. Stimulants may unmask tics in individuals with coexisting Tourette's syndrome.

Adverse Reactions Frequency not defined.

Central nervous system: Insomnia, dizziness, drowsiness, mental depression, increased irritability, seizures, precipitation of Tourette's syndrome, hallucinations, headache, movement disorders

Dermatologic: Rash

Endocrine & metabolic: Suppression of growth in children

Gastrointestinal: Anorexia, weight loss, stomach pain, nausea

Hematologic: Aplastic anemia

Hepatic: Increased liver enzyme (usually reversible upon discontinuation), hepatitis, jaundice, hepatic failure

Overdosage/Toxicology

Signs and symptoms: Tachycardia, hallucinations, agitation

Treatment:

There is no specific antidote for intoxication and the bulk of the treatment is supportive

Hyperactivity and agitation usually respond to reduced sensory input or benzodiazepines, however, with extreme agitation haloperidol (2-5 mg I.M. for adults) may be required

Hyperthermia is best treated with external cooling measures, or when severe or unresponsive, muscle paralysis with pancuronium may be needed

Drug Interactions

Anticonvulsants: Pemoline may decrease seizure threshold; efficacy of anticonvulsants may be decreased

CNS depressants: Effects may be additive; use caution when pemoline is used with other CNS acting medications

Ethanol/Nutrition/Herb Interactions Ethanol: Avoid ethanol (may increase CNS depression).

Mechanism of Action Blocks the reuptake mechanism of dopaminergic neurons, appears to act at the cerebral cortex and subcortical structures; CNS and respiratory stimulant with weak sympathomimetic effects; actions may be mediated via increase in CNS dopamine

Pharmacodynamics/Kinetics

Peak effect: 4 hours

Duration: 8 hours

Protein binding: 50%

Metabolism: Partially by the liver

Half-life:

Children: 7-8.6 hours

Adults: 12 hours

Time to peak serum concentration: Oral: Within 2-4 hours

Elimination: In urine; only negligible amounts can be detected in feces

Usual Dosage Children ≥6 years: Oral: Initial: 37.5 mg given once daily in the morning, increase by 18.75 mg/day at weekly intervals; usual effective dose range: 56.25-75 mg/day; maximum: 112.5 mg/day; dosage range: 0.5-3 mg/kg/24 hours; significant benefit may not be evident until third or fourth week of administration

Dosing adjustment/comments in renal impairment: Cl_{cr} <50 mL/minute: Avoid use

Administration Administer medication in the morning.

Monitoring Parameters Liver enzymes (baseline and every 2 weeks)

Patient Information Avoid caffeine; avoid alcoholic beverages; last daily dose should be given several hours before retiring; do not abruptly discontinue; prolonged use may cause dependence

Nursing Implications Administer medication in the morning

Additional Information Treatment of ADHD should include "Drug Holidays" or periodic discontinuation of stimulant medication in order to assess the patient's requirements and to decrease tolerance and limit suppression of linear growth and weight. The labeling for Cylert® includes recommendations for liver function monitoring and a Patient Information Consent Form.

Dosage Forms
Tablet: 18.75 mg, 37.5 mg, 75 mg
Tablet, chewable: 37.5 mg

Pennyroyal Oil

Synonyms *Mentha pulegium*

Pharmacologic Category Herb

Use Insect repellent; inducing delayed menses; rubefacient; its used primarily by natural health advocates (not FDA approved for stated use); digestive disorders; liver and gallbladder disorders; gout; colds; skin diseases (used externally)

Adverse Reactions
Cardiovascular: Hypotension
Central nervous system: Confusion, delirium, agitation, hallucinations (auditory and visual), seizures (within 3 hours)
Endocrine & metabolic: Abortifacient
Gastrointestinal: Nausea, vomiting, abdominal pain
Genitourinary: Menstrual bleeding
Hematologic: Hemolytic anemia, disseminated intravascular coagulation
Hepatic: Hepatic failure, centrilobular necrosis
Renal: Renal failure, hematuria, acute tubular necrosis
Respiratory: Epistaxis

Overdosage/Toxicology
Decontamination: Due to aspiration risk, do **not** induce emesis; lavage (within 1 hour) is recommended; activated charcoal (with cathartic) may be useful
Treatment: Supportive therapy; N-acetylcysteine (loading dose: 140 mg/kg, then 70 mg/kg every 4 hours) should be administered within the first few hours postingestion for ingestions >10 mL; benzodiazepines can be used for seizures

Usual Dosage
Oil dose used for above purposes: 0.12-0.6 mL
Fatal dose: 15 mL

Additional Information Not reviewed by Commission E; mint-like odor; pulegone may deplete glutathione stores in the liver; a yellow oil; hepatotoxicity has occurred after drinking teas from the herb; should not be taken internally; postmortem pulegone and menthofuran levels in a fatality were 18 ng/mL and 1 ng/mL respectively; a menthofuran level of 40 ng/mL obtained 10 hours postingestion associated with mild toxicity

Pentobarbital (pen toe BAR bi tal)

Related Information
Anxiolytic/Hypnotic Use in Long-Term Care Facilities *on page 562*
Federal OBRA Regulations Recommended Maximum Doses *on page 583*
Patient Information - Anxiolytics & Sedative Hypnotics (Barbiturates) *on page 485*

U.S. Brand Names Nembutal®

Canadian Brand Names Nova Rectal®

Synonyms Pentobarbital Sodium

Pharmacologic Category Anticonvulsant, Barbiturate; Barbiturate

Generic Available Yes

Use Sedative/hypnotic; preanesthetic; high-dose barbiturate coma for treatment of increased intracranial pressure or status epilepticus unresponsive to other therapy
(Continued)

Pentobarbital *(Continued)*

Unlabeled/Investigational Use Tolerance test during withdrawal of sedative hypnotics

Restrictions C-II (capsules, injection); C-III (suppositories)

Pregnancy Risk Factor D

Contraindications Hypersensitivity to barbiturates or any component of the formulation; marked hepatic impairment; dyspnea or airway obstruction; porphyria; pregnancy

Warnings/Precautions Tolerance to hypnotic effect can occur; do not use for >2 weeks to treat insomnia. Potential for drug dependency exists, abrupt cessation may precipitate withdrawal, including status epilepticus in epileptic patients. Do not administer to patients in acute pain. Use caution in elderly, debilitated, renally impaired, hepatic dysfunction, or pediatric patients. May cause paradoxical responses, including agitation and hyperactivity, particularly in acute pain and pediatric patients. Use with caution in patients with depression or suicidal tendencies, or in patients with a history of drug abuse. Tolerance, psychological and physical dependence may occur with prolonged use.

May cause CNS depression, which may impair physical or mental abilities. Patients must be cautioned about performing tasks which require mental alertness (ie, operating machinery or driving). Effects with other sedative drugs or ethanol may be potentiated. Use of this agent as a hypnotic in the elderly is not recommended due to its long half-life and potential for physical and psychological dependence.

May cause respiratory depression or hypotension, particularly when administered intravenously. Use with caution in hemodynamically unstable patients or patients with respiratory disease. High doses (loading doses of 15-35 mg/kg given over 1-2 hours) have been utilized to induce pentobarbital coma, but these higher doses often cause hypotension requiring vasopressor therapy.

Adverse Reactions Frequency not defined.

Cardiovascular: Bradycardia, hypotension, syncope

Central nervous system: Drowsiness, lethargy, CNS excitation or depression, impaired judgment, "hangover" effect, confusion, somnolence, agitation, hyperkinesia, ataxia, nervousness, headache, insomnia, nightmares, hallucinations, anxiety, dizziness

Dermatologic: Rash, exfoliative dermatitis, Stevens-Johnson syndrome

Gastrointestinal: Nausea, vomiting, constipation

Hematologic: Agranulocytosis, thrombocytopenia, megaloblastic anemia

Local: Pain at injection site, thrombophlebitis with I.V. use

Renal: Oliguria

Respiratory: Laryngospasm, respiratory depression, apnea (especially with rapid I.V. use), hypoventilation, apnea

Miscellaneous: Gangrene with inadvertent intra-arterial injection

Overdosage/Toxicology

Signs and symptoms: Unsteady gait, slurred speech, confusion, jaundice, hypothermia, hypotension, respiratory depression, coma

Treatment: If hypotension occurs, administer I.V. fluids and place the patient in the Trendelenburg position. If unresponsive, an I.V. vasopressor (eg, dopamine, epinephrine) may be required. Forced alkaline diuresis is of no value in the treatment of intoxications with short-acting barbiturates. Charcoal hemoperfusion or hemodialysis may be useful in the harder to treat intoxications, especially in the presence of very high serum barbiturate levels when the patient is in a coma, shock, or renal failure.

Drug Interactions Note: Barbiturates are enzyme inducers; patients should be monitored when these drugs are started or stopped for a decreased or increased therapeutic effect respectively

Acetaminophen: Barbiturates may enhance the hepatotoxic potential of acetaminophen overdoses

Antiarrhythmics: Barbiturates may increase the metabolism of antiarrhythmics, decreasing their clinical effect; includes disopyramide, propafenone, and quinidine

Anticonvulsants: Barbiturates may increase the metabolism of anticonvulsants; includes ethosuximide, felbamate (possibly), lamotrigine, phenytoin, tiagabine, topiramate, and zonisamide; does not appear to affect gabapentin or levetiracetam

Antineoplastics: Limited evidence suggests that enzyme-inducing anticonvulsant therapy may reduce the effectiveness of some chemotherapy regimens (specifically in ALL); teniposide and methotrexate may be cleared more rapidly in these patients

Antipsychotics: Barbiturates may enhance the metabolism (decrease the efficacy) of antipsychotics; monitor for altered response; dose adjustment may be needed

Beta-blockers: Metabolism of beta-blockers may be increased and clinical effect decreased; atenolol and nadolol are unlikely to interact given their renal elimination

Calcium channel blockers: Barbiturates may enhance the metabolism of calcium channel blockers, decreasing their clinical effect

Chloramphenicol: Barbiturates may increase the metabolism of chloramphenicol and chloramphenicol may inhibit barbiturate metabolism; monitor for altered response

Cimetidine: Barbiturates may enhance the metabolism of cimetidine, decreasing its clinical effect

CNS depressants: Sedative effects and/or respiratory depression with barbiturates may be additive with other CNS depressants; monitor for increased effect; includes ethanol, sedatives, antidepressants, narcotic analgesics, and benzodiazepines

Corticosteroids: Barbiturates may enhance the metabolism of corticosteroids, decreasing their clinical effect

Cyclosporine: Levels may be decreased by barbiturates; monitor

Doxycycline: Barbiturates may enhance the metabolism of doxycycline, decreasing its clinical effect; higher dosages may be required

Estrogens: Barbiturates may increase the metabolism of estrogens and reduce their efficacy

Felbamate may inhibit the metabolism of barbiturates and barbiturates may increase the metabolism of felbamate

Griseofulvin: Barbiturates may impair the absorption of griseofulvin, and griseofulvin metabolism may be increased by barbiturates, decreasing clinical effect

Guanfacine: Effect may be decreased by barbiturates

Immunosuppressants: Barbiturates may enhance the metabolism of immunosuppressants, decreasing its clinical effect; includes both cyclosporine and tacrolimus

Loop diuretics: Metabolism may be increased and clinical effects decreased; established for furosemide, effect with other loop diuretics not established

MAO inhibitors: Metabolism of barbiturates may be inhibited, increasing clinical effect or toxicity of the barbiturates

Methadone: Barbiturates may enhance the metabolism of methadone resulting in methadone withdrawal

Methoxyflurane: Barbiturates may enhance the nephrotoxic effects of methoxyflurane

Oral contraceptives: Barbiturates may enhance the metabolism of oral contraceptives, decreasing their clinical effect; an alternative method of contraception should be considered

Theophylline: Barbiturates may increase metabolism of theophylline derivatives and decrease their clinical effect

Tricyclic antidepressants: Barbiturates may increase metabolism of tricyclic antidepressants and decrease their clinical effect; sedative effects may be additive

Valproic acid: Metabolism of barbiturates may be inhibited by valproic acid; monitor for excessive sedation; a dose reduction may be needed

(Continued)

Pentobarbital *(Continued)*

Warfarin: Barbiturates inhibit the hypoprothrombinemic effects of oral anticoagulants via increased metabolism; this combination should generally be avoided

Ethanol/Nutrition/Herb Interactions

Ethanol: Avoid ethanol (may increase CNS depression).

Food: Food may decrease the rate but not the extent of oral absorption.

Stability Protect from freezing; aqueous solutions are not stable, commercially available vehicle (containing propylene glycol) is more stable; low pH may cause precipitate; use only clear solution

Mechanism of Action Short-acting barbiturate with sedative, hypnotic, and anticonvulsant properties. Barbiturates depress the sensory cortex, decrease motor activity, alter cerebellar function, and produce drowsiness, sedation, and hypnosis. In high doses, barbiturates exhibit anticonvulsant activity; barbiturates produce dose-dependent respiratory depression.

Pharmacodynamics/Kinetics

Onset of action:

Oral, rectal: 15-60 minutes

I.M.: Within 10-15 minutes

I.V.: Within 1 minute

Duration:

Oral, rectal: 1-4 hours

I.V.: 15 minutes

Distribution: V_d:

Children: 0.8 L/kg

Adults: 1 L/kg

Protein binding: 35% to 55%

Metabolism: Extensively in liver via hydroxylation and oxidation pathways

Half-life, terminal:

Children: 25 hours

Adults, normal: 22 hours; range: 35-50 hours

Elimination: <1% excreted unchanged renally

Usual Dosage

Children:

Sedative: Oral: 2-6 mg/kg/day divided in 3 doses; maximum: 100 mg/day

Hypnotic: I.M.: 2-6 mg/kg; maximum: 100 mg/dose

Sedative/hypnotic: Rectal:

2 months to 1 year (10-20 lb): 30 mg

1-4 years (20-40 lb): 30-60 mg

5-12 years (40-80 lb): 60 mg

12-14 years (80-110 lb): 60-120 mg

or

<4 years: 3-6 mg/kg/dose

>4 years: 1.5-3 mg/kg/dose

Preoperative/preprocedure sedation: ≥6 months:

Oral, I.M., rectal: 2-6 mg/kg; maximum: 100 mg/dose

I.V.: 1-3 mg/kg to a maximum of 100 mg until asleep

Conscious sedation prior to a procedure: Children 5-12 years: I.V.: 2 mg/kg 5-10 minutes before procedures, may repeat one time

Adolescents: Conscious sedation: Oral, I.V.: 100 mg prior to a procedure

Children and Adults: Barbiturate coma in head injury patients: I.V.: Loading dose: 5-10 mg/kg given slowly over 1-2 hours; monitor blood pressure and respiratory rate; Maintenance infusion: Initial: 1 mg/kg/hour; may increase to 2-3 mg/kg/hour; maintain burst suppression on EEG

Status epilepticus: I.V.: **Note**: Intubation required; monitor hemodynamics

Children: Loading dose: 5-15 mg/kg given slowly over 1-2 hours; maintenance infusion: 0.5-5 mg/kg/hour

Adults: Loading dose: 2-15 mg/kg given slowly over 1-2 hours; maintenance infusion: 0.5-3 mg/kg/hour

Adults:
Hypnotic:
Oral: 100-200 mg at bedtime or 20 mg 3-4 times/day for daytime sedation
I.M.: 150-200 mg
I.V.: Initial: 100 mg, may repeat every 1-3 minutes up to 200-500 mg total dose
Rectal: 120-200 mg at bedtime
Preoperative sedation: I.M.: 150-200 mg
Tolerance testing: 200 mg every 2 hours until signs of intoxication are exhibited at any time during the 2 hours after the dose; maximum dose: 1000 mg

Dosing adjustment in hepatic impairment: Reduce dosage in patients with severe liver dysfunction

Administration Pentobarbital may be administered by deep I.M. or slow I.V. injection. I.M.: No more than 5 mL (250 mg) should be injected at any one site because of possible tissue irritation I.V. push doses can be given undiluted, but should be administered no faster than 50 mg/minute; parenteral solutions are highly alkaline; avoid extravasation; avoid rapid I.V. administration >50 mg/minute; avoid intra-arterial injection

Monitoring Parameters Respiratory status (for conscious sedation, includes pulse oximetry), cardiovascular status, CNS status; cardiac monitor and blood pressure monitor required

Reference Range
Therapeutic:
Hypnotic: 1-5 µg/mL (SI: 4-22 µmol/L)
Coma: 10-50 µg/mL (SI: 88-221 µmol/L)
Toxic: >10 µg/mL (SI: >44 µmol/L)

Test Interactions ↑ ammonia (B); ↓ bilirubin (S)

Patient Information Avoid the use of alcohol and other CNS depressants; avoid driving and other hazardous tasks; avoid abrupt discontinuation; may cause physical and psychological dependence; do not alter dose without notifying physician

Nursing Implications Avoid extravasation; institute safety measures to avoid injuries; has many incompatibilities when given I.V.; monitor blood pressure closely with I.V. administration

Additional Information Sodium content of 1 mL injection: 5 mg (0.2 mEq)

Dosage Forms
Capsule, as sodium (C-II): 50 mg, 100 mg
Injection, as sodium (C-II): 50 mg/mL (20 mL, 50 mL)
Suppository, rectal (C-III): 60 mg, 200 mg

♦ **Pentobarbital Sodium** see Pentobarbital on page 289

♦ **Pentothal (Can)** see Thiopental on page 390

♦ **Pentothal® Sodium** see Thiopental on page 390

Pergolide (PER go lide)

Related Information
Discontinuation of Psychotropic Drugs - Withdrawal Symptoms and Recommendations on page 582

U.S. Brand Names Permax®

Canadian Brand Names Permax

Synonyms Pergolide Mesylate

Pharmacologic Category Anti-Parkinson's Agent (Dopamine Agonist); Ergot Derivative

Generic Available No

Use Adjunctive treatment to levodopa/carbidopa in the management of Parkinson's disease

Unlabeled/Investigational Use Tourette's disorder, chronic motor or vocal tic disorder

Pregnancy Risk Factor B

Contraindications Hypersensitivity to pergolide mesylate, other ergot derivatives, or any component of the formulation
(Continued)

Pergolide (Continued)

Warnings/Precautions Symptomatic hypotension occurs in 10% of patients; use with caution in patients with a history of cardiac arrhythmias, hallucinations, or mental illness

Adverse Reactions

>10%:

Central nervous system: Dizziness, somnolence, confusion, hallucinations, dystonia

Gastrointestinal: Nausea, constipation

Neuromuscular & skeletal: Dyskinesia

Respiratory: Rhinitis

1% to 10%:

Cardiovascular: Myocardial infarction, postural hypotension, syncope, arrhythmias, peripheral edema, vasodilation, palpitations, chest pain, hypertension

Central nervous system: Chills, insomnia, anxiety, psychosis, EPS, incoordination

Dermatologic: Rash

Gastrointestinal: Diarrhea, abdominal pain, xerostomia, anorexia, weight gain, dyspepsia, taste perversion

Hematologic: Anemia

Neuromuscular & skeletal: Weakness, myalgia, tremor, NMS (with rapid dose reduction), pain

Ocular: Abnormal vision, diplopia

Respiratory: Dyspnea, epistaxis

Miscellaneous: Flu syndrome, hiccups

<1% (Limited to important or life-threatening symptoms): Pericarditis, pericardial effusion, pleural effusion, pleural fibrosis, pleuritis, pneumothorax, retroperitoneal fibrosis, vasculitis

Overdosage/Toxicology

Signs and symptoms: Vomiting, hypotension, agitation, hallucinations, ventricular extrasystoles, possible seizures; data on overdose is limited;

Treatment: Supportive and may require antiarrhythmias and/or neuroleptics for agitation; hypotension, when unresponsive to I.V. fluids or Trendelenburg positioning, often responds to norepinephrine infusions started at 0.1-0.2 mcg/kg/minute followed by a titrated infusion. If signs of CNS stimulation are present, a neuroleptic may be indicated; antiarrhythmics may be indicated, monitor EKG; activated charcoal is useful to prevent further absorption and to hasten elimination

Drug Interactions

Antipsychotics: May diminish the effects of pergolide (due to dopamine antagonism); these combinations should generally be avoided

Entacapone: Fibrotic complications (retroperitoneal or pulmonary fibrosis) have been associated with combinations of entacapone and bromocriptine

Highly protein-bound drugs: May cause displacement/increased effect; use caution with other highly plasma protein bound drugs

Metoclopramide: May diminish the effects of pergolide (due to dopamine antagonism); concurrent therapy should generally be avoided

Ethanol/Nutrition/Herb Interactions Ethanol: Avoid ethanol (may cause CNS depression).

Mechanism of Action Pergolide is a semisynthetic ergot alkaloid similar to bromocriptine but stated to be more potent (10-1000 times) and longer-acting; it is a centrally-active dopamine agonist stimulating both D_1 and D_2 receptors. Pergolide is believed to exert its therapeutic effect by directly stimulating postsynaptic dopamine receptors in the nigrostriatal system.

Pharmacodynamics/Kinetics

Absorption: Oral: Well absorbed

Protein binding: Plasma 90%

Metabolism: Extensive in the liver (on first-pass)

Elimination: ~50% excreted in urine and 50% in feces

Usual Dosage When adding pergolide to levodopa/carbidopa, the dose of the latter can usually and should be decreased. Patients no longer responsive to bromocriptine may benefit by being switched to pergolide. Oral:

Children and Adolescents: Tourette's disorder, chronic motor or vocal disorder (unlabeled uses): Up to 300 mcg/day

Adults: Parkinson's disease: Start with 0.05 mg/day for 2 days, then increase dosage by 0.1 or 0.15 mg/day every 3 days over next 12 days, increase dose by 0.25 mg/day every 3 days until optimal therapeutic dose is achieved, up to 5 mg/day maximum; usual dosage range: 2-3 mg/day in 3 divided doses

Child/Adolescent Considerations Twenty-four children 7-17 years of age with Tourette's disorder, chronic motor tic disorder, or chronic vocal tic disorder were treated with up to 300 mcg/day (Gilbert, 2000).

Monitoring Parameters Blood pressure (both sitting/supine and standing), symptoms of parkinsonism, dyskinesias, mental status

Patient Information May cause hypotension, arise slowly from prolonged sitting or lying; take with food or meals to lessen GI upset, may cause drowsiness and impair judgment and coordination; report any unusual CNS symptoms, palpitations, chest pain, or involuntary movements to physician

Nursing Implications Monitor closely for orthostasis and other adverse effects; raise bed rails and institute safety measures; aid patient with ambulation, may cause postural hypotension and drowsiness

Dosage Forms Tablet, as mesylate: 0.05 mg, 0.25 mg, 1 mg

- ◆ **Pergolide Mesylate** *see Pergolide on page 293*
- ◆ **Periactin**® *see Cyproheptadine on page 97*
- ◆ **Peridol (Can)** *see Haloperidol on page 172*
- ◆ **Permax**® *see Pergolide on page 293*
- ◆ **Permitil**® *see Fluphenazine on page 151*

Perphenazine (per FEN a zeen)

Related Information

Antipsychotic Agents Comparison Chart *on page 557*
Antipsychotic Medication Guidelines *on page 559*
Discontinuation of Psychotropic Drugs - Withdrawal Symptoms and Recommendations *on page 582*
Federal OBRA Regulations Recommended Maximum Doses *on page 583*
Patient Information - Antipsychotics (General) *on page 466*

U.S. Brand Names Trilafon®

Canadian Brand Names Apo®-Perphenazine; PMS-Perphenazine

Pharmacologic Category Antipsychotic Agent, Phenothiazine, Piperazine

Generic Available Yes

Use Treatment of severe schizophrenia; nausea and vomiting

Unlabeled/Investigational Use Alcohol withdrawal; dementia in elderly; Tourette's syndrome; Huntington's chorea; spasmodic torticollis; Reye's syndrome; psychosis

Pregnancy Risk Factor C

Contraindications Hypersensitivity to perphenazine or any component of the formulation (cross-reactivity between phenothiazines may occur); severe CNS depression; subcortical brain damage; bone marrow suppression; blood dyscrasias; coma

Warnings/Precautions May cause hypotension, particularly with parenteral administration. May be sedating, use with caution in disorders where CNS depression is a feature. Use with caution in Parkinson's disease. Caution in patients with hemodynamic instability; predisposition to seizures; severe cardiac, hepatic, renal, or respiratory disease. Esophageal dysmotility and aspiration have been associated with antipsychotic use - use with caution in patients at risk of pneumonia (ie, Alzheimer's disease). Caution in breast cancer or other prolactin-dependent tumors (may elevate prolactin levels). May alter temperature regulation or mask toxicity of other drugs due to antiemetic effects. May alter cardiac conduction - life-(Continued)

Perphenazine *(Continued)*

threatening arrhythmias have occurred with therapeutic doses of phenothiazines. May cause orthostatic hypotension - use with caution in patients at risk of this effect or those who would tolerate transient hypotensive episodes (cerebrovascular disease, cardiovascular disease, or other medications which may predispose).

Phenothiazines may cause anticholinergic effects (confusion, agitation, constipation, dry mouth, blurred vision, urinary retention); therefore, they should be used with caution in patients with decreased gastrointestinal motility, urinary retention, BPH, xerostomia, or visual problems. Conditions which also may be exacerbated by cholinergic blockade include narrow-angle glaucoma (screening is recommended) and worsening of myasthenia gravis. Relative to other neuroleptics, perphenazine has a low potency of cholinergic blockade.

May cause extrapyramidal reactions, including pseudoparkinsonism, acute dystonic reactions, akathisia, and tardive dyskinesia (risk of these reactions is moderate-high relative to other neuroleptics). May be associated with neuroleptic malignant syndrome (NMS) or pigmentary retinopathy.

Adverse Reactions Frequency not defined.

Cardiovascular: Hypotension, orthostatic hypotension, hypertension, tachycardia, bradycardia, dizziness, cardiac arrest

Central nervous system: Extrapyramidal symptoms (pseudoparkinsonism, akathisia, dystonias, tardive dyskinesia), dizziness, cerebral edema, seizures, headache, drowsiness, paradoxical excitement, restlessness, hyperactivity, insomnia, neuroleptic malignant syndrome (NMS), impairment of temperature regulation

Dermatologic: Increased sensitivity to sun, rash, discoloration of skin (blue-gray)

Endocrine & metabolic: Hypoglycemia, hyperglycemia, galactorrhea, lactation, breast enlargement, gynecomastia, menstrual irregularity, amenorrhea, SIADH, changes in libido

Gastrointestinal: Constipation, weight gain, vomiting, stomach pain, nausea, xerostomia, salivation, diarrhea, anorexia, ileus

Genitourinary: Difficulty in urination, ejaculatory disturbances, incontinence, polyuria, ejaculating dysfunction, priapism

Hematologic: Agranulocytosis, leukopenia, eosinophilia, hemolytic anemia, thrombocytopenic purpura, pancytopenia

Hepatic: Cholestatic jaundice, hepatotoxicity

Neuromuscular & skeletal: Tremor

Ocular: Pigmentary retinopathy, blurred vision, cornea and lens changes

Respiratory: Nasal congestion

Miscellaneous: Diaphoresis

Overdosage/Toxicology

Signs and symptoms: Deep sleep, dystonia, agitation, coma, abnormal involuntary muscle movements, hypotension, arrhythmias

Treatment:

Following initiation of essential overdose management, toxic symptom treatment and supportive treatment should be initiated

Hypotension usually responds to I.V. fluids or Trendelenburg positioning. If unresponsive to these measures, the use of a parenteral inotrope may be required (eg, norepinephrine 0.1-0.2 mcg/kg/minute titrated to response).

Seizures commonly respond to diazepam (I.V. 5-10 mg bolus in adults every 15 minutes if needed up to a total of 30 mg; I.V. 0.25-0.4 mg/kg/dose up to a total of 10 mg in children) or to phenytoin or phenobarbital

Extrapyramidal symptoms (eg, dystonic reactions) may be managed with diphenhydramine or benztropine mesylate.

Drug Interactions CYP2D6 enzyme substrate; CYP2D6 enzyme inhibitor

Aluminum salts: May decrease the absorption of phenothiazines; monitor

Amphetamines: Efficacy may be diminished by antipsychotics; in addition, amphetamines may increase psychotic symptoms; avoid concurrent use

Anticholinergics: May inhibit the therapeutic response to phenothiazines and excess anticholinergic effects may occur; includes benztropine, trihexyphenidyl, biperiden, and drugs with significant anticholinergic activity (TCAs, antihistamines, disopyramide)

Antihypertensives: Concurrent use of phenothiazines with an antihypertensive may produce additive hypotensive effects (particularly orthostasis)

Bromocriptine: Phenothiazines inhibit the ability of bromocriptine to lower serum prolactin concentrations

CNS depressants: Sedative effects may be additive with phenothiazines; monitor for increased effect; includes barbiturates, benzodiazepines, narcotic analgesics, ethanol, and other sedative agents

CYP2D6 inhibitors: Metabolism of phenothiazines may be decreased; increasing clinical effect or toxicity; inhibitors include amiodarone, cimetidine, delavirdine, fluoxetine, paroxetine, propafenone, quinidine, and ritonavir; monitor for increased effect/toxicity

Enzyme inducers: May enhance the hepatic metabolism of phenothiazines; larger doses may be required; includes rifampin, rifabutin, barbiturates, phenytoin, and cigarette smoking

Epinephrine: Chlorpromazine (and possibly other low potency antipsychotics) may diminish the pressor effects of epinephrine

Guanethidine and guanadrel: Antihypertensive effects may be inhibited by phenothiazines

Levodopa: Phenothiazines may inhibit the antiparkinsonian effect of levodopa; avoid this combination

Lithium: Phenothiazines may produce neurotoxicity with lithium; this is a rare effect

Phenytoin: May reduce serum levels of phenothiazines; phenothiazines may increase phenytoin serum levels

Propranolol: Serum concentrations of phenothiazines may be increased; propranolol also increases phenothiazine concentrations

Polypeptide antibiotics: Rare cases of respiratory paralysis have been reported with concurrent use of phenothiazines

QT_c-prolonging agents: Effects on QT_c interval may be additive with phenothiazines, increasing the risk of malignant arrhythmias; includes type Ia antiarrhythmics, TCAs, and some quinolone antibiotics (sparfloxacin, moxifloxacin, and gatifloxacin)

Sulfadoxine-pyrimethamine: May increase phenothiazine concentrations

Tricyclic antidepressants: Concurrent use may produce increased toxicity or altered therapeutic response

Trazodone: Phenothiazines and trazodone may produce additive hypotensive effects

Valproic acid: Serum levels may be increased by phenothiazines

Ethanol/Nutrition/Herb Interactions

Ethanol: Avoid ethanol (may increase CNS depression).

Herb/Nutraceutical: Avoid kava kava, gotu kola, valerian, St John's wort (may increase CNS depression).

Stability Do not mix with beverages containing caffeine (coffee, cola), tannins (tea), or pectinates (apple juice) since physical incompatibility exists; use ~60 mL diluent for each 5 mL of concentrate; protect all dosage forms from light; clear or slightly yellow solutions may be used; should be dispensed in amber or opaque vials/bottles. Solutions may be diluted or mixed with fruit juices or other liquids but must be administered immediately after mixing; do not prepare bulk dilutions or store bulk dilutions.

Mechanism of Action Blocks postsynaptic mesolimbic dopaminergic receptors in the brain; exhibits alpha-adrenergic blocking effect and depresses the release of hypothalamic and hypophyseal hormones

Pharmacodynamics/Kinetics

Absorption: Oral: Well absorbed

Distribution: Crosses the placenta

Metabolism: In the liver

Half-life: 9 hours

(Continued)

Perphenazine *(Continued)*

Time to peak serum concentration: Within 4-8 hours
Elimination: In urine and bile

Usual Dosage

Children:
Schizophrenia/psychoses:
Oral:
1-6 years: 4-6 mg/day in divided doses
6-12 years: 6 mg/day in divided doses
>12 years: 4-16 mg 2-4 times/day
I.M.: 5 mg every 6 hours
Nausea/vomiting: I.M.: 5 mg every 6 hours

Adults:
Schizophrenia/psychoses:
Oral: 4-16 mg 2-4 times/day not to exceed 64 mg/day
I.M.: 5 mg every 6 hours up to 15 mg/day in ambulatory patients and 30 mg/day in hospitalized patients

Nausea/vomiting:
Oral: 8-16 mg/day in divided doses up to 24 mg/day
I.M.: 5-10 mg every 6 hours as necessary up to 15 mg/day in ambulatory patients and 30 mg/day in hospitalized patients
I.V. (severe): 1 mg at 1- to 2-minute intervals up to a total of 5 mg

Elderly: Behavioral symptoms associated with dementia: Oral: Initial: 2-4 mg 1-2 times/day; increase at 4- to 7-day intervals by 2-4 mg/day. Increase dose intervals (bid, tid, etc) as necessary to control behavior response or side effects. Maximum daily dose: 32 mg; gradual increase (titration) may prevent some side effects or decrease their severity.

Hemodialysis: Not dialyzable (0% to 5%)

Dosing adjustment in hepatic impairment: Dosage reductions should be considered in patients with liver disease although no specific guidelines are available

Administration Dilute oral concentration to at least 2 oz with water, juice, or milk; for I.V. use, injection should be diluted to at least 0.5 mg/mL with NS and given at a rate of 1 mg/minute; observe for tremor and abnormal movements or posturing

Monitoring Parameters Cardiac, blood pressure (hypotension when administering I.M. or I.V.); respiratory status

Reference Range 2-6 nmol/L

Test Interactions ↑ cholesterol (S), ↑ glucose; ↓ uric acid (S)

Patient Information May cause drowsiness, impair judgment and coordination; report any feelings of restlessness or any involuntary movements; avoid alcohol and other CNS depressants; do not alter dose or discontinue without consulting physician

Nursing Implications Monitor for hypotension when administering I.M. or I.V. during the first 3-5 days after initiating therapy or making a dosage adjustment

Dosage Forms
Injection: 5 mg/mL (1 mL)
Tablet: 2 mg, 4 mg, 8 mg, 16 mg

♦ **Perphenazine and Amitriptyline** *see* Amitriptyline and Perphenazine *on page 28*
♦ **Pharmacokinetics of Selective Serotonin-Reuptake Inhibitors (SSRIs)** *see page 590*
♦ **Phendiet®** *see* Phendimetrazine *on page 298*
♦ **Phendiet®-105** *see* Phendimetrazine *on page 298*

Phendimetrazine *(fen dye ME tra zeen)*

U.S. Brand Names Bontril PDM®; Bontril® Slow-Release; Melfiat®; Obezine®; Phendiet®; Phendiet®-105; Prelu-2®
Synonyms Phendimetrazine Tartrate
Pharmacologic Category Anorexiant

Generic Available Yes

Use Appetite suppressant during the first few weeks of dieting to help establish new eating habits; its effectiveness lasts only for short periods (3-12 weeks)

Restrictions C-III

Contraindications Hypersensitivity to phendimetrazine or any component of the formulation

Warnings/Precautions Anorexigens have been reported to be associated with the occurrence of serious regurgitant cardiac valvular disease, including disease of the mitral, aortic, and/or tricuspid valves. Primary pulmonary hypertension (PPH) - a rare, frequently fatal disease of the lungs - has been found to occur with increased frequency in patients receiving anorexigens. There have been reports of PPH and valvular irregularities in users of phendimetrazine tartrate tablets. The safety and effectiveness of the combined use of phendimetrazine with other anorexigens in the treatment of obesity have not been established, and there is no approved use of these products together in the treatment of obesity. Phendimetrazine is approved only as a single agent for short-term use (ie, a few weeks). Stimulants may unmask tics in individuals with coexisting Tourette's syndrome.

Adverse Reactions Frequency not defined.
Cardiovascular: Hypertension, tachycardia, arrhythmias
Central nervous system: Euphoria, nervousness, insomnia, confusion, mental depression, restlessness, headache
Dermatologic: Alopecia
Endocrine & metabolic: Changes in libido
Gastrointestinal: Nausea, vomiting, constipation, diarrhea, abdominal cramps
Genitourinary: Dysuria
Hematologic: Blood dyscrasias
Neuromuscular & skeletal: Tremor, myalgia
Ocular: Blurred vision
Renal: Polyuria
Respiratory: Dyspnea
Miscellaneous: Diaphoresis (increased)

Usual Dosage Adults: Oral:
Regular capsule or tablet: 35 mg 2 or 3 times daily, 1 hour before meals
Sustained release: 105 mg once daily in the morning before breakfast

Patient Information Take with a full glass of water one hour before meals (unless your physician directs otherwise). Tell your physician about unusual or allergic reactions you have had to any medications, especially to phendimetrazine or other appetite suppressants (such as benzphetamine, phenmetrazine, diethylpropion, fenfluramine, mazindol, and phentermine) or to epinephrine, norepinephrine, ephedrine, amphetamines, dextroamphetamine, phenylephrine, phenylpropanolamine, pseudoephedrine, albuterol, metaproterenol, or terbutaline. Before having surgery or other medical or dental treatment, tell your physician or dentist you are taking this drug. Phendimetrazine is related to amphetamine and may be habit-forming when taken for long periods of time (both physical and psychological dependence can occur). You should not increase the dosage of this medication or take it for longer than 12 weeks without first consulting your physician. It is also important that you not stop taking this medication abruptly - fatigue, sleep disorders, mental depression, nausea, vomiting, or stomach cramps or pain could occur. Your physician may, therefore, want to decrease your dosage gradually. Be sure to tell your physician if you are pregnant. Although studies of phendimetrazine in humans have not been conducted, some of the appetite suppressants have been shown to cause side effects in the fetuses of animals that received large doses during pregnancy.

Dosage Forms
Capsule, as tartrate: 35 mg
Capsule, sustained release, as tartrate (Bontril® Slow Release, Melfiat®, Phendiet®-105, Prelu-2®): 105 mg
Tablet, as tartrate (Bontril PDM®, Obenzine®, Phendiet®): 35 mg

♦ **Phendimetrazine Tartrate** *see Phendimetrazine on page 298*

Phenelzine (FEN el zeen)

Related Information

Antidepressant Agents Comparison Chart *on page 553*
Patient Information - Antidepressants (MAOIs) *on page 462*
Teratogenic Risks of Psychotropic Medications *on page 594*
Tyramine Content of Foods *on page 595*

U.S. Brand Names Nardil®

Canadian Brand Names Nardil

Synonyms Phenelzine Sulfate

Pharmacologic Category Antidepressant, Monoamine Oxidase Inhibitor

Generic Available No

Use Symptomatic treatment of atypical, nonendogenous, or neurotic depression

Unlabeled/Investigational Use Selective mutism

Pregnancy Risk Factor C

Contraindications Hypersensitivity to phenelzine or any component of the formulation; uncontrolled hypertension; pheochromocytoma; hepatic disease; congestive heart failure; concurrent use of sympathomimetics (and related compounds), CNS depressants, ethanol, meperidine, bupropion, buspirone, guanethidine, serotonergic drugs (including SSRIs) - do not use within 5 weeks of fluoxetine discontinuation or 2 weeks of other antidepressant discontinuation; general anesthesia, local vasoconstrictors; spinal anesthesia (hypotension may be exaggerated); foods with a high content of tyramine, tryptophan, or dopamine, chocolate, or caffeine (may cause hypertensive crisis)

Warnings/Precautions Safety in children <16 years of age has not been established; use with caution in patients who are hyperactive, hyperexcitable, or who have glaucoma, hyperthyroidism, suicidal tendencies, or diabetes; avoid use of meperidine within 2 weeks of phenelzine use. Hypertensive crisis may occur with tyramine, tryptophan, or dopamine-containing foods. Should not be used in combination with other antidepressants. Hypotensive effects of antihypertensives (beta-blockers, thiazides) may be exaggerated. Use with caution in depressed patients at risk of suicide. May cause orthostatic hypotension - use with caution in patients with hypotension or patients who would not tolerate transient hypotensive episodes (cardiovascular or cerebrovascular disease) - effects may be additive with other agents which cause orthostasis. Has been associated with activation of hypomania and/or mania in bipolar patients. May worsen psychotic symptoms in some patients. Use with caution in patients at risk of seizures, or in patients receiving other drugs which may lower seizure threshold. Toxic reactions have occurred with dextromethorphan. Discontinue at least 48 hours prior to myelography.

The MAO inhibitors are effective and generally well tolerated by older patients. It is the potential interactions with tyramine or tryptophan-containing foods and other drugs, and their effects on blood pressure that have limited their use.

Adverse Reactions Frequency not defined.
Cardiovascular: Orthostatic hypotension, edema
Central nervous system: Dizziness, headache, drowsiness, sleep disturbances, fatigue, hyper-reflexia, twitching, ataxia, mania
Dermatologic: Rash, pruritus
Endocrine & metabolic: Decreased sexual ability (anorgasmia, ejaculatory disturbances, impotence), hypernatremia, hypermetabolic syndrome
Gastrointestinal: Xerostomia, constipation, weight gain
Genitourinary: Urinary retention
Hematologic: Leukopenia
Hepatic: Hepatitis
Neuromuscular & skeletal: Weakness, tremor, myoclonus
Ocular: Blurred vision, glaucoma
Miscellaneous: Diaphoresis

Overdosage/Toxicology

Signs and symptoms: Tachycardia, palpitations, muscle twitching, seizures, insomnia, restlessness, transient hypertension, hypotension, drowsiness, hyperpyrexia, coma

Treatment: Competent supportive care is the most important treatment for an overdose with a monoamine oxidase (MAO) inhibitor. Both hypertension or hypotension can occur with intoxication. Hypotension may respond to I.V. fluids or vasopressors and hypertension usually responds to an alpha-adrenergic blocker. While treating the hypertension, care is warranted to avoid sudden drops in blood pressure, since this may worsen the MAO inhibitor toxicity. Muscle irritability and seizures often respond to diazepam, while hyperthermia is best treated antipyretics and cooling blankets. Cardiac arrhythmias are best treated with phenytoin or procainamide.

Drug Interactions

Amphetamines: MAO inhibitors in combination with amphetamines may result in severe hypertensive reaction; these combinations are best avoided

Anorexiants: Concurrent use of anorexiants may result in serotonin syndrome; these combinations are best avoided; includes dexfenfluramine, fenfluramine, or sibutramine

Barbiturates: MAO inhibitors may inhibit the metabolism of barbiturates and prolong their effect

CNS stimulants: MAO inhibitors in combination with stimulants (methylphenidate) may result in severe hypertensive reaction; these combinations are best avoided

Dextromethorphan: Concurrent use of MAO inhibitors may result in serotonin syndrome; these combinations are best avoided

Disulfiram: MAO inhibitors may produce delirium in patients receiving disulfiram; monitor

Guanadrel and guanethidine: MAO inhibitors inhibit the antihypertensive response to guanadrel or guanethidine; use an alternative antihypertensive agent

Hypoglycemic agents: MAO inhibitors may produce hypoglycemia in patients with diabetes; monitor

Levodopa: MAO inhibitors in combination with levodopa may result in hypertensive reactions; monitor

Lithium: MAO inhibitors in combination with lithium have resulted in malignant hyperpyrexia; this combination is best avoided

Meperidine: May cause serotonin syndrome when combined with an MAO inhibitor; avoid this combination

Nefazodone: Concurrent use of MAO inhibitors may result in serotonin syndrome; these combinations are best avoided

Norepinephrine: MAO inhibitors may increase the pressor response of norepinephrine (effect is generally small); monitor

Reserpine: MAO inhibitors in combination with reserpine may result in hypertensive reactions; monitor

Serotonin agonists: Theoretically may increase the risk of serotonin syndrome; includes sumatriptan, naratriptan, rizatriptan, and zolmitriptan

SSRIs: May cause serotonin syndrome when combined with an MAO inhibitor; avoid this combination

Succinylcholine: MAO inhibitors may prolong the muscle relaxation produced by succinylcholine via decreased plasma pseudocholinesterase

Sympathomimetics (indirect-acting): MAO inhibitors in combination with sympathomimetics such as dopamine, metaraminol, phenylephrine, and decongestants (pseudoephedrine) may result in severe hypertensive reaction; these combinations are best avoided

Tramadol: May increase the risk of seizures and serotonin syndrome in patients receiving an MAO inhibitor

Trazodone: Concurrent use of MAO inhibitors may result in serotonin syndrome; these combinations are best avoided

Tricyclic antidepressants: May cause serotonin syndrome when combined with an MAO inhibitor; avoid this combination

(Continued)

301

Phenelzine *(Continued)*

Tyramine: Foods (eg, cheese) and beverages (eg, ethanol) containing tyramine, should be avoided in patients receiving an MAO inhibitor; hypertensive crisis may result

Venlafaxine: Concurrent use of MAO inhibitors may result in serotonin syndrome; these combinations are best avoided

Ethanol/Nutrition/Herb Interactions

Ethanol: Avoid ethanol (ethanolic beverages containing tyramine may induce a severe hypertensive response).

Food: Clinically severe elevated blood pressure may occur if phenelzine is taken with tyramine-containing foods. Avoid foods containing tryptophan, dopamine, chocolate, or caffeine.

Stability Protect from light

Mechanism of Action Thought to act by increasing endogenous concentrations of norepinephrine, dopamine, and serotonin through inhibition of the enzyme (monoamine oxidase) responsible for the breakdown of these neurotransmitters

Pharmacodynamics/Kinetics

Onset of action: Within 2-4 weeks

Absorption: Oral: Well absorbed

Duration: May continue to have a therapeutic effect and interactions 2 weeks after discontinuing therapy

Elimination: In urine primarily as metabolites and unchanged drug

Usual Dosage Oral:

Children: Selective mutism (unlabeled use): 30-60 mg/day

Adults: Depression: 15 mg 3 times/day; may increase to 60-90 mg/day during early phase of treatment, then reduce to dose for maintenance therapy slowly after maximum benefit is obtained; takes 2-4 weeks for a significant response to occur

Elderly: Depression: Initial: 7.5 mg/day; increase by 7.5-15 mg/day every 3-4 days as tolerated; usual therapeutic dose: 15-60 mg/day in 3-4 divided doses

Child/Adolescent Considerations Four children 5.5-7 years of age, diagnosed with selective mutism were treated with 30-60 mg/day for 24-60 weeks (Golwyn, 1999).

Monitoring Parameters Blood pressure, heart rate, diet, weight, mood (if depressive symptoms)

Test Interactions ↓ glucose

Patient Information Avoid tyramine-containing foods: red wine, cheese (except cottage, ricotta, and cream), smoked or pickled fish, beef or chicken liver, dried sausage, fava or broad bean pods, yeast vitamin supplements; do not begin any prescription or OTC medications without consulting your physician or pharmacist; may take as long as 3 weeks to see effects

Nursing Implications Watch for postural hypotension; monitor blood pressure carefully, especially at therapy onset or if other CNS drugs or cardiovascular drugs are added; check for dietary and drug restriction

Additional Information Pyridoxine deficiency has occurred; symptoms include numbness and edema of hands; may respond to supplementation.

The MAO inhibitors are usually reserved for patients who do not tolerate or respond to other antidepressants. The brain activity of monoamine oxidase increases with age and even more so in patients with Alzheimer's disease. Therefore, the MAO inhibitors may have an increased role in patients with Alzheimer's disease who are depressed. Phenelzine is less stimulating than tranylcypromine.

Dosage Forms Tablet, as sulfate: 15 mg

♦ **Phenelzine Sulfate** *see* Phenelzine *on page 300*

♦ **Phenergan®** *see* Promethazine *on page 337*

Phenobarbital *(fee noe BAR bi tal)*

Related Information

Patient Information - Anxiolytics & Sedative Hypnotics (Barbiturates) *on page 485*

U.S. Brand Names Luminal® Sodium

Canadian Brand Names Barbilixir®

Synonyms Phenobarbital Sodium; Phenobarbitone; Phenylethylmalonylurea

Pharmacologic Category Anticonvulsant, Barbiturate; Barbiturate

Generic Available Yes

Use Management of generalized tonic-clonic (grand mal) and partial seizures; sedative

Unlabeled/Investigational Use Febrile seizures in children; may also be used for prevention and treatment of neonatal hyperbilirubinemia and lowering of bilirubin in chronic cholestasis; neonatal seizures; management of sedative/hypnotic withdrawal

Restrictions C-IV

Pregnancy Risk Factor D

Pregnancy/Breast-Feeding Implications

Clinical effects on the fetus: Crosses the placenta. Cardiac defect reported; hemorrhagic disease of newborn due to fetal vitamin K depletion may occur; may induce maternal folic acid deficiency; withdrawal symptoms observed in infant following delivery. Epilepsy itself, number of medications, genetic factors, or a combination of these probably influence the teratogenicity of anticonvulsant therapy. Benefit:risk ratio usually favors continued use during pregnancy and breast-feeding.

Breast-feeding/Lactation: Crosses into breast milk

Clinical effects on the infant: Sedation; withdrawal with abrupt weaning reported. AAP recommends USE WITH CAUTION.

Contraindications Hypersensitivity to barbiturates or any component of the formulation; marked hepatic impairment; dyspnea or airway obstruction; porphyria; pregnancy

Warnings/Precautions Potential for drug dependency exists, abrupt cessation may precipitate withdrawal, including status epilepticus in epileptic patients. Do not administer to patients in acute pain. Use caution in elderly, debilitated, renally or hepatic dysfunction, and pediatric patients. May cause paradoxical responses, including agitation and hyperactivity, particularly in acute pain and pediatric patients. Use with caution in patients with depression or suicidal tendencies, or in patients with a history of drug abuse. Tolerance, psychological and physical dependence may occur with prolonged use. May cause CNS depression, which may impair physical or mental abilities. Patients must cautioned about performing tasks which require mental alertness (ie, operating machinery or driving). Effects with other sedative drugs or ethanol may be potentiated. May cause respiratory depression or hypotension, particularly when administered intravenously. Use with caution in hemodynamically unstable patients (hypovolemic shock, CHF) or patients with respiratory disease. Due to its long half-life and risk of dependence, phenobarbital is not recommended as a sedative in the elderly. Use has been associated with cognitive deficits in children. Use with caution in patients with hypoadrenalism.

Adverse Reactions Frequency not defined.

Cardiovascular: Bradycardia, hypotension, syncope

Central nervous system: Drowsiness, lethargy, CNS excitation or depression, impaired judgment, "hangover" effect, confusion, somnolence, agitation, hyperkinesia, ataxia, nervousness, headache, insomnia, nightmares, hallucinations, anxiety, dizziness

Dermatologic: Rash, exfoliative dermatitis, Stevens-Johnson syndrome

Gastrointestinal: Nausea, vomiting, constipation

Hematologic: Agranulocytosis, thrombocytopenia, megaloblastic anemia

Local: Pain at injection site, thrombophlebitis with I.V. use

Renal: Oliguria

Respiratory: Laryngospasm, respiratory depression, apnea (especially with rapid I.V. use), hypoventilation

Miscellaneous: Gangrene with inadvertent intra-arterial injection

(Continued)

Phenobarbital *(Continued)*

Overdosage/Toxicology

Signs and symptoms: Unsteady gait, slurred speech, confusion, jaundice, hypothermia, hypotension, respiratory depression, coma

Treatment: If hypotension occurs, administer I.V. fluids and place the patient in the Trendelenburg position. If unresponsive, an I.V. vasopressor (eg, dopamine, epinephrine) may be required.

Repeated oral doses of activated charcoal significantly reduce the half-life of phenobarbital resulting from an enhancement of nonrenal elimination. The usual dose is 0.1-1 g/kg every 4-6 hours for 3-4 days unless the patient has no bowel movement causing the charcoal to remain in the GI tract. Assure adequate hydration and renal function. Urinary alkalinization with I.V. sodium bicarbonate also helps to enhance elimination. Hemodialysis or hemoperfusion is of uncertain value. Patients in stage IV coma due to high serum barbiturate levels may require charcoal hemoperfusion.

Drug Interactions CYP1A2, 2B6, 2C8, 2C9, 2C18, 2C19, 3A3/4, and 3A5-7 enzyme inducer

Note: Barbiturates are enzyme inducers; patients should be monitored when these drugs are started or stopped for a decreased or increased therapeutic effect respectively

Acetaminophen: Barbiturates may enhance the hepatotoxic potential of acetaminophen overdoses

Antiarrhythmics: Barbiturates may increase the metabolism of antiarrhythmics, decreasing their clinical effect; includes disopyramide, propafenone, and quinidine

Anticonvulsants: Barbiturates may increase the metabolism of anticonvulsants; includes ethosuximide, felbamate (possibly), lamotrigine, phenytoin, tiagabine, topiramate, and zonisamide; does not appear to affect gabapentin or levetiracetam

Antineoplastics: Limited evidence suggests that enzyme-inducing anticonvulsant therapy may reduce the effectiveness of some chemotherapy regimens (specifically in ALL); teniposide and methotrexate may be cleared more rapidly in these patients

Antipsychotics: Barbiturates may enhance the metabolism (decrease the efficacy) of antipsychotics; monitor for altered response; dose adjustment may be needed

Beta-blockers: Metabolism of beta-blockers may be increased and clinical effect decreased; atenolol and nadolol are unlikely to interact given their renal elimination

Calcium channel blockers: Barbiturates may enhance the metabolism of calcium channel blockers, decreasing their clinical effect

Chloramphenicol: Barbiturates may increase the metabolism of chloramphenicol and chloramphenicol may inhibit barbiturate metabolism; monitor for altered response

Cimetidine: Barbiturates may enhance the metabolism of cimetidine, decreasing its clinical effect

CNS depressants: Sedative effects and/or respiratory depression with barbiturates may be additive with other CNS depressants; monitor for increased effect; includes ethanol, sedatives, antidepressants, narcotic analgesics, and benzodiazepines

Corticosteroids: Barbiturates may enhance the metabolism of corticosteroids, decreasing their clinical effect

Cyclosporine: Levels may be decreased by barbiturates; monitor

Doxycycline: Barbiturates may enhance the metabolism of doxycycline, decreasing its clinical effect; higher dosages may be required

Estrogens: Barbiturates may increase the metabolism of estrogens and reduce their efficacy

Felbamate may inhibit the metabolism of barbiturates and barbiturates may increase the metabolism of felbamate

Griseofulvin: Barbiturates may impair the absorption of griseofulvin, and griseofulvin metabolism may be increased by barbiturates, decreasing clinical effect

Guanfacine: Effect may be decreased by barbiturates

Immunosuppressants: Barbiturates may enhance the metabolism of immunosuppressants, decreasing its clinical effect; includes both cyclosporine and tacrolimus

Loop diuretics: Metabolism may be increased and clinical effects decreased; established for furosemide, effect with other loop diuretics not established

MAO inhibitors: Metabolism of barbiturates may be inhibited, increasing clinical effect or toxicity of the barbiturates

Methadone: Barbiturates may enhance the metabolism of methadone resulting in methadone withdrawal

Methoxyflurane: Barbiturates may enhance the nephrotoxic effects of methoxyflurane

Oral contraceptives: Barbiturates may enhance the metabolism of oral contraceptives, decreasing their clinical effect; an alternative method of contraception should be considered

Theophylline: Barbiturates may increase metabolism of theophylline derivatives and decrease their clinical effect

Tricyclic antidepressants: Barbiturates may increase metabolism of tricyclic antidepressants and decrease their clinical effect; sedative effects may be additive

Valproic acid: Metabolism of barbiturates may be inhibited by valproic acid; monitor for excessive sedation; a dose reduction may be needed

Warfarin: Barbiturates inhibit the hypoprothrombinemic effects of oral anticoagulants via increased metabolism; this combination should generally be avoided

Ethanol/Nutrition/Herb Interactions

Ethanol: Avoid ethanol (may increase CNS depression).

Food: May cause decrease in vitamin D and calcium.

Herb/Nutraceutical: Avoid evening primrose (seizure threshold decreased). Avoid valerian, St John's wort, kava kava, gotu kola (may increase CNS depression).

Stability Protect elixir from light; not stable in aqueous solutions; use only clear solutions; do not add to acidic solutions, precipitation may occur; I.V. form is **incompatible** with benzquinamide (in syringe), cephalothin, chlorpromazine, hydralazine, hydrocortisone, hydroxyzine, insulin, levorphanol, meperidine, methadone, morphine, norepinephrine, pentazocine, prochlorperazine, promazine, promethazine, ranitidine (in syringe), vancomycin

Mechanism of Action Short-acting barbiturate with sedative, hypnotic, and anticonvulsant properties. Barbiturates depress the sensory cortex, decrease motor activity, alter cerebellar function, and produce drowsiness, sedation, and hypnosis. In high doses, barbiturates exhibit anticonvulsant activity; barbiturates produce dose-dependent respiratory depression.

Pharmacodynamics/Kinetics

Oral:

Onset of hypnosis: Within 20-60 minutes

Duration: 6-10 hours

I.V.:

Onset of action: Within 5 minutes

Peak effect: Within 30 minutes

Duration: 4-10 hours

Absorption: Oral: 70% to 90%

Protein binding: 20% to 45%, decreased in neonates

Metabolism: In the liver via hydroxylation and glucuronide conjugation

Half-life:

Neonates: 45-500 hours

Infants: 20-133 hours

Children: 37-73 hours

Adults: 53-140 hours

Time to peak serum concentration: Oral: Within 1-6 hours

Elimination: 20% to 50% excreted unchanged in urine

(Continued)

Phenobarbital *(Continued)*

Usual Dosage

Children:

Sedation: Oral: 2 mg/kg 3 times/day

Hypnotic: I.M., I.V., S.C.: 3-5 mg/kg at bedtime

Preoperative sedation: Oral, I.M., I.V.: 1-3 mg/kg 1-1.5 hours before procedure

Adults:

Sedation: Oral, I.M.: 30-120 mg/day in 2-3 divided doses

Hypnotic: Oral, I.M., I.V., S.C.: 100-320 mg at bedtime

Preoperative sedation: I.M.: 100-200 mg 1-1.5 hours before procedure

Anticonvulsant: Status epilepticus: **Loading dose:** I.V.:

Infants and Children: 10-20 mg/kg in a single or divided dose; in select patients may administer additional 5 mg/kg/dose every 15-30 minutes until seizure is controlled or a total dose of 40 mg/kg is reached

Adults: 300-800 mg initially followed by 120-240 mg/dose at 20-minute intervals until seizures are controlled or a total dose of 1-2 g

Anticonvulsant maintenance dose: Oral, I.V.:

Infants: 5-8 mg/kg/day in 1-2 divided doses

Children:

1-5 years: 6-8 mg/kg/day in 1-2 divided doses

5-12 years: 4-6 mg/kg/day in 1-2 divided doses

Children >12 years and Adults: 1-3 mg/kg/day in divided doses or 50-100 mg 2-3 times/day

Sedative/hypnotic withdrawal (unlabeled use): Initial daily requirement is determined by substituting phenobarbital 30 mg for every 100 mg pentobarbital used during tolerance testing; then daily requirement is decreased by 10% of initial dose

Dosing interval in renal impairment: Cl_{cr} <10 mL/minute: Administer every 12-16 hours

Hemodialysis: Moderately dialyzable (20% to 50%)

Dosing adjustment/comments in hepatic disease: Increased side effects may occur in severe liver disease; monitor plasma levels and adjust dose accordingly

Dietary Considerations Vitamin D: Loss in vitamin D due to malabsorption; increase intake of foods rich in vitamin D. Supplementation of vitamin D and/or calcium may be necessary.

Administration Avoid rapid I.V. administration >50 mg/minute; avoid intra-arterial injection

Monitoring Parameters Phenobarbital serum concentrations, mental status, CBC, LFTs, seizure activity

Reference Range

Therapeutic:

Infants and children: 15-30 µg/mL (SI: 65-129 µmol/L)

Adults: 20-40 µg/mL (SI: 86-172 µmol/L)

Toxic: >40 µg/mL (SI: >172 µmol/L)

Toxic concentration: Slowness, ataxia, nystagmus: 35-80 µg/mL (SI: 150-344 µmol/L)

Coma with reflexes: 65-117 µg/mL (SI: 279-502 µmol/L)

Coma without reflexes: >100 µg/mL (SI: >430 µmol/L)

Test Interactions ↑ ammonia (B); ↓ bilirubin (S), ↑ copper (S), assay interference of LDH, ↑ LFTs

Patient Information Avoid use of alcohol and other CNS depressants; avoid driving and other hazardous tasks; avoid abrupt discontinuation; may cause physical and psychological dependence; do not alter dose without notifying physician

Nursing Implications Parenteral solutions are highly alkaline; avoid extravasation; institute safety measures to avoid injuries; observe patient for excessive sedation and respiratory depression

Additional Information Injectable solutions contain propylene glycol; sodium content of injection (65 mg, 1 mL): 6 mg (0.3 mEq).

Dosage Forms

Elixir: 20 mg/5 mL (5 mL, 7.5 mL, 15 mL, 120 mL, 473 mL, 946 mL, 4000 mL)

Injection, as sodium: 30 mg/mL (1 mL); 60 mg/mL (1 mL); 65 mg/mL (1 mL); 130 mg/mL (1 mL)

Luminal®: 60 mg/mL (1 mL); 130 mg/mL (1 mL);

Tablet: 15 mg, 16 mg, 30 mg, 32 mg, 60 mg, 65 mg, 100 mg

♦ **Phenobarbital Sodium** *see* Phenobarbital *on page 302*

♦ **Phenobarbitone** *see* Phenobarbital *on page 302*

Phentermine (FEN ter meen)

U.S. Brand Names Adipex-P®; Ionamin®; Zantryl®

Canadian Brand Names Fastin; Ionamin

Synonyms Phentermine Hydrochloride

Pharmacologic Category Anorexiant

Generic Available Yes

Use Short-term adjunct in a regimen of weight reduction based on exercise, behavioral modification, and caloric reduction in the management of exogenous obesity for patients with an initial body mass index $\geq$30 kg/m^2 or $\geq$27 kg/m^2 in the presence of other risk factors (diabetes, hypertension); see Body Mass Index *on page 569* in the Appendix)

Restrictions C-IV

Pregnancy Risk Factor C

Contraindications Hypersensitivity or idiosyncrasy to sympathomimetic amines or any component of the formulation; patients with advanced arteriosclerosis, symptomatic cardiovascular disease, moderate to severe hypertension (stage II or III), hyperthyroidism, glaucoma, agitated states; patients with a history of drug abuse; use during or within 14 days following MAO inhibitor therapy; stimulant medications are contraindicated for use in children with attention-deficit/hyperactivity disorders and concomitant Tourette's syndrome or tics

Warnings/Precautions Use with caution in patients with bipolar disorder, diabetes mellitus, cardiovascular disease, seizure disorders, insomnia, porphyria, or mild hypertension (stage I). May exacerbate symptoms of behavior and thought disorder in psychotic patients. Stimulants may unmask tics in individuals with coexisting Tourette's syndrome. Potential for drug dependency exists - avoid abrupt discontinuation in patients who have received for prolonged periods. Use in weight reduction programs only when alternative therapy has been ineffective. Stimulant use has been associated with growth suppression, and careful monitoring is recommended.

Not recommended for use in children <16 years of age (per manufacturer). Primary pulmonary hypertension (PPH), a rare and frequently fatal pulmonary disease, has been reported to occur in patients receiving a combination of phentermine and fenfluramine or dexfenfluramine. The possibility of an association between PPH and the use of phentermine alone cannot be ruled out.

Adverse Reactions Frequency not defined.

Cardiovascular: Hypertension, palpitations, tachycardia, primary pulmonary hypertension and/or regurgitant cardiac valvular disease

Central nervous system: Euphoria, insomnia, overstimulation, dizziness, dysphoria, headache, restlessness, psychosis

Dermatologic: Urticaria

Endocrine & metabolic: Changes in libido, impotence

Gastrointestinal: Nausea, constipation, xerostomia, unpleasant taste, diarrhea

Hematologic: Blood dyscrasias

Neuromuscular & skeletal: Tremor

Ocular: Blurred vision

Overdosage/Toxicology

Signs and symptoms: Hyperactivity, agitation, hyperthermia, hypertension, seizures

(Continued)

Phentermine (Continued)

Treatment: There is no specific antidote for phentermine intoxication and the bulk of the treatment is supportive. Hyperactivity and agitation usually respond to reduced sensory input, however with extreme agitation haloperidol (2-5 mg I.M. for adults) may be required. Hyperthermia is best treated with external cooling measures, or when severe or unresponsive, muscle paralysis with pancuronium may be needed. Hypertension is usually transient and generally does not require treatment unless severe. For diastolic blood pressures >110 mm Hg, a nitroprusside infusion should be initiated. Seizures usually respond to diazepam IVP and/or phenytoin maintenance regimens.

Drug Interactions

Antihypertensives: Phentermine may decrease the effect of antihypertensive medications

Antipsychotics: Efficacy of anorexiants may be decreased by antipsychotics; in addition, amphetamines or related compounds may induce an increase in psychotic symptoms in some patients

Furazolidone: Amphetamines (and related compounds) may induce hypertensive episodes in patients receiving furazolidone

Guanethidine: Amphetamines (and related compounds) inhibit the antihypertensive response to guanethidine; probably also may occur with guanadrel

Hypoglycemic agents: Dosage may need to be adjusted when phentermine is used in a diabetic receiving a special diet

Linezolid: Due to MAO inhibition (see note on MAO inhibitors), this combination should generally be avoided

MAO inhibitors: Concurrent use may be associated with hypertensive episodes

SSRIs: Concurrent use may be associated with a risk of serotonin syndrome

Mechanism of Action
Phentermine is structurally similar to dextroamphetamine and is comparable to dextroamphetamine as an appetite suppressant, but is generally associated with a lower incidence and severity of CNS side effects. Phentermine, like other anorexiants, stimulates the hypothalamus to result in decreased appetite; anorexiant effects are most likely mediated via norepinephrine and dopamine metabolism. However, other CNS effects or metabolic effects may be involved.

Pharmacodynamics/Kinetics

Absorption: Well absorbed; resin absorbed slower and produces more prolonged clinical effects

Half-life: 20 hours

Elimination: Primarily unchanged in urine

Usual Dosage
Oral:

Children 3-15 years: Obesity: 5-15 mg/day for 4 weeks

Adults: Obesity: 8 mg 3 times/day 30 minutes before meals or food or 15-37.5 mg/day before breakfast or 10-14 hours before retiring

Monitoring Parameters
CNS

Patient Information
Take during day to avoid insomnia; do not discontinue abruptly, may cause physical and psychological dependence with prolonged use

Nursing Implications
Dose should not be given in evening or at bedtime

Dosage Forms

Capsule, as hydrochloride: 15 mg, 18.75 mg, 30 mg, 37.5 mg

Capsule, resin complex, as hydrochloride: 15 mg, 30 mg

Tablet, as hydrochloride: 8 mg, 37.5 mg

- **Phentermine Hydrochloride** see Phentermine on page 307
- **Phenylethylmalonylurea** see Phenobarbital on page 302
- **Phenylisohydantoin** see Pemoline on page 287

Phenytoin (FEN i toyn)

U.S. Brand Names Dilantin®

Canadian Brand Names Tremytoine®

Synonyms Diphenylhydantoin; DPH; Phenytoin Sodium; Phenytoin Sodium, Extended; Phenytoin Sodium, Prompt

Pharmacologic Category Antiarrhythmic Agent, Class I-B; Anticonvulsant, Hydantoin

Generic Available Yes

Use Management of generalized tonic-clonic (grand mal), complex partial seizures; prevention of seizures following head trauma/neurosurgery

Unlabeled/Investigational Use Ventricular arrhythmias, including those associated with digitalis intoxication, prolonged QT interval and surgical repair of congenital heart diseases in children; epidermolysis bullosa

Pregnancy Risk Factor D

Pregnancy/Breast-Feeding Implications

Clinical effects on the fetus: Crosses the placenta. Cardiac defects and multiple other malformations reported; characteristic pattern of malformations called "fetal hydantoin syndrome"; hemorrhagic disease of newborn due to fetal vitamin K depletion, maternal folic acid deficiency may occur. Epilepsy itself, number of medications, genetic factors, or a combination of these probably influence the teratogenicity of anticonvulsant therapy. Benefit:risk ratio usually favors continued use during pregnancy and breast-feeding.

Breast-feeding/lactation: Crosses into breast milk

Clinical effects on the infant: Methemoglobinemia, drowsiness and decreased sucking reported in 1 case. AAP considers **compatible** with breast-feeding.

Contraindications Hypersensitivity to phenytoin, other hydantoins, or any component of the formulation; pregnancy

Warnings/Precautions May increase frequency of petit mal seizures; I.V. form may cause hypotension, skin necrosis at I.V. site; avoid I.V. administration in small veins; use with caution in patients with porphyria; discontinue if rash or lymphadenopathy occurs; use with caution in patients with hepatic dysfunction, sinus bradycardia, SA block, or AV block; use with caution in elderly or debilitated patients, or in any condition associated with low serum albumin levels, which will increase the free fraction of phenytoin in the serum and, therefore, the pharmacologic response. Sedation, confusional states, or cerebellar dysfunction (loss of motor coordination) may occur at higher total serum concentrations, or at lower total serum concentrations when the free fraction of phenytoin is increased. Abrupt withdrawal may precipitate status epilepticus.

Adverse Reactions I.V. effects: Hypotension, bradycardia, cardiac arrhythmias, cardiovascular collapse (especially with rapid I.V. use), venous irritation and pain, thrombophlebitis

Effects not related to plasma phenytoin concentrations: Hypertrichosis, gingival hypertrophy, thickening of facial features, carbohydrate intolerance, folic acid deficiency, peripheral neuropathy, vitamin D deficiency, osteomalacia, systemic lupus erythematosus

Concentration-related effects: Nystagmus, blurred vision, diplopia, ataxia, slurred speech, dizziness, drowsiness, lethargy, coma, rash, fever, nausea, vomiting, gum tenderness, confusion, mood changes, folic acid depletion, osteomalacia, hyperglycemia

Related to elevated concentrations:

>20 mcg/mL: Far lateral nystagmus

>30 mcg/mL: 45° lateral gaze nystagmus and ataxia

>40 mcg/mL: Decreased mentation

>100 mcg/mL: Death

Cardiovascular: Hypotension, bradycardia, cardiac arrhythmias, cardiovascular collapse

Central nervous system: Psychiatric changes, slurred speech, dizziness, drowsiness, headache, insomnia

Dermatologic: Rash

Gastrointestinal: Constipation, nausea, vomiting, gingival hyperplasia, enlargement of lips

Hematologic: Leukopenia, thrombocytopenia, agranulocytosis

(Continued)

Phenytoin *(Continued)*

Hepatic: Hepatitis

Local: Thrombophlebitis

Neuromuscular & skeletal: Tremor, peripheral neuropathy, paresthesia

Ocular: Diplopia, nystagmus, blurred vision

Rarely seen effects: SLE-like syndrome, lymphadenopathy, hepatitis, Stevens-Johnson syndrome, blood dyscrasias, dyskinesias, pseudolymphoma, lymphoma, venous irritation and pain, coarsening of the facial features, hypertrichosis

Overdosage/Toxicology

Signs and symptoms: Unsteady gait, slurred speech, confusion, nausea, hypothermia, fever, hypotension, respiratory depression, coma

Treatment: Supportive for hypotension; treat with I.V. fluids and place patient in Trendelenburg position; seizures may be controlled with diazepam 5-10 mg (0.25-0.4 mg/kg in children)

Drug Interactions
CYP2C9 and 2C19 enzyme substrate; CYP1A2, 2B6, 2C8, 2C9, 2C18, 2C19, 3A3/4, and 3A5-7 enzyme inducer

Acetaminophen: Phenytoin may enhance the hepatotoxic potential of acetaminophen overdoses

Acetazolamide: Concurrent use with phenytoin may result in an increased risk of osteomalacia

Acyclovir: May decrease phenytoin serum levels; limited documentation; monitor

Allopurinol: May increase phenytoin serum concentrations; monitor

Antacids: May decrease absorption of phenytoin; separate oral doses by several hours

Antiarrhythmics: Phenytoin may increase the metabolism of antiarrhythmics, decreasing their clinical effect; includes disopyramide, propafenone, and quinidine; amiodarone also may increase phenytoin concentrations (see CYP inhibitors)

Anticonvulsants: Phenytoin may increase the metabolism of anticonvulsants; includes barbiturates, carbamazepine, ethosuximide, felbamate, lamotrigine, tiagabine, topiramate, and zonisamide; does not appear to affect gabapentin or levetiracetam; felbamate and gabapentin may increase phenytoin levels; monitor

Antineoplastics: Several chemotherapeutic agents have been associated with a decrease in serum phenytoin levels; includes cisplatin, bleomycin, carmustine, methotrexate, and vinblastine; monitor phenytoin serum levels. Limited evidence also suggest that enzyme-inducing anticonvulsant therapy may reduce the effectiveness of some chemotherapy regimens (specifically in ALL). Teniposide and methotrexate may be cleared more rapidly in these patients.

Antipsychotics: Phenytoin may enhance the metabolism (decrease the efficacy) of antipsychotics; monitor for altered response; dose adjustment may be needed; also see note on clozapine

Benzodiazepines: Phenytoin may decrease the serum concentrations of some benzodiazepines; monitor for decreased benzodiazepine effect

Beta-blockers: Metabolism of beta-blockers may be increased and clinical effect decreased; atenolol and nadolol are unlikely to interact given their renal elimination

Calcium channel blockers: Phenytoin may enhance the metabolism of calcium channel blockers, decreasing their clinical effect; nifedipine has been reported to increase phenytoin levels (case report); monitor

Capecitabine: May increase the serum concentrations of phenytoin; monitor

Chloramphenicol: Phenytoin may increase the metabolism of chloramphenicol and chloramphenicol may inhibit phenytoin metabolism; monitor for altered response

Ciprofloxacin: Case reports indicate ciprofloxacin may increase or decrease serum phenytoin concentrations; monitor

Clozapine: May decrease phenytoin serum concentrations; monitor

CNS depressants: Sedative effects may be additive with other CNS depressants; monitor for increased effect; includes ethanol, barbiturates, sedatives, antidepressants, narcotic analgesics, and benzodiazepines

Corticosteroids: Phenytoin may increase the metabolism of corticosteroids, decreasing their clinical effect; also see dexamethasone

Cyclosporine and tacrolimus: Levels may be decreased by phenytoin; monitor

CYP2C8/9 inhibitors: Serum levels and/or toxicity of phenytoin may be increased; inhibitors include amiodarone, cimetidine, fluvoxamine, some NSAIDs, metronidazole, ritonavir, sulfonamides, troglitazone, valproic acid, and zafirlukast; monitor for increased effect/toxicity

CYP2C19 inhibitors: Serum levels of phenytoin may be increased; inhibitors include cimetidine, felbamate, fluconazole, fluoxetine, fluvoxamine, omeprazole, teniposide, tolbutamide, and troglitazone

Dexamethasone: May decrease serum phenytoin due to increased metabolism; monitor

Digoxin: Effects and/or levels of digitalis glycosides may be decreased by phenytoin

Disulfiram: May increase serum phenytoin concentrations; monitor

Dopamine: Phenytoin (I.V.) may increase the effect of dopamine (enhanced hypotension)

Doxycycline: Phenytoin may enhance the metabolism of doxycycline, decreasing its clinical effect; higher dosages may be required

Estrogens: Phenytoin may increase the metabolism of estrogens, decreasing their clinical effect; monitor

Enzyme inducers: The serum levels of phenytoin may be reduced by barbiturates, carbamazepine, chronic ethanol, dexamethasone, and rifampin

Folic acid: Replacement of folic acid has been reported to increase the metabolism of phenytoin, decreasing its serum concentrations and/or increasing seizures

Furosemide: Diuretic effect may be blunted by phenytoin (mechanism unclear); possibly due to decreased furosemide bioavailability

HMG-CoA reductase inhibitors: Phenytoin may increase the metabolism of these agents, reducing their clinical effect; monitor

Itraconazole: Phenytoin may decrease the effect of itraconazole

Levodopa: Phenytoin may inhibit the anti-Parkinson effect of levodopa

Lithium: Concurrent use of phenytoin and lithium has resulted in lithium intoxication

Methadone: Phenytoin may enhance the metabolism of methadone resulting in methadone withdrawal

Methylphenidate: May increase serum phenytoin concentrations; monitor

Neuromuscular blocking agents: Duration of effect may be decreased by phenytoin

Omeprazole: May increase serum phenytoin concentrations; monitor

Oral contraceptives: Phenytoin may enhance the metabolism of oral contraceptives, decreasing their clinical effect; an alternative method of contraception should be considered

Phenylbutazone: May increase phenytoin concentrations; monitor and adjust dosage

Primidone: Phenytoin enhances the conversion of primidone to phenobarbital resulting in elevated phenobarbital serum concentrations

Quetiapine: Serum concentrations may be substantially reduced by phenytoin, potentially resulting in a loss of efficacy; limited documentation; monitor

SSRIs: May increase phenytoin serum concentrations; fluoxetine and fluvoxamine are known to inhibit metabolism via CYP enzymes; sertraline and paroxetine have also been shown to increase concentrations in some patients; monitor

Sucralfate: May reduce the GI absorption of phenytoin; monitor

Theophylline: Phenytoin may increase metabolism of theophylline derivatives and decrease their clinical effect; theophylline may also increase phenytoin concentrations

Thyroid hormones (including levothyroxine): Phenytoin may alter the metabolism of thyroid hormones, reducing its effect; there is limited documentation of this interaction, but monitoring should be considered

Ticlopidine: May increase serum phenytoin concentrations and/or toxicity; monitor

Tricyclic antidepressants: Phenytoin may increase metabolism of tricyclic antidepressants and decrease their clinical effect; sedative effects may be additive; tricyclics may also increase phenytoin concentrations

(Continued)

Phenytoin *(Continued)*

Topiramate: Phenytoin may decrease serum levels of topiramate; topiramate may increase the effect of phenytoin

Trazodone: Serum levels of phenytoin may be increased; limited documentation; monitor

Trimethoprim: May increase serum phenytoin concentrations; monitor

Valproic acid (and sulfisoxazole): May displace phenytoin from binding sites; valproic acid may increase, decrease, or have no effect on phenytoin serum concentrations

Vigabatrin: May reduce phenytoin serum concentrations; monitor

Warfarin: Phenytoin transiently increased the hypothrombinemia response to warfarin initially; this is followed by an inhibition of the hypoprothrombinemic response

Ethanol/Nutrition/Herb Interactions

Ethanol:

Acute use: Avoid or limit ethanol (inhibits metabolism of phenytoin). Watch for sedation.

Chronic use: Avoid or limit ethanol (stimulates metabolism of phenytoin).

Food: Phenytoin serum concentrations may be altered if taken with food. If taken with enteral nutrition, phenytoin serum concentrations may be decreased. Tube feedings decrease bioavailability; hold tube feedings 2 hours before and 2 hours after phenytoin administration. May decrease calcium, folic acid, and vitamin D levels.

Herb/Nutraceutical: Avoid evening primrose (seizure threshold decreased). Avoid valerian, St John's wort, kava kava, gotu kola (may increase CNS depression).

Stability Phenytoin is stable as long as it remains free of haziness and precipitation. Use only clear solutions; parenteral solution may be used as long as there is no precipitate and it is not hazy, slightly yellowed solution may be used. Refrigeration may cause precipitate, sometimes the precipitate is resolved by allowing the solution to reach room temperature again. Drug may precipitate at a pH <11.5. May dilute with normal saline for I.V. infusion; stability is concentration dependent.

Standard diluent: Dose/100 mL NS

Minimum volume: Concentration should be maintained at 1-10 mg/mL secondary to stability problems (stable for 4 hours)

Comments: Maximum rate of infusion: 50 mg/minute

IVPB dose should be administered via an in-line 0.22-5 micron filter because of high potential for precipitation I.V. form is highly **incompatible** with many drugs and solutions such as dextrose in water, some saline solutions, amikacin, bretylium, cephapirin, dobutamine, heparin, insulin, levorphanol, lidocaine, meperidine, metaraminol, morphine, norepinephrine, potassium chloride, vitamin B complex with C

Mechanism of Action Stabilizes neuronal membranes and decreases seizure activity by increasing efflux or decreasing influx of sodium ions across cell membranes in the motor cortex during generation of nerve impulses; prolongs effective refractory period and suppresses ventricular pacemaker automaticity, shortens action potential in the heart

Pharmacodynamics/Kinetics

Absorption: Oral: Slow

Distribution: V_d:

Neonates:

Premature: 1-1.2 L/kg

Full-term: 0.8-0.9 L/kg

Infants: 0.7-0.8 L/kg

Children: 0.7 L/kg

Adults: 0.6-0.7 L/kg

Protein binding:

Neonates: Up to 20% free

Infants: Up to 15% free

Adults: 90% to 95%

Others: Increased free fraction (decreased protein binding)

Patients with hyperbilirubinemia, hypoalbuminemia, uremia: Refer to the following:

Disease states resulting in a decrease in serum albumin concentration: Burns, hepatic cirrhosis, nephrotic syndrome, pregnancy, cystic fibrosis

Disease states resulting in an apparent decrease in affinity of phenytoin for serum albumin: Renal failure, jaundice (severe), other drugs (displacers), hyperbilirubinemia (total bilirubin >15 mg/dL), Cl_{cr} <25 mL/minute (unbound fraction is increased two- to threefold in uremia)

Metabolism: Follows dose-dependent capacity-limited (Michaelis-Menten) pharmacokinetics with increased V_{max} in infants >6 months of age and children versus adults

Bioavailability: Dependent upon formulation administered

Time to peak serum concentration (dependent upon formulation administered): Oral:

Extended-release capsule: Within 4-12 hours

Immediate release preparation: Within 2-3 hours

Elimination: Highly variable clearance dependent upon intrinsic hepatic function and dose administered; increased clearance and decreased serum concentrations with febrile illness; <5% excreted unchanged in urine; major metabolite (via oxidation) HPPA undergoes enterohepatic recycling and elimination in urine as glucuronides

Usual Dosage

Status epilepticus: I.V.:

Infants and Children: Loading dose: 15-20 mg/kg in a single or divided dose; maintenance dose: Initial: 5 mg/kg/day in 2 divided doses; usual doses:

6 months to 3 years: 8-10 mg/kg/day

4-6 years: 7.5-9 mg/kg/day

7-9 years: 7-8 mg/kg/day

10-16 years: 6-7 mg/kg/day, some patients may require every 8 hours dosing

Adults: Loading dose: Manufacturer recommends 10-15 mg/kg, however 15-25 mg/kg has been used clinically; maintenance dose: 300 mg/day or 5-6 mg/kg/day in 3 divided doses or 1-2 divided doses using extended release

Anticonvulsant: Children and Adults: Oral:

Loading dose: 15-20 mg/kg; based on phenytoin serum concentrations and recent dosing history; administer oral loading dose in 3 divided doses given every 2-4 hours to decrease GI adverse effects and to ensure complete oral absorption; maintenance dose: same as I.V.

Neurosurgery (prophylactic): 100-200 mg at approximately 4-hour intervals during surgery and during the immediate postoperative period

Dosing adjustment/comments in renal impairment or hepatic disease: Safe in usual doses in mild liver disease; clearance may be substantially reduced in cirrhosis and plasma level monitoring with dose adjustment advisable. Free phenytoin levels should be monitored closely.

Dietary Considerations

Folic acid: Phenytoin may decrease mucosal uptake of folic acid; to avoid folic acid deficiency and megaloblastic anemia, some clinicians recommend giving patients on anticonvulsants prophylactic doses of folic acid and cyanocobalamin. However, folate supplementation may increase seizures in some patients (dose dependent). Discuss with healthcare provider prior to using any supplements.

Calcium: Hypocalcemia has been reported in patients taking prolonged high-dose therapy with an anticonvulsant. Some clinicians have given an additional 4000 units/week of vitamin D (especially in those receiving poor nutrition and getting no sun exposure) to prevent hypocalcemia.

(Continued)

Phenytoin (Continued)

Vitamin D: Phenytoin interferes with vitamin D metabolism and osteomalacia may result; may need to supplement with vitamin D

Tube feedings: Tube feedings decrease phenytoin absorption. To avoid decreased serum levels with continuous NG feeds, hold feedings for 2 hours prior to and 2 hours after phenytoin administration, if possible. There is a variety of opinions on how to administer phenytoin with enteral feedings. Be **consistent** throughout therapy.

Administration

Phenytoin may be administered by IVP or IVPB administration

I.M. administration is not recommended due to erratic absorption, pain on injection and precipitation of drug at injection site

S.C. administration is not recommended because of the possibility of local tissue damage

The maximum rate of I.V. administration is 50 mg/minute; highly sensitive patients (eg, elderly, patients with pre-existing cardiovascular conditions) should receive phenytoin more slowly (eg, 20 mg/minute)

An in-line 0.22-5 micron filter is recommended for IVPB solutions due to the high potential for precipitation of the solution; avoid extravasation; following I.V. administration, NS should be injected through the same needle or I.V. catheter to prevent irritation

Monitoring Parameters Blood pressure, vital signs (with I.V. use), plasma phenytoin level, CBC, liver function tests

Reference Range Timing of serum samples: Because it is slowly absorbed, peak blood levels may occur 4-8 hours after ingestion of an oral dose. The serum half-life varies with the dosage and the drug follows Michaelis-Menten kinetics. The average adult half-life is about 24 hours. Steady-state concentrations are reached in 5-10 days.

Children and Adults: Toxicity is measured clinically, and some patients require levels outside the suggested therapeutic range

Therapeutic range:
Total phenytoin: 10-20 µg/mL (children and adults), 8-15 µg/mL (neonates)
Concentrations of 5-10 µg/mL may be therapeutic for some patients but concentrations <5 µg/mL are not likely to be effective
50% of patients show decreased frequency of seizures at concentrations >10 µg/mL
86% of patients show decreased frequency of seizures at concentrations >15 µg/mL
Add another anticonvulsant if satisfactory therapeutic response is not achieved with a phenytoin concentration of 20 µg/mL

Free phenytoin: 1-2.5 µg/mL

Toxic: <30-50 µg/mL (SI: <120-200 µmol/L)

Lethal: >100 µg/mL (SI: >400 µmol/L)

When to draw levels: This is dependent on the disease state being treated and the clinical condition of the patient

Key points:
Slow absorption of extended capsules and prolonged half-life minimize fluctuations between peak and trough concentrations, timing of sampling not crucial

Trough concentrations are generally recommended for routine monitoring. Daily levels are not necessary and may result in incorrect dosage adjustments. If it is determined essential to monitor free phenytoin concentrations, concomitant monitoring of total phenytoin concentrations is not necessary and expensive.

After a loading dose: Draw level within 48-96 hours

Rapid achievement: Draw within 2-3 days of therapy initiation to ensure that the patient's metabolism is not remarkably different from that which would be predicted by average literature-derived pharmacokinetic parameters; early levels should be used cautiously in design of new dosing regimens

Second concentration: Draw within 6-7 days with subsequent doses of phenytoin adjusted accordingly

If plasma concentrations have not changed over a 3- to 5-day period, monitoring interval may be increased to once weekly in the acute clinical setting

In stable patients requiring long-term therapy, generally monitor levels at 3- to 12-month intervals

Adjustment of serum concentration: See tables.

Adjustment of Serum Concentration in Patients With Low Serum Albumin

Measured Total Phenytoin Concentration (mcg/mL)	Patient's Serum Albumin (g/dL)			
	3.5	3	2.5	2
	Adjusted Total Phenytoin Concentration (mcg/mL)*			
5	6	7	8	10
10	13	14	17	20
15	19	21	25	30

*Adjusted concentration = measured total concentration ÷ [(0.2 x albumin) + 0.1].

Adjustment of Serum Concentration in Patients With Renal Failure ($Cl_{cr} \leq 10$ mL/min) (Product Information From Parke-Davis)

Measured Total Phenytoin Concentration (mcg/mL)	Patient's Serum Albumin (g/dL)				
	4	3.5	3	2.5	2
	Adjusted Total Phenytoin Concentration (mcg/mL)*				
5	10	11	13	14	17
10	20	22	25	29	33
15	30	33	38	43	50

*Adjusted concentration = measured total concentration ÷ [(0.1 x albumin) + 0.1].

Test Interactions ↑ glucose, alkaline phosphatase (S); ↓ thyroxine (S), calcium (S)

Patient Information Shake oral suspension well prior to each dose; do not change brand or dosage form without consulting physician; do not skip doses, may cause drowsiness, dizziness, ataxia, loss of coordination or judgment; take with food; maintain good oral hygiene

Nursing Implications Maintenance doses usually start 12 hours after loading dose; shake oral suspension well prior to each dose; do not exceed I.V. infusion rate of 1-3 mg/kg/minute or 50 mg/minute; I.V. injections should be followed by normal saline flushes through the same needle or I.V. catheter to avoid local irritation of the vein; avoid extravasation; avoid I.M. use due to erratic absorption, pain on injection, and precipitation of drug at injection site

Additional Information Sodium content of 1 g injection: 88 mg (3.8 mEq)

Dosage Forms
Capsule, extended, as sodium: 30 mg, 100 mg
Capsule, prompt, as sodium: 100 mg
Injection, as sodium: 50 mg/mL (2 mL, 5 mL)
(Continued)

Phenytoin *(Continued)*

Suspension, oral: 125 mg/5 mL (5 mL, 240 mL)

Tablet, chewable: 50 mg

♦ **Phenytoin Sodium** *see* Phenytoin *on page 308*

♦ **Phenytoin Sodium, Extended** *see* Phenytoin *on page 308*

♦ **Phenytoin Sodium, Prompt** *see* Phenytoin *on page 308*

♦ **Phrenilin®** *see* Butalbital Compound *on page 59*

♦ **Phrenilin® Forte** *see* Butalbital Compound *on page 59*

Pimozide *(PI moe zide)*

Related Information

Antipsychotic Agents Comparison Chart *on page 557*

Antipsychotic Medication Guidelines *on page 559*

Discontinuation of Psychotropic Drugs - Withdrawal Symptoms and Recommendations *on page 582*

Patient Information - Antipsychotics (General) *on page 466*

U.S. Brand Names Orap™

Canadian Brand Names Orap

Pharmacologic Category Antipsychotic Agent, Diphenylbutylpiperidine

Generic Available No

Use Suppression of severe motor and phonic tics in patients with Tourette's disorder who have failed to respond satisfactorily to standard treatment

Unlabeled/Investigational Use Psychosis; reported use in individuals with delusions focused on physical symptoms (ie, preoccupation with parasitic infestation); Huntington's chorea

Pregnancy Risk Factor C

Contraindications Hypersensitivity to pimozide or any component of the formulation; severe CNS depression; coma; history of dysrhythmia; prolonged QT syndrome; concurrent use of drugs that are inhibitors of CYP3A3/4, including concurrent use of azole antifungals, macrolide antibiotics (such as clarithromycin or erythromycin), mesoridazine, nefazodone, protease inhibitors (ie, indinavir, nelfinavir, ritonavir, saquinavir), thioridazine, zileuton, and ziprasidone; simple tics other than Tourette's

Warnings/Precautions May cause hypotension, use with caution in patients with autonomic instability. Moderately sedating, use with caution in disorders where CNS depression is a feature. Use with caution in Parkinson's disease. Caution in patients with hemodynamic instability; bone marrow suppression; predisposition to seizures; subcortical brain damage; severe cardiac, hepatic, renal, or respiratory disease. Esophageal dysmotility and aspiration have been associated with antipsychotic use - use with caution in patients at risk of pneumonia (ie, Alzheimer's disease). Caution in breast cancer or other prolactin-dependent tumors (may elevate prolactin levels). May alter temperature regulation or mask toxicity of other drugs due to antiemetic effects. May alter cardiac conduction - sudden unexplained deaths have occurred in patients taking high doses (>10 mg). This may be due to prolongation of the QT interval predisposing patients to ventricular arrhythmias. May cause orthostatic hypotension - use with caution in patients at risk of this effect or those who would tolerate transient hypotensive episodes (cerebrovascular disease, cardiovascular disease, or other medications which may predispose).

May cause anticholinergic effects (confusion, agitation, constipation, dry mouth, blurred vision, urinary retention); therefore, they should be used with caution in patients with decreased gastrointestinal motility, urinary retention, BPH, xerostomia, or visual problems. Conditions which also may be exacerbated by cholinergic blockade include narrow-angle glaucoma (screening is recommended) and worsening of myasthenia gravis. Relative to neuroleptics, pimozide has a moderate potency of cholinergic blockade.

May cause extrapyramidal reactions, including pseudoparkinsonism, acute dystonic reactions, akathisia, and tardive dyskinesia (risk of these reactions is high relative to other neuroleptics). May be associated with neuroleptic malignant syndrome (NMS) or pigmentary retinopathy.

Avoid grapefruit juice due to potential inhibition of pimozide metabolism

Adverse Reactions Frequency not defined.

Cardiovascular: Facial edema, tachycardia, orthostatic hypotension, chest pain, hypertension, palpitations, ventricular arrhythmias, QT prolongation

Central nervous system: Extrapyramidal symptoms (akathisia, akinesia, dystonia, pseudoparkinsonism, tardive dyskinesia), drowsiness, NMS, headache, dizziness, excitement

Dermatologic: Rash

Endocrine & metabolic: Edema of breasts, decreased libido

Gastrointestinal: Constipation, xerostomia, weight gain/loss, nausea, salivation, vomiting, anorexia

Genitourinary: Impotence

Hematologic: Blood dyscrasias

Hepatic: Jaundice

Neuromuscular & skeletal: Weakness, tremor

Ocular: Visual disturbance, decreased accommodation, blurred vision

Miscellaneous: Diaphoresis

Overdosage/Toxicology

Signs and symptoms: Hypotension, respiratory depression, EKG abnormalities, extrapyramidal symptoms

Treatment: Following attempts at decontamination, treatment is supportive and symptomatic. Seizures can be treated with diazepam, phenytoin, or phenobarbital.

Drug Interactions CYP3A3/4 enzyme substrate; CYP1A2 (minor)

Aluminum salts: May decrease the absorption of antipsychotics; monitor

Amphetamines: Efficacy may be diminished by antipsychotics; in addition, amphetamines may increase psychotic symptoms; avoid concurrent use

Anticholinergics: May inhibit the therapeutic response to antipsychotics and excess anticholinergic effects may occur; includes benztropine, trihexyphenidyl, biperiden, and drugs with significant anticholinergic activity (TCAs, antihistamines, disopyramide)

Antihypertensives: Concurrent use of antipsychotics with an antihypertensive may produce additive hypotensive effects (particularly orthostasis)

Bromocriptine: Antipsychotics inhibit the ability of bromocriptine to lower serum prolactin concentrations

CNS depressants: Sedative effects may be additive with antipsychotics; monitor for increased effect; includes barbiturates, benzodiazepines, narcotic analgesics, ethanol, and other sedative agents

CYP3A3/4 inhibitors: Serum level and/or toxicity of some benzodiazepines may be increased; inhibitors include amiodarone, cimetidine, clarithromycin, erythromycin, delavirdine, diltiazem, dirithromycin, disulfiram, fluoxetine, fluvoxamine, grapefruit juice, indinavir, itraconazole, ketoconazole, metronidazole, nefazodone, nevirapine, propoxyphene, quinupristin-dalfopristin, ritonavir, saquinavir, verapamil, zafirlukast, zileuton. May cause life-threatening arrhythmias; avoid these combinations.

Enzyme inducers: May enhance the hepatic metabolism of antipsychotics; larger doses may be required; includes rifampin, rifabutin, barbiturates, phenytoin, and cigarette smoking

Epinephrine: Chlorpromazine (and possibly other low potency antipsychotics) may diminish the pressor effects of epinephrine

Guanethidine and guanadrel: Antihypertensive effects may be inhibited by antipsychotics

Levodopa: Antipsychotics may inhibit the antiparkinsonian effect of levodopa; avoid this combination

Lithium: Antipsychotics may produce neurotoxicity with lithium; this is a rare effect

(Continued)

Pimozide *(Continued)*

Phenytoin: May reduce serum levels of antipsychotics; antipsychotics may increase phenytoin serum levels

Propranolol: Serum concentrations of antipsychotics may be increased; propranolol also increases antipsychotics concentrations

QT_c-prolonging agents: Effects on QT_c interval may be additive with antipsychotics, increasing the risk of malignant arrhythmias; includes type Ia antiarrhythmics, tricyclic antidepressants, and some quinolone antibiotics (sparfloxacin, moxifloxacin, and gatifloxacin)

Sulfadoxine-pyrimethamine: May increase antipsychotics concentrations

Tricyclic antidepressants: Concurrent use may produce increased toxicity or altered therapeutic response (also see note under QT_c prolonging agents)

Trazodone: Antipsychotics and trazodone may produce additive hypotensive effects

Valproic acid: Serum levels may be increased by antipsychotics

Ethanol/Nutrition/Herb Interactions

Food: Pimozide serum concentration may be increased when taken with grapefruit juice; avoid concurrent use.

Ethanol: Avoid ethanol (may increase CNS depression).

Herb/Nutraceutical: St John's wort may decrease pimozide levels. Avoid kava kava, gotu kola, valerian, St John's wort (may increase CNS depression).

Mechanism of Action A potent centrally-acting dopamine-receptor antagonist resulting in its characteristic neuroleptic effects

Pharmacodynamics/Kinetics

Absorption: Oral: 50%

Protein binding: 99%

Metabolism: In the liver with significant first-pass decay

Half-life: 50 hours

Time to peak serum concentration: Within 6-8 hours

Elimination: In urine

Usual Dosage Oral:

Children ≤12 years: Tourette's disorder: Initial: 1-2 mg/day in divided doses; usual range: 2-4 mg/day; do not exceed 10 mg/day (0.2 mg/kg/day)

Children >12 years and Adults: Tourette's disorder: Initial: 1-2 mg/day in divided doses, then increase dosage as needed every other day; range is usually 7-16 mg/day, maximum dose: 20 mg/day or 0.3 mg/kg/day should not be exceeded.

Note: Sudden unexpected deaths have occurred in patients taking doses >10 mg. Therefore, dosages exceeding 10 mg/day are generally not recommended.

Dosing adjustment in hepatic impairment: Reduction of dose is necessary in patients with liver disease

Child/Adolescent Considerations Twenty-two children 7-16 years of age with Tourette's disorder were treated with a mean dose of 3.4 mg/day (Sallee, 1997). Twenty-four patients with Tourette's disorder were treated with 2.9 mg/day (Bruggeman, 2001).

Test Interactions ↑ prolactin (S)

Patient Information Treatment with pimozide exposes the patient to serious risks; a decision to use pimozide chronically in Tourette's disorder is one that deserves full consideration by the patient (or patient's family) as well as by the treating physician. Because the goal of treatment is symptomatic improvement, the patient's view of the need for treatment and assessment of response are critical in evaluating the impact of therapy and weighing its benefits against the risks.

Nursing Implications Perform EKG at baseline and periodically thereafter, and with dose increases; refer to Contraindications for medicines which may predispose patients to fatal cardiac arrhythmias

Additional Information Less sedation but pimozide is more likely to cause acute extrapyramidal symptoms than chlorpromazine.

Dosage Forms Tablet: 1 mg, 2 mg

Pindolol (PIN doe lole)

U.S. Brand Names Visken®

Canadian Brand Names Apo®-Pindol; Gen-Pindolol®; Novo-Pindol®; Nu-Pindol®; Syn-Pindol®

Pharmacologic Category Beta Blocker (with Intrinsic Sympathomimetic Activity)

Generic Available Yes

Use Management of hypertension

Unlabeled/Investigational Use Potential augmenting agent for antidepressants; ventricular arrhythmias/tachycardia, antipsychotic-induced akathisia, situational anxiety; aggressive behavior associated with dementia

Pregnancy Risk Factor B

Contraindications Hypersensitivity to pindolol, beta-blockers, or any component of the formulation; uncompensated congestive heart failure; cardiogenic shock; bradycardia, sinus node dysfunction, or heart block (2nd or 3rd degree) except in patients with a functioning artificial pacemaker; pulmonary edema; severe hyperactive airway disease (asthma or COPD); Raynaud's disease

Warnings/Precautions Administer very cautiously to patients with CHF, asthma, diabetes mellitus, hyperthyroidism. May mask signs and symptoms of thyrotoxicosis. Abrupt withdrawal of the drug should be avoided, drug should be discontinued over 1-2 weeks. Do not use in pregnant or nursing women. May potentiate hypoglycemia in a diabetic patient and mask signs and symptoms. Use with caution in patients with myasthenia gravis or peripheral vascular disease. May cause CNS depression; use caution in patients with a history of psychiatric illness. May potentiate anaphylactic reactions and/or blunt response to epinephrine treatment. Beta-blockers with intrinsic sympathomimetic activity (including pindolol) do not appear to be of benefit in congestive heart failure.

Adverse Reactions

1% to 10%:

Cardiovascular: Chest pain (3%), edema (6%)

Central nervous system: Nightmares/vivid dreams (5%), dizziness (9%), insomnia (10%), fatigue (8%), nervousness (7%), anxiety (<2%)

Dermatologic: Rash, itching (4%)

Gastrointestinal: Nausea (5%), abdominal discomfort (4%)

Neuromuscular & skeletal: Weakness (4%), paresthesia (3%), arthralgia (7%), muscle pain (10%)

Respiratory: Dyspnea (5%)

<1%: Bradycardia, CHF, claudication, confusion, dry eyes, hallucinations, hypotension, impotence, mental depression, palpitations, thrombocytopenia, wheezing

Overdosage/Toxicology

Signs and symptoms: Cardiac disturbances, CNS toxicity, bronchospasm, hypoglycemia and hyperkalemia. The most common cardiac symptoms include hypotension and bradycardia; atrioventricular block, intraventricular conduction disturbances, cardiogenic shock, and asystole may occur with severe overdose, especially with membrane-depressant drugs (eg, propranolol); CNS effects include convulsions, coma, and respiratory arrest is commonly seen with propranolol and other membrane-depressant and lipid-soluble drugs.

Treatment: Includes symptomatic treatment of seizures, hypotension, hyperkalemia and hypoglycemia; bradycardia and hypotension resistant to atropine, isoproterenol or pacing may respond to glucagon; wide QRS defects caused by the membrane-depressant poisoning may respond to hypertonic sodium bicarbonate; repeat-dose charcoal, hemoperfusion, or hemodialysis may be helpful in removal of only those beta-blockers with a small V_d, long half-life or low intrinsic clearance (acebutolol, atenolol, nadolol, sotalol).

Drug Interactions CYP2D6 enzyme substrate

Albuterol (and other beta$_2$ agonists): Effects may be blunted by nonspecific beta-blockers

Alpha-blockers (prazosin, terazosin): Concurrent use of beta-blockers may increase risk of orthostasis

(Continued)

Pindolol *(Continued)*

Calcium channel blockers (diltiazem, verapamil): May have synergistic or additive pharmacological effects when taken concurrently with beta-blockers

Clonidine: Hypertensive crisis after or during withdrawal of either agent

CYP2D6 inhibitors: Serum levels and/or toxicity of some beta-blockers may be increased; inhibitors include amiodarone, cimetidine, delavirdine, fluoxetine, paroxetine, propafenone, quinidine, and ritonavir; monitor for increased effect/toxicity

Drugs which slow AV conduction (digoxin): Effects may be additive with beta-blockers

Epinephrine (including local anesthetics with epinephrine): Pindolol may cause hypertension

Glucagon: Pindolol may blunt the hyperglycemic action

Insulin and oral hypoglycemics: May mask symptoms of hypoglycemia

NSAIDs (ibuprofen, indomethacin, naproxen, piroxicam): May reduce the antihypertensive effects of beta-blockers

Salicylates: May reduce the antihypertensive effects of beta-blockers

Sulfonylureas: Beta-blockers may alter response to hypoglycemic agents

Ethanol/Nutrition/Herb Interactions Herb/Nutraceutical: Avoid dong quai if using for hypertension (has estrogenic activity). Avoid ephedra, yohimbe, ginseng (may worsen hypertension).

Stability Protect from light

Mechanism of Action Blocks both beta$_1$- and beta$_2$-receptors and has mild intrinsic sympathomimetic activity; pindolol has negative inotropic and chronotropic effects and can significantly slow AV nodal conduction. Augmentative action of antidepressants thought to be mediated via a serotonin 1A autoreceptor antagonism.

Pharmacodynamics/Kinetics

Absorption: Oral: Rapid, 50% to 95%

Protein binding: 50%

Metabolism: In the liver (60% to 65%) to conjugates

Half-life: 2.5-4 hours; increased with renal insufficiency, age, and cirrhosis

Time to peak serum concentration: Within 1-2 hours

Elimination: In urine (35% to 50% unchanged drug)

Usual Dosage Oral:

Adults:

Hypertension: Initial: 5 mg twice daily, increase as necessary by 10 mg/day every 3-4 weeks; maximum daily dose: 60 mg

Antidepressant augmentation: 2.5 mg 3 times/day

Elderly: Initial: 5 mg once daily, increase as necessary by 5 mg/day every 3-4 weeks

Dosing adjustment in renal and hepatic impairment: Reduction is necessary in severely impaired

Dietary Considerations May be administered without regard to meals.

Monitoring Parameters Blood pressure, standing and sitting/supine, pulse, respiratory function

Patient Information Adhere to dosage regimen; watch for postural hypotension; abrupt withdrawal of the drug should be avoided; take at the same time each day; may mask diabetes symptoms; do not discontinue medication abruptly; consult pharmacist or physician before taking over-the-counter cold preparations

Nursing Implications Evaluate blood pressure, apical and radial pulses; do not discontinue abruptly

Dosage Forms Tablet: 5 mg, 10 mg

♦ **PIO** see Pemoline on page 287

♦ **Piper methysticum** see Kava on page 186

♦ **Placidyl®** see Ethchlorvynol on page 137

♦ **PMS-Amantadine (Can)** see Amantadine on page 19

- **PMS-Benztropine (Can)** *see* Benztropine *on page 45*
- **PMS-Carbamazepine (Can)** *see* Carbamazepine *on page 61*
- **PMS-Chloral Hydrate (Can)** *see* Chloral Hydrate *on page 69*
- **PMS-Clonazepam (Can)** *see* Clonazepam *on page 85*
- **PMS-Cyproheptadine (Can)** *see* Cyproheptadine *on page 97*
- **PMS-Desipramine (Can)** *see* Desipramine *on page 101*
- **PMS-Diazepam (Can)** *see* Diazepam *on page 110*
- **PMS-Flupam (Can)** *see* Flurazepam *on page 155*
- **PMS-Fluphenazine [Hydrochloride] (Can)** *see* Fluphenazine *on page 151*
- **PMS-Hydroxyzine (Can)** *see* Hydroxyzine *on page 178*
- **PMS-Imipramine (Can)** *see* Imipramine *on page 180*
- **PMS-Levothyroxine Sodium (Can)** *see* Levothyroxine *on page 198*
- **PMS-Lorazepam (Can)** *see* Lorazepam *on page 209*
- **PMS-Methylphenidate (Can)** *see* Methylphenidate *on page 236*
- **PMS-Oxazepam (Can)** *see* Oxazepam *on page 276*
- **PMS-Perphenazine (Can)** *see* Perphenazine *on page 295*
- **PMS-Prochlorperazine (Can)** *see* Prochlorperazine *on page 328*
- **PMS-Procyclidine (Can)** *see* Procyclidine *on page 332*
- **PMS-Thioridazine (Can)** *see* Thioridazine *on page 393*
- **PMS-Trihexyphenidyl (Can)** *see* Trihexyphenidyl *on page 418*

Polygonum multiflorum
Pharmacologic Category Herb
Use Tuberous root (raw or processed) used for vertigo, insomnia, constipation
Adverse Reactions
    Cardiovascular: Palpitations
    Central nervous system: Dizziness, fever
    Dermatologic: Erythema, rash, pruritus
    Gastrointestinal: Nausea, diarrhea
    Hepatic: Hepatitis, jaundice
    Ocular: Blurred vision
    Respiratory: Tachypnea
Overdosage/Toxicology Treatment: Supportive therapy; hepatitis can resolve within 3 weeks upon discontinuation of drug; antihistamines can be used for pruritus
Drug Interactions
    Hypoglycemic agents: Effects may be altered; monitor glucose
    Digoxin: Herb may promote hypokalemia, increasing risk of toxicity
Additional Information A climbing evergreen plant native in Japan

- **Poor Mans Treacle** *see* Garlic *on page 166*
- **Poptillo** *see* Ephedra *on page 131*
- **P. quinquefolium L.** *see* Ginseng *on page 168*

Pramipexole *(pra mi PEX ole)*
Related Information
    Patient Information - Miscellaneous Medications *on page 495*
U.S. Brand Names Mirapex®
Canadian Brand Names Mirapex
Pharmacologic Category Anti-Parkinson's Agent (Dopamine Agonist)
Generic Available No
Use Treatment of the signs and symptoms of idiopathic Parkinson's disease
Unlabeled/Investigational Use Treatment of depression
Pregnancy Risk Factor C
Contraindications Hypersensitivity to pramipexole or any component of the formulation
(Continued)

321

Pramipexole *(Continued)*

Warnings/Precautions Caution should be taken in patients with renal insufficiency and in patients with pre-existing dyskinesias. May cause orthostatic hypotension; Parkinson's disease patients appear to have an impaired capacity to respond to a postural challenge. Use with caution in patients at risk of hypotension (such as those receiving antihypertensive drugs) or where transient hypotensive episodes would be poorly tolerated (cardiovascular disease or cerebrovascular disease). Parkinson's patients being treated with dopaminergic agonists ordinarily require careful monitoring for signs and symptoms of postural hypotension, especially during dose escalation, and should be informed of this risk. May cause hallucinations, particularly in older patients. Pathologic degenerative changes were observed in the retinas of albino rats during studies with this agent, but were not observed in the retinas of pigmented rats or in other species. The significance of these data for humans remains uncertain.

Although not reported for pramipexole, other dopaminergic agents have been associated with a syndrome resembling neuroleptic malignant syndrome on withdrawal or significant dosage reduction after long-term use. Dopaminergic agents from the ergot class have also been associated with fibrotic complications, such as retroperitoneum, lungs, and pleura.

Pramipexole has been associated with somnolence, particularly at higher dosages (>1.5 mg/day). In addition, patients have been reported to fall asleep during activities of daily living, including driving, while taking this medication. Whether these patients exhibited somnolence prior to these events is not clear. Patients should be advised of this issue and factors which may increase risk (sleep disorders, other sedating medications, or concomitant medications which increase pramipexole concentrations) and instructed to report daytime somnolence or sleepiness to the prescriber. Patients should use caution in performing activities which require alertness (driving or operating machinery), and to avoid other medications which may cause CNS depression, including ethanol.

Adverse Reactions
>10%:
  Cardiovascular: Postural hypotension
  Central nervous system: Asthenia, dizziness, somnolence, insomnia, hallucinations, abnormal dreams
  Gastrointestinal: Nausea, constipation
  Neuromuscular & skeletal: Weakness, dyskinesia, EPS
1% to 10%:
  Cardiovascular: Edema, postural hypotension, syncope, tachycardia, chest pain
  Central nervous system: Malaise, confusion, amnesia, dystonias, akathisia, thinking abnormalities, myoclonus, hyperesthesia, gait abnormalities, hypertonia, paranoia
  Endocrine & metabolic: Decreased libido
  Gastrointestinal: Anorexia, weight loss, xerostomia
  Genitourinary: Urinary frequency (up to 6%), impotence
  Neuromuscular & skeletal: Muscle twitching, leg cramps, arthritis, bursitis
  Ocular: Vision abnormalities (3%)
  Respiratory: Dyspnea, rhinitis
<1%: Elevated liver transaminase levels
Percentage unknown, dose related: Falling asleep during activities of daily living

Drug Interactions
  Antipsychotics: May decrease the efficiency of pramipexole due to dopamine antagonism
  Cationic drugs: Drugs secreted by the cationic transport system (diltiazem, triamterene, verapamil, quinidine, quinine, ranitidine) decrease the clearance of pramipexole by ~20%
  Cimetidine: May increase serum concentrations; cimetidine in combination with pramipexole produced a 50% increase in AUC and a 40% increase in half-life

Metoclopramide: May decrease the efficiency of pramipexole due to dopamine antagonism

Ethanol/Nutrition/Herb Interactions
Ethanol: Avoid ethanol (may increase CNS depression).
Food: Food intake does not affect the extent of drug absorption, although the time to maximal plasma concentration is delayed by 60 minutes when taken with a meal.
Herb/Nutraceutical: Avoid valerian, St John's wort, SAMe, kava kava (may increase risk of serotonin syndrome and/or excessive sedation).

Mechanism of Action Pramipexole is a nonergot dopamine agonist with specificity for the D_2 subfamily dopamine receptor, and has also been shown to bind to D_3 and D_4 receptors. By binding to these receptors, it is thought that pramipexole can stimulate dopamine activity on the nerves of the striatum and substantia nigra.

Pharmacodynamics/Kinetics
Protein binding: 15%
Bioavailability: 90%
Half-life: ~8 hours (12-14 hours in the elderly)
Time to peak serum concentration: Within 2 hours
Elimination: Urine, 90% recovered as unmetabolized drug

Usual Dosage Adults: Oral: Initial: 0.375 mg/day given in 3 divided doses, increase gradually by 0.125 mg/dose every 5-7 days; range: 1.5-4.5 mg/day

Administration Doses should be titrated gradually in all patients to avoid the onset of intolerable side effects. The dosage should be increased to achieve a maximum therapeutic effect, balanced against the side effects of dyskinesia, hallucinations, somnolence, and dry mouth.

Monitoring Parameters Monitor for improvement in symptoms of Parkinson's disease (eg, mentation, behavior, daily living activities, motor examinations), blood pressure, body weight changes, and heart rate

Patient Information Ask your physician or pharmacist before taking any other medicine, including over-the-counter products; especially important are other medicines that could make you sleepy such as sleeping pills, tranquilizers, some cold and allergy medicines, narcotic pain killers, or medicines that relax muscles. Avoid alcohol. Use caution in performing activities that require alertness (driving or operating machinery); can cause significant drowsiness.

Dosage Forms Tablet: 0.125 mg, 0.25 mg, 0.5 mg, 1 mg, 1.5 mg

Prazepam (PRA ze pam)

Related Information
Benzodiazepines Comparison Chart *on page 566*
Federal OBRA Regulations Recommended Maximum Doses *on page 583*
Patient Information - Anxiolytics & Sedative Hypnotics (Benzodiazepines) *on page 483*

Pharmacologic Category Benzodiazepine

Generic Available Yes

Use Treatment of anxiety

Unlabeled/Investigational Use Alcohol withdrawal; duodenal ulcer; narcotic addiction; spasticity; partial seizures

Pregnancy Risk Factor D

Contraindications Hypersensitivity to prazepam or any component of the formulation (cross-sensitivity with other benzodiazepines may exist); narrow-angle glaucoma; pregnancy

Warnings/Precautions Use with caution in elderly or debilitated patients, patients with hepatic disease (including alcoholics), or renal impairment. Use with caution in patients with respiratory disease, or impaired gag reflex. Avoid use in patients with sleep apnea.

Causes CNS depression (dose-related) resulting in sedation, dizziness, confusion, or ataxia which may impair physical and mental capabilities. Patients must be cautioned about performing tasks which require mental alertness (operating
(Continued)

Prazepam *(Continued)*

machinery or driving). Use with caution in patients receiving other CNS depressants or psychoactive agents. Effects with other sedative drugs or ethanol may be potentiated. Benzodiazepines have been associated with falls and traumatic injury and should be used with extreme caution in patients who are at risk of these events (especially the elderly).

Use caution in patients with depression, particularly if suicidal risk may be present. Use with caution in patients with a history of drug dependence. Benzodiazepines have been associated with dependence and acute withdrawal symptoms on discontinuation or reduction in dose. Acute withdrawal, including seizures, may be precipitated after administration of flumazenil to patients receiving long-term benzodiazepine therapy.

Benzodiazepines have been associated with anterograde amnesia. Paradoxical reactions, including hyperactive or aggressive behavior have been reported with benzodiazepines, particularly in adolescent/pediatric or psychiatric patients. Does not have analgesic, antidepressant, or antipsychotic properties.

Adverse Reactions
Cardiovascular: Hypotension

Central nervous system: Drowsiness, fatigue, impaired coordination, lightheadedness, memory impairment, insomnia, depression, headache, anxiety, confusion, nervousness, syncope, dizziness, akathisia, drowsiness, ataxia, lightheadedness, vivid dreams

Dermatologic: Rash, pruritus

Endocrine & metabolic: Decreased libido, menstrual irregularities

Gastrointestinal: Xerostomia, constipation, diarrhea, decreased salivation, nausea, vomiting, increased or decreased appetite, increased salivation, weight gain/loss

Hematologic: Blood dyscrasias

Neuromuscular & skeletal: Dysarthria, tremor, muscle cramps, rigidity, weakness, reflex slowing

Ocular: Blurred vision, increased lenticular pressure

Otic: Tinnitus

Respiratory: Nasal congestion, hyperventilation

Miscellaneous: Diaphoresis, drug dependence

Overdosage/Toxicology
Signs and symptoms: Somnolence, confusion, coma, hypoactive reflexes, dyspnea, hypotension, slurred speech, impaired coordination

Treatment: Treatment for benzodiazepine overdose is supportive. Rarely is mechanical ventilation required. Flumazenil has been shown to selectively block the binding of benzodiazepines to CNS receptors, resulting in a reversal of benzodiazepine-induced CNS depression, but not respiratory depression

Drug Interactions
CNS depressants: Sedative effects and/or respiratory depression may be additive with CNS depressants; includes ethanol, barbiturates, narcotic analgesics, and other sedative agents; monitor for increased effect

CYP inhibitors: May increase serum levels/toxicity of prazepam; includes cimetidine, ciprofloxacin, clarithromycin, clozapine, CNS depressants, diltiazem, disulfiram, digoxin, erythromycin, ethanol, fluconazole, fluoxetine, fluvoxamine, grapefruit juice, isoniazid, itraconazole, ketoconazole, labetalol, levodopa, loxapine, metoprolol, metronidazole, miconazole, nefazodone, omeprazole, troleandomycin, valproic acid, verapamil; monitor for altered benzodiazepine response

Enzyme inducers: Metabolism of some benzodiazepines may be increased, decreasing their therapeutic effect; consider using an alternative sedative/hypnotic agent; potential inducers include phenobarbital, phenytoin, carbamazepine, rifampin, and rifabutin

Oral contraceptives: May decrease the clearance of some benzodiazepines (those which undergo oxidative metabolism); monitor for increased benzodiazepine effect

Theophylline: May partially antagonize some of the effects of benzodiazepines; monitor for decreased response; may require higher doses for sedation

Ethanol/Nutrition/Herb Interactions

Ethanol: Avoid ethanol (may increase CNS depression).

Herb/Nutraceutical: Avoid valerian, St John's wort, kava kava, gotu kola (may increase CNS depression).

Mechanism of Action Binds to stereospecific benzodiazepine receptors on the postsynaptic GABA neuron at several sites within the central nervous system, including the limbic system, reticular formation. Enhancement of the inhibitory effect of GABA on neuronal excitability results by increased neuronal membrane permeability to chloride ions. This shift in chloride ions results in hyperpolarization (a less excitable state) and stabilization.

Pharmacodynamics/Kinetics

Peak action: Within 6 hours

Duration: 48 hours

Metabolism: First-pass hepatic metabolism

Half-life:

Parent drug: 78 minutes

Desmethyldiazepam: 30-100 hours

Elimination: Renal excretion of unchanged drug and primarily N-desmethyldiazepam (active)

Usual Dosage Adults: Oral: 30 mg/day in divided doses, may increase gradually to a maximum of 60 mg/day

Monitoring Parameters Respiratory and cardiovascular status

Patient Information Avoid alcohol and other CNS depressants; avoid activities needing good psychomotor coordination until CNS effects are known; drug may cause physical or psychological dependence; avoid abrupt discontinuation after prolonged use

Additional Information Prazepam offers no significant advantage over other benzodiazepines.

Dosage Forms

Capsule: 5 mg, 10 mg, 20 mg

Tablet: 5 mg, 10 mg

♦ **Prelu-2**® *see* Phendimetrazine *on page 298*

♦ **Pre-Sed**® *see* Hexobarbital *on page 176*

♦ **Primaclone** *see* Primidone *on page 325*

Primidone (PRI mi done)

Related Information

Patient Information - Anxiolytics & Sedative Hypnotics (Barbiturates) *on page 485*

U.S. Brand Names Mysoline®

Canadian Brand Names Apo®-Primidone; Sertan®

Synonyms Desoxyphenobarbital; Primaclone

Pharmacologic Category Anticonvulsant, Miscellaneous; Barbiturate

Generic Available Yes: Tablet

Use Management of grand mal, psychomotor, and focal seizures

Unlabeled/Investigational Use Benign familial tremor (essential tremor)

Pregnancy Risk Factor D

Pregnancy/Breast-Feeding Implications

Clinical effects on the fetus: Crosses the placenta. Dysmorphic facial features; hemorrhagic disease of newborn due to fetal vitamin K depletion, maternal folic acid deficiency may occur. Epilepsy itself, number of medications, genetic factors, or a combination of these probably influence the teratogenicity of anticonvulsant therapy. Benefit:risk ratio usually favors continued use during pregnancy and breast-feeding.

Breast-feeding/lactation: Crosses into breast milk

(Continued)

Primidone (Continued)

Clinical effects on the infant: Sedation; feeding problems reported. AAP recommends USE WITH CAUTION.

Contraindications Hypersensitivity to primidone, phenobarbital, or any component of the formulation; porphyria; pregnancy

Warnings/Precautions Use with caution in patients with renal or hepatic impairment, pulmonary insufficiency; abrupt withdrawal may precipitate status epilepticus. Potential for drug dependency exists. Do not administer to patients in acute pain. Use caution in elderly, debilitated, or pediatric patients - may cause paradoxical responses. May cause CNS depression, which may impair physical or mental abilities. Patients must cautioned about performing tasks which require mental alertness (ie, operating machinery or driving). Effects with other sedative drugs or ethanol may be potentiated. Use with caution in patients with depression or suicidal tendencies, or in patients with a history of drug abuse. Tolerance or psychological and physical dependence may occur with prolonged use. Primidone's metabolite, phenobarbital, has been associated with cognitive deficits in children. Use with caution in patients with hypoadrenalism.

Adverse Reactions

Central nervous system: Drowsiness, vertigo, ataxia, lethargy, behavior change, fatigue, hyperirritability

Dermatologic: Rash

Gastrointestinal: Nausea, vomiting, anorexia

Genitourinary: Impotence

Hematologic: Agranulocytopenia, agranulocytosis, anemia

Ocular: Diplopia, nystagmus

Overdosage/Toxicology

Signs and symptoms: Unsteady gait, slurred speech, confusion, jaundice, hypothermia, fever, hypotension, coma, respiratory arrest

Treatment: Assure adequate hydration and renal function. Urinary alkalinization with I.V. sodium bicarbonate also helps to enhance elimination. Repeated oral doses of activated charcoal significantly reduces the half-life of primidone resulting from an enhancement of nonrenal elimination. The usual dose is 0.1-1 g/kg every 4-6 hours for 3-4 days unless the patient has no bowel movement causing the charcoal to remain in the GI tract. Hemodialysis or hemoperfusion is of uncertain value. Patients in stage IV coma due to high serum drug levels may require charcoal hemoperfusion.

Drug Interactions CYP1A2, 2B6, 2C, 2C8, 3A3/4, and 3A5-7 enzyme inducer.
Note: Primidone is metabolically converted to phenobarbital. Barbiturates are cytochrome P450 enzyme inducers. Patients should be monitored when these drugs are started or stopped for a decreased or increased therapeutic effect respectively.

Acetaminophen: Barbiturates may enhance the hepatotoxic potential of acetaminophen overdoses

Antiarrhythmics: Barbiturates may increase the metabolism of antiarrhythmics, decreasing their clinical effect; includes disopyramide, propafenone, and quinidine

Anticonvulsants: Barbiturates may increase the metabolism of anticonvulsants; includes ethosuximide, felbamate (possibly), lamotrigine, phenytoin, tiagabine, topiramate, and zonisamide; does not appear to affect gabapentin or levetiracetam

Antineoplastics: Limited evidence suggests that enzyme-inducing anticonvulsant therapy may reduce the effectiveness of some chemotherapy regimens (specifically in ALL); teniposide and methotrexate may be cleared more rapidly in these patients

Antipsychotics: Barbiturates may enhance the metabolism (decrease the efficacy) of antipsychotics; monitor for altered response; dose adjustment may be needed

Beta-blockers: Metabolism of beta-blockers may be increased and clinical effect decreased; atenolol and nadolol are unlikely to interact given their renal elimination

Calcium channel blockers: Barbiturates may enhance the metabolism of calcium channel blockers, decreasing their clinical effect

Chloramphenicol: Barbiturates may increase the metabolism of chloramphenicol and chloramphenicol may inhibit barbiturate metabolism; monitor for altered response

Cimetidine: Barbiturates may enhance the metabolism of cimetidine, decreasing its clinical effect

CNS depressants: Sedative effects and/or respiratory depression with barbiturates may be additive with other CNS depressants; monitor for increased effect. Includes ethanol, sedatives, antidepressants, narcotic analgesics, and benzodiazepines

Corticosteroids: Barbiturates may enhance the metabolism of corticosteroids, decreasing their clinical effect

Cyclosporine: Levels may be decreased by barbiturates; monitor

Doxycycline: Barbiturates may enhance the metabolism of doxycycline, decreasing its clinical effect; higher dosages may be required

Estrogens: Barbiturates may increase the metabolism of estrogens and reduce their efficacy

Felbamate may inhibit the metabolism of barbiturates and barbiturates may increase the metabolism of felbamate

Griseofulvin: Barbiturates may impair the absorption of griseofulvin, and griseofulvin metabolism may be increased by barbiturates, decreasing clinical effect

Guanfacine: Effect may be decreased by barbiturates

Immunosuppressants: Barbiturates may enhance the metabolism of immunosuppressants, decreasing its clinical effect; includes both cyclosporine and tacrolimus

Loop diuretics: Metabolism may be increased and clinical effects decreased; established for furosemide, effect with other loop diuretics not established

MAO inhibitors: Metabolism of barbiturates may be inhibited, increasing clinical effect or toxicity of the barbiturates

Methadone: Barbiturates may enhance the metabolism of methadone resulting in methadone withdrawal

Methoxyflurane: Barbiturates may enhance the nephrotoxic effects of methoxyflurane

Oral contraceptives: Barbiturates may enhance the metabolism of oral contraceptives, decreasing their clinical effect; an alternative method of contraception should be considered

Theophylline: Barbiturates may increase metabolism of theophylline derivatives and decrease their clinical effect

Tricyclic antidepressants: Barbiturates may increase metabolism of tricyclic antidepressants and decrease their clinical effect; sedative effects may be additive

Valproic acid: Metabolism of barbiturates may be inhibited by valproic acid; monitor for excessive sedation; a dose reduction may be needed

Warfarin: Barbiturates inhibit the hypoprothrombinemic effects of oral anticoagulants via increased metabolism; this combination should generally be avoided

Ethanol/Nutrition/Herb Interactions

Ethanol: Avoid ethanol (may increase CNS depression).

Food: Protein-deficient diets increase duration of action of primidone.

Herb/Nutraceutical: Avoid valerian, St John's wort, kava kava, gotu kola (may increase CNS depression).

Stability Protect from light

Mechanism of Action Decreases neuron excitability, raises seizure threshold similar to phenobarbital; primidone has two active metabolites, phenobarbital and phenylethylmalonamide (PEMA); PEMA may enhance the activity of phenobarbital

Pharmacodynamics/Kinetics

Distribution: V_d: 2-3 L/kg in adults

Protein binding: 99%

Metabolism: In the liver to phenobarbital (active) and phenylethylmalonamide (PEMA)

Bioavailability: 60% to 80%

(Continued)

Primidone (Continued)

Half-life (age dependent):
Primidone: 10-12 hours
PEMA: 16 hours
Phenobarbital: 52-118 hours
Time to peak serum concentration: Oral: Within 4 hours
Elimination: Urinary excretion of both active metabolites and unchanged primidone (15% to 25%)

Usual Dosage Oral:
Children <8 years: Initial: 50-125 mg/day given at bedtime; increase by 50-125 mg/day increments every 3-7 days; usual dose: 10-25 mg/kg/day in divided doses 3-4 times/day
Children ≥8 years and Adults: Initial: 125-250 mg/day at bedtime; increase by 125-250 mg/day every 3-7 days; usual dose: 750-1500 mg/day in divided doses 3-4 times/day with maximum dosage of 2 g/day

Dosing interval in renal impairment:
Cl_{cr} 50-80 mL/minute: Administer every 8 hours
Cl_{cr} 10-50 mL/minute: Administer every 8-12 hours
Cl_{cr} <10 mL/minute: Administer every 12-24 hours
Hemodialysis: Moderately dialyzable (20% to 50%); administer dose postdialysis or administer supplemental 30% dose

Dietary Considerations Folic acid: Low erythrocyte and CSF folate concentrations. Megaloblastic anemia has been reported. To avoid folic acid deficiency and megaloblastic anemia, some clinicians recommend giving patients on anticonvulsants prophylactic doses of folic acid and cyanocobalamin.

Monitoring Parameters Serum primidone and phenobarbital concentration, CBC, neurological status. Due to CNS effects, monitor closely when initiating drug in elderly. Monitor CBC at 6-month intervals to compare with baseline obtained at start of therapy. Since elderly metabolize phenobarbital at a slower rate than younger adults, it is suggested to measure both primidone and phenobarbital levels together.

Reference Range Therapeutic: Children <5 years: 7-10 µg/mL (SI: 32-46 µmol/L); Adults: 5-12 µg/mL (SI: 23-55 µmol/L); toxic effects rarely present with levels <10 µg/mL (SI: 46 µmol/L) if phenobarbital concentrations are low. Dosage of primidone is adjusted with reference mostly to the phenobarbital level; Toxic: >15 µg/mL (SI: >69 µmol/L)

Test Interactions ↑ alkaline phosphatase (S); ↓ calcium (S)

Patient Information May cause drowsiness, impair judgment and coordination; do not abruptly discontinue or change dosage without notifying physician; can take with food to avoid GI upset

Nursing Implications Observe patient for excessive sedation; institute safety measures

Dosage Forms
Suspension, oral: 250 mg/5 mL (240 mL)
Tablet: 50 mg, 250 mg

Prochlorperazine (proe klor PER a zeen)

Related Information
Antipsychotic Medication Guidelines on page 559
Patient Information - Antipsychotics (General) on page 466
U.S. Brand Names Compazine®; Compro™
Canadian Brand Names Nu-Prochlor®; PMS-Prochlorperazine; Prorazin®; Stemetil®
Synonyms Prochlorperazine Edisylate; Prochlorperazine Maleate
Pharmacologic Category Antipsychotic Agent, Phenothiazine, Piperazine
Generic Available Yes: Injection and tablet
Use Management of nausea and vomiting; psychosis; anxiety; treatment of schizophrenia; short-term treatment of nonpsychotic anxiety

Unlabeled/Investigational Use Dementia behavior

Pregnancy Risk Factor C

Pregnancy/Breast-Feeding Implications

Clinical effects on the fetus: Crosses the placenta. Isolated reports of congenital anomalies, however some included exposures to other drugs. Available evidence with use of occasional low doses suggests safe use during pregnancy.

Breast-feeding/lactation: No data available. AAP considers **compatible** with breast-feeding.

Contraindications Hypersensitivity to prochlorperazine or any component of the formulation (cross-reactivity between phenothiazines may occur); severe CNS depression; coma; bone marrow suppression; should not be used in children <2 years of age or <10 kg

Warnings/Precautions May be sedating; use with caution in disorders where CNS depression is a feature. May impair physical or mental abilities; patients must cautioned about performing tasks which require mental alertness (ie, operating machinery or driving). Effects with other sedative drugs or ethanol may be potentiated. Avoid use in Reye's syndrome. Use with caution in Parkinson's disease; hemodynamic instability; bone marrow suppression; predisposition to seizures; subcortical brain damage; and in severe cardiac, hepatic, renal or respiratory disease. Caution in breast cancer or other prolactin-dependent tumors (may elevate prolactin levels). May alter temperature regulation or mask toxicity of other drugs due to antiemetic effects. May alter cardiac conduction - life threatening arrhythmias have occurred with therapeutic doses of phenothiazines. May cause orthostatic hypotension; use with caution in patients at risk of hypotension or where transient hypotensive episodes would be poorly tolerated (cardiovascular disease or cerebrovascular disease). Hypotension may occur following administration, particularly when parenteral form is used or in high dosages.

Phenothiazines may cause anticholinergic effects (constipation, dry mouth, blurred vision, urinary retention); therefore, they should be used with caution in patients with decreased gastrointestinal motility, urinary retention, BPH, xerostomia, or visual problems. Conditions which also may be exacerbated by cholinergic blockade include narrow-angle glaucoma (screening is recommended) and worsening of myasthenia gravis. May cause extrapyramidal reactions, including pseudoparkinsonism, acute dystonic reactions, akathisia and tardive dyskinesia. May be associated with neuroleptic malignant syndrome (NMS).

Adverse Reactions Frequency not defined.

Cardiovascular: Hypotension, orthostatic hypotension, hypertension, tachycardia, bradycardia, dizziness, cardiac arrest

Central nervous system: Extrapyramidal symptoms (pseudoparkinsonism, akathisia, dystonias, tardive dyskinesia), dizziness, cerebral edema, seizures, headache, drowsiness, paradoxical excitement, restlessness, hyperactivity, insomnia, neuroleptic malignant syndrome (NMS), impairment of temperature regulation

Dermatologic: Increased sensitivity to sun, rash, discoloration of skin (blue-gray)

Endocrine & metabolic: Hypoglycemia, hyperglycemia, galactorrhea, lactation, breast enlargement, gynecomastia, menstrual irregularity, amenorrhea, SIADH, changes in libido

Gastrointestinal: Constipation, weight gain, vomiting, stomach pain, nausea, xerostomia, salivation, diarrhea, anorexia, ileus

Genitourinary: Difficulty in urination, ejaculatory disturbances, incontinence, polyuria, ejaculating dysfunction, priapism

Hematologic: Agranulocytosis, leukopenia, eosinophilia, hemolytic anemia, thrombocytopenic purpura, pancytopenia

Hepatic: Cholestatic jaundice, hepatotoxicity

Neuromuscular & skeletal: Tremor

Ocular: Pigmentary retinopathy, blurred vision, cornea and lens changes

Respiratory: Nasal congestion

Miscellaneous: Diaphoresis

(Continued)

Prochlorperazine *(Continued)*

Overdosage/Toxicology

Signs and symptoms: Deep sleep, coma, extrapyramidal symptoms, abnormal involuntary muscle movements, hypotension

Treatment:

Following initiation of essential overdose management, toxic symptom treatment and supportive treatment should be initiated.

Hypotension usually responds to I.V. fluids or Trendelenburg positioning. If unresponsive to these measures, the use of a parenteral inotrope may be required (eg, norepinephrine 0.1-0.2 mcg/kg/minute titrated to response).

Seizures commonly respond to diazepam (I.V. 5-10 mg bolus in adults every 15 minutes if needed up to a total of 30 mg; I.V. 0.25-0.4 mg/kg/dose up to a total of 10 mg in children) or to phenytoin or phenobarbital.

Also critical cardiac arrhythmias often respond to I.V. phenytoin (15 mg/kg up to 1 gram), while other antiarrhythmics can be used.

Extrapyramidal symptoms (eg, dystonic reactions) may require management with diphenhydramine 1-2 mg/kg (adults) up to a maximum of 50 mg I.M. or I.V. slow push followed by a maintenance dose for 48-72 hours. Alternatively, benztropine mesylate I.V. 1-2 mg (adults) may be effective. These agents are generally effective within 2-5 minutes.

Drug Interactions Possible CYP2D6 enzyme substrate

Aluminum salts: May decrease the absorption of phenothiazines; monitor

Amphetamines: Efficacy may be diminished by antipsychotics; in addition, amphetamines may increase psychotic symptoms; avoid concurrent use

Anticholinergics: May inhibit the therapeutic response to phenothiazines and excess anticholinergic effects may occur; includes benztropine, trihexyphenidyl, biperiden, and drugs with significant anticholinergic activity (TCAs, antihistamines, disopyramide)

Antihypertensives: Concurrent use of phenothiazines with an antihypertensive may produce additive hypotensive effects (particularly orthostasis)

Bromocriptine: Phenothiazines inhibit the ability of bromocriptine to lower serum prolactin concentrations

CNS depressants: Sedative effects may be additive with phenothiazines; monitor for increased effect; includes barbiturates, benzodiazepines, narcotic analgesics, ethanol and other sedative agents

CYP2D6 inhibitors: Metabolism of phenothiazines may be decreased, increasing clinical effect or toxicity; inhibitors include amiodarone, cimetidine, delavirdine, fluoxetine, paroxetine, propafenone, quinidine, and ritonavir; monitor for increased effect/toxicity

Enzyme inducers: May enhance the hepatic metabolism of phenothiazines; larger doses may be required; includes rifampin, rifabutin, barbiturates, phenytoin, and cigarette smoking

Epinephrine: Chlorpromazine (and possibly other low potency antipsychotics) may diminish the pressor effects of epinephrine

Guanethidine and guanadrel: Antihypertensive effects may be inhibited by phenothiazines

Levodopa: Phenothiazines may inhibit the antiparkinsonian effect of levodopa; avoid this combination

Lithium: Phenothiazines may produce neurotoxicity with lithium; this is a rare effect

Phenytoin: May reduce serum levels of phenothiazines; phenothiazines may increase phenytoin serum levels

Propranolol: Serum concentrations of phenothiazines may be increased; propranolol also increases phenothiazine concentrations

Polypeptide antibiotics: Rare cases of respiratory paralysis have been reported with concurrent use of phenothiazines

QT_c-prolonging agents: Effects on QT_c interval may be additive with phenothiazines, increasing the risk of malignant arrhythmias; includes type Ia antiarrhythmics, TCAs, and some quinolone antibiotics (sparfloxacin, moxifloxacin, and gatifloxacin)

Sulfadoxine-pyrimethamine: May increase phenothiazine concentrations

Tricyclic antidepressants: Concurrent use may produce increased toxicity or altered therapeutic response

Trazodone: Phenothiazines and trazodone may produce additive hypotensive effects

Valproic acid: Serum levels may be increased by phenothiazines

Ethanol/Nutrition/Herb Interactions

Ethanol: Avoid ethanol (may increase CNS depression).

Food: Limit caffeine.

Herb/Nutraceutical: Avoid dong quai, St John's wort (may also cause photosensitization). Avoid kava kava, gotu kola, valerian, St John's wort (may increase CNS depression).

Stability Protect from light; clear or slightly yellow solutions may be used; **incompatible** when mixed with aminophylline, amphotericin B, ampicillin, calcium salts, cephalothin, foscarnet (Y-site), furosemide, hydrocortisone, hydromorphone, methohexital, midazolam, penicillin G, pentobarbital, phenobarbital, thiopental

Mechanism of Action Blocks postsynaptic mesolimbic dopaminergic D_1 and D_2 receptors in the brain, including the medullary chemoreceptor trigger zone; exhibits a strong alpha-adrenergic and anticholinergic blocking effect and depresses the release of hypothalamic and hypophyseal hormones; believed to depress the reticular activating system, thus affecting basal metabolism, body temperature, wakefulness, vasomotor tone and emesis

Pharmacodynamics/Kinetics

Onset of effect:

Oral: Within 30-40 minutes

I.M.: Within 10-20 minutes

Rectal: Within 60 minutes

Duration: Persists longest with I.M. and oral extended-release doses (12 hours); shortest following rectal and immediate release oral administration (3-4 hours)

Distribution: Crosses the placenta; appears in breast milk

Metabolism: Hepatic

Half-life: 23 hours

Elimination: Primarily by hepatic metabolism

Usual Dosage

Antiemetic: Children (not recommended in children <10 kg or <2 years):

Oral, rectal:

>10 kg: 0.4 mg/kg/24 hours in 3-4 divided doses; **or**

9-14 kg: 2.5 mg every 12-24 hours as needed; maximum: 7.5 mg/day

14-18 kg: 2.5 mg every 8-12 hours as needed; maximum: 10 mg/day

18-39 kg: 2.5 mg every 8 hours or 5 mg every 12 hours as needed; maximum: 15 mg/day

I.M.: 0.1-0.15 mg/kg/dose; usual: 0.13 mg/kg/dose; change to oral as soon as possible

Antiemetic: Adults:

Oral:

Tablet: 5-10 mg 3-4 times/day; usual maximum: 40 mg/day

Capsule, sustained action: 15 mg upon arising or 10 mg every 12 hours

I.M.: 5-10 mg every 3-4 hours; usual maximum: 40 mg/day

I.V.: 2.5-10 mg; maximum 10 mg/dose or 40 mg/day; may repeat dose every 3-4 hours as needed

Rectal: 25 mg twice daily

Surgical nausea/vomiting: Adults:

I.M.: 5-10 mg 1-2 hours before induction; may repeat once if necessary

I.V.: 5-10 mg 15-30 minutes before induction; may repeat once if necessary

Antipsychotic:

Children 2-12 years (not recommended in children <10 kg or <2 years):

Oral, rectal: 2.5 mg 2-3 times/day; increase dosage as needed to maximum daily dose of 20 mg for 2-5 years and 25 mg for 6-12 years

I.M.: 0.13 mg/kg/dose; change to oral as soon as possible

(Continued)

Prochlorperazine *(Continued)*

Adults:

Oral: 5-10 mg 3-4 times/day; doses up to 150 mg/day may be required in some patients for treatment of severe disturbances

I.M.: 10-20 mg every 4-6 hours may be required in some patients for treatment of severe disturbances; change to oral as soon as possible

Nonpsychotic anxiety: Adults: Not >20 mg/day for no longer than 12 weeks

Elderly: Behavioral symptoms associated with dementia: Initial: 2.5-5 mg 1-2 times/day; increase dose at 4- to 7-day intervals by 2.5-5 mg/day; increase dosing intervals (twice daily, 3 times/day, etc) as necessary to control response or side effects; maximum daily dose should probably not exceed 75 mg in elderly; gradual increases (titration) may prevent some side effects or decrease their severity

Hemodialysis: Not dialyzable (0% to 5%)

Dietary Considerations Increase dietary intake of riboflavin; should be administered with food or water.

Administration May be administered orally, I.M., or I.V.:

Oral: Avoid skin contact with oral solution; contact dermatitis has occurred.

I.M. should be administered into the upper outer quadrant of the buttock; avoid skin contact with injection solution; contact dermatitis has occurred

I.V. may be administered IVP or IVPB; IVP should be administered at a concentration of 1 mg/mL at a rate of 1 mg/minute; avoid skin contact with injection solution; contact dermatitis has occurred

Monitoring Parameters CBC with differential and periodic ophthalmic exams (if chronically used)

Test Interactions False-positives for phenylketonuria, urinary amylase, uroporphyrins, urobilinogen

Patient Information May cause drowsiness, impair judgment and coordination; may cause photosensitivity; avoid excessive sunlight; notify physician of involuntary movements or feelings of restlessness

Nursing Implications Avoid skin contact with oral solution or injection, contact dermatitis has occurred; observe for extrapyramidal symptoms

Additional Information Not recommended as an antipsychotic due to inferior efficacy compared to other phenothiazines.

Dosage Forms

Capsule, sustained action, as maleate: 10 mg, 15 mg, 30 mg

Injection, as edisylate: 5 mg/mL (2 mL, 10 mL)

Suppository, rectal: 2.5 mg, 5 mg, 25 mg (12/box)

Syrup, as edisylate: 5 mg/5 mL (120 mL)

Tablet, as maleate: 5 mg, 10 mg, 25 mg

♦ **Prochlorperazine Edisylate** *see* Prochlorperazine *on page 328*

♦ **Prochlorperazine Maleate** *see* Prochlorperazine *on page 328*

♦ **Procyclid (Can)** *see* Procyclidine *on page 332*

Procyclidine *(proe SYE kli deen)*

Related Information

Antiparkinsonian Agents Comparison Chart *on page 556*

Patient Information - Agents for Treatment of Extrapyramidal Symptoms *on page 493*

U.S. Brand Names Kemadrin®

Canadian Brand Names PMS-Procyclidine; Procyclid

Synonyms Procyclidine Hydrochloride

Pharmacologic Category Anticholinergic Agent; Anti-Parkinson's Agent (Anticholinergic)

Generic Available No

Use Relieves symptoms of parkinsonian syndrome and drug-induced extrapyramidal symptoms

Pregnancy Risk Factor C

Contraindications Angle-closure glaucoma; safe use in children not established

Warnings/Precautions Use with caution in hot weather or during exercise. Elderly patients frequently develop increased sensitivity and require strict dosage regulation - side effects may be more severe in elderly patients with atherosclerotic changes. Use with caution in patients with tachycardia, cardiac arrhythmias, hypertension, hypotension, prostatic hypertrophy (especially in the elderly) or any tendency toward urinary retention, liver or kidney disorders or obstructive disease of the GI or GU tract. When given in large doses or to susceptible patients, may cause weakness and inability to move particular muscle groups.

Adverse Reactions

Cardiovascular: Tachycardia, palpitations

Central nervous system: Confusion, drowsiness, headache, loss of memory, fatigue, ataxia, giddiness, lightheadedness

Dermatologic: Dry skin, increased sensitivity to light, rash

Gastrointestinal: Constipation, xerostomia, dry throat, nausea, vomiting, epigastric distress

Genitourinary: Difficult urination

Neuromuscular & skeletal: Weakness

Ocular: Increased intraocular pain, blurred vision, mydriasis

Respiratory: Dry nose

Miscellaneous: Diaphoresis (decreased)

Overdosage/Toxicology

Signs and symptoms: Disorientation, hallucinations, delusions, blurred vision, dysphagia, absent bowel sounds, hyperthermia, hypertension, urinary retention; anticholinergic toxicity is caused by strong binding of the drug to cholinergic receptors; anticholinesterase inhibitors reduce acetylcholinesterase, the enzyme that breaks down acetylcholine and thereby allows acetylcholine to accumulate and compete for receptor binding with the offending anticholinergic

Treatment: For anticholinergic overdose with severe life-threatening symptoms, physostigmine 1-2 mg (0.5 or 0.02 mg/kg for children) S.C. or I.V., slowly may be given to reverse these effects.

Drug Interactions

Amantadine, rimantadine: Central and/or peripheral anticholinergic syndrome can occur when administered with amantadine or rimantadine

Anticholinergic agents: Central and/or peripheral anticholinergic syndrome can occur when administered with narcotic analgesics, phenothiazines and other antipsychotics (especially with high anticholinergic activity), tricyclic antidepressants, quinidine and some other antiarrhythmics, and antihistamines

Atenolol: Anticholinergics may increase the bioavailability of atenolol (and possibly other beta-blockers); monitor for increased effect

Cholinergic agents: Anticholinergics may antagonize the therapeutic effect of cholinergic agents; includes tacrine and donepezil

Digoxin: Anticholinergics may decrease gastric degradation and increase the amount of digoxin absorbed by delaying gastric emptying

Levodopa: Anticholinergics may increase gastric degradation and decrease the amount of levodopa absorbed by delaying gastric emptying

Neuroleptics: Anticholinergics may antagonize the therapeutic effects of neuroleptics

Ethanol/Nutrition/Herb Interactions Ethanol: Avoid ethanol.

Mechanism of Action Thought to act by blocking excess acetylcholine at cerebral synapses; many of its effects are due to its pharmacologic similarities with atropine; it exerts an antispasmodic effect on smooth muscle, is a potent mydriatic; inhibits salivation

Pharmacodynamics/Kinetics

Onset of effect: Oral: Within 30-40 minutes

Duration: 4-6 hours

Usual Dosage Adults: Oral: 2.5 mg 3 times/day after meals; if tolerated, gradually increase dose, maximum of 20 mg/day if necessary

(Continued)

Procyclidine *(Continued)*

Dosing adjustment in hepatic impairment: Decrease dose to a twice daily dosing regimen

Dietary Considerations Should be administered after meals to minimize stomach upset.

Administration Should be administered after meals to minimize stomach upset.

Monitoring Parameters Symptoms of EPS or Parkinson's disease, pulse, anticholinergic effects (ie, CNS, bowel and bladder function)

Patient Information Take after meals; do not discontinue drug abruptly; notify physician if adverse GI effects, fever or heat intolerance occurs; may cause drowsiness; avoid alcohol; adequate fluid intake or sugar free gum or hard candy may help dry mouth; adequate fluid and exercise may help constipation

Nursing Implications Do not discontinue drug abruptly

Dosage Forms Tablet, as hydrochloride: 5 mg

- ◆ **Procyclidine Hydrochloride** *see Procyclidine on page 332*
- ◆ **Prolixin**® *see Fluphenazine on page 151*
- ◆ **Prolixin Decanoate**® *see Fluphenazine on page 151*
- ◆ **Prolixin Enanthate**® *see Fluphenazine on page 151*
- ◆ **Pro-Lorazepam**® (Can) *see Lorazepam on page 209*

Promazine *(PROE ma zeen)*

Related Information

Antipsychotic Agents Comparison Chart *on page 557*
Antipsychotic Medication Guidelines *on page 559*
Discontinuation of Psychotropic Drugs - Withdrawal Symptoms and Recommendations *on page 582*
Federal OBRA Regulations Recommended Maximum Doses *on page 583*
Patient Information - Antipsychotics (General) *on page 466*

U.S. Brand Names Sparine®

Synonyms Promazine Hydrochloride

Pharmacologic Category Antipsychotic Agent, Phenothiazine, Aliphatic

Generic Available No

Use Management of manifestations of psychotic disorders

Unlabeled/Investigational Use Nausea and vomiting; preoperative sedation

Pregnancy Risk Factor C

Contraindications Hypersensitivity to promazine or any component of the formulation (cross-reactivity between phenothiazines may occur); severe CNS depression, bone marrow suppression and coma; intra-arterial injection of the parenteral formulation

Warnings/Precautions Moderately sedating, use with caution in disorders where CNS depression is a feature. Use with caution in Parkinson's disease. Caution in patients with hemodynamic instability; bone marrow suppression; predisposition to seizures; subcortical brain damage; severe cardiac, hepatic, renal, or respiratory disease. Esophageal dysmotility and aspiration have been associated with antipsychotic use - use with caution in patients at risk of pneumonia (ie, Alzheimer's disease). Caution in breast cancer or other prolactin-dependent tumors (may elevate prolactin levels). May alter temperature regulation or mask toxicity of other drugs due to antiemetic effects. May alter cardiac conduction - life-threatening arrhythmias have occurred with therapeutic doses of phenothiazines. May cause orthostatic hypotension - use with caution in patients at risk of this effect or those who would tolerate transient hypotensive episodes (cerebrovascular disease, cardiovascular disease, or other medications which may predispose).

Phenothiazines may cause anticholinergic effects (confusion, agitation, constipation, dry mouth, blurred vision, urinary retention); therefore, they should be used with caution in patients with decreased gastrointestinal motility, urinary retention, BPH, xerostomia, or visual problems. Conditions which also may be exacerbated by cholinergic blockade include narrow-angle glaucoma (screening is recommended) and worsening of myasthenia gravis. Relative to other neuroleptics, promazine has a high potency of cholinergic blockade.

May cause extrapyramidal reactions, including pseudoparkinsonism, acute dystonic reactions, akathisia, and tardive dyskinesia (risk of these reactions is moderate relative to other neuroleptics). May be associated with neuroleptic malignant syndrome (NMS) or pigmentary retinopathy.

Adverse Reactions

Cardiovascular: Postural hypotension, tachycardia, dizziness, nonspecific QT changes

Central nervous system: Drowsiness, dystonias, akathisia, pseudoparkinsonism, tardive dyskinesia, neuroleptic malignant syndrome, seizures

Dermatologic: Photosensitivity, dermatitis, skin pigmentation (slate gray)

Endocrine & metabolic: Lactation, breast engorgement, false-positive pregnancy test, amenorrhea, gynecomastia, hyper- or hypoglycemia

Gastrointestinal: Xerostomia, constipation, nausea

Genitourinary: Urinary retention, ejaculatory disorder, impotence

Hematologic: Agranulocytosis, eosinophilia, leukopenia, hemolytic anemia, aplastic anemia, thrombocytopenic purpura

Hepatic: Jaundice

Ocular: Blurred vision, corneal and lenticular changes, epithelial keratopathy, pigmentary retinopathy

Overdosage/Toxicology

Signs and symptoms: Deep sleep, coma, extrapyramidal symptoms, abnormal involuntary muscle movements, hypotension

Treatment:

Following initiation of essential overdose management, toxic symptom treatment and supportive treatment should be initiated

Hypotension usually responds to I.V. fluids and Trendelenburg positioning. If unresponsive to these measures, the use of a parenteral inotrope may be required (eg, norepinephrine 0.1-0.2 mcg/kg/minute titrated to response).

Seizures commonly respond to diazepam (I.V. 5-10 mg bolus in adults every 15 minutes if needed up to a total of 30 mg; I.V. 0.25-0.4 mg/kg/dose up to a total of 10 mg in children) or to phenytoin or phenobarbital

Also critical cardiac arrhythmics often respond to I.V. phenytoin (15 mg/kg up to 1 gram), while other antiarrhythmics can be used

Neuroleptics often cause extrapyramidal symptoms (eg, dystonic reactions) requiring management with diphenhydramine 1-2 mg/kg (adults) up to a maximum of 50 mg I.M. or I.V. slow push followed by a maintenance dose for 48-72 hours. Alternatively, benztropine mesylate I.V. 1-2 mg (adults) may be effective. These agents are generally effective within 2-5 minutes.

Drug Interactions

Aluminum salts: May decrease the absorption of phenothiazines; monitor

Amphetamines: Efficacy may be diminished by antipsychotics; in addition, amphetamines may increase psychotic symptoms; avoid concurrent use

Anticholinergics: May inhibit the therapeutic response to phenothiazines and excess anticholinergic effects may occur; includes benztropine, trihexyphenidyl, biperiden, and drugs with significant anticholinergic activity (TCAs, antihistamines, disopyramide)

Antihypertensives: Concurrent use of phenothiazines with an antihypertensive may produce additive hypotensive effects (particularly orthostasis)

Bromocriptine: Phenothiazines inhibit the ability of bromocriptine to lower serum prolactin concentrations

CNS depressants: Sedative effects may be additive with phenothiazines; monitor for increased effect; includes barbiturates, benzodiazepines, narcotic analgesics, ethanol, and other sedative agents

CYP2D6 inhibitors: Metabolism of phenothiazines may be decreased; increasing clinical effect or toxicity; inhibitors include amiodarone, cimetidine, delavirdine, (Continued)

Promazine *(Continued)*

fluoxetine, paroxetine, propafenone, quinidine, and ritonavir; monitor for increased effect/toxicity

Enzyme inducers: May enhance the hepatic metabolism of phenothiazines; larger doses may be required; includes rifampin, rifabutin, barbiturates, phenytoin, and cigarette smoking

Epinephrine: Chlorpromazine (and possibly other low potency antipsychotics) may diminish the pressor effects of epinephrine

Guanethidine and guanadrel: Antihypertensive effects may be inhibited by phenothiazines

Levodopa: Phenothiazines may inhibit the antiparkinsonian effect of levodopa; avoid this combination

Lithium: Phenothiazines may produce neurotoxicity with lithium; this is a rare effect

Phenytoin: May reduce serum levels of phenothiazines; phenothiazines may increase phenytoin serum levels

Propranolol: Serum concentrations of phenothiazines may be increased; propranolol also increases phenothiazine concentrations

Polypeptide antibiotics: Rare cases of respiratory paralysis have been reported with concurrent use of phenothiazines

QT_c-prolonging agents: Effects on QT_c interval may be additive with phenothiazines, increasing the risk of malignant arrhythmias; includes type Ia antiarrhythmics, TCAs, and some quinolone antibiotics (sparfloxacin, moxifloxacin, and gatifloxacin)

Sulfadoxine-pyrimethamine: May increase phenothiazine concentrations

Tricyclic antidepressants: Concurrent use may produce increased toxicity or altered therapeutic response

Trazodone: Phenothiazines and trazodone may produce additive hypotensive effects

Valproic acid: Serum levels may be increased by phenothiazines

Ethanol/Nutrition/Herb Interactions Ethanol: Avoid ethanol (may increase CNS depression).

Stability Protect all dosage forms from light, clear or slightly yellow solutions may be used; should be dispensed in amber or opaque vials/bottles.

Injection: **Incompatible** when mixed with aminophylline, dimenhydrinate, methohexital, nafcillin, penicillin G, pentobarbital, phenobarbital, sodium bicarbonate, thiopental

Mechanism of Action Blocks postsynaptic mesolimbic dopaminergic D_1 and D_2 receptors in the brain; exhibits a strong alpha-adrenergic blocking and anticholinergic effect; depresses the release of hypothalamic and hypophyseal hormones; believed to depress the reticular activating system thus affecting basal metabolism, body temperature, wakefulness, vasomotor tone, and emesis

Pharmacodynamics/Kinetics The specific pharmacokinetics of promazine are poorly established but probably resemble those of other phenothiazines.

Absorption: Phenothiazines are only partially absorbed; great variability in plasma levels resulting from a given dose

Metabolism: Extensively in the liver

Half-life: Most phenothiazines have long half-lives in the range of 24 hours or more

Usual Dosage Oral, I.M.:

Children >12 years: Psychosis: 10-25 mg every 4-6 hours

Adults:

Psychosis: 10-200 mg every 4-6 hours not to exceed 1000 mg/day

Antiemetic (unlabeled use): 25-50 mg every 4-6 hours as needed

Hemodialysis: Not dialyzable (0% to 5%)

Administration I.M. injections should be deep injections; if giving I.V., dilute to at least 25 mg/mL and administer slowly

Monitoring Parameters Orthostatic blood pressure, tremors, gait changes, abnormal movement in trunk, neck, buccal area or extremities; monitor target behaviors for which the agent is given; monitor hepatic function (especially if fever with flu-like symptoms)

Test Interactions ↑ cholesterol (S), ↑ glucose; ↓ uric acid (S)

Patient Information May cause drowsiness, impair judgment and coordination; may cause photosensitivity; avoid excessive sunlight; notify physician of involuntary movements or feelings of restlessness

Nursing Implications Watch for hypotension

Additional Information Coadministration of two or more antipsychotics does not improve clinical response and may increase the potential for adverse effects. Not recommended as an antipsychotic due to inferior efficacy compared to other phenothiazines.

Dosage Forms
Injection, as hydrochloride: 50 mg/mL (10 mL)
Tablet, as hydrochloride: 25 mg, 50 mg

♦ **Promazine Hydrochloride** *see* Promazine *on page 334*

Promethazine (proe METH a zeen)

U.S. Brand Names Anergan®; Phenergan®

Canadian Brand Names Histantil

Synonyms Promethazine Hydrochloride

Pharmacologic Category Antiemetic

Generic Available Yes

Use Symptomatic treatment of various allergic conditions; antiemetic; motion sickness; sedative; analgesic adjunct for control of postoperative pain; anesthetic adjunct

Pregnancy Risk Factor C

Pregnancy/Breast-Feeding Implications
Clinical effects on the fetus: Crosses the placenta. Possible respiratory depression if drug is administered near time of delivery; behavioral changes, EEG alterations, impaired platelet aggregation reported with use during labor. Available evidence with use of occasional low doses suggests safe use during pregnancy.
Breast-feeding/lactation: No data available. AAP makes NO RECOMMENDATION.

Contraindications Hypersensitivity to promethazine or any component of the formulation (cross-reactivity between phenothiazines may occur); severe CNS depression; coma; intra-arterial or subcutaneous injection

Warnings/Precautions May be sedating; use with caution in disorders where CNS depression is a feature. May impair physical or mental abilities; patients must be cautioned about performing tasks which require mental alertness (ie, operating machinery or driving). Effects with other sedative drugs or ethanol may be potentiated. Avoid use in Reye's syndrome. Use with caution in Parkinson's disease; hemodynamic instability; bone marrow suppression; predisposition to seizures; subcortical brain damage; and in severe cardiac, hepatic, renal, or respiratory disease. Caution in breast cancer or other prolactin-dependent tumors (may elevate prolactin levels). May alter temperature regulation or mask toxicity of other drugs due to antiemetic effects. May alter cardiac conduction (life-threatening arrhythmias have occurred with therapeutic doses of phenothiazines). May cause orthostatic hypotension; use with caution in patients at risk of hypotension or where transient hypotensive episodes would be poorly tolerated (cardiovascular disease or cerebrovascular disease).

Phenothiazines may cause anticholinergic effects (constipation, dry mouth, blurred vision, urinary retention); therefore, they should be used with caution in patients with decreased gastrointestinal motility, urinary retention, BPH, xerostomia, or visual problems. Conditions which also may be exacerbated by cholinergic blockade include narrow-angle glaucoma (screening is recommended) and worsening of myasthenia gravis. May cause extrapyramidal reactions, including pseudoparkinsonism, acute dystonic reactions, akathisia, and tardive dyskinesia. May be associated with neuroleptic malignant syndrome (NMS). Ampuls contain sodium metabisulfite.
(Continued)

Promethazine *(Continued)*

Adverse Reactions

Cardiovascular: Postural hypotension, tachycardia, dizziness, nonspecific QT changes

Central nervous system: Drowsiness, dystonias, akathisia, pseudoparkinsonism, tardive dyskinesia, neuroleptic malignant syndrome, seizures

Dermatologic: Photosensitivity, dermatitis, skin pigmentation (slate gray)

Endocrine & metabolic: Lactation, breast engorgement, false-positive pregnancy test, amenorrhea, gynecomastia, hyper- or hypoglycemia

Gastrointestinal: Xerostomia, constipation, nausea

Genitourinary: Urinary retention, ejaculatory disorder, impotence

Hematologic: Agranulocytosis, eosinophilia, leukopenia, hemolytic anemia, aplastic anemia, thrombocytopenic purpura

Hepatic: Jaundice

Ocular: Blurred vision, corneal and lenticular changes, epithelial keratopathy, pigmentary retinopathy

Overdosage/Toxicology

Signs and symptoms: CNS depression, respiratory depression, possible CNS stimulation, dry mouth, fixed and dilated pupils, hypotension

Treatment:

Following initiation of essential overdose management, toxic symptom treatment and supportive treatment should be initiated

Hypotension usually responds to I.V. fluids or Trendelenburg positioning. If unresponsive to these measures, norepinephrine 0.1-0.2 mcg/kg/minute titrated to response may be tried.

Seizures commonly respond to diazepam (I.V. 5-10 mg bolus in adults every 15 minutes if needed up to a total of 30 mg; I.V. 0.25-0.4 mg/kg/dose up to a total of 10 mg in children) or to phenytoin or phenobarbital

Also critical cardiac arrhythmias often respond to I.V. phenytoin (15 mg/kg up to 1 gram), while other antiarrhythmics can be used

Neuroleptics often cause extrapyramidal symptoms (eg, dystonic reactions) requiring management with diphenhydramine 1-2 mg/kg (adults) up to a maximum of 50 mg I.M. or I.V. slow push followed by a maintenance dose for 48-72 hours. Alternatively, benztropine mesylate I.V. 1-2 mg (adults) may be effective. These agents are generally effective within 2-5 minutes.

Drug Interactions CYP2D6 enzyme substrate

Aluminum salts: May decrease the absorption of phenothiazines; monitor

Amphetamines: Efficacy may be diminished by antipsychotics; in addition, amphetamines may increase psychotic symptoms; avoid concurrent use

Anticholinergics: May inhibit the therapeutic response to phenothiazines and excess anticholinergic effects may occur; includes benztropine, trihexyphenidyl, biperiden, and drugs with significant anticholinergic activity (TCAs, antihistamines, disopyramide)

Antihypertensives: Concurrent use of phenothiazines with an antihypertensive may produce additive hypotensive effects (particularly orthostasis)

Bromocriptine: Phenothiazines inhibit the ability of bromocriptine to lower serum prolactin concentrations

CNS depressants: Sedative effects may be additive with phenothiazines; monitor for increased effect; includes barbiturates, benzodiazepines, narcotic analgesics, ethanol, and other sedative agents

CYP2D6 inhibitors: Metabolism of phenothiazines may be decreased; increasing clinical effect or toxicity; inhibitors include amiodarone, cimetidine, delavirdine, fluoxetine, paroxetine, propafenone, quinidine, and ritonavir; monitor for increased effect/toxicity

Enzyme inducers: May enhance the hepatic metabolism of phenothiazines; larger doses may be required; includes rifampin, rifabutin, barbiturates, phenytoin, and cigarette smoking

Epinephrine: Chlorpromazine (and possibly other low potency antipsychotics) may diminish the pressor effects of epinephrine

Guanethidine and guanadrel: Antihypertensive effects may be inhibited by pheno-thiazines

Levodopa: Phenothiazines may inhibit the antiparkinsonian effect of levodopa; avoid this combination

Lithium: Phenothiazines may produce neurotoxicity with lithium; this is a rare effect

Phenytoin: May reduce serum levels of phenothiazines; phenothiazines may increase phenytoin serum levels

Propranolol: Serum concentrations of phenothiazines may be increased; propran-olol also increases phenothiazine concentrations

Polypeptide antibiotics: Rare cases of respiratory paralysis have been reported with concurrent use of phenothiazines

QT_c-prolonging agents: Effects on QT_c interval may be additive with phenothi-azines, increasing the risk of malignant arrhythmias; includes type Ia antiar-rhythmics, TCAs, and some quinolone antibiotics (sparfloxacin, moxifloxacin, and gatifloxacin)

Sulfadoxine-pyrimethamine: May increase phenothiazine concentrations

Tricyclic antidepressants: Concurrent use may produce increased toxicity or altered therapeutic response

Trazodone: Phenothiazines and trazodone may produce additive hypotensive effects

Valproic acid: Serum levels may be increased by phenothiazines

Ethanol/Nutrition/Herb Interactions

Ethanol: Avoid ethanol (may increase CNS depression).

Herb/Nutraceutical: Avoid valerian, St John's wort, kava kava, gotu kola (may increase CNS depression).

Stability Protect from light and from freezing; **compatible** (when comixed in the same syringe) with atropine, chlorpromazine, diphenhydramine, droperidol, fentanyl, glycopyrrolate, hydromorphone, hydroxyzine hydrochloride, meperidine, midazolam, nalbuphine, pentazocine, prochlorperazine, scopolamine; **incompat-ible** when mixed with aminophylline, cefoperazone (Y-site), chloramphenicol, dimenhydrinate (same syringe), foscarnet (Y-site), furosemide, heparin, hydrocorti-sone, methohexital, penicillin G, pentobarbital, phenobarbital, thiopental

Mechanism of Action Blocks postsynaptic mesolimbic dopaminergic receptors in the brain; exhibits a strong alpha-adrenergic blocking effect and depresses the release of hypothalamic and hypophyseal hormones; competes with histamine for the H_1-receptor; reduces stimuli to the brainstem reticular system

Pharmacodynamics/Kinetics

Onset of effect: I.V.: Within 20 minutes (3-5 minutes with I.V. injection)

Duration: 2-6 hours

Metabolism: In the liver

Half-life: 16-19 hours

Peak effect: C_{max}: 9.04 mg/mL (suppository); 19.3 mg/mL (syrup)

Time to maximum serum concentration: 4.4 hours (syrup); 6.7-8.6 hours (supposi-tories)

Elimination: Principally as inactive metabolites in urine and in feces

Usual Dosage

Children:

Antihistamine: Oral, rectal: 0.1 mg/kg/dose every 6 hours during the day and 0.5 mg/kg/dose at bedtime as needed

Antiemetic: Oral, I.M., I.V., rectal: 0.25-1 mg/kg 4-6 times/day as needed

Motion sickness: Oral, rectal: 0.5 mg/kg/dose 30 minutes to 1 hour before depar-ture, then every 12 hours as needed

Sedation: Oral, I.M., I.V., rectal: 0.5-1 mg/kg/dose every 6 hours as needed

Adults:

Antihistamine (including allergic reactions to blood or plasma):

Oral, rectal: 12.5 mg 3 times/day and 25 mg at bedtime

I.M., I.V.: 25 mg, may repeat in 2 hours when necessary; switch to oral route as soon as feasible

Antiemetic: Oral, I.M., I.V., rectal: 12.5-25 mg every 4 hours as needed

(Continued)

Promethazine *(Continued)*

Motion sickness: Oral, rectal: 25 mg 30-60 minutes before departure, then every 12 hours as needed

Sedation: Oral, I.M., I.V., rectal: 25-50 mg/dose

Hemodialysis: Not dialyzable (0% to 5%)

Dietary Considerations Increase dietary intake of riboflavin; should be administered with food or water.

Administration Avoid I.V. use; if necessary, may dilute to a maximum concentration of 25 mg/mL and infuse at a maximum rate of 25 mg/minute; rapid I.V. administration may produce a transient fall in blood pressure

Monitoring Parameters Relief of symptoms, mental status

Test Interactions Alters the flare response in intradermal allergen tests

Patient Information May cause drowsiness, impair judgment and coordination; may cause photosensitivity; avoid excessive sunlight; notify physician of involuntary movements or feelings of restlessness

Nursing Implications Avoid S.C. administration, promethazine is a chemical irritation which may produce necrosis; avoid I.V. use; if necessary, may dilute to a maximum concentration of 25 mg/mL and infuse at a maximum rate of 25 mg/minute

Dosage Forms

Injection, as hydrochloride: 25 mg/mL (1 mL, 10 mL); 50 mg/mL (1 mL, 10 mL)

Suppository, rectal, as hydrochloride: 12.5 mg, 25 mg, 50 mg

Syrup, as hydrochloride: 6.25 mg/5 mL (5 mL, 120 mL, 480 mL, 4000 mL); 25 mg/5 mL (120 mL, 480 mL, 4000 mL)

Tablet, as hydrochloride: 12.5 mg, 25 mg, 50 mg

♦ **Promethazine Hydrochloride** *see Promethazine on page 337*

Propranolol *(proe PRAN oh lole)*

Related Information

Clozapine-Induced Side Effects *on page 568*

Nonbenzodiazepine Anxiolytics and Hypnotics *on page 589*

U.S. Brand Names Inderal®; Inderal® LA

Canadian Brand Names Apo®-Propranolol; Detensol®; Nu-Propranolol®

Synonyms Propranolol Hydrochloride

Pharmacologic Category Beta Blocker, Nonselective

Generic Available Yes

Use Management of hypertension; angina pectoris; pheochromocytoma; essential tremor; tetralogy of Fallot cyanotic spells; arrhythmias (such as atrial fibrillation and flutter, A-V nodal re-entrant tachycardias, and catecholamine-induced arrhythmias); prevention of myocardial infarction; migraine headache; symptomatic treatment of hypertrophic subaortic stenosis

Unlabeled/Investigational Use Tremor due to Parkinson's disease; alcohol withdrawal; aggressive behavior; antipsychotic-induced akathisia; prevention of bleeding esophageal varices; anxiety; schizophrenia; acute panic; gastric bleeding in portal hypertension

Pregnancy Risk Factor C (manufacturer); D (2nd and 3rd trimesters - expert analysis)

Pregnancy/Breast-Feeding Implications

Clinical effects on the fetus: Crosses the placenta. IUGR, hypoglycemia, bradycardia, respiratory depression, hyperbilirubinemia, polycythemia, polydactyly reported. IUGR probably related to maternal hypertension. Preterm labor has been reported. Available evidence suggests safe use during pregnancy and breast-feeding. Monitor breast-fed infant for symptoms of beta-blockade.

Breast-feeding/lactation: Crosses into breast milk. AAP considers **compatible** with breast-feeding.

Contraindications Hypersensitivity to propranolol, beta-blockers, or any component of the formulation; uncompensated congestive heart failure (unless the failure is due to tachyarrhythmias being treated with propranolol), cardiogenic shock, bradycardia or heart block (2nd or 3rd degree), pulmonary edema, severe hyperactive airway disease (asthma or COPD), Raynaud's disease; pregnancy (2nd and 3rd trimesters)

Warnings/Precautions Administer cautiously in compensated heart failure and monitor for a worsening of the condition (efficacy of propranolol in CHF has not been demonstrated). Avoid abrupt discontinuation in patients with a history of CAD; slowly wean while monitoring for signs and symptoms of ischemia. Use caution in patient with PVD. Use caution with concurrent use of beta-blockers and either verapamil or diltiazem; bradycardia or heart block can occur. Avoid concurrent I.V. use of both agents. Use cautiously in diabetics because it can mask prominent hypoglycemic symptoms. Can mask signs of thyrotoxicosis. Can cause fetal harm when administered in pregnancy. Use cautiously in hepatic dysfunction (dosage adjustment required). Use care with anesthetic agents which decrease myocardial function.

Adverse Reactions

Cardiovascular: Bradycardia, congestive heart failure, reduced peripheral circulation, chest pain, hypotension, impaired myocardial contractility, worsening of AV conduction disturbance, cardiogenic shock, Raynaud's syndrome, mesenteric thrombosis (rare)

Central nervous system: Mental depression, lightheadedness, amnesia, emotional lability, confusion, hallucinations, dizziness, insomnia, fatigue, vivid dreams, lethargy, cold extremities, vertigo, syncope, cognitive dysfunction, psychosis, hypersomnolence

Dermatologic: Rash, alopecia, exfoliative dermatitis, psoriasiform eruptions, eczematous eruptions, hyperkeratosis, nail changes, pruritus, urticaria, ulcerative lichenoid, contact dermatitis

Endocrine & metabolic: Hypoglycemia, hyperglycemia, hyperlipidemia, hyperkalemia

Gastrointestinal: Diarrhea, nausea, vomiting, stomach discomfort, constipation, anorexia

Genitourinary: Impotence, proteinuria (rare), oliguria (rare), interstitial nephritis (rare), Peyronie's disease

Hematologic: Agranulocytosis, thrombocytopenia, thrombocytopenic purpura

Neuromuscular & skeletal: Weakness, carpal tunnel syndrome (rare), paresthesias, myotonus, polyarthritis, arthropathy

Respiratory: Wheezing, pharyngitis, bronchospasm, pulmonary edema

Ocular: Hyperemia of the conjunctiva, decreased tear production, decreased visual acuity, mydriasis

Miscellaneous: Lupus-like syndrome (rare)

Overdosage/Toxicology

Signs and symptoms: Severe hypotension, bradycardia, heart failure and bronchospasm, hypoglycemia

Treatment: Sympathomimetics (eg, epinephrine or dopamine), glucagon, or a pacemaker can be used to treat the toxic bradycardia, asystole, and/or hypotension. Initially, fluids may be the best treatment for hypotension.

Drug Interactions CYP1A2, 2C18, 2C19, and 2D6 enzyme substrate

Albuterol (and other beta$_2$-agonists): Effects may be blunted by nonspecific beta-blockers

Alpha-blockers (prazosin, terazosin): Concurrent use of beta-blockers may increase risk of orthostasis

Cimetidine increases the plasma concentration of propranolol and its pharmacodynamic effects may be increased

Clonidine: Hypertensive crisis after or during withdrawal of either agent

CYP1A2 inhibitors: Metabolism of propranolol may be decreased; increasing clinical effect or toxicity; inhibitors include cimetidine, ciprofloxacin, fluvoxamine, isoniazid, ritonavir, and zileuton.

CYP2C19 inhibitors: Serum levels of some beta-blockers may be increased; inhibitors include cimetidine, felbamate, fluconazole, fluoxetine, fluvoxamine, omeprazole, teniposide, tolbutamide, and troglitazone

(Continued)

Propranolol *(Continued)*

CYP2D6 inhibitors: Serum levels and/or toxicity of some beta-blockers may be increased; inhibitors include amiodarone, cimetidine, delavirdine, fluoxetine, paroxetine, propafenone, quinidine, and ritonavir; monitor for increased effect/toxicity

Drugs which slow AV conduction (digoxin): Effects may be additive with beta-blockers

Epinephrine (including local anesthetics with epinephrine): Propranolol may cause hypertension

Flecainide: Pharmacological activity of both agents may be increased when used concurrently

Fluoxetine may inhibit the metabolism of propranolol, resulting in cardiac toxicity

Glucagon: Propranolol may blunt hyperglycemic action

Haloperidol: Hypotensive effects may be potentiated

Hydralazine: The bioavailability propranolol (rapid release) and hydralazine may be enhanced with concurrent dosing

Insulin: Propranolol inhibits recovery and may cause hypertension and bradycardia following insulin-induced hypoglycemia; also masks the tachycardia that usually accompanies insulin-induced hypoglycemia

NSAIDs (ibuprofen, indomethacin, naproxen, piroxicam) may reduce the antihypertensive effects of beta-blockers

Salicylates may reduce the antihypertensive effects of beta-blockers

Sulfonylureas: Beta-blockers may alter response to hypoglycemic agents

Verapamil or diltiazem may have synergistic or additive pharmacological effects when taken concurrently with beta-blockers; avoid concurrent I.V. use of both

Ethanol/Nutrition/Herb Interactions

Food: Propranolol serum levels may be increased if taken with food. Protein-rich foods may increase bioavailability; a change in diet from high carbohydrate/low protein to low carbohydrate/high protein may result in increased oral clearance.

Herb/Nutraceutical: Avoid dong quai if using for hypertension (has estrogenic activity). Avoid ephedra, yohimbe, ginseng (may worsen hypertension or arrhythmia). Avoid natural licorice (causes sodium and water retention and increases potassium loss). Avoid garlic (may have increased antihypertensive effect).

Stability Compatible in saline, **incompatible** with HCO_3^-; protect injection from light; solutions have maximum stability at pH of 3 and decompose rapidly in alkaline pH; propranolol is stable for 24 hours at room temperature in D_5W or NS

Mechanism of Action Nonselective beta-adrenergic blocker (class II antiarrhythmic); competitively blocks response to beta$_1$- and beta$_2$-adrenergic stimulation which results in decreases in heart rate, myocardial contractility, blood pressure, and myocardial oxygen demand

Pharmacodynamics/Kinetics

Onset of beta-blockade: Oral: Within 1-2 hours

Duration: ~6 hours

Distribution: V_d: 3.9 L/kg in adults; crosses the placenta; small amounts appear in breast milk

Protein binding:
Newborns: 68%
Adults: 93%

Metabolism: Extensive first-pass effect; metabolized in the liver to active and inactive compounds

Bioavailability: 30% to 40%; oral bioavailability may be increased in Down syndrome children

Half-life:
Neonates and Infants: Possible increased half-life
Children: 3.9-6.4 hours
Adults: 4-6 hours

Elimination: Primarily in urine (96% to 99%)

Usual Dosage

Tachyarrhythmias:

Oral:

Children: Initial: 0.5-1 mg/kg/day in divided doses every 6-8 hours; titrate dosage upward every 3-7 days; usual dose: 2-4 mg/kg/day; higher doses may be needed; do not exceed 16 mg/kg/day or 60 mg/day

Adults: 10-30 mg/dose every 6-8 hours

Elderly: Initial: 10 mg twice daily; increase dosage every 3-7 days; usual dosage range: 10-320 mg given in 2 divided doses

I.V.:

Children: 0.01-0.1 mg/kg slow IVP over 10 minutes; maximum dose: 1 mg

Adults: 1 mg/dose slow IVP; repeat every 5 minutes up to a total of 5 mg

Hypertension: Oral:

Children: Initial: 0.5-1 mg/kg/day in divided doses every 6-12 hours; increase gradually every 3-7 days; maximum: 2 mg/kg/24 hours

Adults: Initial: 40 mg twice daily; increase dosage every 3-7 days; usual dose: ≤320 mg divided in 2-3 doses/day; maximum daily dose: 640 mg

Long-acting formulation: Initial: 80 mg once daily; usual maintenance: 120-160 mg once daily; maximum daily dose: 640 mg

Migraine headache prophylaxis: Oral:

Children: 0.6-1.5 mg/kg/day **or**

≤35 kg: 10-20 mg 3 times/day

>35 kg: 20-40 mg 3 times/day

Adults: Initial: 80 mg/day divided every 6-8 hours; increase by 20-40 mg/dose every 3-4 weeks to a maximum of 160-240 mg/day given in divided doses every 6-8 hours; if satisfactory response not achieved within 6 weeks of starting therapy, drug should be withdrawn gradually over several weeks

Long-acting formulation: Initial: 80 mg once daily; effective dose range: 160-240 mg once daily

Tetralogy spells: Children:

Oral: 1-2 mg/kg/day every 6 hours as needed, may increase by 1 mg/kg/day to a maximum of 5 mg/kg/day, or if refractory may increase slowly to a maximum of 10-15 mg/kg/day

I.V.: 0.15-0.25 mg/kg/dose slow IVP; may repeat in 15 minutes

Thyrotoxicosis:

Adolescents and Adults: Oral: 10-40 mg/dose every 6 hours

Adults: I.V.: 1-3 mg/dose slow IVP as a single dose

Adults: Oral:

Akathisia: 30-120 mg/day in 2-3 divided doses

Angina: 80-320 mg/day in doses divided 2-4 times/day

Long-acting formulation: Initial: 80 mg once daily; maximum dose: 320 mg once daily

Essential tremor: 20-40 mg twice daily initially; maintenance doses: usually 120-320 mg/day

Hypertrophic subaortic stenosis: 20-40 mg 3-4 times/day

Long-acting formulation: 80-160 mg once daily

Myocardial infarction prophylaxis: 180-240 mg/day in 3-4 divided doses

Pheochromocytoma: 30-60 mg/day in divided doses

Dosing adjustment in renal impairment:

Cl_{cr} 31-40 mL/minute: Administer every 24-36 hours or administer 50% of normal dose

Cl_{cr} 10-30 mL/minute: Administer every 24-48 hours or administer 50% of normal dose

Cl_{cr} <10 mL/minute: Administer every 40-60 hours or administer 25% of normal dose

Hemodialysis: Not dialyzable (0% to 5%); supplemental dose is not necessary

Peritoneal dialysis: Supplemental dose is not necessary

(Continued)

Propranolol *(Continued)*

Dosing adjustment/comments in hepatic disease: Marked slowing of heart rate may occur in cirrhosis with conventional doses; low initial dose and regular heart rate monitoring

Dietary Considerations Administer with food.

Administration I.V. administration should not exceed 1 mg/minute; I.V. dose much smaller than oral dose

Monitoring Parameters Blood pressure, EKG, heart rate, CNS and cardiac effects

Reference Range Therapeutic: 50-100 ng/mL (SI: 190-390 nmol/L) at end of dose interval

Test Interactions ↑ thyroxine (S)

Patient Information Do not discontinue abruptly; notify physician if CHF symptoms become worse; take at the same time each day; may mask diabetes symptoms; sweating will continue

Nursing Implications Patient's therapeutic response may be evaluated by looking at blood pressure, apical and radial pulses, fluid I & O, daily weight, respirations, and circulation in extremities before and during therapy. Do not crush long acting forms.

Additional Information Not indicated for hypertensive emergencies. Do not abruptly discontinue therapy, taper dosage gradually over 2 weeks.

Dosage Forms
Capsule, long-acting, as hydrochloride: 60 mg, 80 mg, 120 mg, 160 mg
Injection, as hydrochloride: 1 mg/mL (1 mL)
Solution, oral, as hydrochloride: 4 mg/mL (5 mL, 500 mL); 8 mg/mL (5 mL, 500 mL) [strawberry-mint flavor]
Solution, oral concentrate, as hydrochloride: 80 mg/mL (30 mL)
Tablet, hydrochloride: 10 mg, 20 mg, 40 mg, 60 mg, 80 mg, 90 mg

♦ **Propranolol Hydrochloride** *see Propranolol on page 340*

♦ **2-Propylpentanoic Acid** *see Valproic Acid and Derivatives on page 425*

♦ **2-Propylvaleric Acid** *see Valproic Acid and Derivatives on page 425*

♦ **Prorazin® (Can)** *see Prochlorperazine on page 328*

♦ **ProSom™** *see Estazolam on page 135*

♦ **ProStep® Patch** *see Nicotine on page 264*

♦ **Prostigmin®** *see Neostigmine on page 262*

Protriptyline *(proe TRIP ti leen)*

Related Information
Antidepressant Agents Comparison Chart *on page 553*
Discontinuation of Psychotropic Drugs - Withdrawal Symptoms and Recommendations *on page 582*
Federal OBRA Regulations Recommended Maximum Doses *on page 583*
Patient Information - Antidepressants (TCAs) *on page 454*

U.S. Brand Names Vivactil®

Canadian Brand Names Triptil®

Synonyms Protriptyline Hydrochloride

Pharmacologic Category Antidepressant, Tricyclic (Secondary Amine)

Generic Available Yes

Use Treatment of depression

Pregnancy Risk Factor C

Contraindications Hypersensitivity to protriptyline (cross-reactivity to other cyclic antidepressants may occur) or any component of the formulation; use of MAO inhibitors within 14 days; use of cisapride; use in a patient during the acute recovery phase of MI

Warnings/Precautions May cause sedation, resulting in impaired performance of tasks requiring alertness (ie, operating machinery or driving). Sedative effects may be additive with other CNS depressants and/or ethanol. The degree of sedation is low relative to other antidepressants. May worsen psychosis in some patients or precipitate a shift to mania or hypomania in patients with bipolar disease. In addition, may aggravate aggressive behavior. May increase the risks associated with electroconvulsive therapy. This agent should be discontinued, when possible, prior to elective surgery. Therapy should not be abruptly discontinued in patients receiving high doses for prolonged periods. May alter glucose regulation - use with caution in patients with diabetes.

May cause orthostatic hypotension (risk is moderate relative to other antidepressants) - use with caution in patients at risk of hypotension or in patients where transient hypotensive episodes would be poorly tolerated (cardiovascular disease or cerebrovascular disease). The degree of anticholinergic blockade produced by this agent is moderate relative to other cyclic antidepressants, however, caution should still be used in patients with urinary retention, benign prostatic hypertrophy, narrow-angle glaucoma, xerostomia, visual problems, constipation, or history of bowel obstruction.

Use caution in patients with depression, particularly if suicidal risk may be present. Use with caution in patients with a history of cardiovascular disease (including previous MI, stroke, tachycardia, or conduction abnormalities). The risk of conduction abnormalities with this agent is moderate-high relative to other antidepressants. Use caution in patients with a previous seizure disorder or condition predisposing to seizures such as brain damage, alcoholism, or concurrent therapy with other drugs which lower the seizure threshold. Use with caution in hyperthyroid patients or those receiving thyroid supplementation. Use with caution in patients with hepatic or renal dysfunction and in elderly patients.

Adverse Reactions

Cardiovascular: Arrhythmias, hypotension, myocardial infarction, stroke, heart block, hypertension, tachycardia, palpitations

Central nervous system: Dizziness, drowsiness, headache, confusion, delirium, hallucinations, restlessness, insomnia, nightmares, fatigue, delusions, anxiety, agitation, hypomania, exacerbation of psychosis, panic, seizures, incoordination, ataxia, EPS

Dermatologic: Alopecia, photosensitivity, rash, petechiae, urticaria, itching

Endocrine & metabolic: Breast enlargement, galactorrhea, SIADH, gynecomastia, increased or decreased libido

Gastrointestinal: Xerostomia, constipation, unpleasant taste, weight gain/loss, increased appetite, nausea, diarrhea, heartburn, vomiting, anorexia, trouble with gums, decreased lower esophageal sphincter tone may cause GE reflux

Genitourinary: Difficult urination, impotence, testicular edema

Hematologic: Agranulocytosis, leukopenia, eosinophilia, thrombocytopenia, purpura

Hepatic: Cholestatic jaundice, increased liver enzymes

Neuromuscular & skeletal: Fine muscle tremors, weakness, tremor, numbness, tingling

Ocular: Blurred vision, eye pain, increased intraocular pressure

Otic: Tinnitus

Miscellaneous: Diaphoresis (excessive), allergic reactions

Overdosage/Toxicology

Signs and symptoms: Confusion, hallucinations, urinary retention, hypotension, tachycardia, seizures, hyperthermia

Treatment:

Following initiation of essential overdose management, toxic symptoms should be treated

Ventricular arrhythmias often respond to systemic alkalinization (sodium bicarbonate 0.5-2 mEq/kg I.V.). Arrhythmias unresponsive to this therapy may respond to lidocaine 1 mg/kg I.V. followed by a titrated infusion. Physostigmine (1-2 mg I.V. slowly for adults or 0.5 mg I.V. slowly for children) may be indicated in reversing cardiac arrhythmias that are life-threatening.

Seizures usually respond to diazepam I.V. boluses (5-10 mg for adults up to 30 mg or 0.25-0.4 mg/kg/dose for children up to 10 mg/dose). If seizures are unresponsive or recur, phenytoin or phenobarbital may be required.

(Continued)

Protriptyline *(Continued)*

Drug Interactions CYP2D6 enzyme substrate

Altretamine: Concurrent use may cause orthostatic hypertension

Amphetamines: TCAs may enhance the effect of amphetamines; monitor for adverse CV effects

Anticholinergics: Combined use with TCAs may produce additive anticholinergic effects

Antihypertensives: Cyclic antidepressants may inhibit the antihypertensive response to bethanidine, clonidine, debrisoquin, guanadrel, guanethidine, guanabenz, guanfacine; monitor BP; consider alternate antihypertensive agent

Beta-agonists: When combined with TCAs may predispose patients to cardiac arrhythmias

Bupropion: May increase the levels of tricyclic antidepressants; based on limited information; monitor response

Carbamazepine: Tricyclic antidepressants may increase carbamazepine levels; monitor

Cholestyramine and colestipol: May bind TCAs and reduce their absorption; monitor for altered response

Clonidine: Abrupt discontinuation of clonidine may cause hypertensive crisis, cyclic antidepressants may enhance the response

CNS depressants: Sedative effects may be additive with TCAs; monitor for increased effect; includes benzodiazepines, barbiturates, antipsychotics, ethanol, and other sedative medications

Epinephrine (and other direct alpha-agonists): Pressor response to I.V. epinephrine, norepinephrine, and phenylephrine may be enhanced in patients receiving TCAs (**Note:** Effect is unlikely with epinephrine or levonordefrin dosages typically administered as infiltration in combination with local anesthetics)

Fenfluramine: May increase tricyclic antidepressant levels/effects

Hypoglycemic agents (including insulin): TCAs may enhance the hypoglycemic effects of tolazamide, chlorpropamide, or insulin; monitor for changes in blood glucose levels; reported with chlorpropamide, tolazamide, and insulin

Levodopa: tricyclic antidepressants may decrease the absorption (bioavailability) of levodopa; rare hypertensive episodes have also been attributed to this combination

Linezolid: Hyperpyrexia, hypertension, tachycardia, confusion, seizures, and **deaths have been reported** with agents which inhibit MAO (serotonin syndrome); this combination should be avoided

Lithium: Concurrent use with a TCA may increase the risk for neurotoxicity

MAO inhibitors: Hyperpyrexia, hypertension, tachycardia, confusion, seizures, and **deaths have been reported** (serotonin syndrome); this combination should be avoided

Methylphenidate: Metabolism of tricyclic antidepressants may be decreased

Phenothiazines: Serum concentrations of some TCAs may be increased; in addition, TCAs may increase concentration of phenothiazines; monitor for altered clinical response

QT_c-prolonging agents: Concurrent use of tricyclic agents with other drugs which may prolong QT_c interval may increase the risk of potentially fatal arrhythmias; includes type Ia and type III antiarrhythmics agents, selected quinolones (sparfloxacin, gatifloxacin, moxifloxacin, grepafloxacin), cisapride, and other agents

Sucralfate: Absorption of tricyclic antidepressants may be reduced with coadministration

Sympathomimetics, indirect-acting: Tricyclic antidepressants may result in a decreased sensitivity to indirect-acting sympathomimetics; includes dopamine and ephedrine; also see interaction with epinephrine (and direct-acting sympathomimetics)

Tramadol: Tramadol's risk of seizures may be increased with TCAs

Valproic acid: May increase serum concentrations/adverse effects of some tricyclic antidepressants

Warfarin (and other oral anticoagulants): Tricyclic antidepressants may increase the anticoagulant effect in patients stabilized on warfarin; monitor INR

Ethanol/Nutrition/Herb Interactions

Ethanol: Avoid ethanol (may increase CNS depression).

Food: Grapefruit juice may inhibit the metabolism of some TCAs and clinical toxicity may result.

Herb/Nutraceutical: Avoid valerian, St John's wort, SAMe, kava kava (may increase risk of serotonin syndrome and/or excessive sedation).

Mechanism of Action Increases the synaptic concentration of serotonin and/or norepinephrine in the central nervous system by inhibition of their reuptake by the presynaptic neuronal membrane

Pharmacodynamics/Kinetics

Distribution: Crosses the placenta

Protein binding: 92%

Metabolism: Undergoes first-pass metabolism (10% to 25%); extensively metabolized in the liver by N-oxidation, hydroxylation and glucuronidation

Half-life: 54-92 hours, averaging 74 hours

Time to peak serum concentration: Oral: Within 24-30 hours

Elimination: In urine

Usual Dosage Oral:

Adolescents: 15-20 mg/day

Adults: 15-60 mg in 3-4 divided doses

Elderly: 15-20 mg/day

Dietary Considerations May be administered with food to decrease GI distress.

Administration Make any dosage increase in the morning dose

Monitoring Parameters Monitor for cardiac abnormalities in elderly patients receiving doses >20 mg

Reference Range Therapeutic: 70-250 ng/mL (SI: 266-950 nmol/L); Toxic: >500 ng/mL (SI: >1900 nmol/L)

Test Interactions ↑ glucose

Patient Information Avoid unnecessary exposure to sunlight; do not discontinue abruptly; take dose in morning to avoid insomnia

Nursing Implications Offer patient sugarless hard candy or gum for dry mouth

Dosage Forms Tablet, as hydrochloride: 5 mg, 10 mg

♦ **Protriptyline Hydrochloride** *see* Protriptyline *on page 344*

♦ **Provigil®** *see* Modafinil *on page 247*

♦ **Prozac®** *see* Fluoxetine *on page 146*

♦ **Prozac® Weekly™** *see* Fluoxetine *on page 146*

♦ **P. trifolius L.** *see* Ginseng *on page 168*

♦ **Purple Coneflower** *see* Echinacea *on page 129*

Quazepam (KWAY ze pam)

Related Information

Anxiolytic/Hypnotic Use in Long-Term Care Facilities *on page 562*

Benzodiazepines Comparison Chart *on page 566*

Patient Information - Anxiolytics & Sedative Hypnotics (Benzodiazepines) *on page 483*

U.S. Brand Names Doral®

Pharmacologic Category Benzodiazepine

Generic Available No

Use Treatment of insomnia

Restrictions C-IV

Pregnancy Risk Factor X

Contraindications Hypersensitivity to quazepam or any component of the formulation (cross-sensitivity with other benzodiazepines may exist); narrow-angle glaucoma (not in product labeling, however, benzodiazepines are contraindicated); pregnancy

(Continued)

Quazepam *(Continued)*

Warnings/Precautions Should be used only after evaluation of potential causes of sleep disturbance. Failure of sleep disturbance to resolve after 7-10 days may indicate psychiatric or medical illness. A worsening of insomnia or the emergence of new abnormalities of thought or behavior may represent unrecognized psychiatric or medical illness and requires immediate and careful evaluation. Use with caution in elderly or debilitated patients, patients with hepatic disease (including alcoholics), or renal impairment. Use with caution in patients with respiratory disease or impaired gag reflex. Avoid use in patients with sleep apnea.

Causes CNS depression (dose-related) resulting in sedation, dizziness, confusion, or ataxia which may impair physical and mental capabilities. Patients must be cautioned about performing tasks which require mental alertness (operating machinery or driving). Use with caution in patients receiving other CNS depressants or psychoactive agents. Effects with other sedative drugs or ethanol may be potentiated. Benzodiazepines have been associated with falls and traumatic injury and should be used with extreme caution in patients who are at risk of these events (especially the elderly).

Use caution in patients with depression, particularly if suicidal risk may be present. Use with caution in patients with a history of drug dependence. Benzodiazepines have been associated with dependence and acute withdrawal symptoms on discontinuation or reduction in dose. Acute withdrawal, including seizures, may be precipitated after administration of flumazenil to patients receiving long-term benzodiazepine therapy.

Benzodiazepines have been associated with anterograde amnesia. Paradoxical reactions, including hyperactive or aggressive behavior have been reported with benzodiazepines, particularly in adolescent/pediatric or psychiatric patients. Does not have analgesic, antidepressant, or antipsychotic properties.

Adverse Reactions Frequency not defined.

Cardiovascular: Palpitations

Central nervous system: Drowsiness, fatigue, ataxia, memory impairment, anxiety, depression, headache, confusion, nervousness, dizziness, incoordination, hypo- and hyperkinesia, agitation, euphoria, paranoid reaction, nightmares, abnormal thinking

Dermatologic: Dermatitis, pruritus, rash

Endocrine & metabolic: Decreased libido, menstrual irregularities

Gastrointestinal: Xerostomia, constipation, diarrhea, dyspepsia, anorexia, abnormal taste perception, nausea, vomiting, increased or decreased appetite, abdominal pain

Genitourinary: Impotence, incontinence

Hematologic: Blood dyscrasias

Neuromuscular & skeletal: Dysarthria, rigidity, tremor, muscle cramps, reflex slowing

Ocular: Blurred vision

Miscellaneous: Drug dependence

Overdosage/Toxicology

Signs and symptoms: Somnolence, confusion, coma, hypoactive reflexes, dyspnea, hypotension, slurred speech, impaired coordination

Treatment:

Treatment for benzodiazepine overdose is supportive; rarely is mechanical ventilation required

Flumazenil has been shown to selectively block the binding of benzodiazepines to CNS receptors, resulting in a reversal of benzodiazepine-induced CNS depression, but not respiratory depression

Drug Interactions

CNS depressants: Sedative effects and/or respiratory depression may be additive with CNS depressants; includes ethanol, barbiturates, narcotic analgesics, and other sedative agents; monitor for increased effect

Cytochrome P450 inhibitors: May increase levels and effects of quazepam; may include fluvoxamine, isoniazid, itraconazole, ketoconazole, labetalol, loxapine, metoprolol, metronidazole, miconazole, nefazodone, omeprazole, troleandomycin, valproic acid, verapamil, grapefruit juice

Enzyme inducers: Metabolism of some benzodiazepines may be increased, decreasing their therapeutic effect; consider using an alternative sedative/ hypnotic agent; potential inducers include phenobarbital, phenytoin, carbamazepine, rifampin, and rifabutin

Levodopa: Therapeutic effects may be diminished in some patients following the addition of a benzodiazepine; limited/inconsistent data

Oral contraceptives: May decrease the clearance of some benzodiazepines (those which undergo oxidative metabolism); monitor for increased benzodiazepine effect

Theophylline: May partially antagonize some of the effects of benzodiazepines; monitor for decreased response; may require higher doses for sedation

Ethanol/Nutrition/Herb Interactions Ethanol: Avoid ethanol (may increase CNS depression).

Mechanism of Action Binds to stereospecific benzodiazepine receptors on the postsynaptic GABA neuron at several sites within the central nervous system, including the limbic system, reticular formation. Enhancement of the inhibitory effect of GABA on neuronal excitability results by increased neuronal membrane permeability to chloride ions. This shift in chloride ions results in hyperpolarization (a less excitable state) and stabilization.

Pharmacodynamics/Kinetics
Absorption: Oral: Rapid
Protein binding: 95%
Metabolism: In the liver to at least one active compound
Half-life:
Parent drug: 25-41 hours
Active metabolite: 40-114 hours

Usual Dosage Adults: Oral: Initial: 15 mg at bedtime, in some patients the dose may be reduced to 7.5 mg after a few nights

Dosing adjustment in hepatic impairment: Dose reduction may be necessary

Monitoring Parameters Respiratory and cardiovascular status

Patient Information Avoid alcohol and other CNS depressants; avoid activities needing good psychomotor coordination until CNS effects are known; drug may cause physical or psychological dependence; avoid abrupt discontinuation after prolonged use

Nursing Implications
Provide safety measures (ie, side rails, night light, call button); remove smoking materials from area; supervise ambulation
Monitor respiratory and cardiovascular status

Additional Information More likely than short-acting benzodiazepine to cause daytime sedation and fatigue; is classified as a long-acting benzodiazepine hypnotic (eg, flurazepam), this long duration of action may prevent withdrawal symptoms when therapy is discontinued. Abrupt discontinuation after sustained use (generally >10 days) may cause withdrawal symptoms.

Dosage Forms Tablet: 7.5 mg, 15 mg

Quetiapine (kwe TYE a peen)
Related Information
U.S. Brand Names Seroquel®
(Continued)

Quetiapine *(Continued)*

Canadian Brand Names Seroquel

Synonyms Quetiapine Fumarate

Pharmacologic Category Antipsychotic Agent, Dibenzothiazepine

Generic Available No

Use Treatment of schizophrenia

Unlabeled/Investigational Use Treatment of mania, bipolar disorder (children and adults); autism, psychosis (children)

Pregnancy Risk Factor C

Contraindications Hypersensitivity to quetiapine or any component of the formulation; severe CNS depression; bone marrow suppression; blood dyscrasias; severe hepatic disease; coma

Warnings/Precautions Has been noted to cause cataracts in animals, although quetiapine-associated cataracts have not been observed in humans; lens examination on initiation of therapy and every 6 months is recommended. May be sedating, use with caution in disorders where CNS depression is a feature. Use with caution in Parkinson's disease. Caution in patients with hemodynamic instability; prior myocardial infarction or ischemic heart disease; hypercholesterolemia; thyroid disease; predisposition to seizures; subcortical brain damage; hepatic impairment; severe cardiac, renal, or respiratory disease. May alter temperature regulation or mask toxicity of other drugs due to antiemetic effects. May alter cardiac conduction - life-threatening arrhythmias have occurred with therapeutic doses of antipsychotics. May cause orthostatic hypotension - use with caution in patients at risk of this effect or those who would tolerate transient hypotensive episodes (cerebrovascular disease, cardiovascular disease, or other medications which may predispose). Esophageal dysmotility and aspiration have been associated with antipsychotic use - use with caution in patients at risk of pneumonia (ie, Alzheimer's disease).

May cause anticholinergic effects (confusion, agitation, constipation, dry mouth, blurred vision, urinary retention); therefore, they should be used with caution in patients with decreased gastrointestinal motility, urinary retention, BPH, xerostomia, or visual problems. Conditions which also may be exacerbated by cholinergic blockade include narrow-angle glaucoma (screening is recommended) and worsening of myasthenia gravis. Relative to other antipsychotics, quetiapine has a moderate potency of cholinergic blockade. The risk of extrapyramidal symptoms, tardive dyskinesia, and neuroleptic malignant syndrome in association with quetiapine is very low relative to other antipsychotics.

Adverse Reactions

>10%:
   Central nervous system: Headache, somnolence
   Gastrointestinal: Weight gain

1% to 10%:
   Cardiovascular: Postural hypotension, tachycardia, palpitations
   Central nervous system: Dizziness
   Dermatologic: Rash
   Gastrointestinal: Abdominal pain, constipation, xerostomia, dyspepsia, anorexia
   Hematologic: Leukopenia
   Neuromuscular & skeletal: Dysarthria, back pain, weakness
   Respiratory: Rhinitis, pharyngitis, cough, dyspnea
   Miscellaneous: Diaphoresis

<1%: Abnormal dreams, anemia, bradycardia, diabetes, elevated alkaline phosphatase, elevated GGT, epistaxis, hyperlipidemia, hypothyroidism, increased appetite, increased salivation, involuntary movements, leukocytosis, QT prolongation, rash, tardive dyskinesia, vertigo

Drug Interactions CYP3A4, 2D6 (minor); 2C9 (minor) enzyme substrate

Antihypertensives: Concurrent use with an antihypertensive may produce additive hypotensive effects (particularly orthostasis)

Cimetidine: May decrease quetiapine's clearance by 20%; increasing serum concentrations

CNS depressants: Quetiapine may enhance the sedative effects of other CNS depressants; includes antidepressants, benzodiazepines, barbiturates, ethanol, narcotic analgesics, and other sedative agents; monitor for increased effect

CYP3A3/4 inhibitors: Serum level and/or toxicity of quetiapine may be increased; inhibitors include amiodarone, cimetidine, clarithromycin, erythromycin, delavirdine, diltiazem, dirithromycin, disulfiram, fluoxetine, fluvoxamine, grapefruit juice, indinavir, itraconazole, ketoconazole, metronidazole, nefazodone, nevirapine, propoxyphene, quinupristin-dalfopristin, ritonavir, saquinavir, verapamil, zafirlukast, zileuton; monitor for altered response

Enzyme inducers: May increase the metabolism of quetiapine, reducing serum levels and effect; enzyme inducers include carbamazepine, barbiturates, and rifampin; also see note on phenytoin

Levodopa: Quetiapine may inhibit the antiparkinsonian effect of levodopa; avoid this combination

Lorazepam: Metabolism of lorazepam may be reduced by quetiapine; clearance is reduced 20% in the presence of quetiapine; monitor for increased sedative effect

Phenytoin: Metabolism/clearance of quetiapine may be increased; fivefold changes have been noted

Thioridazine: May increase clearance of quetiapine, decreasing serum concentrations; clearance may be increased by 65%

Ethanol/Nutrition/Herb Interactions

Ethanol: Avoid ethanol (may cause excessive impairment in cognition/motor function).

Food: In healthy volunteers, administration of quetiapine with food resulted in an increase in the peak serum concentration and AUC (each by ~15%) compared to the fasting state.

Herb/Nutraceutical: St John's wort may decrease quetiapine levels. Avoid valerian, St John's wort, kava kava, gotu kola (may increase CNS depression).

Mechanism of Action Mechanism of action of quetiapine, as with other antipsychotic drugs, is unknown. However, it has been proposed that this drug's antipsychotic activity is mediated through a combination of dopamine type 2 (D_2) and serotonin type 2 ($5-HT_2$) antagonism. However, it is an antagonist at multiple neurotransmitter receptors in the brain: serotonin $5-HT_{1A}$ and $5-HT_2$, dopamine D_1 and D_2, histamine H_1, and adrenergic alpha$_1$- and alpha$_2$-receptors; but appears to have no appreciable affinity at cholinergic muscarinic and benzodiazepine receptors.

Antagonism at receptors other than dopamine and $5-HT_2$ with similar receptor affinities may explain some of the other effects of quetiapine. The drug's antagonism of histamine H_1-receptors may explain the somnolence observed with it. The drug's antagonism of adrenergic alpha$_1$-receptors may explain the orthostatic hypotension observed with it.

Pharmacodynamics/Kinetics

Absorption: Accumulation is predictable upon multiple dosing

Distribution: Steady-state concentrations are expected to be achieved within 2 days of dosing; unlikely to interfere with the metabolism of drugs metabolized by cytochrome P450 enzymes

Metabolism: Both metabolites are pharmacologically inactive

Half-life, mean terminal: ~6 hours

Time to peak plasma concentrations: 1.5 hours

Elimination: Mainly via hepatic metabolism

Usual Dosage Oral:

Children and Adolescents:

Autism (unlabeled use): 100-350 mg/day (1.6-5.2 mg/kg/day)

Psychosis and mania (unlabeled use): Initial: 25 mg twice daily, titrate as necessary to 450 mg/day

Adults: Schizophrenia/psychoses: Initial: 25 mg twice daily; increase in increments of 25-50 mg 2-3 times/day on the second and third day, if tolerated, to a target

(Continued)

Quetiapine *(Continued)*

dose of 300-400 mg in 2-3 divided doses by day 4. Make further adjustments as needed at intervals of at least 2 days in adjustments of 25-50 mg twice daily. Usual maintenance range: 300-800 mg/day

Elderly: 40% lower mean oral clearance of quetiapine in adults >65 years of age; higher plasma levels expected and, therefore, dosage adjustment may be needed; elderly patients usually require 50-200 mg/day

Dosing comments in hepatic insufficiency: 30% lower mean oral clearance of quetiapine than normal subjects; higher plasma levels expected in hepatically impaired subjects; dosage adjustment may be needed

Child/Adolescent Considerations Six children with autistic disorder (mean age: 10.9 years) received 100-350 mg/day (1.6-5.2 mg/kg/day; Martin, 1999). Ten patients with DSM-IV chronic or intermittent psychotic disorders (12.3-15.9 years of age) received quetiapine twice daily starting at 25 mg and reaching 400 mg by day 20. The trial ended on day 23 (McConville, 2000). Thirty manic or mixed bipolar I adolescents (12-18 years of age) received quetiapine 25 mg twice daily with titration to 450 mg/day by day 7 (DelBello, 2001).

Dietary Considerations Can be taken with or without food.

Monitoring Parameters Patients should have eyes checked for cataracts every 6 months while on this medication

Patient Information May cause drowsiness, dizziness, and/or headache; might increase risk of cataracts

Nursing Implications Seroquel® has a very low incidence of extrapyramidal symptoms such as restlessness and abnormal movement; is at least as effective as conventional antipsychotics (ie, Haldol®)

Additional Information Quetiapine has a very low incidence of extrapyramidal symptoms such as restlessness and abnormal movement, and is at least as effective as conventional antipsychotics.

Dosage Forms Tablet: 25 mg, 100 mg, 200 mg, 300 mg

♦ **Quetiapine Fumarate** *see Quetiapine on page 349*
♦ **Quinalbarbitone Sodium** *see Secobarbital on page 367*
♦ **Racemic Amphetamine Sulfate** *see Amphetamine on page 40*
♦ **Radix** *see Valerian on page 425*
♦ **Red Valerian** *see Valerian on page 425*
♦ **Remeron®** *see Mirtazapine on page 244*
♦ **Remeron® SolTab™** *see Mirtazapine on page 244*
♦ **Reminyl®** *see Galantamine on page 163*
♦ **Repan®** *see Butalbital Compound on page 59*
♦ **Requip®** *see Ropinirole on page 361*

Reserpine *(re SER peen)*

U.S. Brand Names Serpalan®

Canadian Brand Names Novo-Reserpine®; Srpa il®

Pharmacologic Category Rauwolfia Alkaloid

Generic Available Yes

Use Management of mild to moderate hypertension

Unlabeled/Investigational Use Management of tardive dyskinesia

Pregnancy Risk Factor C

Contraindications Hypersensitivity to reserpine or any component of the formulation; active peptic ulcer disease; ulcerative colitis; history of mental depression (especially with suicidal tendencies); MAO inhibitors

Warnings/Precautions Discontinue reserpine 7 days before electroshock therapy; use with caution in patients with impaired renal function, inflammatory bowel disease, asthma, gallstones, or history of peptic ulcer disease, and the elderly. At high doses, significant mental depression, anxiety, or psychosis may occur (uncommon at dosages <0.25 mg/day). May cause orthostatic hypotension; use with caution in patients at risk of hypotension or in patients where transient hypotensive episodes would be poorly tolerated (cardiovascular disease or cerebrovascular disease). Some products may contain tartrazine.

Adverse Reactions Frequency not defined.

Cardiovascular: Peripheral edema, arrhythmias, bradycardia, chest pain, PVC, hypotension

Central nervous system: Dizziness, headache, nightmares, nervousness, drowsiness, fatigue, mental depression, parkinsonism, dull sensorium, syncope, paradoxical anxiety

Dermatologic: Rash, pruritus, flushing of skin

Gastrointestinal: Anorexia, diarrhea, dry mouth, nausea, vomiting, increased salivation, weight gain, increased gastric acid secretion

Genitourinary: Impotence, decreased libido

Hematologic: Thrombocytopenia purpura

Ocular: Blurred vision

Respiratory: Nasal congestion, dyspnea, epistaxis

Overdosage/Toxicology

Signs and symptoms: Hypotension, bradycardia, CNS depression, sedation, coma, hypothermia, miosis, tremors, diarrhea, vomiting

Treatment: Hypotension usually responds to I.V. fluids or Trendelenburg positioning. If unresponsive to these measures, the use of a parenteral inotrope may be required (eg, norepinephrine 0.1-0.2 mcg/kg/minute titrated to response). Anticholinergic agents may be useful in reducing the parkinsonian effects and bradycardia.

Drug Interactions

CNS depressants, ethanol: Additive CNS effects may occur.

Digitalis glycosides: Concomitant administration may predispose some patients to cardiac arrhythmias.

Diuretics, antihypertensives: Hypotensive effects may be increased.

Levodopa: Effects of levodopa may be decreased with concomitant administration.

MAO inhibitors: Reserpine may cause hypertensive reactions; use an alternative antihypertensive. Theoretically, risk is decreased if reserpine is administered several days prior to MAO inhibitors.

Quinidine, procainamide: Cardiac depressant effects may be increased.

Sympathomimetics: Theoretically, effects may be increased/prolonged; monitor.

Tricyclic antidepressants: Antihypertensive effects may de decreased with concomitant administration of TCAs.

Ethanol/Nutrition/Herb Interactions

Ethanol: Avoid ethanol (may increase CNS depression).

Herb/Nutraceutical: Avoid dong quai if using for hypertension (has estrogenic activity). Avoid ephedra, yohimbe (may worsen hypertension). Avoid valerian, St John's wort, kava kava, gotu kola (may increase CNS depression). Avoid garlic (may have increased antihypertensive effect).

Stability Protect oral dosage forms from light

Mechanism of Action Reduces blood pressure via depletion of sympathetic biogenic amines (norepinephrine and dopamine); this also commonly results in sedative effects

Pharmacodynamics/Kinetics

Onset of antihypertensive effect: Within 3-6 days

Duration: 2-6 weeks

Absorption: Oral: ~40%

Distribution: Crosses the placenta; appears in breast milk

Protein binding: 96%

Metabolism: Extensively in the liver, >90%

Half-life: 50-100 hours

Elimination: Principal excretion in feces (30% to 60%) and small amounts in urine (10%)

Usual Dosage Note: When used for management of hypertension, full antihypertensive effects may take as long as 3 weeks.

(Continued)

Reserpine *(Continued)*

Oral:
Children: Hypertension: 0.01-0.02 mg/kg/24 hours divided every 12 hours; maximum dose: 0.25 mg/day (not recommended in children)

Adults:
Hypertension: 0.1-0.25 mg/day in 1-2 doses; initial: 0.5 mg/day for 1-2 weeks; maintenance: reduce to 0.1-0.25 mg/day;
Psychiatric: Initial: 0.5 mg/day; usual range: 0.1-1 mg
Elderly: Initial: 0.05 mg once daily, increasing by 0.05 mg every week as necessary

Dosing adjustment in renal impairment: Cl$_{cr}$ <10 mL/minute: Avoid use

Dialysis: Not removed by hemo or peritoneal dialysis; supplemental dose is not necessary

Monitoring Parameters Blood pressure, standing and sitting/supine

Test Interactions ↓ catecholamines (U)

Patient Information Take with food or milk; impotency is reversible; notify physician if a weight gain of more than 5 lb has taken place during therapy; may cause drowsiness, impair judgment and coordination

Nursing Implications Observe for mental depression and alert family members to report any symptoms

Additional Information Adverse effects are usually dose related, mild, and infrequent when administered for the management of hypertension.

Dosage Forms Tablet: 0.1 mg, 0.25 mg

♦ **Restall®** *see* Hydroxyzine *on page 178*

♦ **Restoril®** *see* Temazepam *on page 388*

♦ **Revex®** *see* Nalmefene *on page 252*

♦ **ReVia®** *see* Naltrexone *on page 256*

♦ **Rhotrimine® (Can)** *see* Trimipramine *on page 421*

♦ **Risperdal®** *see* Risperidone *on page 354*

Risperidone *(ris PER i done)*

Related Information

Antipsychotic Agents Comparison Chart *on page 557*
Antipsychotic Medication Guidelines *on page 559*
Atypical Antipsychotics *on page 565*
Discontinuation of Psychotropic Drugs - Withdrawal Symptoms and Recommendations *on page 582*
Federal OBRA Regulations Recommended Maximum Doses *on page 583*
Liquid Compatibility With Antipsychotics and Mood Stabilizers *on page 587*
Patient Information - Antipsychotics (General) *on page 466*

U.S. Brand Names Risperdal®

Canadian Brand Names Risperdal

Pharmacologic Category Antipsychotic Agent, Benzisoxazole

Generic Available No

Use Management of psychotic disorders (eg, schizophrenia)

Unlabeled/Investigational Use Behavioral symptoms associated with dementia in elderly; treatment of bipolar disorder, mania, Tourette's disorder; treatment of pervasive developmental disorder and autism in children and adolescents

Pregnancy Risk Factor C

Contraindications Hypersensitivity to risperidone or any component of the formulation

Warnings/Precautions Low to moderately sedating, use with caution in disorders where CNS depression is a feature. Use with caution in Parkinson's disease. Caution in patients with hemodynamic instability; bone marrow suppression; predisposition to seizures; subcortical brain damage; severe cardiac, hepatic, or respiratory disease. Use with caution in renal dysfunction. Esophageal dysmotility and aspiration have been associated with antipsychotic use - use with caution in patients at risk of aspiration pneumonia (ie, Alzheimer's disease). Caution in breast cancer or other prolactin-dependent tumors (may elevate prolactin levels). May alter temperature regulation or mask toxicity of other drugs due to antiemetic effects. May alter cardiac conduction (low risk relative to other neuroleptics) - life-threatening arrhythmias have occurred with therapeutic doses of neuroleptics. Avoid in patients with QT prolongation. Use with caution in elderly patients or in patients who would not tolerate transient hypotensive episodes (cerebrovascular or cardiovascular disease) due to potential for orthostasis.

May cause anticholinergic effects (confusion, agitation, constipation, dry mouth, blurred vision, urinary retention); therefore, they should be used with caution in patients with decreased gastrointestinal motility, urinary retention, BPH, xerostomia, or visual problems. Conditions which also may be exacerbated by cholinergic blockade include narrow-angle glaucoma (screening is recommended) and worsening of myasthenia gravis. Relative to other neuroleptics, risperidone has a low potency of cholinergic blockade.

May cause extrapyramidal reactions, including pseudoparkinsonism, acute dystonic reactions, akathisia, and tardive dyskinesia (risk of these reactions is low relative to other neuroleptics, and is dose-dependent). May be associated with neuroleptic malignant syndrome (NMS) or pigmentary retinopathy.

Adverse Reactions
Frequency not defined: Dysphagia, esophageal dysmotility

>10%: Central nervous system: Insomnia, agitation, anxiety, headache

1% to 10%:

Cardiovascular: Hypotension (especially orthostatic), tachycardia

Central nervous system: Sedation, dizziness, restlessness, anxiety, extrapyramidal reactions (dose dependent); dystonic reactions, pseudoparkinson, tardive dyskinesia, neuroleptic malignant syndrome, altered central temperature regulation

Dermatologic: Photosensitivity (rare), rash, dry skin

Endocrine & metabolic: Amenorrhea, galactorrhea, gynecomastia, sexual dysfunction

Gastrointestinal: Constipation, GI upset, xerostomia, dyspepsia, vomiting, abdominal pain, nausea, anorexia, weight gain

Genitourinary: Polyuria

Ocular: Abnormal vision

Respiratory: Rhinitis, coughing, sinusitis, pharyngitis, dyspnea

Overdosage/Toxicology
Signs and symptoms: Drowsiness, sedation, tachycardia, hypotension, extrapyramidal symptoms; one case involved decreased sodium and potassium and prolonged Q-T and widened QRS

Treatment: Establish and maintain airway to ensure adequate oxygenation and ventilation; consider gastric lavage and activated charcoal together with a laxative; monitor cardiovascular status, including EKG to detect arrhythmias; do not treat arrhythmias with disopyramide, procainamide, or quinidine as these potentiate the Q-T prolonging the effects of risperidone; do not use epinephrine or norepinephrine for hypotension as the beta stimulation may worsen this symptom; anticholinergics may be required for severe extrapyramidal side effects

Drug Interactions CYP2D6 enzyme substrate and weak inhibitor; CYP3A4 substrate

Antihypertensives: Risperidone may enhance the hypotensive effects of antihypertensive agents

Clozapine: Decreases clearance of risperidone, increasing its serum concentrations

CYP2D6 inhibitors: Metabolism of risperidone may be decreased; increasing clinical effect or toxicity; inhibitors include amiodarone, cimetidine, delavirdine, fluoxetine, paroxetine, propafenone, quinidine, and ritonavir; monitor for increased effect/toxicity

(Continued)

Risperidone *(Continued)*

CYP3A3/4 inhibitors: May increase serum concentrations of risperidone; inhibitors include amiodarone, cimetidine, clarithromycin, erythromycin, delavirdine, diltiazem, dirithromycin, disulfiram, fluoxetine, fluvoxamine, grapefruit juice, indinavir, itraconazole, ketoconazole, metronidazole, nefazodone, nevirapine, propoxyphene, quinupristin-dalfopristin, ritonavir, saquinavir, verapamil, zafirlukast, zileuton; monitor for altered response

Enzyme inducers: May increase the metabolism of risperidone, reducing serum levels and effect; enzyme inducers include carbamazepine, barbiturates, phenytoin and rifampin; see note on carbamazepine

Levodopa: At high doses (>6 mg/day), risperidone may inhibit the antiparkinsonian effect of levodopa; avoid this combination when high doses are used

Valproic acid: Generalized edema has been reported as a consequence of concurrent therapy (case report)

Ethanol/Nutrition/Herb Interactions

Ethanol: Avoid ethanol (may increase CNS depression).

Herb/Nutraceutical: Avoid kava kava, gotu kola, valerian, St John's wort (may increase CNS depression).

Mechanism of Action Risperidone is a benzisoxazole derivative, mixed serotonin-dopamine antagonist; binds to 5-HT_2-receptors in the CNS and in the periphery with a very high affinity; binds to dopamine-D_2 receptors with less affinity. The binding affinity to the dopamine-D_2 receptor is 20 times lower than the 5-HT_2 affinity. The addition of serotonin antagonism to dopamine antagonism (classic neuroleptic mechanism) is thought to improve negative symptoms of psychoses and reduce the incidence of extrapyramidal side effects. Alpha$_1$, alpha$_2$ adrenergic, and histaminergic receptors are also antagonized with high affinity. Risperidone has low to moderate affinity for 5-HT_{1c}, 5-HT_{1d}, and 5-HT_{1A} receptors, weak affinity for D_1 and no affinity for muscarinics or beta$_1$ and beta$_2$ receptors

Pharmacodynamics/Kinetics

Absorption: Oral: Rapid

Metabolism: Extensive by cytochrome P450

Protein binding: Plasma: 90%

Half-life: 24 hours (risperidone and its active metabolite)

Time to peak: Peak plasma concentrations within 1 hour

Usual Dosage Oral:

Children and Adolescents:

Pervasive developmental disorder (unlabeled use): Initial: 0.25 mg twice daily, titrate up 0.25 mg/day every 5-7 days; optimal dose range: 0.75-3 mg/day

Autism (unlabeled use): Initial: 0.25 mg at bedtime, titrate to 1 mg/day (0.1 mg/kg/day)

Schizophrenia: Initial: 0.5 mg twice daily, titrate as necessary up to 2-6 mg/day

Bipolar disorder (unlabeled use): 0.5-3 mg/day

Tourette's disorder (unlabeled use): 2-4 mg/day

Adults: Recommended starting dose: 0.5-1 mg twice daily; slowly increase to the optimum range of 3-6 mg/day; may be given as a single daily dose once maintenance dose is achieved; daily dosages >10 mg does not appear to confer any additional benefit, and the incidence of extrapyramidal reactions is higher than with lower doses

Elderly: A starting dose of 0.25-1 mg in 1-2 divided doses, and titration should progress slowly. Additional monitoring of renal function and orthostatic blood pressure may be warranted. If once-a-day dosing in the elderly or debilitated patient is considered, a twice daily regimen should be used to titrate to the target dose, and this dose should be maintained for 2-3 days prior to attempts to switch to a once-daily regimen.

Dosing adjustment in renal, hepatic impairment: Starting dose of 0.25-0.5 mg twice daily is advisable

Child/Adolescent Considerations Fourteen children and adolescents 9-17 years of age were treated for pervasive developmental disorder with 0.25 mg twice daily initially and titrated up 0.25 mg/day every 5-7 days. Optimal dose ranged from

0.75-1 mg/day (Fisman, 1996). Eighteen children 10.2 ± 3.7 years of age with pervasive developmental disorders improved with an optimal dose of 1.8 ± 1 mg/day (McDougle, 1997). Six children 7-14 years of age with pervasive developmental disorder received the mean optimal dose of 2.7 mg/day for 5.2 months (Perry, 1997). Twenty children and adolescents with developmental disorders 8-17 years of age refractory to previous psychotropics were treated with 1.5-10 mg/day (Hardan, 1996).

Six children 5-9 years of age with autistic disorder were treated with 0.25 mg at bedtime (mean: 1.1 mg at week 8) (Findling, 1997). Ten boys 4.5-10.8 years of age with autistic disorder were initiated on 0.5 mg daily and titrated to 6 mg/day or 0.1 mg/kg/day (Nicolson, 1998).

Ten adolescents 11-18 years of age with schizophrenia were treated with a mean dose of 6.6 mg (4-10 mg/day) (Armenteros, 1997). Eleven children and adolescents 5.5-16 years of age with mood disorders and aggressive behaviors who responded inadequately to several mood stabilizing agents received 0.75-2.5 mg/day (Schreier, 1998).

Twenty-eight children 10.4 ± 3.8 years of age with bipolar disorder received a mean dose of 1.7 ± 1.3 mg/day over an average of 6.1 ± 8.5 months (Frazier, 1999). Twenty-six children 10-18 years of age (19 with borderline IQ and 5 with mild mental retardation) who were hospitalized for treatment of psychiatric disorders associated with aggressive behavior, were treated with 0.5-4 mg/day for 2-12 months (Buitelaar, 2000). Ten children with conduct disorder received a total daily dose 1.5-3 mg/day depending on their weight (Findling, 2000).

Twenty-four patients with Tourette's disorder were treated with a mean daily dose of 3.8 mg (Bruggeman, 2001).

Administration Oral solution can be mixed with water, coffee, orange juice, or low-fat milk, but is not compatible with cola or tea

Monitoring Parameters Monitor for extrapyramidal effects, orthostatic blood pressure changes for 3-5 days after starting or increasing dose

Patient Information May cause drowsiness

Nursing Implications Monitor and observe for extrapyramidal effects, orthostatic blood pressure changes for 3-5 days after starting or increasing dose

Dosage Forms
Solution, oral: 1 mg/mL (30 mL)
Tablet: 0.25 mg, 0.5 mg, 1 mg, 2 mg, 3 mg, 4 mg

♦ **Ritalin**® *see* Methylphenidate *on page 236*

♦ **Ritalin-SR**® *see* Methylphenidate *on page 236*

Rivastigmine (ri va STIG meen)

Related Information
Patient Information - Agents for the Treatment of Alzheimer's Disease *on page 491*

U.S. Brand Names Exelon®

Canadian Brand Names Exelon

Synonyms ENA 713; SDZ ENA 713

Pharmacologic Category Acetylcholinesterase Inhibitor (Central)

Generic Available No

Use Mild to moderate dementia from Alzheimer's disease

Pregnancy Risk Factor B

Pregnancy/Breast-Feeding Implications There are no adequate studies in pregnant women. Should be used only if the benefit outweighs the potential risk to the fetus. It is unknown if rivastigmine is excreted in human breast milk. There is no indication for use in nursing mothers.

Contraindications Hypersensitivity to rivastigmine, other carbamate derivatives, or any component of the formulation

Warnings/Precautions Significant nausea, vomiting, anorexia, and weight loss are associated with use; occurs more frequently in women and during the titration

(Continued)

Rivastigmine *(Continued)*

phase. If treatment is interrupted for more than several days, reinstate at the lowest daily dose. Use caution in patients with a history of peptic ulcer disease or concurrent NSAID use. Caution in patients undergoing anesthesia who will receive succinylcholine-type muscle relaxation, patients with sick sinus syndrome, bradycardia or supraventricular conduction conditions, urinary obstruction, seizure disorders, or pulmonary conditions such as asthma or COPD. There are no trials evaluating the safety and efficacy in children.

Adverse Reactions

>10%:

Central nervous system: Dizziness (21%), headache (17%)

Gastrointestinal: Nausea (47%), vomiting (31%), diarrhea (19%), anorexia (17%), abdominal pain (13%)

2% to 10%:

Cardiovascular: Syncope (3%), hypertension (3%)

Central nervous system: Fatigue (9%), insomnia (9%), confusion (8%), depression (6%), anxiety (5%), malaise (5%), somnolence (5%), hallucinations (4%), aggressiveness (3%)

Gastrointestinal: Dyspepsia (9%), constipation (5%), flatulence (4%), weight loss (3%), eructation (2%)

Genitourinary: Urinary tract infection (7%)

Neuromuscular & skeletal: Weakness (6%), tremor (4%)

Respiratory: Rhinitis (4%)

Miscellaneous: Increased diaphoresis (4%), flu-like syndrome (3%)

>2% (but frequency equal to placebo): Chest pain, peripheral edema, vertigo, back pain, arthralgia, pain, bone fracture, agitation, nervousness, delusion, paranoid reaction, upper respiratory tract infections, infection, coughing, pharyngitis, bronchitis, rash, urinary incontinence.

<2% (Limited to important or life-threatening symptoms; reactions may be at a similar frequency to placebo): Fever, edema, allergy, periorbital or facial edema, hypothermia, hypotension, postural hypotension, cardiac failure, ataxia, convulsions, apraxia, aphasia, dysphonia, hyperkinesia, hypertonia, hypokinesia, migraine, neuralgia, peripheral neuropathy, hypothyroidism, peptic ulcer, gastroesophageal reflux, GI hemorrhage, intestinal obstruction, pancreatitis, colitis, atrial fibrillation, bradycardia, AV block, bundle branch block, sick sinus syndrome, cardiac arrest, supraventricular tachycardia, tachycardia, abnormal hepatic function, cholecystitis, dehydration, arthritis, angina pectoris, myocardial infarction, epistaxis, hematoma, thrombocytopenia, purpura, delirium, emotional lability, psychosis, anemia, bronchospasm, apnea, rashes (maculopapular, eczema, bullous, exfoliative, psoriaform, erythematous), urticaria, acute renal failure, peripheral ischemia, pulmonary embolism, thrombosis, thrombophlebitis, intracranial hemorrhage, conjunctival hemorrhage, diplopia, glaucoma, lymphadenopathy, leukocytosis.

Postmarketing and/or case reports: Stevens-Johnson syndrome, severe vomiting with esophageal rupture (following inappropriate reinitiation of dose)

Overdosage/Toxicology In cases of asymptomatic overdoses, rivastigmine should be held for 24 hours. Cholinergic crisis, caused by significant acetylcholinesterase inhibition, is characterized by severe nausea, vomiting, salivation, sweating, bradycardia, hypotension, respiratory depression, collapse, and convulsions. Treatment is supportive and symptomatic. Dialysis would not be helpful.

Drug Interactions

Anticholinergics: Effects may be reduced with rivastigmine

Beta-blockers without ISA activity: May increase risk of bradycardia

Calcium channel blockers (diltiazem or verapamil): May increase risk of bradycardia

Cholinergic agonists: Effects may be increased with rivastigmine

Cigarette use increases the clearance of rivastigmine by 23%

Digoxin: Increased risk of bradycardia with concurrent use

Neuromuscular blockers: Depolarizing neuromuscular blocking agents effects may be increased with rivastigmine

NSAIDs: Although not seen in clinical studies, patients may be at increased risk for peptic ulcers or gastrointestinal bleeding with concomitant use; monitor

Ethanol/Nutrition/Herb Interactions

Cigarette use: Increases the clearance of rivastigmine by 23%.

Ethanol: Avoid ethanol (due to risk of sedation; may increase GI irritation).

Food: Food delays absorption by 90 minutes, lowers C_{max} by 30% and increases AUC by 30%.

Stability Store below 25°C (77°F); store solution in an upright position and protect from freezing

Mechanism of Action A deficiency of cortical acetylcholine is thought to account for some of the symptoms of Alzheimer's disease; rivastigmine increases acetylcholine in the central nervous system through reversible inhibition of its hydrolysis by cholinesterase

Pharmacodynamics/Kinetics

Absorption: Rapid and complete within 1 hour when administered in the fasting state

Distribution: V_d: 1.8-2.7 L/kg

Protein binding: 40%

Metabolism: Extensively metabolized by cholinesterase-mediated hydrolysis in the brain. The metabolite undergoes N-demethylation and/or sulfate conjugation in the liver. Cytochrome P450 minimally involved. Linear kinetics at 3 mg twice daily, but nonlinear at higher doses.

Bioavailability: 40%

Half-life: 1.5 hours

Time to peak: 1 hour

Elimination: 97% recovered in urine as metabolites; 0.4% in feces

Usual Dosage Adults: Mild to moderate Alzheimer's dementia: Oral: Initial: 1.5 mg twice daily to start; if dose is tolerated for at least 2 weeks then it may be increased to 3 mg twice daily; increases to 4.5 mg twice daily and 6 mg twice daily should only be attempted after at least 2 weeks at the previous dose; maximum dose: 6 mg twice daily. If adverse events such as nausea, vomiting, abdominal pain, or loss of appetite occur, the patient should be instructed to discontinue treatment for several doses then restart at the same or next lower dosage level; antiemetics have been used to control GI symptoms. If treatment is interrupted for longer than several days, restart the treatment at the lowest dose and titrate as previously described.

Elderly: Clearance is significantly lower in patients older than 60 years of age, but dosage adjustments are not recommended. Titrate dose to individual's tolerance.

Dosage adjustment in renal impairment: Dosage adjustments are not recommended, however, titrate the dose to the individual's tolerance.

Dosage adjustment in hepatic impairment: Clearance is significantly reduced in mild to moderately impaired patients. Although dosage adjustments are not recommended, use lowest possible dose and titrate according to individual's tolerance. May consider waiting >2 weeks between dosage adjustments.

Dietary Considerations Take with meals.

Monitoring Parameters Cognitive function at periodic intervals

Patient Information Take with meals at breakfast and dinner. Swallow capsule whole. Do not chew, break, or crush capsule. A liquid (solution) is available for patients who cannot swallow capsules. Monitor for nausea, vomiting, loss of appetite, or weight loss; notify healthcare provider if any of these occur. See instructions for use of oral solution. Can swallow solution directly from syringe or mix with water, juice, or soda. Stir well and drink all of mixture within 4 hours of mixing. Do not mix with other liquids. Avoid concurrent ethanol use.

Nursing Implications Educate patient or caregiver about medicine.

Dosage Forms

Capsule, as tartrate: 1.5 mg, 3 mg, 4.5 mg, 6 mg

(Continued)

Rivastigmine *(Continued)*

Solution, oral, as tartrate: 2 mg/mL (120 mL)

♦ **Rivotril® (Can)** *see Clonazepam on page 85*

Rizatriptan *(rye za TRIP tan)*

Related Information

Patient Information - Miscellaneous Medications - Antimigraine Medications *on page 521*

U.S. Brand Names Maxalt®; Maxalt-MLT™

Canadian Brand Names Maxalt

Synonyms MK462

Pharmacologic Category Serotonin 5-HT$_{1D}$ Receptor Agonist

Generic Available No

Use Acute treatment of migraine with or without aura

Pregnancy Risk Factor C

Contraindications Hypersensitivity to rizatriptan or any component of the formulation; documented ischemic heart disease or Prinzmetal's angina; uncontrolled hypertension; basilar or hemiplegic migraine; during or within 2 weeks of MAO inhibitors; during or within 24 hours of treatment with another 5-HT$_1$ agonist, or an ergot-containing or ergot-type medication (eg, methysergide, dihydroergotamine)

Warnings/Precautions Use only in patients with a clear diagnosis of migraine; use with caution in elderly or patients with hepatic or renal impairment, history of hypersensitivity to sumatriptan or adverse effects from sumatriptan, and in patients at risk of coronary artery disease (as predicted by presence of risk factors) unless cardiovascular evaluation provides evidence that the patient is free of cardiovascular disease. In patients with risk factors for coronary artery disease, following adequate evaluation to establish the absence of coronary artery disease, the initial dose should be administered in a setting where response may be evaluated (physician's office or similarly staffed setting). EKG monitoring may be considered. Do not use with ergotamines. May increase blood pressure transiently; may cause coronary vasospasm (less than sumatriptan); avoid in patients with signs/symptoms suggestive of reduced arterial flow (ischemic bowel, Raynaud's) which could be exacerbated by vasospasm. Phenylketonurics (tablets contain phenylalanine).

Patients who experience sensations of chest pain/pressure/tightness or symptoms suggestive of angina following dosing should be evaluated for coronary artery disease or Prinzmetal's angina before receiving additional doses.

Caution in dialysis patients or hepatically impaired. Reconsider diagnosis of migraine if no response to initial dose. Long-term effects on vision have not been evaluated.

Adverse Reactions

1% to 10%:

Cardiovascular: Systolic/diastolic blood pressure increases (5-10 mm Hg), chest pain (5%), palpitation

Central nervous system: Dizziness, drowsiness, fatigue (13% to 30%, dose related)

Dermatologic: Skin flushing

Endocrine & metabolic: Mild increase in growth hormone, hot flashes

Gastrointestinal: Nausea, abdominal pain, dry mouth (<5%)

Respiratory: Dyspnea

<1%: Akinesia, angina, arrhythmia, arthralgia, blurred vision, bradykinesia, decreased mental activity, diaphoresis, diarrhea, dry eyes, eye pain, facial edema, bradycardia, chills, hangover, heat sensitivity muscle weakness, myalgia, nasopharyngeal irritation, neck pain/stiffness, neurological/psychiatric abnormalities, pharyngitis, polyuria, pruritus, syncope, tachycardia, tinnitus

Postmarketing and/or case reports: Myocardial ischemia, myocardial infarction, stroke, toxic epidermal necrolysis, dysgeusia

Drug Interactions Use within 24 hours of another selective 5-HT$_1$ agonist or ergot-containing drug should be avoided due to possible additive vasoconstriction

MAO inhibitors and nonselective MAO inhibitors increase concentration of rizatriptan

Propranolol: Plasma concentration of rizatriptan increased 70%

SSRIs: Rarely, concurrent use results in weakness and incoordination; monitor closely

Ethanol/Nutrition/Herb Interactions Food: Food delays absorption.

Stability Store in blister pack until administration

Mechanism of Action Selective agonist for serotonin (5-HT$_{1d}$ receptor) in cranial arteries to cause vasoconstriction and reduce sterile inflammation associated with antidromic neuronal transmission correlating with relief of migraine

Usual Dosage Note: In patients with risk factors for coronary artery disease, following adequate evaluation to establish the absence of coronary artery disease, the initial dose should be administered in a setting where response may be evaluated (physician's office or similarly staffed setting). EKG monitoring may be considered.

Oral: 5-10 mg, repeat after 2 hours if significant relief is not attained; maximum: 30 mg in a 24-hour period (use 5 mg dose in patients receiving propranolol with a maximum of 15 mg in 24 hours)

Note: For orally-disintegrating tablets (Maxalt-MLT™): Patient should be instructed to place tablet on tongue and allow to dissolve. Dissolved tablet will be swallowed with saliva.

Dietary Considerations Orally-disintegrating tablet contains phenylalanine (1.05 mg per 5 mg tablet, 2.10 mg per 10 mg tablet).

Monitoring Parameters Headache severity, signs/symptoms suggestive of angina; consider monitoring blood pressure, heart rate, and/or EKG with first dose in patients with likelihood of unrecognized coronary disease, such as patients with significant hypertension, hypercholesterolemia, obese patients, diabetics, smokers with other risk factors or strong family history of coronary artery disease

Patient Information Administration of orally disintegrating tablets: Do not open blister pack before using. Open with dry hands. Do not crush, chew, or swallow tablet; allow to dissolve on tongue. Take as prescribed; do not increase dosing schedule. May repeat one time after 2 hours, if first dose is ineffective. Do not ever take more than two doses without consulting prescriber. You may experience dizziness or drowsiness (use caution when driving, climbing stairs, or engaging in tasks requiring alertness until response to drug is known); skin flushing or hot flashes (cool clothes or a cool environment may help); mild abdominal discomfort or nausea or vomiting. Report severe dizziness, acute headache, chest pain or palpitation, stiff or painful neck or facial swelling, muscle weakness or pain, changes in mental acuity, blurred vision, eye pain, or excessive perspiration or urination.

Dosage Forms

Tablet, as benzoate (Maxalt®): 5 mg, 10 mg

Tablet, orally disintegrating (Maxalt-MLT™): 5 mg, 10 mg

♦ **Romazicon**™ *see Flumazenil on page 143*

Ropinirole *(roe PIN i role)*

Related Information

Patient Information - Miscellaneous Medications *on page 495*

U.S. Brand Names Requip®

Canadian Brand Names Requip

Synonyms Ropinirole Hydrochloride

Pharmacologic Category Anti-Parkinson's Agent (Dopamine Agonist)

Generic Available No

Use Treatment of idiopathic Parkinson's disease; in patients with early Parkinson's disease who were not receiving concomitant levodopa therapy as well as in patients with advanced disease on concomitant levodopa

(Continued)

Ropinirole *(Continued)*

Pregnancy Risk Factor C

Contraindications Hypersensitivity to ropinirole or any component of the formulation

Warnings/Precautions Syncope, sometimes associated with bradycardia, was observed in association with ropinirole in both early Parkinson's disease (without levodopa) patients and advanced Parkinson's disease (with levodopa) patients. Dopamine agonists appear to impair the systemic regulation of blood pressure resulting in postural hypotension, especially during dose escalation. Parkinson's disease patients appear to have an impaired capacity to respond to a postural challenge; use with caution in patients at risk of hypotension (ie, those receiving antihypertensive drugs) or where transient hypotensive episodes would be poorly tolerated (cardiovascular disease or cerebrovascular disease). Parkinson's patients being treated with dopaminergic agonists ordinarily require careful monitoring for signs and symptoms of postural hypotension, especially during dose escalation, and should be informed of this risk. May cause hallucinations. Use with caution in patients with pre-existing dyskinesia, severe hepatic or renal dysfunction.

Patients treated with ropinirole have reported falling asleep while engaging in activities of daily living. Discontinue if significant daytime sleepiness or episodes of falling asleep occur. Pathologic degenerative changes were observed in the retinas of albino rats during studies with this agent, but were not observed in the retinas of albino mice or in other species. The significance of these data for humans remains uncertain.

Although not reported for ropinirole, other dopaminergic agents have been associated with a syndrome resembling neuroleptic malignant syndrome on withdrawal or significant dosage reduction after long-term use. Dopaminergic agents from the ergot class have been associated with fibrotic complications, such as retroperitoneum, lungs, and pleura. No clear association with nonergot agents (ropinirole) has been established.

Adverse Reactions

Early Parkinson's disease (without levodopa):

>10%:

Cardiovascular: Syncope (12%)

Central nervous system: Dizziness (40%), somnolence (40%), fatigue (11%)

Gastrointestinal: Nausea (60%), vomiting (12%)

Miscellaneous: Viral infection (11%)

1% to 10%:

Cardiovascular: Dependent/leg edema (6% to 7%), orthostasis (6%), hypertension (5%), chest pain (4%), flushing (3%), palpitations (3%), peripheral ischemia (3%), hypotension (2%), tachycardia (2%)

Central nervous system: Pain (8%), confusion (5%), hallucinations (5%, dose related), hypoesthesia (4%), amnesia (3%), malaise (3%), vertigo (2%), yawning (3%)

Gastrointestinal: Constipation (>5%), dyspepsia (10%), abdominal pain (6%), xerostomia (5%), anorexia (4%), flatulence (3%)

Genitourinary: Urinary tract infection (5%), impotence (3%)

Hepatic: Elevated alkaline phosphatase (3%)

Neuromuscular & skeletal: Weakness (6%)

Ocular: Abnormal vision (6%), xerophthalmia (2%)

Respiratory: Pharyngitis (6%), rhinitis (4%), sinusitis (4%), dyspnea (3%)

Miscellaneous: Diaphoresis (increased) (6%)

Advanced Parkinson's disease (with levodopa):

>10%:

Central nervous system: Dizziness (26%), somnolence (20%), headache (17%)

Gastrointestinal: Nausea (30%)

Neuromuscular & skeletal: Dyskinesias (34%)

1% to 10%:

Cardiovascular: Syncope (3%), hypotension (2%)

Central nervous system: Hallucinations (10%, dose related), aggravated parkinsonism, confusion (9%), pain (5%), paresis (3%), amnesia (5%), anxiety (6%), abnormal dreaming (3%), insomnia

Gastrointestinal: Abdominal pain (9%), vomiting (7%), constipation (6%), diarrhea (5%), dysphagia (2%), flatulence (2%), increased salivation (2%), xerostomia, weight loss (2%)

Genitourinary: Urinary tract infections

Hematologic: Anemia (2%)

Neuromuscular & skeletal: Falls (10%), arthralgia (7%), tremor (6%), hypokinesia (5%), paresthesia (5%), arthritis (3%)

Respiratory: Upper respiratory tract infection (9%), dyspnea (3%)

Miscellaneous: Injury, increased diaphoresis (7%), viral infection, increased drug level (7%)

Other adverse effects (all phase 2/3 trials):

1% to 10%:

Central nervous system: Neuralgia (>1%)

Renal: Elevated BUN (>1%)

<1% (Limited to important or life-threatening symptoms): Abnormal coordination, acidosis, agitation, angina, aphasia, asthma, bradycardia, bundle branch block, cardiac arrest, cardiac failure, cholecystitis, choreoathetosis, coma, delirium, delusion, dementia, diabetes mellitus, dysphonia, eosinophilia, extrapyramidal symptoms, gangrene, gastrointestinal hemorrhage, gastrointestinal ulceration, glaucoma, goiter, gynecomastia, hyperbilirubinemia, hyperkalemia, hyperthyroidism, hypoglycemia, hyponatremia, hypothyroidism, leukopenia, lymphopenia, limb embolism, manic reaction, pancreatitis, paralysis, paranoid reaction, peripheral neuropathy, photosensitivity, pleural effusion, pulmonary edema, pulmonary embolism, rash, renal calculus, renal failure (acute), seizures, sepsis, SIADH, stomatitis, stupor, suicide attempt, tachycardia, thrombocytopenia, thrombosis, tinnitus, torticollis, urticaria, ventricular tachycardia

Overdosage/Toxicology No reports of intentional overdose; symptoms reported with accidental overdosage were agitation, increased dyskinesia, sedation, orthostatic hypotension, chest pain, confusion, nausea, and vomiting. It is anticipated that the symptoms of overdose will be related to its dopaminergic activity. General supportive measures are recommended. Vital signs should be maintained, if necessary. Removal of any unabsorbed material (eg, by gastric lavage) should be considered.

Drug Interactions CYP1A2 enzyme substrate

Antipsychotics: May reduce the effect of ropinirole due to dopamine antagonism

Ciprofloxacin: May inhibit the metabolism of ropinirole; consider using ofloxacin or lomefloxacin; also may occur with enoxacin

CYP1A2 inhibitors: May increase serum concentrations of ropinirole; inhibitors include cimetidine, ciprofloxacin, erythromycin, fluvoxamine, isoniazid, ritonavir, and zileuton.

Enzyme inducers: May increase the metabolism or ropinirole, reducing serum concentrations and/or effect; inducers include barbiturates, carbamazepine, phenytoin, rifampin, cigarette smoking, and rifabutin

Estrogens: May reduce the metabolism of ropinirole; dosage adjustments may be needed; clearance may be reduced by 36%

Metoclopramide: May reduce the effect of ropinirole due to dopamine antagonism

Ethanol/Nutrition/Herb Interactions

Ethanol: Avoid ethanol (may increase CNS depression).

Herb/Nutraceutical: Avoid kava kava, gotu kola, valerian, St John's wort (may increase CNS depression).

Mechanism of Action Ropinirole has a high relative *in vitro* specificity and full intrinsic activity at the D_2 and D_3 dopamine receptor subtypes, binding with higher affinity to D_3 than to D_2 or D_4 receptor subtypes; relevance of D_3 receptor binding in Parkinson's disease is unknown. Ropinirole has moderate *in vitro* affinity for opioid (Continued)

Ropinirole *(Continued)*

receptors. Ropinirole and its metabolites have negligible *in vitro* affinity for dopamine D_1, 5-HT$_1$, 5-HT$_2$, benzodiazepine, GABA, muscarinic, alpha$_1$-, alpha$_2$-, and beta-adrenoreceptors. Although precise mechanism of action of ropinirole is unknown, it is believed to be due to stimulation of postsynaptic dopamine D_2-type receptors within the caudate-putamen in the brain. Ropinirole caused decreases in systolic and diastolic blood pressure at doses >0.25 mg. The mechanism of ropinirole-induced postural hypotension is believed to be due to D_2-mediated blunting of the noradrenergic response to standing and subsequent decrease in peripheral vascular resistance.

Pharmacodynamics/Kinetics

Absorption: Not affected by food; T_{max} increased by 2.5 hours when drug taken with a meal; absolute bioavailability was 55%, indicating first-pass effect; relative bioavailability from tablet compared to oral solution is 85%

Distribution: V_d: 525 L; removal of drug by hemodialysis is unlikely

Metabolism: Extensively by liver to inactive metabolites; steady-state concentrations are expected to be achieved within 2 days of dosing; CYP1A2 was the major enzyme responsible for metabolism of ropinirole

Half-life, elimination: ~6 hours

Time to peak concentration: ~1-2 hours

Usual Dosage Adults: Oral: The dosage should be increased to achieve a maximum therapeutic effect, balanced against the principal side effects of nausea, dizziness, somnolence and dyskinesia

Recommended starting dose is 0.25 mg 3 times/day; based on individual patient response, the dosage should be titrated with weekly increments as described below:
- Week 1: 0.25 mg 3 times/day; total daily dose: 0.75 mg
- Week 2: 0.5 mg 3 times/day; total daily dose: 1.5 mg
- Week 3: 0.75 mg 3 times/day; total daily dose: 2.25 mg
- Week 4: 1 mg 3 times/day; total daily dose: 3 mg

After week 4, if necessary, daily dosage may be increased by 1.5 mg per day on a weekly basis up to a dose of 9 mg/day, and then by up to 3 mg/day weekly to a total of 24 mg/day

Dietary Considerations May be taken with or without food.

Patient Information Ropinirole can be taken with or without food. Hallucinations can occur and elderly are at a higher risk than younger patients with Parkinson's disease. Postural hypotension may develop with or without symptoms such as dizziness, nausea, syncope, and sometimes sweating. Hypotension and/or orthostatic symptoms may occur more frequently during initial therapy or with an increase in dose at any time. Use caution when rising rapidly after sitting or lying down, especially after having done so for prolonged periods and especially at the initiation of treatment with ropinirole. Because of additive sedative effects and the possibility of falling asleep while engaging in activities of daily living, caution should be used when taking CNS depressants (eg, benzodiazepines, antipsychotics, antidepressants) in combination with ropinirole.

Nursing Implications Hallucinations can occur and elderly are at a higher risk than younger patients with Parkinson's disease. Postural hypotension may develop with or without symptoms such as dizziness, nausea, syncope, and sometimes sweating. Hypotension and/or orthostatic symptoms may occur more frequently during initial therapy or with an increase in dose at any time. Use caution when rising rapidly after sitting or lying down, especially after having done so for prolonged periods and especially at the initiation of treatment with ropinirole. Because of additive sedative effects, caution should be used when taking CNS depressants (eg, benzodiazepines, antipsychotics, antidepressants) in combination with ropinirole.

Additional Information If therapy with a drug known to be a potent inhibitor of CYP1A2 is stopped or started during treatment with ropinirole, adjustment of ropinirole dose may be required. Ropinirole binds to melanin-containing tissues (ie, eyes, skin) in pigmented rats. After a single dose, long-term retention of drug was demonstrated, with a half-life in the eye of 20 days; not known if ropinirole accumulates in these tissues over time.

Dosage Forms Tablet: 0.25 mg, 0.5 mg, 1 mg, 2 mg, 4 mg, 5 mg

♦ **Ropinirole Hydrochloride** *see* Ropinirole *on page 361*

♦ **Rosin Rose** *see* St John's Wort *on page 382*

Rue

Synonyms Herb-of-Grace; *Ruta gravedens*

Pharmacologic Category Herb

Use Antispasmodic; abortifacient; emmenagogue; topical insect repellent; earache; toothache; skin inflammation; contraceptive

Pregnancy Risk Factor Contraindicated

Adverse Reactions Per Commission E:

Dermatologic: Oil can cause contact dermatitis; phototoxic reactions causing dermatoses have been noted

Hepatic: Severe liver damage

Renal: Kidney damage herb contains furans coumarins which have phototoxic and mutagenic actions

Therapeutic dosages can have these effects:

Central nervous system: Melancholic moods, sleep disorders, fatigue, dizziness

Neuromuscular & skeletal: Spasms

Juice of fresh leaves can lead to:

Cardiovascular: Low pulse

Central nervous system: Fainting, sleepiness

Endocrine & metabolic: Abortion

Gastrointestinal: Painful irritations of stomach and intestines, swelling of tongue

Miscellaneous: Clammy skin

Overdosage/Toxicology

Signs and symptoms: Nausea, vomiting, emesis upon ingestion; volatile oil may be an irritant and can cause hepatic and renal abnormalities; topical administration of fresh leaves can cause dermal erythema, blistering, and photosensitization

Fatal dose: ~100 mL of the oil or 4 ounces of fresh leaves

Decontamination:

Oral: Lavage (within 1 hour)/activated charcoal with cathartic

Dermal: Wash with soap and water; avoid sunlight

Additional Information See Commission E; rue oil is used as an abortifacient; it is a pale yellow oil (density: 0.8) which is not water soluble; the plant (which is native to Europe but found worldwide) is an evergreen shrub which can grow to 2-3 feet with yellow flowers blooming in summer

♦ **Rustic Treacle** *see* Garlic *on page 166*

♦ *Ruta gravedens* *see* Rue *on page 365*

Sabah Vegetable

Pharmacologic Category Herb

Use Has been used (at a daily dose of 150 g) for weight reduction and vision protection

Adverse Reactions

Cardiovascular: Palpitations, prolonged Q-T interval, torsade de pointes, chest tightness

Central nervous system: Insomnia, anxiety, fatigue, dizziness

Dermatologic: Rashes

Endocrine & metabolic: Hypokalemia

Gastrointestinal: Anorexia

Neuromuscular & skeletal: Tremor

Respiratory: Dyspnea, hypoxia, cough, tachypnea, obstructive lung disease, bronchiolitis obliterans (may all develop after 4 months of use), wheezing and rales may also occur

(Continued)

Sabah Vegetable *(Continued)*

Overdosage/Toxicology

Decontamination: Ipecac (within 30 minutes)/activated charcoal with cathartic is useful

Treatment: Supportive therapy; lorazepam or diazepam 10-20 mg (0.25-0.4 mg/kg for children) is helpful for seizures; I.V. fluids and alpha-adrenergic pressors should be used for hypotension; sodium bicarbonate (1 mEq/kg) is useful to treat acidosis. Multiple dosing of activated charcoal may be useful.

Additional Information Not sold in U.S. market; commonly found in Malaysia, Thailand, India, Taiwan; shrub-like plant which can grow up to 1.5 meters high

♦ *Sabal serrulata* see Saw Palmetto *on page 367*

♦ *Sabaslis serrulatae* see Saw Palmetto *on page 367*

SAMe (S-adenosylmethionine)

Pharmacologic Category Nutritional Supplement

Use Depression; fibromyalgia; Alzheimer's disease; cardiovascular disease; insomnia; liver disease (cirrhosis, cholestasis, hepatitis); osteoarthritis

Adverse Reactions Xerostomia, nausea, restless, anxiety, hypomania, mania

Drug Interactions

Antidepressants (SSRI and cyclic agents): May potentiate effect and/or toxicity; monitor

Linezolid: Effect/toxicity may be enhanced; avoid concurrent administration

MAO inhibitors: May potentiate activity and/or toxicities; avoid concurrent use

Serotonergic compounds: May increase risk of serotonin syndrome when concurrently; avoid combinations

Mechanism of Action S-adenosyl methionine is involved in several primary biochemical pathways. It functions as a methyl donor in synthetic pathways which form nucleic acids (DNA and RNA), proteins, phospholipids, and neurotransmitters. SAMe's role in phospholipid synthesis may influence membrane fluidity. It has also been noted to protect neuronal anoxia and promote myelination of nerve fibers. It is involved in trans-sulfuration reactions, regulating formation of sulfur-containing amino acids such as cysteine, glutathione, and taurine. Of note, glutathione is an important antioxidant, involved in the detoxification of a number of physiologic and environmental toxins. SAMe is also a cofactor in the synthesis of polyamines, which include spermidine, putrescine, and spermine. Polyamines are essential for cellular growth and differentiation by virtue of their effects on gene expression, protein phosphorylation, neuron regeneration, and the DNA repair.

Usual Dosage Range: 200-1600 mg/day; adult RDI, ODA, and RDA have not been established; most common dosage: 400 mg/day

Patient Information Consult prescriber before combining SAMe with other antidepressants, tryptophan, or 5-HTP

Additional Information SAMe is formed from the essential amino acid methionine. It is a cofactor in three important biochemical pathways, and is synthesized throughout the body. Due to the nature and scope of biochemical reactions that it regulates, SAMe has been investigated for its effect on a wide variety of health problems and disease conditions.

Dosage Forms Capsule, tablets, and intravenous solution

♦ **Sanorex®** see Mazindol *on page 220*

♦ **Sarafem™** see Fluoxetine *on page 146*

♦ *Sassafras albidum* see Sassafras Oil *on page 366*

Sassafras Oil

Synonyms Sassafras albidum

Pharmacologic Category Herb

Use Banned by FDA in food since 1960; has been used as a mild counterirritant on the skin (ie, for lice or insect bites); should not be ingested

Adverse Reactions (Primarily related to sassafras oil and safrole)
Cardiovascular: Tachycardia, flushing, hypotension, sinus tachycardia
Central nervous system: Anxiety, hallucinations, vertigo, aphasia
Dermatologic: Contact dermatitis
Gastrointestinal: Vomiting
Hepatic: Fatty changes of the liver, hepatic necrosis
Ocular: Mydriasis
Miscellaneous: Diaphoresis
Little documentation of adverse effects due to ingestion of herbal tea

Overdosage/Toxicology
Decontamination: Emesis (within 30 minutes) can be considered for ingestion >5 mL if airway is protected; activated charcoal with cathartic can be used
Treatment: Supportive therapy; hypotension can be treated with intravenous crystalloid (10-20 mL/kg) and placement in Trendelenburg position; dopamine or norepinephrine can be used for refractory cases

Usual Dosage Sassafras tea can contain as much as 200 mg (3 mg/kg) of safrole
Lethal dose: ~5 mL
Toxic dose: 0.66 mg/kg is considered to be toxic to humans based on rodent studies

Patient Information Considered unsafe by the FDA

Additional Information Not reviewed by Commission E; specific gravity: 1.07; a yellow liquid which may also contain eugenol, pinene, and d-camphor

Saw Palmetto

Synonyms Palmetto Scrub; *Sabal serrulata*; *Sabaslis serrulatae*; *Serenoa repens*
Pharmacologic Category Herb
Use Benign prostatic hyperplasia
Contraindications Pregnancy and breast-feeding
Adverse Reactions
Central nervous system: Headache
Endocrine & metabolic: Gynecomastia
Gastrointestinal: Stomach problems (in rare cases) per Commission E
Overdosage/Toxicology
Signs and symptoms: Diarrhea
Decontamination: Ipecac within 30 minutes or lavage (within 1 hour)/activated charcoal with cathartic
Usual Dosage Adults: Dried fruit: 0.5-1 g 3 times/day
Additional Information A fan palm plant growing up to 10 feet tall on the southern Atlantic coast; the red or brownish black berries, when ripe, are used in herbal medicine; this product has no effect on PSA or testosterone levels

♦ **Scury Root, American Coneflower** *see* Echinacea *on page 129*

♦ **SDZ ENA 713** *see* Rivastigmine *on page 357*

♦ **Sea Grape** *see* Ephedra *on page 131*

Secobarbital (see koe BAR bi tal)

Related Information
Anxiolytic/Hypnotic Use in Long-Term Care Facilities *on page 562*
Federal OBRA Regulations Recommended Maximum Doses *on page 583*
Patient Information - Anxiolytics & Sedative Hypnotics (Barbiturates) *on page 485*

U.S. Brand Names Seconal™
Canadian Brand Names Novo-Secobarb®
Synonyms Quinalbarbitone Sodium; Secobarbital Sodium
Pharmacologic Category Barbiturate
Generic Available Yes
Use Preanesthetic agent; short-term treatment of insomnia
Restrictions C-II
Pregnancy Risk Factor D
(Continued)

Secobarbital *(Continued)*

Contraindications Hypersensitivity to barbiturates or any component of the formulation; marked hepatic impairment; dyspnea or airway obstruction; porphyria; pregnancy

Warnings/Precautions Should be used only after evaluation of potential causes of sleep disturbance. Failure of sleep disturbance to resolve after 7-10 days may indicate psychiatric or medical illness. Potential for drug dependency exists, abrupt cessation may precipitate withdrawal, including status epilepticus in epileptic patients. Do not administer to patients in acute pain. Use caution in elderly, debilitated, renally impaired, or pediatric patients. May cause paradoxical responses, including agitation and hyperactivity, particularly in acute pain and pediatric patients. Use with caution in patients with depression or suicidal tendencies, or in patients with a history of drug abuse. Tolerance, psychological and physical dependence may occur with prolonged use. Use with caution in patients with hepatic function impairment. May cause CNS depression, which may impair physical or mental abilities. Patients must cautioned about performing tasks which require mental alertness (ie, operating machinery or driving). Effects with other sedative drugs or ethanol may be potentiated. May cause respiratory depression or hypotension, Use with caution in hemodynamically unstable patients or patients with respiratory disease.

Adverse Reactions Frequency not defined.

Cardiovascular: Hypotension

Central nervous system: Dizziness, lightheadedness, "hangover" effect, drowsiness, CNS depression, fever, confusion, mental depression, unusual excitement, nervousness, faint feeling, headache, insomnia, nightmares, hallucinations

Dermatologic: Exfoliative dermatitis, rash, Stevens-Johnson syndrome

Gastrointestinal: Nausea, vomiting, constipation

Hematologic: Agranulocytosis, megaloblastic anemia, thrombocytopenia, thrombophlebitis, urticaria apnea

Local: Pain at injection site

Respiratory: Respiratory depression, laryngospasm

Overdosage/Toxicology

Signs and symptoms: Unsteady gait, slurred speech, confusion, jaundice, hypothermia, fever, hypotension, respiratory depression, coma

Treatment: If hypotension occurs, administer I.V. fluids and place the patient in the Trendelenburg position. If unresponsive, an I.V. vasopressor (eg, dopamine, epinephrine) may be required. Charcoal hemoperfusion or hemodialysis may be useful in the harder to treat intoxications, especially in the presence of very high serum barbiturate levels when the patient is in shock, coma, or renal failure. Forced alkaline diuresis is of no value in the treatment of intoxications with short-acting barbiturates.

Drug Interactions CYP2C9, 3A3/4, and 3A5-7 enzyme inducer

Note: Barbiturates are enzyme inducers; patients should be monitored when these drugs are started or stopped for a decreased or increased therapeutic effect respectively

Acetaminophen: Barbiturates may enhance the hepatotoxic potential of acetaminophen overdoses

Antiarrhythmics: Barbiturates may increase the metabolism of antiarrhythmics, decreasing their clinical effect; includes disopyramide, propafenone, and quinidine

Anticonvulsants: Barbiturates may increase the metabolism of anticonvulsants; includes ethosuximide, felbamate (possibly), lamotrigine, phenytoin, tiagabine, topiramate, and zonisamide; does not appear to affect gabapentin or levetiracetam

Antineoplastics: Limited evidence suggests that enzyme-inducing anticonvulsant therapy may reduce the effectiveness of some chemotherapy regimens (specifically in ALL); teniposide and methotrexate may be cleared more rapidly in these patients

Antipsychotics: Barbiturates may enhance the metabolism (decrease the efficacy) of antipsychotics; monitor for altered response; dose adjustment may be needed

Beta-blockers: Metabolism of beta-blockers may be increased and clinical effect decreased; atenolol and nadolol are unlikely to interact given their renal elimination

Calcium channel blockers: Barbiturates may enhance the metabolism of calcium channel blockers, decreasing their clinical effect

Chloramphenicol: Barbiturates may increase the metabolism of chloramphenicol and chloramphenicol may inhibit barbiturate metabolism; monitor for altered response

Cimetidine: Barbiturates may enhance the metabolism of cimetidine, decreasing its clinical effect

CNS depressants: Sedative effects and/or respiratory depression with barbiturates may be additive with other CNS depressants; monitor for increased effect; includes ethanol, sedatives, antidepressants, narcotic analgesics, and benzodiazepines

Corticosteroids: Barbiturates may enhance the metabolism of corticosteroids, decreasing their clinical effect

Cyclosporine: Levels may be decreased by barbiturates; monitor

Doxycycline: Barbiturates may enhance the metabolism of doxycycline, decreasing its clinical effect; higher dosages may be required

Estrogens: Barbiturates may increase the metabolism of estrogens and reduce their efficacy

Felbamate may inhibit the metabolism of barbiturates and barbiturates may increase the metabolism of felbamate

Griseofulvin: Barbiturates may impair the absorption of griseofulvin, and griseofulvin metabolism may be increased by barbiturates, decreasing clinical effect

Guanfacine: Effect may be decreased by barbiturates

Immunosuppressants: Barbiturates may enhance the metabolism of immunosuppressants, decreasing its clinical effect; includes both cyclosporine and tacrolimus

Loop diuretics: Metabolism may be increased and clinical effects decreased; established for furosemide, effect with other loop diuretics not established

MAO inhibitors: Metabolism of barbiturates may be inhibited, increasing clinical effect or toxicity of the barbiturates

Methadone: Barbiturates may enhance the metabolism of methadone resulting in methadone withdrawal

Methoxyflurane: Barbiturates may enhance the nephrotoxic effects of methoxyflurane

Oral contraceptives: Barbiturates may enhance the metabolism of oral contraceptives, decreasing their clinical effect; an alternative method of contraception should be considered

Theophylline: Barbiturates may increase metabolism of theophylline derivatives and decrease their clinical effect

Tricyclic antidepressants: Barbiturates may increase metabolism of tricyclic antidepressants and decrease their clinical effect; sedative effects may be additive

Valproic acid: Metabolism of barbiturates may be inhibited by valproic acid; monitor for excessive sedation; a dose reduction may be needed

Warfarin: Barbiturates inhibit the hypoprothrombinemic effects of oral anticoagulants via increased metabolism; this combination should generally be avoided

Ethanol/Nutrition/Herb Interactions

Ethanol: Avoid ethanol (may increase CNS depression).

Herb/Nutraceutical: Avoid valerian, St John's wort, kava kava, gotu kola (may increase CNS depression).

Mechanism of Action Depresses CNS activity by binding to barbiturate site at GABA-receptor complex enhancing GABA activity, depressing reticular activity system; higher doses may be gabamimetic

Pharmacodynamics/Kinetics

Onset of hypnosis: Oral: 15-30 minutes; I.M.: 7-10 minutes; I.V. injection: 1-3 minutes

(Continued)

Secobarbital *(Continued)*

Duration: Oral: 3-4 hours with 100 mg dose; I.V.: ~15 minutes
Distribution: 1.5 L/kg; crosses the placenta; appears in breast milk
Protein binding: 45% to 60%
Metabolism: In the liver by microsomal enzyme system
Half-life: 15-40 hours, mean: 28 hours
Time to peak serum concentration: Within 2-4 hours
Elimination: Renally as inactive metabolites and small amounts as unchanged drug

Usual Dosage Oral:

Children:

Preoperative sedation: 2-6 mg/kg (maximum dose: 100 mg/dose) 1-2 hours before procedure
Sedation: 6 mg/kg/day divided every 8 hours

Adults:

Hypnotic: Usual: 100 mg/dose at bedtime; range 100-200 mg/dose
Preoperative sedation: 100-300 mg 1-2 hours before procedure

Monitoring Parameters Blood pressure, heart rate, respiratory rate, CNS status

Patient Information Avoid the use of alcohol and other CNS depressants; avoid driving and other hazardous tasks; avoid abrupt discontinuation; may cause physical and psychological dependence; do not alter dose without notifying physician

Dosage Forms Capsule, as sodium: 100 mg

♦ **Secobarbital and Amobarbital** *see* Amobarbital and Secobarbital *on page 34*

♦ **Secobarbital Sodium** *see* Secobarbital *on page 367*

♦ **Seconal**™ *see* Secobarbital *on page 367*

♦ **Sedapap-10**® **Triad**® *see* Butalbital Compound *on page 59*

Selegiline *(seh LEDGE ah leen)*

Related Information

Patient Information - Antidepressants (MAOIs) *on page 462*
Patient Information - Miscellaneous Medications *on page 495*

U.S. Brand Names Atapryl®; Eldepryl®; Selpak®

Canadian Brand Names Novo-Selegiline®

Synonyms Deprenyl; L-Deprenyl; Selegiline Hydrochloride

Pharmacologic Category Antidepressant, Monoamine Oxidase Inhibitor; Anti-Parkinson's Agent (Monoamine Oxidase Inhibitor)

Generic Available Yes

Use Adjunct in the management of parkinsonian patients in which levodopa/carbidopa therapy is deteriorating

Unlabeled/Investigational Use Early Parkinson's disease; attention-deficit/hyperactivity disorder (ADHD); negative symptoms of schizophrenia; extrapyramidal symptoms; depression; Alzheimer's disease (studies have shown some improvement in behavioral and cognitive performance)

Pregnancy Risk Factor C

Contraindications Hypersensitivity to selegiline or any component of the formulation; concomitant use of meperidine

Warnings/Precautions Increased risk of nonselective MAO inhibition occurs with doses >10 mg/day; it is a monoamine oxidase inhibitor type "B", there should not be a problem with tyramine-containing products as long as the typical doses are employed, however, rare reactions have been reported. Use with tricyclic antidepressants and SSRIs has also been associated with rare reactions and should generally be avoided. Addition to levodopa therapy may result in exacerbation of levodopa adverse effects, requiring a reduction in levodopa dosage.

Adverse Reactions

Cardiovascular: Orthostatic hypotension, hypertension, arrhythmias, palpitations, angina, tachycardia, peripheral edema, bradycardia, syncope
Central nervous system: Hallucinations, dizziness, confusion, anxiety, depression, drowsiness, behavior/mood changes, dreams/nightmares, fatigue, delusions

Dermatologic: Rash, photosensitivity

Gastrointestinal: Xerostomia, nausea, vomiting, constipation, weight loss, anorexia, diarrhea, heartburn

Genitourinary: Nocturia, prostatic hypertrophy, urinary retention, sexual dysfunction

Neuromuscular & skeletal: Tremor, chorea, loss of balance, restlessness, bradykinesia

Ocular: Blepharospasm, blurred vision

Miscellaneous: Diaphoresis (increased)

Overdosage/Toxicology

Signs and symptoms: Tachycardia, palpitations, muscle twitching, seizures

Treatment: Competent supportive care is the most important treatment; both hypertension or hypotension can occur with intoxication. Hypotension may respond to I.V. fluids or vasopressors, and hypertension usually responds to an alpha-adrenergic blocker. While treating the hypertension, care is warranted to avoid sudden drops in blood pressure, since this may worsen the MAO inhibitor toxicity. Muscle irritability and seizures often respond to diazepam, while hyperthermia is best treated antipyretics and cooling blankets. Cardiac arrhythmias are best treated with phenytoin or procainamide.

Drug Interactions CYP2D6 enzyme substrate

Note: Many drug interactions involving selegiline are theoretical, primarily based on interactions with nonspecific MAO inhibitors; at doses <10 mg/day, the risk of these interactions with selegiline may be very low

Amphetamines: MAO inhibitors in combination with amphetamines may result in severe hypertensive reaction or serotonin syndrome; these combinations are best avoided

Anorexiants: Concurrent use of selegiline (high dose) in combination with CNS stimulants or anorexiants may result in serotonin syndrome; these combinations are best avoided; includes dexfenfluramine, fenfluramine, or sibutramine

Barbiturates: MAO inhibitors may inhibit the metabolism of barbiturates and prolong their effect

CNS stimulants: MAO inhibitors in combination with stimulants (methylphenidate) may result in serotonin syndrome; these combinations are best avoided

CYP2D6 inhibitors: Theoretically, inhibitors may decrease hepatic metabolism of selegiline, increasing serum concentrations; inhibitors include amiodarone, cimetidine, delavirdine, fluoxetine, paroxetine, propafenone, quinidine, and ritonavir; monitor for increased effect/toxicity

Dextromethorphan: Concurrent use of selegiline (high dose) may result in serotonin syndrome; these combinations are best avoided

Disulfiram: MAO inhibitors may produce delirium in patients receiving disulfiram; monitor

Enzyme inducers: May increase the metabolism of selegiline, reducing serum levels and effect; enzyme inducers include carbamazepine, barbiturates, phenytoin, and rifampin

Guanadrel and guanethidine: MAO inhibitors inhibit the antihypertensive response to guanadrel or guanethidine; use an alternative antihypertensive agent

Hypoglycemic agents: MAO inhibitors may produce hypoglycemia in patients with diabetes; monitor

Levodopa: MAO inhibitors in combination with levodopa may result in hypertensive reactions; monitor

Lithium: MAO inhibitors in combination with lithium have resulted in malignant hyperpyrexia; this combination is best avoided

Meperidine: Concurrent use of selegiline (high dose) may result in serotonin syndrome; these combinations are best avoided

Nefazodone: Concurrent use of selegiline (high dose) may result in serotonin syndrome; these combinations are best avoided

Norepinephrine: MAO inhibitors may increase the pressor response of norepinephrine (effect is generally small); monitor

Oral contraceptives: Increased selegiline levels have been noted with concurrent administration; monitor

(Continued)

Selegiline *(Continued)*

Reserpine: MAO inhibitors in combination with reserpine may result in hypertensive reactions; monitor

SSRIs: Concurrent use of selegiline with an SSRI may result in mania or hypertension; it is generally best to avoid these combinations

Sympathomimetics (indirect-acting): MAO inhibitors in combination with sympathomimetics such as dopamine, metaraminol, phenylephrine, and decongestants (pseudoephedrine) may result in severe hypertensive reaction; these combinations are best avoided

Succinylcholine: MAO inhibitors may prolong the muscle relaxation produced by succinylcholine via decreased plasma pseudocholinesterase

Tramadol: May increase the risk of seizures and serotonin syndrome in patients receiving an MAO inhibitor

Trazodone: Concurrent use of selegiline (high dose) may result in serotonin syndrome; these combinations are best avoided

Tricyclic antidepressants: May cause serotonin syndrome when combined with an MAO inhibitor; avoid this combination

Tyramine: Selegiline (>10 mg/day) in combination with tyramine (cheese, ethanol) may increase the pressor response; avoid high tyramine-containing foods in patients receiving >10 mg/day of selegiline

Venlafaxine: Concurrent use of selegiline (high dose) may result in serotonin syndrome; these combinations are best avoided

Ethanol/Nutrition/Herb Interactions

Ethanol: Avoid ethanol. Avoid beverages containing tyramine (wine [Chianti and hearty red] and beer).

Food: Selegiline may cause sudden and severe high blood pressure when taken with food high in tyramine (cheeses, sour cream, yogurt, pickled herring, chicken liver, canned figs, raisins, bananas, avocados, soy sauce, broad bean pods, yeast extracts, meats prepared with tenderizers, and many foods aged to improve flavor). Small amounts of caffeine may produce irregular heartbeat or high blood pressure and can interact with this medication for up to 2 weeks after stopping its use.

Herb/Nutraceutical: Avoid valerian, St John's wort, SAMe, kava kava (may increase risk of serotonin syndrome and/or excessive sedation).

Mechanism of Action Potent monoamine oxidase (MAO) type-B inhibitor; MAO type-B plays a major role in the metabolism of dopamine; selegiline may also increase dopaminergic activity by interfering with dopamine reuptake at the synapse

Pharmacodynamics/Kinetics

Onset of therapeutic effects: Within 1 hour

Duration: 24-72 hours

Half-life: 10 hours

Metabolism: In the liver to amphetamine and methamphetamine

Usual Dosage Oral:

Children and Adolescents: ADHD (unlabeled use): 5-15 mg/day

Adults: Parkinson's disease: 5 mg twice daily with breakfast and lunch or 10 mg in the morning

Elderly: Parkinson's disease: Initial: 5 mg in the morning, may increase to a total of 10 mg/day

Child/Adolescent Considerations Twenty-nine children 6-18 years of age (mean: 11.2 years) with ADHD refractory to conventional treatments received an average daily dose of 8.1 mg (5-15 mg/day) for an average of 6.7 months (Jankovic, 1993).

Monitoring Parameters Blood pressure, symptoms of parkinsonism

Patient Information Do not exceed daily doses of 10 mg; report to physician any involuntary movements or CNS agitation

Nursing Implications Monoamine oxidase inhibitor type "B"; there should **not** be a problem with tyramine-containing products as long as the typical doses are employed

Additional Information When adding selegiline to levodopa/carbidopa the dose of the latter can usually be decreased. Studies are investigating the use of selegiline in early Parkinson's disease to slow the progression of the disease.

Dosage Forms
Capsule, as hydrochloride (Eldepryl®): 5 mg
Tablet, as hydrochloride: 5 mg

♦ **Selegiline Hydrochloride** see Selegiline on page 370

♦ **Selpak®** see Selegiline on page 370

♦ **Senexon® [OTC]** see Senna on page 373

Senna

U.S. Brand Names Black Draught® [OTC]; Senexon® [OTC]; Senna-Gen® [OTC]; Senokot® [OTC]; X-Prep® Liquid [OTC]

Synonyms C. angustifolia; Cassia acutifolia; Senna Alexandria

Pharmacologic Category Herb

Use Short-term treatment of constipation; evacuate the colon for bowel or rectal examinations

Contraindications Per Commission E: Intestinal obstruction, acute intestinal inflammation (eg, Crohn's disease), colitis ulcerosa, appendicitis, abdominal pain of unknown origin, children <12 years, and pregnancy

Adverse Reactions
Cardiovascular: Palpitations
Central nervous system: Tetany, dizziness
Dermatologic: Finger clubbing (reversible)
Endocrine & metabolic: Hypokalemia
Gastrointestinal: Vomiting (with fresh plant leaves or pods), diarrhea, abdominal cramping, nausea, melanosis coli (reversible), cachexia
Genitourinary: red discoloration in alkaline urine (yellow-brown in acidic urine)
Hepatic: Hepatitis
Renal: Oliguria, proteinuria
Respiratory: Dyspnea

Per Commission E:
Endocrine & metabolic: Long-term use/abuse can cause electrolyte imbalance
Gastrointestinal: In single incidents, cramp-like discomforts of G.I. tract requiring a reduction in dosage

Overdosage/Toxicology Decontamination: Do **not** induce emesis; lavage (within 1 hour)/activated charcoal can be used

Drug Interactions Per Commission E: Potentiation of cardiac glycosides (with long-term use) is possible due to loss in potassium; effect on antiarrhythmics is possible; potassium deficiency can be increased by simultaneous application of thiazide diuretics, corticosteroids, and licorice root

Usual Dosage
Children: Oral:
>6 years: 10-20 mg/kg/dose at bedtime; maximum daily dose: 872 mg
6-12 years, >27 kg: 1 tablet at bedtime, up to 4 tablets/day **or** ½ teaspoonful of granules (326 mg/tsp) at bedtime (up to 2 teaspoonfuls/day)
Liquid:
2-5 years: 5-10 mL at bedtime
6-15 years: 10-15 mL at bedtime
Suppository: ½ at bedtime
Syrup:
1 month to 1 year: 1.25-2.5 mL at bedtime up to 5 mL/day
1-5 years: 2.5-5 mL at bedtime up to 10 mL/day
5-10 years: 5-10 mL at bedtime up to 20 mL/day
Adults:
Granules (326 mg/teaspoon): 1 teaspoonful at bedtime, not to exceed 2 teaspoonfuls twice daily
Liquid: 15-30 mL with meals and at bedtime
(Continued)

Senna *(Continued)*

Suppository: 1 at bedtime, may repeat once in 2 hours
Syrup: 2-3 teaspoonfuls at bedtime, not to exceed 30 mL/day
Tablet: 187 mg: 2 tablets at bedtime, not to exceed 8 tablets/day
Tablet: 374 mg: 1 at bedtime, up to 4/day; 600 mg: 2 tablets at bedtime, up to 3 tablets/day

Patient Information May discolor urine or feces (yellow, brown, pink, red, or violet); may cause dependence with prolonged or excessive use

Additional Information Both leaf and fruits ("pods") are use; avoid prolonged use; may increase potency and toxicity of digitalis; the plant is found in North Africa and India; a low branching shrub with large yellow leaves on the top of the plant are harvested; compatible for breast-feeding; hypersensitivity to the ingredients; contraindications in fecal impaction, bowel obstruction, and abdominal pain

♦ **Senna Alexandria** *see Senna on page 373*
♦ **Senna-Gen® [OTC]** *see Senna on page 373*
♦ **Senokot® [OTC]** *see Senna on page 373*
♦ **Serax®** *see Oxazepam on page 276*
♦ *Serenoa repens* *see Saw Palmetto on page 367*
♦ **Serentil®** *see Mesoridazine on page 224*
♦ **Seroquel®** *see Quetiapine on page 349*
♦ **Serotonin Syndrome** *see page 591*
♦ **Serpalan®** *see Reserpine on page 352*
♦ **Sertan® (Can)** *see Primidone on page 325*

Sertraline *(SER tra leen)*

Related Information

Antidepressant Agents Comparison Chart *on page 553*
Discontinuation of Psychotropic Drugs - Withdrawal Symptoms and Recommendations *on page 582*
Patient Information - Antidepressants (SSRIs) *on page 452*
Pharmacokinetics of Selective Serotonin-Reuptake Inhibitors (SSRIs) *on page 590*
Teratogenic Risks of Psychotropic Medications *on page 594*

U.S. Brand Names Zoloft®

Canadian Brand Names Zoloft

Synonyms Sertraline Hydrochloride

Pharmacologic Category Antidepressant, Selective Serotonin Reuptake Inhibitor

Generic Available No

Use Treatment of major depression; obsessive-compulsive disorder (OCD); panic disorder; post-traumatic stress disorder

Unlabeled/Investigational Use Eating disorders; anxiety disorders; premenstrual disorders; impulse control disorders

Pregnancy Risk Factor C

Contraindications Hypersensitivity to sertraline or any component of the formulation; use of MAO inhibitors within 14 days; concurrent use of sertraline oral concentrate with disulfiram is contraindicated

Warnings/Precautions Potential for severe reaction when used with MAO inhibitors - serotonin syndrome (hyperthermia, muscular rigidity, mental status changes/agitation, autonomic instability) may occur. May precipitate a shift to mania or hypomania in patients with bipolar disease. Has a very low potential to impair cognitive or motor performance. However, caution patients regarding activities requiring alertness until response to sertraline is known. Does not appear to potentiate the effects of alcohol, however, alcohol use is not advised. Use caution in patients with depression, particularly if suicidal risk may be present. Use caution in patients with a previous seizure disorder or condition predisposing to seizures such as brain damage, alcoholism, or concurrent therapy with other drugs which lower the seizure threshold. Use with caution in patients with hepatic or renal dysfunction and in elderly patients. May cause hyponatremia/SIADH. Use with caution in patients with renal insufficiency or other concurrent illness (due to limited experience). Sertraline acts as a mild uricosuric - use with caution in patients at risk of uric acid nephropathy. Use with caution in patients at risk of bleeding or receiving anticoagulant therapy - may cause impairment in platelet aggregation. Use with caution in patients where weight loss is undesirable. May cause or exacerbate sexual dysfunction. Use oral concentrate formulation with caution in patients with latex sensitivity; dropper dispenser contains dry natural rubber.

Adverse Reactions

>10%:

Central nervous system: Insomnia, somnolence, dizziness, headache, fatigue

Gastrointestinal: Xerostomia, diarrhea, nausea

Genitourinary: Ejaculatory disturbances

1% to 10%:

Cardiovascular: Palpitations

Central nervous system: Agitation, anxiety, nervousness

Dermatologic: Rash

Endocrine & metabolic: Decreased libido

Gastrointestinal: Constipation, anorexia, dyspepsia, flatulence, vomiting

Genitourinary: Micturition disorders

Neuromuscular & skeletal: Tremors, paresthesia

Ocular: Visual difficulty, abnormal vision

Otic: Tinnitus

Miscellaneous: Diaphoresis (increased)

Postmarketing and/or case reports: Abdominal pain, acute renal failure, agranulocytosis, anaphylactoid reaction, angioedema, aplastic anemia, atrial arrhythmias, AV block, blindness, bradycardia, cataract, extrapyramidal symptoms, galactorrhea, hepatic failure. hepatitis, hepatomegaly, hyperglycemia, hyperprolactinemia, hypothyroidism, increased bilirubin, increased transaminases, increased PT/INR, jaundice, leukopenia, lupus-like syndrome, neuroleptic malignant syndrome, oculogyric crisis, serotonin syndrome, SIADH, Stevens-Johnson syndrome (and other severe dermatologic reactions), optic neuritis, pancreatitis (rare), photosensitivity, psychosis, pulmonary hypertension, QT_c prolongation, serum sickness, thrombocytopenia, vasculitis, ventricular tachycardia (including torsade de pointes), vomiting

Overdosage/Toxicology

Signs and symptoms: Serious toxicity has not yet been reported, monitor cardiovascular, gastrointestinal, and hepatic functions

Treatment: There are no specific antidotes for sertraline overdose; treatment should be aimed first at decontamination, then symptomatic and supportive care

Drug Interactions CYP3A3/4 and CYP2D6 (minor) enzyme substrate; CYP1A2 (weak), 2C9, 2C19, 2D6 (weak) and 3A3/4 enzyme inhibitor

Amphetamines: SSRIs may increase the sensitivity to amphetamines, and amphetamines may increase the risk of serotonin syndrome

Benzodiazepines: Sertraline may inhibit the metabolism of alprazolam and diazepam resulting in elevated serum levels; monitor for increased sedation and psychomotor impairment

Buspirone: Sertraline inhibits the reuptake of serotonin; combined use with a serotonin agonist (buspirone) may cause serotonin syndrome

Carbamazepine: Sertraline may inhibit the metabolism of carbamazepine resulting in increased carbamazepine levels and toxicity; monitor for altered carbamazepine response

Clozapine: Sertraline may increase serum levels of clozapine; monitor for increased effect/toxicity

Cyclosporine: Sertraline may increase serum levels of cyclosporine (and possibly tacrolimus); monitor

Cyproheptadine: May inhibit the effects of serotonin reuptake inhibitors (fluoxetine); monitor for altered antidepressant response; cyproheptadine acts as a serotonin agonist

(Continued)

Sertraline *(Continued)*

Dextromethorphan: Some SSRIs inhibit the metabolism of dextromethorphan; visual hallucinations occurred; monitor for serotonin syndrome

Erythromycin: Serotonin syndrome has been reported when added to sertraline; limited documentation

Haloperidol: Serum concentrations may be increased by sertraline (small increase); monitor

HMG-CoA reductase inhibitors: Sertraline may inhibit the metabolism of lovastatin and simvastatin (metabolized by CYP3A3/4) resulting in myositis and rhabdomyolysis; although its inhibition is weak, these combinations are best avoided

Lamotrigine: Toxicity has been reported following the addition of sertraline; monitor

Lithium: Patients receiving SSRIs and lithium have developed neurotoxicity; if combination is used; monitor for neurotoxicity

Loop diuretics: Sertraline may cause hyponatremia; additive hyponatremic effects may be seen with combined use of a loop diuretic (bumetanide, furosemide, torsemide); monitor for hyponatremia

MAO inhibitors: Sertraline should not be used with nonselective MAO inhibitors (isocarboxazid, phenelzine); fatal reactions have been reported; this combination should be avoided

Meperidine: Concurrent use may result in serotonin syndrome; these combinations are best avoided

Nefazodone: May increase the risk of serotonin syndrome

Phenothiazines: sertraline may inhibit metabolism of thioridazine or mesoridazine, potentially leading to malignant ventricular arrhythmias. Avoid concurrent use.

Phenytoin: Sertraline inhibits the metabolism of phenytoin and may result in phenytoin toxicity; monitor for phenytoin toxicity (ataxia, confusion, dizziness, nystagmus, involuntary muscle movement)

Selegiline: SSRIs have been reported to cause mania or hypertension when combined with selegiline; this combination is best avoided. Concurrent use with SSRIs has been reported to cause serotonin syndrome. As a MAO type-B inhibitor, the risk of serotonin syndrome may be less than with nonselective MAO inhibitors.

Sibutramine: May increase the risk of serotonin syndrome with SSRIs

SSRIs: Combined use with other drugs which inhibit the reuptake may cause serotonin syndrome

Sumatriptan (and other serotonin agonists): Concurrent use may result in toxicity; weakness, hyper-reflexia, and incoordination have been observed with sumatriptan and SSRIs. In addition, concurrent use may theoretically increase the risk of serotonin syndrome; includes sumatriptan, naratriptan, rizatriptan, and zolmitriptan.

Sympathomimetics: May increase the risk of serotonin syndrome with SSRIs

Tramadol: Sertraline combined with tramadol (serotonergic effects) may cause serotonin syndrome; monitor

Trazodone: Sertraline may inhibit the metabolism of trazodone resulting in increased toxicity; monitor

Tricyclic antidepressants: Sertraline may inhibit the metabolism of tricyclic antidepressants (amitriptyline, desipramine, imipramine, nortriptyline) resulting is elevated serum levels; if combination is warranted, a low dose of TCA (10-25 mg/day) should be utilized

Tryptophan: Sertraline may inhibit the reuptake of serotonin; combination with tryptophan, a serotonin precursor, may cause agitation and restlessness; this combination is best avoided

Venlafaxine: Sertraline may increase the risk of serotonin syndrome

Warfarin: Sertraline may alter the hypoprothrombinemic response to warfarin; monitor

Zolpidem: Onset of hypnosis may be shortened in patients receiving sertraline; monitor

Ethanol/Nutrition/Herb Interactions

Ethanol: Avoid ethanol (may increase CNS depression).

Food: Sertraline average peak serum levels may be increased if taken with food.

Herb/Nutraceutical: Avoid valerian, St John's wort, kava kava, gotu kola (may increase CNS depression).

Stability Tablets should be stored at controlled room temperature (15°C to 30°C or 59°F to 86°F)

Mechanism of Action Antidepressant with selective inhibitory effects on presynaptic serotonin (5-HT) reuptake and only very weak effects on norepinephrine and dopamine neuronal uptake

Pharmacodynamics/Kinetics

Absorption: Slow

Protein binding: High

Metabolism: Extensive

Half-life:

Parent: 24 hours

Metabolites: 66 hours

Elimination: In both urine and feces

Usual Dosage Oral:

Children and Adolescents: Depression/OCD: 25-200 mg/day

Adults:

Depression/OCD: Oral: Initial: 50 mg/day (see "Note")

Panic disorder/post-traumatic stress disorder: Oral: Initial 25 mg once daily; increased after 1 week to 50 mg once daily (see "Note")

Note: May increase by 50 mg/day increments at intervals of not less than 1 week if tolerated to 100 mg/day; additional increases may be necessary; maximum: 200 mg/day. If somnolence is noted, give at bedtime.

Elderly: Depression/OCD: Start treatment with 25 mg/day in the morning and increase by 25 mg/day increments every 2-3 days if tolerated to 50-100 mg/day; additional increases may be necessary; maximum dose: 200 mg/day

Hemodialysis: Not removed by hemodialysis

Dosage comments in hepatic impairment: Sertraline is extensively metabolized by the liver; caution should be used in patients with hepatic impairment

Child/Adolescent Considerations Twenty-nine children 6-12 years of age and 32 adolescents 13-17 years of age with major depression, obsessive-compulsive disorder, or both, received 25-200 mg/day (Alderman, 1998). Fifty-three children 6-12 years of age and 39 adolescents 13-17 years of age with obsessive-compulsive disorder received up to 200 mg/day (March, 1998).

Administration Oral concentrate: Must be diluted before use. Immediately before administration, use the dropper provided to measure the required amount of concentrate; mix with 4 ounces (½ cup) of water, ginger ale, lemon/lime soda, lemonade, or orange juice **only**. Do not mix with any other liquids than these. The dose should be taken immediately after mixing; do not mix in advance. A slight haze may appear after mixing; this is normal. **Note:** Use with caution in patients with latex sensitivity; dropper dispenser contains dry natural rubber.

Monitoring Parameters Uric acid, liver function, CBC; monitor nutritional intake and weight

Test Interactions Minor ↑ triglycerides (S), ↑ LFTs, ↓ uric acid (S)

Patient Information If you are currently on another antidepressant drug, please notify your physician. Although sertraline has not been shown to increase the effects of alcohol, it is recommended that you refrain from drinking while on this medication. If you are pregnant or intend becoming pregnant while on this drug, please alert your physician to this fact.

Nursing Implications If patient becomes anxious or overstimulated, notify physician; if somnolent, administer dose at bedtime; offer hard, sugarless candy or ice chips for dry mouth. Monitor nutritional intake and weight

Additional Information Buspirone (15-60 mg/day) may be useful in treatment of sexual dysfunction during treatment with a selective serotonin reuptake inhibitor. May exacerbate tics in Tourette's syndrome.

Dosage Forms

Solution, oral concentrate: 20 mg/mL (60 mL)

(Continued)

Sertraline *(Continued)*

Tablet, as hydrochloride: 25 mg, 50 mg, 100 mg

♦ **Sertraline Hydrochloride** *see* Sertraline *on page 374*

♦ **Serzone**® *see* Nefazodone *on page 259*

Sibutramine *(si BYOO tra meen)*

Related Information
Patient Information - Miscellaneous Medications *on page 495*

U.S. Brand Names Meridia®

Synonyms Sibutramine Hydrochloride Monohydrate

Pharmacologic Category Anorexiant

Generic Available No

Use Management of obesity, including weight loss and maintenance of weight loss, and should be used in conjunction with a reduced calorie diet

Restrictions C-IV; Recommended only for obese patients with a body mass index ≥30 kg/m^2 or ≥27 kg/m^2 in the presence of other risk factors such as hypertension, diabetes, and/or dyslipidemia

Pregnancy Risk Factor C

Contraindications Hypersensitivity to sibutramine or any component of the formulation; during or within 2 weeks of MAO inhibitors (eg, phenelzine, selegiline) or concomitant centrally-acting appetite suppressants; anorexia nervosa; uncontrolled or poorly controlled hypertension; congestive heart failure; coronary heart disease; conduction disorders (arrhythmias); stroke; concurrent use of serotonergic agents (eg, SSRIs sumatriptan, dihydroergotamine, dextromethorphan, meperidine, pentazocine, fentanyl, lithium)

Warnings/Precautions Use with caution in severe renal impairment or severe hepatic dysfunction, seizure disorder, hypertension, gallstones, narrow-angle glaucoma, nursing mothers, elderly patients. Primary pulmonary hypertension (PPH), a rare and frequently fatal pulmonary disease, has been reported to occur in patients receiving other agents with serotonergic activity which have been used as anorexiants. Although not reported in clinical trials, it is possible that sibutramine may share this potential, and patients should be monitored closely. Stimulants may unmask tics in individuals with coexisting Tourette's syndrome.

Adverse Reactions
>10%

Central nervous system: Headache, insomnia

Gastrointestinal: Anorexia, xerostomia, constipation

Respiratory: Rhinitis

1% to 10%

Cardiovascular: Tachycardia, vasodilation, hypertension, palpitations, chest pain, edema

Central nervous system: Migraine, dizziness, nervousness, anxiety, depression, somnolence, CNS stimulation, emotional liability

Dermatologic: Rash

Endocrine & metabolic: Dysmenorrhea

Gastrointestinal: Increased appetite, nausea, dyspepsia, gastritis, vomiting, taste perversion, abdominal pain

Neuromuscular & skeletal: Weakness, arthralgia, back pain

Respiratory: Pharyngitis, sinusitis, cough, laryngitis

Miscellaneous: Diaphoresis, flu-like syndrome, allergic reactions, thirst

Postmarketing reports (frequency unknown - limited to important or life-threatening): Anaphylactic shock, anaphylactoid reaction, angina, arrhythmia, atrial fibrillation, congestive heart failure, cardiac arrest, syncope, torsade de pointes, transient ischemic attack, stroke, ventricular dysrhythmias, cholecystitis, cholelithiasis, GI hemorrhage, intestinal obstruction, goiter, hyperthyroidism, hypothyroidism, mania, serotonin syndrome, vascular headache, alopecia, increased intraocular pressure, photosensitivity, impotence

Overdosage/Toxicology Treatment: There is no specific antidote; treatment should consist of general supportive measures employed in the management of overdosage. Cautious use of beta-blockers to control elevated blood pressure and tachycardia may be indicated; the benefits of forced diuresis and hemodialysis remain unknown.

Drug Interactions CYP3A3/4 enzyme substrate

Buspirone: Concurrent use may result in serotonin syndrome; these combinations are best avoided

CNS stimulants: May increase potential for sibutramine-associated cardiovascular complications or serotonergic effects; includes decongestants, centrally-acting weight loss products, amphetamines, and amphetamine-like compounds

CYP3A3/4 inhibitors: Serum level and/or toxicity of sibutramine may be increased; inhibitors include amiodarone, cimetidine, clarithromycin, erythromycin, delavirdine, diltiazem, dirithromycin, disulfiram, fluoxetine, fluvoxamine, grapefruit juice, indinavir, itraconazole, ketoconazole, metronidazole, nefazodone, nevirapine, propoxyphene, quinupristin-dalfopristin, ritonavir, saquinavir, verapamil, zafirlukast, zileuton; monitor for altered response

Dihydroergotamine: Concurrent use may result in serotonin syndrome; these combinations are best avoided

Dextromethorphan: Concurrent use may result in serotonin syndrome; these combinations are best avoided

Lithium: Concurrent use may result in serotonin syndrome; these combinations are best avoided

MAO inhibitors: Sibutramine should not be used with nonselective MAO inhibitors (isocarboxazid, phenelzine) due to a theoretical risk of serotonin syndrome

Meperidine: Concurrent use may result in serotonin syndrome; these combinations are best avoided

Nefazodone: Concurrent use may result in serotonin syndrome; these combinations are best avoided

Serotonergic agents: Concurrent use may result in serotonin syndrome; includes selective serotonin reuptake inhibitors (eg, sumatriptan, lithium, tryptophan), some opioid/analgesics (eg, meperidine, tramadol), and venlafaxine

SSRIs: Combined use with other drugs which inhibit the reuptake (sibutramine) may cause serotonin syndrome; avoid these combinations

Serotonin agonists: Theoretically may increase the risk of serotonin syndrome; includes sumatriptan, naratriptan, rizatriptan, and zolmitriptan

Tramadol: Sertraline combined with tramadol (serotonergic effects) may cause serotonin syndrome; monitor

Trazodone: Sertraline may inhibit the metabolism of trazodone resulting in increased toxicity; monitor

Tricyclic antidepressants: Sertraline may inhibit the metabolism of tricyclic antidepressants (amitriptyline, desipramine, imipramine, nortriptyline) resulting in elevated serum levels; if combination is warranted, a low dose of TCA (10-25 mg/day) should be utilized

Tryptophan: Sertraline may inhibit the reuptake of serotonin; combination with tryptophan, a serotonin precursor, may cause agitation and restlessness; this combination is best avoided

Venlafaxine: Combined use with sibutramine may increase the risk of serotonin syndrome

Ethanol/Nutrition/Herb Interactions

Ethanol: Avoid excess ethanol ingestion.

Herb/Nutraceutical: St John's wort may decrease sibutramine levels.

Mechanism of Action Sibutramine blocks the neuronal uptake of norepinephrine and, to a lesser extent, serotonin and dopamine

Usual Dosage Adults ≥16 years: Initial: 10 mg once daily; after 4 weeks may titrate up to 15 mg once daily as needed and tolerated (may be used for up to 2 years, per manufacturer labeling)

Dietary Considerations Sibutramine, as an appetite suppressant, is the most effective when combined with a low calorie diet and behavior modification counseling.

(Continued)

Sibutramine *(Continued)*

Monitoring Parameters Do initial blood pressure and heart rate evaluation and then monitor regularly during therapy. If patient has sustained increases in either blood pressure or pulse rate, consider discontinuing or reducing the dose of the drug.

Patient Information Maintain proper medical follow-up and inform physician of any potential concomitant medications including over-the-counter products you are taking, especially weight loss products, antidepressants, antimigraine drugs, decongestants, lithium, tryptophan, antitussives, or ergot derivatives

Additional Information Physicians should carefully evaluate patients for history of drug abuse and follow such patients closely, observing them for signs of misuse or abuse (eg, development of tolerance, excessive increases of doses, drug seeking behavior).

Unlike dexfenfluramine and fenfluramine, the medication does not cause the release of serotonin from neurons. Tests done on humans show no evidence of valvular heart disease and experiments done on animals show no evidence of the neurotoxicity which was found in similar testing using animals treated with fenfluramine and dexfenfluramine; has minimal potential for abuse.

Dosage Forms Capsule, as hydrochloride: 5 mg, 10 mg, 15 mg

♦ **Sibutramine Hydrochloride Monohydrate** *see Sibutramine on page 378*

♦ **Siladryl® [OTC]** *see Diphenhydramine on page 116*

Sildenafil *(sil DEN a fil)*

U.S. Brand Names Viagra®

Canadian Brand Names Viagra

Synonyms UK 92480

Pharmacologic Category Phosphodiesterase Enzyme Inhibitor

Generic Available No

Use Treatment of erectile dysfunction

Unlabeled/Investigational Use Psychotropic-induced sexual dysfunction

Pregnancy Risk Factor B

Contraindications Hypersensitivity to sildenafil or any component of the formulation; concurrent use of organic nitrates (nitroglycerin) in any form (potentiates the hypotensive effects)

Warnings/Precautions There is a degree of cardiac risk associated with sexual activity; therefore, physicians may wish to consider the cardiovascular status of their patients prior to initiating any treatment for erectile dysfunction. Agents for the treatment of erectile dysfunction should be used with caution in patients with anatomical deformation of the penis (angulation, cavernosal fibrosis, or Peyronie's disease), or in patients who have conditions which may predispose them to priapism (sickle cell anemia, multiple myeloma, leukemia).

The safety and efficacy of sildenafil with other treatments for erectile dysfunction have not been studied and are, therefore, not recommended as combination therapy.

A minority of patients with retinitis pigmentosa have generic disorders of retinal phosphodiesterases. There is no safety information on the administration of sildenafil to these patients and sildenafil should be administered with caution.

Adverse Reactions

>10%:

Central nervous system: Headache

Note: Dyspepsia and abnormal vision (blurred or increased sensitivity to light) occurred at an incidence of >10% with doses of 100 mg.

1% to 10%:

Cardiovascular: Flushing

Central nervous system: Dizziness

Dermatologic: Rash

Genitourinary: Urinary tract infection

Ophthalmic: Abnormal vision (blurred or increased sensitivity to light)

Respiratory: Nasal congestion

<2% (Limited to important of life-threatening symptoms): Shock, allergic reaction, angina pectoris, AV block, migraine, syncope, hypotension, postural hypotension, myocardial ischemia, cerebral thrombosis, cardiac arrest, heart failure, cardiomyopathy, colitis, rectal hemorrhage, edema, gout, hyperglycemia, neuralgia, vertigo, asthma, dyspnea, exfoliative dermatitis, eye hemorrhage, cataract, anorgasmia, seizures, priapism

Overdosage/Toxicology Signs and symptoms: In studies with healthy volunteers of single doses up to 800 mg, adverse events were similar to those seen at lower doses but incidence rates were increased

Drug Interactions CYP3A3/4 enzyme substrate (major); CYP2C9 enzyme substrate (minor)

Concurrent use of sildenafil and nitroglycerin (or any other nitrate) is contraindicated due to the potential for severe, potentially fatal, hypotensive responses

Increased effect/toxicity: Cimetidine, erythromycin, ketoconazole, itraconazole, mibefradil, nitroglycerin, protease inhibitors. A reduction in sildenafil's dose is recommended when used with ritonavir or indinavir (protease inhibitors); no more than 25 mg per dose, no more than 25 mg in 48 hours.

Decreased effect: Rifampin

Ethanol/Nutrition/Herb Interactions

Food: Amount and rate of absorption of sildenafil is reduced when taken with a high-fat meal. Serum concentrations/toxicity may be increased with grapefruit juice; avoid concurrent use.

Herb/Nutraceutical: St John's wort may decrease sildenafil levels.

Stability Store tablets at controlled room temperature 15°C to 30°C (59°F to 86°F)

Mechanism of Action Does not directly cause penile erections, but affects the response to sexual stimulation. The physiologic mechanism of erection of the penis involves release of nitric oxide (NO) in the corpus cavernosum during sexual stimulation. NO then activates the enzyme guanylate cyclase, which results in increased levels of cyclic guanosine monophosphate (cGMP), producing smooth muscle relaxation and inflow of blood to the corpus cavernosum. Sildenafil enhances the effect of NO by inhibiting phosphodiesterase type 5 (PDE5), which is responsible for degradation of cGMP in the corpus cavernosum; when sexual stimulation causes local release of NO, inhibition of PDE5 by sildenafil causes increased levels of cGMP in the corpus cavernosum, resulting in smooth muscle relaxation and inflow of blood to the corpus cavernosum; at recommended doses, it has no effect in the absence of sexual stimulation.

Usual Dosage Adults: Oral: For most patients, the recommended dose is 50 mg taken as needed, approximately 1 hour before sexual activity. However, sildenafil may be taken anywhere from 30 minutes to 4 hours before sexual activity. Based on effectiveness and tolerance, the dose may be increased to a maximum recommended dose of 100 mg or decreased to 25 mg. The maximum recommended dosing frequency is once daily.

Dosage adjustment for patients >65 years of age, hepatic impairment (cirrhosis), severe renal impairment (creatinine clearance <30 mL/minute), or concomitant use of potent cytochrome P450 3A4 inhibitors (erythromycin, ketoconazole, itraconazole): Higher plasma levels have been associated which may result in increase in efficacy and adverse effects and a starting dose of 25 mg should be considered

Administration Administer 30 minutes to 4 hours before sexual activity (optimally 1 hour before)

Patient Information Inform prescriber of all other medications you are taking; serious side effects can result when sildenafil is used with nitrates and some other medications. Do not combine sildenafil with other approaches to treating erectile dysfunction without consulting prescriber. Note that sildenafil provides no protection against sexually transmitted diseases, including HIV. You may experience headache, flushing, or abnormal vision (blurred or increased sensitivity to light); use caution when driving at night or in poorly lit environments. Report immediately

(Continued)

Sildenafil *(Continued)*

acute allergic reactions, chest pain or palpitations, persistent dizziness, sign of urinary tract infection, rash, respiratory difficulties, genital swelling, or other adverse reactions.

Dosage Forms Tablet, as citrate: 25 mg, 50 mg, 100 mg

St John's Wort

Synonyms Amber Touch-and-Feel; Goatweed; *Hypercium perforatum*; Klamath Weed; Rosin Rose

Pharmacologic Category Herb

Use Mild to moderate depression; also used traditionally for treatment of stress, anxiety, insomnia; used topically for vitiligo; also a popular drug for AIDS patients due to possible antiretroviral activity; used topically for wound healing

Per Commission E: Psychovegetative disorders, depressive moods, anxiety and/or nervous unrest; oily preparations for dyspeptic complaints; oily preparations externally for treatment of post-therapy of acute and contused injuries, myalgia, first degree burns

Contraindications St. John's wort is contraindicated in pregnancy (based on animal studies); children <2 years of age (not confirmed in animal models, *in vitro* only); endogenous depression

Adverse Reactions

Cardiovascular: Sinus tachycardia

Dermatologic: Photosensitization is possible, especially in fair-skinned persons (per Commission E)

Gastrointestinal: Stomach pains, abdominal pain

Miscellaneous: May exacerbate bipolar disorder by causing mania

Overdosage/Toxicology

Signs and symptoms: Photosensitivity/rash, drowsiness, fever, tachycardia, pruritus, diarrhea, nausea

Decontamination: Lavage (within 1hour)/activated charcoal with cathartic

Drug Interactions

Note: St John's wort has been proposed to be a CYP3A4 inducer; however, some evidence suggests reported drug interactions may result from inhibition of the p-glycoprotein drug transporter

Antidepressants: Avoid use with SSRIs or other antidepressants

Cyclosporine: Effect/levels may be decreased; contraindicated

CYP3A3/4 substrates: Effect levels may be reduced by St John's wort; avoid concurrent administration or monitor closely for diminished effect; includes oral contraceptives

Digoxin: AUC decreased 25% and trough C_{max} concentration decreased by 33% and 26% respectively after 15 days of concurrent use

Indinavir (and potentially other protease inhibitors): Effects may be decreased; contraindicated

Linezolid: Effect/toxicity may be potentiated; theoretically, serotonin syndrome may result

MAO inhibitors: Effect/toxicity may be potentiated; theoretically, serotonin syndrome may result

Usual Dosage Based on hypericin extract content

Oral: 300 mg 3 times daily (not to be used longer than 8 weeks)

Herb: 2-4 g 3 times daily

Liquid extract: 2-4 mL 3 times/day

Tincture: 2-4 mL 3 times/day

Topical: Crushed leaves and flowers are applied to affected area after cleansing with soap and water

Per Commission E: 2-4 g drug (dried herb) or 0.2-1 mg of total hypericin in other forms of drug application

Additional Information

VIMRxgn is a synthetic hypericin for HIV treatment; leaves and tops of *Hypericum perforatum* plant used in herbal medicine. St John's wort is a perennial that reaches 2 feet tall with the aroma similar to turpentine; golden yellow flowers bloom in early summer. Young plant is almost as toxic as the mature plant. Hypericin inhibits both type A and type B monoamine oxidase; contraindications in endogenous depression, pregnancy, children <2 years of age (not confirmed in animal models, *in vitro* only).

Sumatriptan (SOO ma trip tan)

Related Information

Patient Information - Miscellaneous Medications - Antimigraine Medications *on page 521*

U.S. Brand Names Imitrex®

Canadian Brand Names Imitrex

Pharmacologic Category Serotonin 5-HT$_{1D}$ Receptor Agonist

Generic Available No

Use Acute treatment of migraine with or without aura

Sumatriptan injection: Acute treatment of cluster headache episodes

Pregnancy Risk Factor C

Pregnancy/Breast-Feeding Implications There are no adequate and well-controlled studies using sumatriptan in pregnant women. Use only if potential benefit to the mother outweighs the potential risk to the fetus. Sumatriptan is excreted in human breast milk. Use caution if administered to a nursing woman.

Contraindications Hypersensitivity to sumatriptan or any component of the formulation; patients with ischemic heart disease or signs or symptoms of ischemic heart disease (including Prinzmetal's angina, angina pectoris, myocardial infarction, silent myocardial ischemia); cerebrovascular syndromes (including strokes, transient ischemic attacks); peripheral vascular syndromes (including ischemic bowel disease); uncontrolled hypertension; use within 24 hours of ergotamine derivatives; use with in 24 hours of another 5-HT$_1$ agonist; concurrent administration or within 2 weeks of discontinuing an MAO inhibitor, specifically MAO-A inhibitors; management of hemiplegic or basilar migraine; prophylactic treatment of migraine; severe hepatic impairment; not for I.V. administration

(Continued)

Sumatriptan *(Continued)*

Warnings/Precautions Sumatriptan is indicated only in patients ≥18 years of age with a clear diagnosis of migraine or cluster headache.

Cardiac events (coronary artery vasospasm, transient ischemia, myocardial infarction, ventricular tachycardia/fibrillation, cardiac arrest and death), cerebral/subarachnoid hemorrhage and stroke have been reported with 5-HT$_1$ agonist administration.

Do not give to patients with risk factors for CAD until a cardiovascular evaluation has been performed; if evaluation is satisfactory, the healthcare provider should administer the first dose and cardiovascular status should be periodically evaluated.

Significant elevation in blood pressure, including hypertensive crisis, has also been reported on rare occasions in patients with and without a history of hypertension. Vasospasm-related reactions have been reported other than coronary artery vasospasm. Peripheral vascular ischemia and colonic ischemia with abdominal pain and bloody diarrhea have occurred.

Use with caution in patients with history of seizure disorder. Safety and efficacy in pediatric patients have not been established.

Adverse Reactions

>10%:

Central nervous system: Dizziness (injection 12%), warm/hot sensation (injection 11%)

Gastrointestinal: Bad taste (nasal spray 13% to 24%), nausea (nasal spray 11% to 13%), vomiting (nasal spray 11% to 13%)

Local: Injection: Pain at the injection site (59%)

Neuromuscular & skeletal: Tingling (injection 13%)

1% to 10%:

Cardiovascular: Chest pain/tightness/heaviness/pressure (injection 2% to 3%, tablet 1% to 2%)

Central nervous system: Burning (injection 7%), dizziness (nasal spray 1% to 2%, tablet >1%), feeling of heaviness (injection 7%), flushing (injection 7%), pressure sensation (injection 7%), feeling of tightness (injection 5%), numbness (injection 5%), drowsiness (injection 3%, tablet >1%), malaise/fatigue (tablet 2% to 3%, injection 1%), feeling strange (injection 2%), headache (injection 2%, tablet >1%), tight feeling in head (injection 2%), nonspecified pain (tablet 1% to 2%, placebo 1%), vertigo (tablet <1% to 2%, nasal spray 1% to 2%), migraine (tablet >1%), sleepiness (tablet >1%), cold sensation (injection 1%), anxiety (injection 1%)

Gastrointestinal: Nausea (tablet >1%), vomiting (tablet >1%), hyposalivation (tablet >1%), abdominal discomfort (injection 1%), dysphagia (injection 1%)

Neuromuscular & skeletal: Neck, throat, and jaw pain/tightness/pressure (injection 2% to 5%, tablet 2% to 3%), mouth/tongue discomfort (injection 5%), paresthesia (tablet 3% to 5%), weakness (injection 5%), myalgia (injection 2%), muscle cramps (injection 1%)

Ocular: Vision alterations (injection 1%)

Respiratory: Nasal disorder/discomfort (nasal spray 2% to 4%, injection 2%), throat discomfort (injection 3%, nasal spray 1% to 2%)

Miscellaneous: Warm/cold sensation (tablet 2% to 3%, placebo 2%), nonspecified pressure/tightness/heaviness (tablet 1% to 3%, placebo 2%), diaphoresis (injection 2%)

<1%: Postmarketing and uncontrolled studies (limited to important or life-threatening symptoms): Abdominal aortic aneurysm, abdominal discomfort, abnormal menstrual cycle, abnormal/elevated liver function tests, accommodation disorders, acute renal failure, agitation, anemia, angioneurotic edema, arrhythmia, atrial fibrillation, bronchospasm, cerebral ischemia, cerebrovascular accident, convulsions, death, decreased appetite, dental pain, diarrhea, dyspeptic symptoms, dysphagia, dystonic reaction, EKG changes, fluid disturbances (including retention), flushing, gastrointestinal pain, hallucinations, heart block, hematuria, hemolytic anemia, hiccoughs, hypersensitivity reactions, increased intracranial

pressure, increased TSH, intestinal obstruction, ischemic colitis, joint ache, muscle stiffness, nose/throat hemorrhage, numbness of tongue, pancytopenia, paresthesia, phlebitis, photosensitivity, Prinzmetal's angina, pruritus, psychomotor disorders, pulmonary embolism, rash, Raynaud syndrome, sensation changes, severe anaphylaxis/anaphylactoid reactions, shock, subarachnoid hemorrhage, swallowing disorders, syncope, thrombocytopenia, thrombophlebitis, thrombosis, transient myocardial ischemia, xerostomia

Drug Interactions

Ergot-containing drugs: Prolong vasospastic reactions; do not use sumatriptan or ergot-containing drugs within 24 hours of each other.

MAO inhibitors (MAO-A inhibitors, nonspecific MAO inhibitors): Reduce sumatriptan clearance; concurrent use is contraindicated; wait at least 2 weeks after discontinuing MAO-A inhibitor to start sumatriptan.

Selegiline: Selegiline is a selective MAO type-B inhibitor; while not specifically contraindicated, combination may best be avoided until further study.

SSRIs: Can lead to symptoms of hyper-reflexia, weakness, and incoordination; monitor.

Stability Store at 2°C to 20°C (36°F to 86°F); protect from light

Mechanism of Action Selective agonist for serotonin (5-HT$_{1d}$ receptor) in cranial arteries to cause vasoconstriction and reduces sterile inflammation associated with antidromic neuronal transmission correlating with relief of migraine

Usual Dosage Adults:

Oral: A single dose of 25 mg, 50 mg, or 100 mg (taken with fluids). If a satisfactory response has not been obtained at 2 hours, a second dose may be administered. Results from clinical trials show that initial doses of 50 mg and 100 mg are more effective than doses of 25 mg, and that 100 mg doses do not provide a greater effect than 50 mg and may have increased incidence of side effects. Although doses of up to 300 mg/day have been studied, the total daily dose should not exceed 200 mg. The safety of treating an average of >4 headaches in a 30-day period have not been established.

Intranasal: A single dose of 5 mg, 10 mg, or 20 mg administered in one nostril. A 10 mg dose may be achieved by administering a single 5 mg dose in each nostril. If headache returns, the dose may be repeated once after 2 hours, not to exceed a total daily dose of 40 mg. The safety of treating an average of >4 headaches in a 30-day period has not been established.

S.C.: 6 mg; a second injection may be administered at least 1 hour after the initial dose, but not more than 2 injections in a 24-hour period. If side effects are dose-limiting, lower doses may be used.

Dosage adjustment in renal impairment: Dosage adjustment not necessary

Dosage adjustment in hepatic impairment: Bioavailability of oral sumatriptan is increased with liver disease. If treatment is needed, do not exceed single doses of 50 mg. The nasal spray has not been studied in patients with hepatic impairment, however, because the spray does not undergo first-pass metabolism, levels would not be expected to alter. Use of all dosage forms is contraindicated with severe hepatic impairment.

Elderly: Due to increased risk of CAD, decreased hepatic function, and more pronounced blood pressure increases, use of the tablet dosage form in elderly patients is not recommended. Use of the nasal spray has not been studied in the elderly. Pharmacokinetics of injectable sumatriptan in the elderly are similar to healthy patients.

Administration

Oral: Should be taken with fluids as soon as symptoms to appear

Do not administer I.V.; may cause coronary vasospasm

Patient Information Take at first sign of migraine attack. This drug is to be used to relieve your migraine, not to prevent or reduce number of attacks.

Oral: If headache returns or is not fully resolved after first dose, the dose may be repeated after 2 hours. **Do not exceed 200 mg in 24 hours.** Take whole with fluids.

(Continued)

Sumatriptan *(Continued)*

S.C.: If headache returns or is not fully resolved after first dose, the dose may be repeated after 1 hour. **Do not exceed two injections in 24 hours. Do not take within 24 hours of any other migraine medication without first consulting prescriber.**

Nasal: Administer dose into one nostril. If headache returns or is not fully resolved after the first dose, the dose may be repeated after 2 hours. Do not exceed 40 mg in 24 hours.

All dosage forms: Do not take within 24 hours of any other migraine medication without first consulting prescriber. You may experience some dizziness (use caution); hot flashes (cool room may help); nausea or vomiting (frequent small meals, frequent mouth care, sucking lozenges, or chewing gum may help); pain at injection site (lasts about 1 hour, will resolve); or excess sweating (will resolve). Report chest tightness or pain; excessive drowsiness; acute abdominal pain; skin rash or burning sensation; muscle weakness, soreness, or numbness; or respiratory difficulty.

Nursing Implications Pain at injection site lasts <1 hour

Dosage Forms

Injection: 12 mg/mL (0.5 mL, 2 mL)

Solution, intranasal [spray]: 5 mg (100 µL unit dose spray device); 20 mg (100 µL unit dose spray device)

Tablet: 25 mg, 50 mg

♦ **Surmontil®** *see* Trimipramine *on page 421*

♦ **Sweet Root** *see* Licorice *on page 201*

♦ **Symadine®** *see* Amantadine *on page 19*

♦ **Symmetrel®** *see* Amantadine *on page 19*

♦ **Syn-Pindol® (Can)** *see* Pindolol *on page 319*

♦ **Synthroid®** *see* Levothyroxine *on page 198*

♦ **T₃ Sodium** *see* Liothyronine *on page 202*

♦ **T₄** *see* Levothyroxine *on page 198*

Tacrine *(TAK reen)*

Related Information

Patient Information - Agents for the Treatment of Alzheimer's Disease *on page 491*

U.S. Brand Names Cognex®

Synonyms Tacrine Hydrochloride; Tetrahydroaminoacrine; THA

Pharmacologic Category Acetylcholinesterase Inhibitor (Central)

Generic Available No

Use Treatment of mild to moderate dementia of the Alzheimer's type

Pregnancy Risk Factor C

Contraindications Hypersensitivity to tacrine, acridine derivatives, or any component of the formulation; patients previously treated with tacrine who developed jaundice

Warnings/Precautions The use of tacrine has been associated with elevations in serum transaminases; serum transaminases (specifically ALT) must be monitored throughout therapy; use extreme caution in patients with current evidence of a history of abnormal liver function tests; use caution in patients with urinary tract obstruction (bladder outlet obstruction or prostatic hypertrophy), asthma, and sick-sinus syndrome (tacrine may cause bradycardia). Also, patients with cardiovascular disease, asthma, or peptic ulcer should use cautiously. Use with caution in patients with a history of seizures. May cause nausea, vomiting, or loose stools. Abrupt discontinuation or dosage decrease may worsen cognitive function. May be associated with neutropenia.

Adverse Reactions

>10%

Central nervous system: Headache, dizziness

Gastrointestinal: Nausea, vomiting, diarrhea
Miscellaneous: Elevated transaminases

1% to 10%
Cardiovascular: Flushing
Central nervous system: Confusion, ataxia, insomnia, somnolence, depression, anxiety, fatigue
Dermatologic: Rash
Gastrointestinal: Dyspepsia, anorexia, abdominal pain, flatulence, constipation, weight loss
Neuromuscular & skeletal: Myalgia, tremor
Respiratory: Rhinitis

Overdosage/Toxicology
Treatment: General supportive measures; can cause a cholinergic crisis characterized by severe nausea, vomiting, salivation, sweating, bradycardia, hypotension, collapse, and convulsions; increased muscle weakness is a possibility and may result in death if respiratory muscles are involved

Tertiary anticholinergics, such as atropine, may be used as an antidote for overdosage. I.V. atropine sulfate titrated to effect is recommended; initial dose of 10-20 mg I.V. with subsequent doses based upon clinical response. Atypical increases in blood pressure and heart rate have been reported with other cholinomimetics when coadministered with quaternary anticholinergics such as glycopyrrolate.

Drug Interactions CYP1A2 enzyme substrate; CYP1A2 inhibitor
Anticholinergic agents: Tacrine may antagonize the therapeutic effect of anticholinergic agents (benztropine, trihexphenidyl); a peripherally-acting agent (glycopyrrolate) has been reported to reduce tacrine-associated gastrointestinal complaints
Beta-blockers: Tacrine in combination with beta blockers may produce additive bradycardia
Calcium channel blockers: Tacrine in combination with heart rate lowering calcium channel blockers (diltiazem and verapamil) may produce additive bradycardia
Cholinergic agents: Tacrine in combination with other cholinergic agents (eg, ambenonium, edrophonium, neostigmine, pyridostigmine, bethanechol), will likely produce additive cholinergic effects
CYP1A2 inhibitors: May increase tacrine concentrations; includes cimetidine, ciprofloxacin, isoniazid, fluvoxamine, ritonavir and zileuton; cigarette smoking may also share this effect
Digoxin: Tacrine, in combination with digoxin, may produce additive bradycardia
Haloperidol: Tacrine may worsen Parkinson's disease and inhibit the effects of haloperidol.
Levodopa: Tacrine may worsen Parkinson's disease and inhibit the effects of levodopa
Neuromuscular blocking agents (nondepolarizing): Theoretically, tacrine may antagonize the effect of nondepolarizing neuromuscular blocking agents
Succinylcholine: Tacrine may prolong the effect of succinylcholine
Theophylline: Tacrine may inhibit the metabolism of theophylline resulting in elevated plasma levels; dose adjustment will likely be needed

Ethanol/Nutrition/Herb Interactions Food: Food decreases bioavailability.

Mechanism of Action Centrally-acting cholinesterase inhibitor. It elevates acetylcholine in cerebral cortex by slowing the degradation of acetylcholine.

Pharmacodynamics/Kinetics
Peak plasma concentrations: 1-2 hours
Plasma bound: 55%
Metabolism: Cytochrome P450 enzyme system in the liver (CYP1A2)
Half-life, elimination: 2-4 hours, steady-state achieved in 24-36 hours

Usual Dosage Adults: Initial: 10 mg 4 times/day; may increase by 40 mg/day adjusted every 6 weeks; maximum: 160 mg/day; best administered separate from meal times.
Dose adjustment based upon transaminase elevations:
ALT ≤3 x ULN*: Continue titration
(Continued)

Tacrine *(Continued)*

ALT >3 to ≤5 x ULN*: Decrease dose by 40 mg/day, resume when ALT returns to normal

ALT >5 x ULN*: Stop treatment, may rechallenge upon return of ALT to normal

*ULN = upper limit of normal

Patients with clinical jaundice confirmed by elevated total bilirubin (>3 mg/dL) should not be rechallenged with tacrine

Dietary Considerations Give with food if GI side effects are intolerable.

Monitoring Parameters ALT (SGPT) levels and other liver enzymes weekly for at least the first 18 weeks, then monitor once every 3 months

Reference Range In clinical trials, serum concentrations >20 ng/mL were associated with a much higher risk of development of symptomatic adverse effects

Patient Information Effect of tacrine therapy is thought to depend upon its administration at regular intervals, as directed; possibility of adverse effects such as those occurring in close temporal association with the initiation of treatment or an increase in dose (ie, nausea, vomiting, loose stools, diarrhea) and those with a delayed onset (ie, rash, jaundice, changes in the color of stool); inform physician of the emergence of new events or any increase in the severity of existing adverse effects; abrupt discontinuation of the drug or a large reduction in total daily dose (80 mg/day or more) may cause a decline in cognitive function and behavioral disturbances; unsupervised increases in the dose may also have serious consequences; do not change dose without consulting physician

Nursing Implications Monitor ALT levels and other liver enzymes weekly for at least the first 18 weeks, then monitor once every 3 months

Dosage Forms Capsule, as hydrochloride: 10 mg, 20 mg, 30 mg, 40 mg

- ♦ **Tacrine Hydrochloride** *see Tacrine on page 386*
- ♦ *Tanacetum parthenium* *see Feverfew on page 143*
- ♦ **Tarasan (Can)** *see Chlorprothixene on page 78*
- ♦ **Tasmar®** *see Tolcapone on page 401*
- ♦ **Tegretol®** *see Carbamazepine on page 61*
- ♦ **Tegretol®-XR** *see Carbamazepine on page 61*

Temazepam *(te MAZ e pam)*

Related Information

Anxiolytic/Hypnotic Use in Long-Term Care Facilities *on page 562*
Benzodiazepines Comparison Chart *on page 566*
Federal OBRA Regulations Recommended Maximum Doses *on page 583*
Patient Information - Anxiolytics & Sedative Hypnotics (Benzodiazepines) *on page 483*

U.S. Brand Names Restoril®

Canadian Brand Names Apo®-Temazepam

Pharmacologic Category Benzodiazepine

Generic Available Yes

Use Short-term treatment of insomnia

Unlabeled/Investigational Use Treatment of anxiety; adjunct in the treatment of depression; management of panic attacks

Restrictions C-IV

Pregnancy Risk Factor X

Contraindications Hypersensitivity to temazepam or any component of the formulation (cross-sensitivity with other benzodiazepines may exist); narrow-angle glaucoma (not in product labeling, however, benzodiazepines are contraindicated); pregnancy

Warnings/Precautions Should be used only after evaluation of potential causes of sleep disturbance. Failure of sleep disturbance to resolve after 7-10 days may indicate psychiatric or medical illness. A worsening of insomnia or the emergence of new abnormalities of thought or behavior may represent unrecognized psychiatric or medical illness and requires immediate and careful evaluation.

Use with caution in elderly or debilitated patients, patients with hepatic disease (including alcoholics), or renal impairment. Use with caution in patients with respiratory disease, or impaired gag reflex. Avoid use inpatients with sleep apnea.

Causes CNS depression (dose-related) resulting in sedation, dizziness, confusion, or ataxia which may impair physical and mental capabilities. Patients must be cautioned about performing tasks which require mental alertness (ie, operating machinery or driving). Use with caution in patients receiving other CNS depressants or psychoactive agents. Effects with other sedative drugs or ethanol may be potentiated. Benzodiazepines have been associated with falls and traumatic injury and should be used with extreme caution in patients who are at risk of these events (especially the elderly).

Use caution in patients with depression, particularly if suicidal risk may be present. Use with caution in patients with a history of drug dependence. Benzodiazepines have been associated with dependence and acute withdrawal symptoms on discontinuation or reduction in dose (may occur after as little as 10 days). Acute withdrawal, including seizures, may be precipitated after administration of flumazenil to patients receiving long-term benzodiazepine therapy.

Benzodiazepines have been associated with anterograde amnesia. Paradoxical reactions, including hyperactive or aggressive behavior, have been reported with benzodiazepines, particularly in adolescent/pediatric or psychiatric patients. Does not have analgesic, antidepressant, or antipsychotic properties.

Adverse Reactions

1% to 10%:

Central nervous system: Confusion, dizziness, drowsiness, fatigue, anxiety, headache, lethargy, hangover, euphoria, vertigo

Dermatologic: Rash

Endocrine & metabolic: Decreased libido

Gastrointestinal: Diarrhea

Neuromuscular & skeletal: Dysarthria, weakness

Otic: Blurred vision

Miscellaneous: Diaphoresis

<1%: Amnesia, anorexia, ataxia, back pain, blood dyscrasias, drug dependence, increased dreaming, menstrual irregularities, palpitations, paradoxical reactions, reflex slowing, tremor, vomiting

Overdosage/Toxicology

Signs and symptoms: Somnolence, confusion, coma, hypoactive reflexes, dyspnea, hypotension, slurred speech, impaired coordination

Treatment: Supportive; rarely is mechanical ventilation required. Flumazenil has been shown to selectively block the binding of benzodiazepines to CNS receptors, resulting in a reversal of benzodiazepine-induced CNS depression.

Drug Interactions CYP3A3/4 enzyme substrate

CNS depressants: Sedative effects and/or respiratory depression may be additive with CNS depressants; includes ethanol, barbiturates, narcotic analgesics, and other sedative agents; monitor for increased effect

CYP3A3/4 inhibitors: Serum level and/or toxicity of some benzodiazepines may be increased; inhibitors include amiodarone, cimetidine, clarithromycin, erythromycin, delavirdine, diltiazem, dirithromycin, disulfiram, fluoxetine, fluvoxamine, grapefruit juice, indinavir, itraconazole, ketoconazole, nefazodone, nevirapine, propoxyphene, quinupristin-dalfopristin, ritonavir, saquinavir, verapamil, zafirlukast, zileuton; monitor for altered benzodiazepine response

Enzyme inducers: Metabolism of some benzodiazepines may be increased, decreasing their therapeutic effect; consider using an alternative sedative/hypnotic agent; potential inducers include phenobarbital, phenytoin, carbamazepine, rifampin, and rifabutin

Levodopa: Therapeutic effects may be diminished in some patients following the addition of a benzodiazepine; limited/inconsistent data

(Continued)

Temazepam *(Continued)*

Oral contraceptives: May decrease the clearance of some benzodiazepines (those which undergo oxidative metabolism); monitor for increased benzodiazepine effect

Theophylline: May partially antagonize some of the effects of benzodiazepines; monitor for decreased response; may require higher doses for sedation

Ethanol/Nutrition/Herb Interactions

Ethanol: Avoid ethanol (may increase CNS depression).

Food: Serum levels may be increased by grapefruit juice.

Herb/Nutraceutical: St John's wort may decrease temazepam levels. Avoid valerian, St John's wort, kava kava, gotu kola (may increase CNS depression).

Mechanism of Action Binds to stereospecific benzodiazepine receptors on the postsynaptic GABA neuron at several sites within the central nervous system, including the limbic system, reticular formation. Enhancement of the inhibitory effect of GABA on neuronal excitability results by increased neuronal membrane permeability to chloride ions. This shift in chloride ions results in hyperpolarization (a less excitable state) and stabilization.

Pharmacodynamics/Kinetics

Distribution: V_d: 1.4

Protein binding: 96%

Metabolism: In the liver (phase II)

Half-life: 9.5-12.4 hours

Time to peak serum concentration: Within 2-3 hours

Elimination: 80% to 90% excreted in urine as inactive metabolites

Usual Dosage Oral:

Adults: 15-30 mg at bedtime

Elderly or debilitated patients: 15 mg

Monitoring Parameters Respiratory and cardiovascular status

Reference Range Therapeutic: 26 ng/mL after 24 hours

Patient Information Avoid alcohol and other CNS depressants; avoid activities needing good psychomotor coordination until CNS effects are known; drug may cause physical or psychological dependence; avoid abrupt discontinuation after prolonged use

Nursing Implications Provide safety measures (ie, side rails, night light, and call button); remove smoking materials from area; supervise ambulation

Additional Information Abrupt discontinuation after sustained use (generally >10 days) may cause withdrawal symptoms.

Dosage Forms Capsule: 7.5 mg, 15 mg, 30 mg

♦ **Tenuate**® *see* Diethylpropion *on page 114*

♦ **Tenuate**® **Dospan**® *see* Diethylpropion *on page 114*

♦ **Teratogenic Risks of Psychotropic Medications** *see page 594*

♦ **Terfluzine (Can)** *see* Trifluoperazine *on page 413*

♦ **Tetrahydroaminoacrine** *see* Tacrine *on page 386*

♦ **Teucrium chamaedrys** *see* Germander *on page 166*

♦ **THA** *see* Tacrine *on page 386*

Thiopental *(thye oh PEN tal)*

Related Information

Patient Information - Anxiolytics & Sedative Hypnotics (Barbiturates) *on page 485*

U.S. Brand Names Pentothal® Sodium

Canadian Brand Names Pentothal

Synonyms Thiopental Sodium

Pharmacologic Category Anticonvulsant, Barbiturate; Barbiturate; General Anesthetic

Generic Available Yes

Use Induction of anesthesia; adjunct for intubation in head injury patients; control of convulsive states; treatment of elevated intracranial pressure

Restrictions C-III

Pregnancy Risk Factor C

Contraindications Hypersensitivity to thiopental, barbiturates, or any component of the formulation; status asthmaticus; severe cardiovascular disease; porphyria (variegate or acute intermittent); inflammatory bowel disease or lower gastrointestinal neoplasm (rectal gel); should not be administered by intra-arterial injection

Warnings/Precautions Laryngospasm or bronchospasms may occur; use with extreme caution in patients with reactive airway diseases (asthma or COPD). Use with caution when the hypnotic may be prolonged or potentiated (excessive premedication, Addison's disease, hepatic or renal dysfunction, myxedema, increased blood urea, severe anemia, or myasthenia gravis). Potential for drug dependency exists, abrupt cessation may precipitate withdrawal, including status epilepticus in epileptic patients. Do not administer to patients in acute pain. Use caution in patients with unstable aneurysms, cardiovascular disease, renal impairment, or hepatic disease. Use caution in elderly, debilitated, or pediatric patients. May cause paradoxical responses, including agitation and hyperactivity, particularly in acute pain and pediatric patients. Effects with other sedative drugs or ethanol may be potentiated. May cause respiratory depression or hypotension. Use with caution in hemodynamically unstable patients (hypotension or shock) or patients with respiratory disease. Repeated dosing or continuous infusions may cause cumulative effects. Extravasation or intra-arterial injection causes necrosis due to pH of 10.6; ensure patient has intravenous access.

Adverse Reactions

Cardiovascular: Bradycardia, hypotension, syncope

Central nervous system: Drowsiness, lethargy, CNS excitation or depression, impaired judgment, "hangover" effect, confusion, somnolence, agitation, hyperkinesia, ataxia, nervousness, headache, insomnia, nightmares, hallucinations, anxiety, dizziness

Dermatologic: Rash, exfoliative dermatitis, Stevens-Johnson syndrome

Gastrointestinal: Nausea, vomiting, constipation

Hematologic: Agranulocytosis, thrombocytopenia, megaloblastic anemia

Local: Pain at injection site, thrombophlebitis with I.V. use

Renal: Oliguria

Respiratory: Laryngospasm, respiratory depression, apnea (especially with rapid I.V. use), hypoventilation, apnea

Miscellaneous: Gangrene with inadvertent intra-arterial injection

Overdosage/Toxicology

Signs and symptoms: Respiratory depression, hypotension, shock

Treatment: Hypotension should respond to I.V. fluids and placement of patient in Trendelenburg position; if necessary, pressors such as norepinephrine may be used; patient may require ventilatory support

Drug Interactions In chronic use, barbiturates are potent inducers of CYP isoenzymes resulting in multiple interactions with medication groups. When used for limited periods, thiopental is not likely to interact via this mechanism.

CNS depressants: Sedative effects and/or respiratory depression with barbiturates may be additive with other CNS depressants; monitor for increased effect; includes ethanol, sedatives, antidepressants, narcotic analgesics, and benzodiazepines

Felbamate may inhibit the metabolism of barbiturates and barbiturates may increase the metabolism of felbamate

Methoxyflurane: Barbiturates may enhance the nephrotoxic effects of methoxyflurane

Stability Reconstituted solutions remain stable for 3 days at room temperature and 7 days when refrigerated; solutions are alkaline and **incompatible** with drugs with acidic pH, such as succinylcholine, atropine sulfate, etc. I.V. form is **incompatible** when mixed with amikacin, benzquinamide, chlorpromazine, codeine, dimenhydrinate, diphenhydramine, glycopyrrolate, hydromorphone, insulin, levorphanol, (Continued)

Thiopental *(Continued)*

meperidine, metaraminol, morphine, norepinephrine, penicillin G, prochlorperazine, succinylcholine, tetracycline

Mechanism of Action Short-acting barbiturate with sedative, hypnotic, and anticonvulsant properties. Barbiturates depress the sensory cortex, decrease motor activity, alter cerebellar function, and produce drowsiness, sedation, and hypnosis. In high doses, barbiturates exhibit anticonvulsant activity; barbiturates produce dose-dependent respiratory depression.

Pharmacodynamics/Kinetics

Onset of action: I.V.: Anesthesia occurs in 30-60 seconds

Duration: 5-30 minutes

Distribution: V_d: 1.4 L/kg

Protein binding: 72% to 86%

Metabolism: In the liver primarily to inactive metabolites but pentobarbital is also formed

Half-life: 3-11.5 hours, decreased in children vs adults

Usual Dosage

I.V.:

Induction anesthesia:

Infants: 5-8 mg/kg

Children 1-12 years: 5-6 mg/kg

Adults: 3-5 mg/kg

Maintenance anesthesia:

Children: 1 mg/kg as needed

Adults: 25-100 mg as needed

Increased intracranial pressure: Children and Adults: 1.5-5 mg/kg/dose; repeat as needed to control intracranial pressure

Seizures:

Children: 2-3 mg/kg/dose; repeat as needed

Adults: 75-250 mg/dose; repeat as needed

Rectal administration (patient should be NPO for no less than 3 hours prior to administration):

Suggested initial doses of thiopental rectal suspension are:

<3 months: 15 mg/kg/dose

>3 months: 25 mg/kg/dose

Note: The age of a premature infant should be adjusted to reflect the age that the infant would have been if full-term (eg, an infant, now age 4 months, who was 2 months premature should be considered to be a 2-month old infant). Doses should be rounded downward to the nearest 50 mg increment to allow for accurate measurement of the dose

Inactive or debilitated patients and patients recently medicated with other sedatives (eg, chloral hydrate, meperidine, chlorpromazine, and promethazine), may require smaller doses than usual

If the patient is not sedated within 15-20 minutes, a single repeat dose of thiopental can be given. The single repeat doses are:

<3 months: <7.5 mg/kg/dose

>3 months: 15 mg/kg/dose

Adults weighing >90 kg should not receive >3 g as a total dose (initial plus repeat doses)

Children weighing >34 kg should not receive >1 g as a total dose (initial plus repeat doses)

Neither adults nor children should receive more than one course of thiopental rectal suspension (initial dose plus repeat dose) per 24-hour period

Dosing adjustment in renal impairment: Cl_{cr} <10 mL/minute: Administer at 75% of normal dose

Note: Accumulation may occur with chronic dosing due to lipid solubility; prolonged recovery may result from redistribution of thiopental from fat stores

Administration Rapid I.V. injection may cause hypotension or decreased cardiac output

Monitoring Parameters Respiratory rate, heart rate, blood pressure

Reference Range Therapeutic: Hypnotic: 1-5 µg/mL (SI: 4.1-20.7 µmol/L); Coma: 30-100 µg/mL (SI: 124-413 µmol/L); Anesthesia: 7-130 µg/mL (SI: 29-536 µmol/L); Toxic: >10 µg/mL (SI: >41 µmol/L)

Test Interactions ↑ potassium (S)

Nursing Implications Monitor vital signs every 3-5 minutes; monitor for respiratory distress; place patient in Sim's position if vomiting, to prevent from aspirating vomitus; avoid extravasation, necrosis may occur

Additional Information Sodium content of 1 g (injection): 86.8 mg (3.8 mEq). Thiopental switches from linear to nonlinear pharmacokinetics following prolonged continuous infusions.

Dosage Forms
Injection, as sodium: 250 mg, 400 mg, 500 mg, 1 g, 2.5 g, 5 g
Suspension, rectal, as sodium: 400 mg/g (2 g)

♦ **Thiopental Sodium** *see* Thiopental *on page 390*

Thioridazine (thye oh RID a zeen)

Related Information
Antipsychotic Agents Comparison Chart *on page 557*
Antipsychotic Medication Guidelines *on page 559*
Discontinuation of Psychotropic Drugs - Withdrawal Symptoms and Recommendations *on page 582*
Federal OBRA Regulations Recommended Maximum Doses *on page 583*
Liquid Compatibility With Antipsychotics and Mood Stabilizers *on page 587*
Patient Information - Antipsychotics (General) *on page 466*

U.S. Brand Names Mellaril®

Canadian Brand Names Apo®-Thioridazine; Novo-Ridazine®; PMS-Thioridazine

Synonyms Thioridazine Hydrochloride

Pharmacologic Category Antipsychotic Agent, Phenothiazine, Piperidine

Generic Available Yes

Use Management of schizophrenic patients who fail to respond adequately to treatment with other antipsychotic drugs, either because of insufficient effectiveness or the inability to achieve an effective dose due to intolerable adverse effects from those medications

Unlabeled/Investigational Use Psychosis

Pregnancy Risk Factor C

Contraindications Hypersensitivity to thioridazine or any component of the formulation (cross-reactivity between phenothiazines may occur); severe CNS depression; circulatory collapse; severe hypotension; bone marrow suppression; blood dyscrasias; coma; in combination with other drugs that are known to prolong the QT_c interval; in patients with congenital long QT syndrome or a history of cardiac arrhythmias; concurrent use with medications that inhibit the metabolism of thioridazine (fluoxetine, paroxetine, fluvoxamine, propranolol, pindolol); patients known to have genetic defect leading to reduced levels of activity of CYP2D6

Warnings/Precautions Thioridazine has dose-related effects on ventricular repolarization leading to QT_c prolongation, a potentially life-threatening effect. Therefore, it should be reserved for patients with schizophrenia who have failed to respond to adequate levels of other antipsychotic drugs. May cause orthostatic hypotension - use with caution in patients at risk of this effect or those who would tolerate transient hypotensive episodes (cerebrovascular disease, cardiovascular disease, or other medications which may predispose).

Highly sedating, use with caution in disorders where CNS depression is a feature. Use with caution in Parkinson's disease. Caution in patients with hemodynamic instability; bone marrow suppression; predisposition to seizures; subcortical brain damage; severe cardiac, hepatic, renal, or respiratory disease. Esophageal dysmotility and aspiration have been associated with antipsychotic use - use with
(Continued)

393

Thioridazine (Continued)

caution in patients at risk of pneumonia (ie, Alzheimer's disease). Caution in breast cancer or other prolactin-dependent tumors (may elevate prolactin levels). May alter temperature regulation or mask toxicity of other drugs due to antiemetic effects.

Phenothiazines may cause anticholinergic effects (confusion, agitation, constipation, dry mouth, blurred vision, urinary retention); therefore, they should be used with caution in patients with decreased gastrointestinal motility, urinary retention, BPH, xerostomia, or visual problems. Conditions which also may be exacerbated by cholinergic blockade include narrow-angle glaucoma (screening is recommended) and worsening of myasthenia gravis. Relative to other neuroleptics, thioridazine has a high potency of cholinergic blockade.

May cause extrapyramidal reactions, including pseudoparkinsonism, acute dystonic reactions, akathisia, and tardive dyskinesia (risk of these reactions is low relative to other neuroleptics). May be associated with neuroleptic malignant syndrome (NMS). Doses exceeding recommended doses may cause pigmentary retinopathy.

Adverse Reactions

Cardiovascular: Hypotension, orthostatic hypotension, peripheral edema, EKG changes

Central nervous system: EPS (pseudoparkinsonism, akathisia, dystonias, tardive dyskinesia), dizziness, drowsiness, neuroleptic malignant syndrome (NMS), impairment of temperature regulation, lowering of seizures threshold, seizure

Dermatologic: Increased sensitivity to sun, rash, discoloration of skin (blue-gray)

Endocrine & metabolic: Changes in menstrual cycle, changes in libido, breast pain, galactorrhea, amenorrhea

Gastrointestinal: Constipation, weight gain, nausea, vomiting, stomach pain, xerostomia, nausea, vomiting, diarrhea

Genitourinary: Difficulty in urination, ejaculatory disturbances, urinary retention, priapism

Hematologic: Agranulocytosis, leukopenia

Hepatic: Cholestatic jaundice, hepatotoxicity

Neuromuscular & skeletal: Tremor

Ocular: Pigmentary retinopathy, blurred vision, cornea and lens changes

Respiratory: Nasal congestion

Overdosage/Toxicology

Signs and symptoms: Deep sleep, coma, extrapyramidal symptoms, abnormal involuntary muscle movements, hypotension, arrhythmias

Treatment:

Following initiation of essential overdose management, toxic symptom treatment and supportive treatment should be initiated

Hypotension usually responds to I.V. fluids or Trendelenburg positioning. If unresponsive to these measures, the use of a parenteral inotrope may be required (eg, norepinephrine 0.1-0.2 mcg/kg/minute titrated to response); do not use epinephrine or dopamine.

Seizures commonly respond to diazepam (I.V. 5-10 mg bolus in adults every 15 minutes if needed up to a total of 30 mg; I.V. 0.25-0.4 mg/kg/dose up to a total of 10 mg in children) or to phenytoin. Avoid barbiturates; may potentiate respiratory depression.

Neuroleptics often cause extrapyramidal symptoms (eg, dystonic reactions) requiring management with diphenhydramine 1-2 mg/kg (adults) up to a maximum of 50 mg I.M. or I.V. slow push followed by a maintenance dose for 48-72 hours. Alternatively, benztropine mesylate I.V. 1-2 mg (adults) may be effective. These agents are generally effective within 2-5 minutes.

Drug Interactions

CYP1A2 and 2D6 enzyme substrate; CYP2D6 enzyme inhibitor

Aluminum salts: May decrease the absorption of phenothiazines; monitor

Amphetamines: Efficacy may be diminished by antipsychotics; in addition, amphetamines may increase psychotic symptoms; avoid concurrent use

Anticholinergics: May inhibit the therapeutic response to phenothiazines and excess anticholinergic effects may occur; includes benztropine, trihexyphenidyl, biperiden, and drugs with significant anticholinergic activity (TCAs, antihistamines, disopyramide)

Antihypertensives: Concurrent use of phenothiazines with an antihypertensive may produce additive hypotensive effects (particularly orthostasis)

Beta-blockers: May increase the risk of arrhythmia; propranolol and pindolol are **contraindicated**

Bromocriptine: Phenothiazines inhibit the ability of bromocriptine to lower serum prolactin concentrations

Carvedilol: Serum concentrations may be increased, leading to hypotension and bradycardia; avoid concurrent use

CNS depressants: Sedative effects may be additive with phenothiazines; monitor for increased effect; includes barbiturates, benzodiazepines, narcotic analgesics, ethanol, and other sedative agents

CYP1A2 inhibitors: Metabolism of phenothiazines may be decreased; increasing clinical effect or toxicity. Inhibitors include cimetidine, ciprofloxacin, fluvoxamine, isoniazid, ritonavir, and zileuton. Concurrent use with fluvoxamine is contraindicated.

CYP2D6 inhibitors: Metabolism of phenothiazines may be decreased; increasing clinical effect or toxicity. Inhibitors include amiodarone, cimetidine, delavirdine, fluoxetine, paroxetine, propafenone, quinidine, and ritonavir; monitor for increased effect/toxicity. **Thioridazine is contraindicated with inhibitors of this enzyme, including fluoxetine and paroxetine.**

Enzyme inducers: May enhance the hepatic metabolism of phenothiazines; larger doses may be required; includes rifampin, rifabutin, barbiturates, phenytoin, and cigarette smoking

Epinephrine: Chlorpromazine (and possibly other low potency antipsychotics) may diminish the pressor effects of epinephrine

Guanethidine and guanadrel: Antihypertensive effects may be inhibited by phenothiazines

Levodopa: Phenothiazines may inhibit the antiparkinsonian effect of levodopa; avoid this combination

Lithium: Phenothiazines may produce neurotoxicity with lithium; this is a rare effect

Phenytoin: May reduce serum levels of phenothiazines; phenothiazines may increase phenytoin serum levels

Polypeptide antibiotics: Rare cases of respiratory paralysis have been reported with concurrent use of phenothiazines

Potassium-depleting agents: May increase the risk of serious arrhythmias with thioridazine; includes many diuretics, aminoglycosides, and amphotericin; monitor serum potassium closely

Propranolol: Serum concentrations of phenothiazines may be increased; propranolol also increases phenothiazine concentrations; may also occur with pindolol. **These agents are contraindicated with thioridazine.**

QT_c-prolonging agents: Effects on QT_c interval may be additive with phenothiazines, increasing the risk of malignant arrhythmias; includes type Ia antiarrhythmics, TCAs, and some quinolone antibiotics (sparfloxacin, moxifloxacin and gatifloxacin). **These agents are contraindicated with thioridazine.**

Sulfadoxine-pyrimethamine: May increase phenothiazine concentrations

Trazodone: Phenothiazines and trazodone may produce additive hypotensive effects

Tricyclic antidepressants: Concurrent use may produce increased toxicity or altered therapeutic response

Valproic acid: Serum levels may be increased by phenothiazines

Ethanol/Nutrition/Herb Interactions

Ethanol: Avoid ethanol (may increase CNS depression).

Herb/Nutraceutical: Avoid kava kava, valerian, St John's wort, gotu kola (may increase CNS depression). Avoid dong quai, St John's wort (may also cause photosensitization).

Stability Protect all dosage forms from light

(Continued)

Thioridazine (Continued)

Mechanism of Action Blocks postsynaptic mesolimbic dopaminergic receptors in the brain; exhibits a strong alpha-adrenergic blocking effect and depresses the release of hypothalamic and hypophyseal hormones

Pharmacodynamics/Kinetics
Duration of action: 4-5 days
Half-life: 21-25 hours
Time to peak serum concentration: Within 1 hour

Usual Dosage Oral:

Children >2-12 years: Range: 0.5-3 mg/kg/day in 2-3 divided doses; usual: 1 mg/kg/day; maximum: 3 mg/kg/day

Behavior problems: Initial: 10 mg 2-3 times/day, increase gradually

Severe psychoses: Initial: 25 mg 2-3 times/day, increase gradually

Children >12 years and Adults:

Schizophrenia/psychoses: Initial: 50-100 mg 3 times/day with gradual increments as needed and tolerated; maximum: 800 mg/day in 2-4 divided doses; if >65 years, initial dose: 10 mg 3 times/day

Depressive disorders/dementia: Initial: 25 mg 3 times/day; maintenance dose: 20-200 mg/day

Elderly: Behavioral symptoms associated with dementia: Oral: Initial: 10-25 mg 1-2 times/day; increase at 4- to 7-day intervals by 10-25 mg/day; increase dose intervals (qd, bid, etc) as necessary to control response or side effects. Maximum daily dose: 400 mg; gradual increases (titration) may prevent some side effects or decrease their severity.

Hemodialysis: Not dialyzable (0% to 5%)

Administration Oral concentrate must be diluted in 2-4 oz of liquid (eg, water, fruit juice, carbonated drinks, milk, or pudding) before administration. Do not take antacid within 2 hours of taking drug. Thioridazine concentrate is not compatible with carbamazepine suspension; schedule dosing at least 1-2 hours apart from each other. **Note:** Avoid skin contact with oral suspension or solution; may cause contact dermatitis.

Monitoring Parameters Baseline and periodic EKG and serum potassium; periodic eye exam, CBC with differential, blood pressure, liver enzyme tests; do not initiate if QT_c >450 msec

Reference Range Toxic: >1 mg/mL; lethal: 2-8 mg/dL

Test Interactions False-positives for phenylketonuria, urinary amylase, uroporphyrins, urobilinogen

Patient Information Oral concentrate must be diluted in 2-4 oz of liquid (water, fruit juice, carbonated drinks, milk, or pudding); do not take antacid within 1 hour of taking drug; avoid excess sun exposure; may cause drowsiness, restlessness, avoid alcohol and other CNS depressants; do not alter dosage or discontinue without consulting physician; yearly eye exams are necessary; might discolor urine (pink or reddish brown)

Nursing Implications Avoid skin contact with oral suspension or solution; may cause contact dermatitis

Dosage Forms

Solution, oral concentrate, as hydrochloride: 30 mg/mL (120 mL); 100 mg/mL (3.4 mL, 120 mL)

Tablet, as hydrochloride: 10 mg, 15 mg, 25 mg, 50 mg, 100 mg, 150 mg, 200 mg

♦ **Thioridazine Hydrochloride** see Thioridazine on page 393

Thiothixene (thye oh THIKS een)
Related Information

Liquid Compatibility With Antipsychotics and Mood Stabilizers *on page 587*
Patient Information - Antipsychotics (General) *on page 466*

U.S. Brand Names Navane®

Canadian Brand Names Navane

Synonyms Tiotixene

Pharmacologic Category Antipsychotic Agent, Thioxanthene Derivative

Generic Available Yes

Use Management of psychotic disorders

Pregnancy Risk Factor C

Contraindications Hypersensitivity to thiothixene or any component of the formulation; severe CNS depression; circulatory collapse; blood dyscrasias; coma

Warnings/Precautions May be sedating, use with caution in disorders where CNS depression is a feature. Use with caution in Parkinson's disease. Caution in patients with hemodynamic instability; predisposition to seizures; subcortical brain damage; bone marrow suppression; severe cardiac, hepatic, renal, or respiratory disease. Esophageal dysmotility and aspiration have been associated with antipsychotic use - use with caution in patients at risk of pneumonia (ie, Alzheimer's disease). Caution in breast cancer or other prolactin-dependent tumors (may elevate prolactin levels). May alter temperature regulation or mask toxicity of other drugs due to antiemetic effects. May alter cardiac conduction - life-threatening arrhythmias have occurred with therapeutic doses of neuroleptics. May cause orthostatic hypotension - use with caution in patients at risk of this effect or those who would tolerate transient hypotensive episodes (cerebrovascular disease, cardiovascular disease, or other medications which may predispose).

May cause anticholinergic effects (confusion, agitation, constipation, dry mouth, blurred vision, urinary retention); therefore, they should be used with caution in patients with decreased gastrointestinal motility, urinary retention, BPH, xerostomia, or visual problems. Conditions which also may be exacerbated by cholinergic blockade include narrow-angle glaucoma (screening is recommended) and worsening of myasthenia gravis. Relative to other neuroleptics, thiothixene has a low potency of cholinergic blockade.

May cause extrapyramidal reactions, including pseudoparkinsonism, acute dystonic reactions, akathisia, and tardive dyskinesia (risk of these reactions is high relative to other neuroleptics). May be associated with neuroleptic malignant syndrome (NMS) or pigmentary retinopathy.

Adverse Reactions

Cardiovascular: Hypotension, tachycardia, syncope, nonspecific EKG changes

Central nervous system: Extrapyramidal symptoms (pseudoparkinsonism, akathisia, dystonias, lightheadedness, tardive dyskinesia), dizziness, drowsiness, restlessness, agitation, insomnia

Dermatologic: Discoloration of skin (blue-gray), rash, pruritus, urticaria, photosensitivity

Endocrine & metabolic: Changes in menstrual cycle, changes in libido, breast pain, galactorrhea, lactation, amenorrhea, gynecomastia, hyperglycemia, hypoglycemia

Gastrointestinal: Weight gain, nausea, vomiting, stomach pain, constipation, xerostomia, increased salivation

Genitourinary: Difficulty in urination, ejaculatory disturbances, impotence

Hematologic: Leukopenia, leukocytes

Neuromuscular & skeletal: Tremors

Ocular: Pigmentary retinopathy, blurred vision

Respiratory: Nasal congestion

Miscellaneous: Diaphoresis

Overdosage/Toxicology

Signs and symptoms: Muscle twitching, drowsiness, dizziness, rigidity, tremor, hypotension, cardiac arrhythmias

(Continued)

Thiothixene *(Continued)*

Treatment:

Following initiation of essential overdose management, toxic symptom treatment and supportive treatment should be initiated

Hypotension usually responds to I.V. fluids or Trendelenburg positioning. If unresponsive to these measures, the use of a parenteral inotrope may be required (eg, norepinephrine 0.1-0.2 mcg/kg/minute titrated to response).

Seizures commonly respond to diazepam (I.V. 5-10 mg bolus in adults every 15 minutes if needed up to a total of 30 mg; I.V. 0.25-0.4 mg/kg/dose up to a total of 10 mg in children) or to phenytoin or phenobarbital.

Neuroleptics often cause extrapyramidal symptoms (eg, dystonic reactions) requiring management with diphenhydramine 1-2 mg/kg (adults) up to a maximum of 50 mg I.M. or I.V. slow push followed by a maintenance dose for 48-72 hours. Alternatively, benztropine mesylate I.V. 1-2 mg (adults) may be effective. These agents are generally effective within 2-5 minutes.

Drug Interactions CYP1A2 enzyme substrate

Aluminum salts: May decrease the absorption of antipsychotics; monitor

Amphetamines: Efficacy may be diminished by antipsychotics; in addition, amphetamines may increase psychotic symptoms; avoid concurrent use

Anticholinergics: May inhibit the therapeutic response to antipsychotics and excess anticholinergic effects may occur; includes benztropine, trihexyphenidyl, biperiden, and drugs with significant anticholinergic activity (TCAs, antihistamines, disopyramide)

Antihypertensives: Concurrent use of antipsychotics with an antihypertensive may produce additive hypotensive effects (particularly orthostasis)

Bromocriptine: Antipsychotics inhibit the ability of bromocriptine to lower serum prolactin concentrations

CNS depressants: Sedative effects may be additive with antipsychotics; monitor for increased effect; includes barbiturates, benzodiazepines, narcotic analgesics, ethanol, and other sedative agents

CYP1A2 inhibitors: Serum levels may be increased; inhibitors include cimetidine, ciprofloxacin, fluvoxamine, isoniazid, ritonavir, and zileuton

Enzyme inducers: May enhance the hepatic metabolism of antipsychotics; larger doses may be required; includes rifampin, rifabutin, barbiturates, phenytoin, and cigarette smoking

Epinephrine: Chlorpromazine (and possibly other low potency antipsychotics) may diminish the pressor effects of epinephrine

Guanethidine and guanadrel: Antihypertensive effects may be inhibited by antipsychotics

Levodopa: Antipsychotics may inhibit the antiparkinsonian effect of levodopa; avoid this combination

Lithium: Antipsychotics may produce neurotoxicity with lithium; this is a rare effect

Phenytoin: May reduce serum levels of antipsychotics; antipsychotics may increase phenytoin serum levels

Propranolol: Serum concentrations of antipsychotics may be increased; propranolol also increases antipsychotics concentrations

QT_c-prolonging agents: Effects on QT_c interval may be additive with antipsychotics, increasing the risk of malignant arrhythmias; includes type Ia antiarrhythmics, TCAs, and some quinolone antibiotics (sparfloxacin, moxifloxacin, and gatifloxacin)

Sulfadoxine-pyrimethamine: May increase antipsychotics concentrations

Trazodone: Antipsychotics and trazodone may produce additive hypotensive effects

Tricyclic antidepressants: Concurrent use may produce increased toxicity or altered therapeutic response

Valproic acid: Serum levels may be increased by antipsychotics

Ethanol/Nutrition/Herb Interactions

Ethanol: Avoid ethanol (may increase CNS depression)

Herb/Nutraceutical: Avoid kava kava, valerian, St John's wort, gotu kola (may increase CNS depression).

Stability Refrigerate powder for injection. Reconstituted powder for injection is stable at room temperature for 48 hours.

Mechanism of Action Elicits antipsychotic activity by postsynaptic blockade of CNS dopamine receptors resulting in inhibition of dopamine-mediated effects; also has alpha-adrenergic blocking activity

Pharmacodynamics/Kinetics

Metabolism: Extensive in the liver

Half-life: >24 hours with chronic use

Usual Dosage

Children <12 years: Schizophrenia/psychoses: Oral: 0.25 mg/kg/24 hours in divided doses (dose not well established)

Children >12 years and Adults: Mild to moderate psychosis:

Oral: 2 mg 3 times/day, up to 20-30 mg/day; more severe psychosis: Initial: 5 mg 2 times/day, may increase gradually, if necessary; maximum: 60 mg/day

I.M.: 4 mg 2-4 times/day, increase dose gradually; usual: 16-20 mg/day; maximum: 30 mg/day; change to oral dose as soon as able

Rapid tranquilization of the agitated patient (administered every 30-60 minutes):

Oral: 5-10 mg

I.M.: 10-20 mg

Average total dose for tranquilization: 15-30 mg

Hemodialysis: Not dialyzable (0% to 5%)

Monitoring Parameters Orthostatic blood pressures; tremors, gait changes, abnormal movement in trunk, neck, buccal area or extremities; monitor target behaviors for which the agent is given

Test Interactions ↑ cholesterol (S), ↑ glucose; ↓ uric acid (S); may cause false-positive pregnancy test

Patient Information May cause drowsiness, restlessness, avoid alcohol and other CNS depressants; do not alter dosage or discontinue without consulting physician

Nursing Implications Observe for extrapyramidal effects; concentrate should be mixed in juice before administration

Additional Information Coadministration of two or more antipsychotics does not improve clinical response and may increase the potential for adverse effects.

Dosage Forms

Capsule: 1 mg, 2 mg, 5 mg, 10 mg, 20 mg

Powder for injection, as hydrochloride: 5 mg/mL (2 mL)

Solution, oral concentrate, as hydrochloride: 5 mg/mL (30 mL, 120 mL)

♦ **Thorazine®** see Chlorpromazine on page 74

♦ **Thyrox®** see Levothyroxine on page 198

Tiagabine (tye AJ a bene)

U.S. Brand Names Gabitril®

Synonyms Tiagabine Hydrochloride

Pharmacologic Category Anticonvulsant, Miscellaneous

Generic Available No

Use Adjunctive therapy in adults and children ≥12 years of age in the treatment of partial seizures

Unlabeled/Investigational Use Bipolar disorder

Pregnancy Risk Factor C

Contraindications Hypersensitivity to tiagabine or any component of the formulation

Warnings/Precautions Anticonvulsants should not be discontinued abruptly because of the possibility of increasing seizure frequency; tiagabine should be withdrawn gradually to minimize the potential of increased seizure frequency, unless safety concerns require a more rapid withdrawal. Rarely, nonconvulsive status epilepticus has been reported following abrupt discontinuation or dosage reduction.

(Continued)

Tiagabine *(Continued)*

Use with caution in patients with hepatic impairment. Experience in patients not receiving enzyme-inducing drugs has been limited - caution should be used in treating any patient who is not receiving one of these medications. Weakness, sedation, and confusion may occur with tiagabine use. Patients must cautioned about performing tasks which require mental alertness (ie, operating machinery or driving). Effects with other sedative drugs or ethanol may be potentiated. May cause potentially serious rash, including Stevens-Johnson syndrome.

Adverse Reactions

>10%:

Central nervous system: Dizziness, somnolence

Gastrointestinal: Nausea

Neuromuscular & skeletal: Weakness

1% to 10%:

Central nervous system: Nervousness, difficulty with concentration, insomnia, ataxia, confusion, speech disorder, depression, emotional lability, abnormal gait, hostility

Dermatologic: Rash, pruritus

Gastrointestinal: Diarrhea, vomiting, increased appetite

Neuromuscular & skeletal: Tremor, paresthesia

Ocular: Nystagmus

Otic: Hearing impairment

Respiratory: Pharyngitis, cough

Overdosage/Toxicology Somnolence, impaired consciousness, agitation, confusion, speech difficulty, hostility, depression, weakness, myoclonus, and seizures may occur. Treatment is supportive.

Drug Interactions CYP2D6 and 3A3/4 enzyme substrate

CNS depressants: Sedative effects may be additive with other CNS depressants; monitor for increased effect; includes ethanol, sedatives, antidepressants, narcotic analgesics, other anticonvulsants, and benzodiazepines

CYP2D6 inhibitors: Serum levels and/or toxicity of tiagabine may be increased; inhibitors include amiodarone, cimetidine, delavirdine, fluoxetine, paroxetine, propafenone, quinidine, and ritonavir; monitor for increased effect/toxicity

CYP3A3/4 inhibitors: Serum level and/or toxicity of tiagabine may be increased; inhibitors include amiodarone, cimetidine, clarithromycin, erythromycin, delavirdine, diltiazem, dirithromycin, disulfiram, fluoxetine, fluvoxamine, grapefruit juice, indinavir, itraconazole, ketoconazole, nevirapine, propoxyphene, quinupristin-dalfopristin, ritonavir, saquinavir, verapamil, zafirlukast, zileuton; monitor for altered effects

Enzyme inducers: May increase the metabolism of tiagabine resulting in decreased effect. Primidone, phenobarbital, phenytoin, and carbamazepine increase tiagabine clearance by 60%

Valproate: Increased free tiagabine concentrations by 40%

Ethanol/Nutrition/Herb Interactions

Ethanol: Avoid ethanol (may increase CNS depression).

Food: Food reduces the rate but not the extent of absorption.

Herb/Nutraceutical: St John's wort may decrease tiagabine levels. Avoid valerian, St John's wort, kava kava, gotu kola (may increase CNS depression).

Mechanism of Action The exact mechanism by which tiagabine exerts antiseizure activity is not definitively known; however, *in vitro* experiments demonstrate that it enhances the activity of gamma aminobutyric acid (GABA), the major neuroinhibitory transmitter in the nervous system; it is thought that binding to the GABA uptake carrier inhibits the uptake of GABA into presynaptic neurons, allowing an increased amount of GABA to be available to postsynaptic neurons; based on *in vitro* studies, tiagabine does not inhibit the uptake of dopamine, norepinephrine, serotonin, glutamate, or choline

Pharmacodynamics/Kinetics

Absorption: Rapid (within 1 hour); food prolongs absorption

Protein binding: 96%

Half-life: 6.7 hours

Usual Dosage Oral (administer with food):

Children 12-18 years: 4 mg once daily for 1 week; may increase to 8 mg daily in 2 divided doses for 1 week; then may increase by 4-8 mg weekly to response or up to 32 mg daily in 2-4 divided doses

Adults: 4 mg once daily for 1 week; may increase by 4-8 mg weekly to response or up to 56 mg daily in 2-4 divided doses

Dietary Considerations Take with food.

Monitoring Parameters A reduction in seizure frequency is indicative of therapeutic response to tiagabine in patients with partial seizures; complete blood counts, renal function tests, liver function tests, and routine blood chemistry should be monitored periodically during therapy

Reference Range Maximal plasma level after a 24 mg/dose: 552 ng/mL

Patient Information Use exactly as directed by mouth with food, usually beginning at 4 mg once daily, and usually in addition to other antiepilepsy drugs. The dose will be increased based on age and medial condition, up to 2-4 times/day. Do not interrupt or discontinue treatment without consulting your physician or pharmacist. If told to stop this medication, it should be discontinued gradually.

Dosage Forms Tablet: 2 mg, 4 mg, 12 mg, 16 mg, 20 mg

♦ **Tiagabine Hydrochloride** *see* Tiagabine *on page 399*

♦ **Tiotixene** *see* Thiothixene *on page 396*

♦ **Tofranil®** *see* Imipramine *on page 180*

♦ **Tofranil-PM®** *see* Imipramine *on page 180*

Tolcapone (TOLE ka pone)

U.S. Brand Names Tasmar®

Pharmacologic Category Anti-Parkinson's Agent (COMT Inhibitor)

Generic Available No

Use Adjunct to levodopa and carbidopa for the treatment of signs and symptoms of idiopathic Parkinson's disease

Pregnancy Risk Factor C

Contraindications Hypersensitivity to tolcapone or any component of the formulation

Warnings/Precautions Due to reports of fatal liver injury associated with use of this drug, the manufacturer is advising that tolcapone be reserved for use only in patients who do not have severe movement abnormalities and who do not respond to or who are not appropriate candidates for other available treatments. Use with caution in patients with pre-existing dyskinesias, hepatic impairment, or severe renal impairment. May cause orthostatic hypotension; Parkinson's disease patients appear to have an impaired capacity to respond to a postural challenge; use with caution in patients at risk of hypotension (such as those receiving antihypertensive drugs) or where transient hypotensive episodes would be poorly tolerated (cardiovascular disease or cerebrovascular disease). Parkinson's patients being treated with dopaminergic agonists ordinarily require careful monitoring for signs and symptoms of postural hypotension, especially during dose escalation, and should be informed of this risk. May cause hallucinations, which may improve with reduction in levodopa therapy. Use with caution in patients with lower gastrointestinal disease or an increased risk of dehydration - tolcapone has been associated with delayed development of diarrhea (onset after 2-12 weeks).

It is not recommended that patients receive tolcapone concomitantly with nonselective MAO inhibitors (see Drug Interactions). Selegiline is a selective MAO type-B inhibitor and can be taken with tolcapone.

Although not reported for tolcapone, other dopaminergic agents have been associated with a syndrome resembling neuroleptic malignant syndrome on withdrawal or significant dosage reduction after long-term use. Dopaminergic agents from the ergot class have also been associated with fibrotic complications, such as retroperitoneum, lungs, and pleura.

(Continued)

Tolcapone *(Continued)*

Adverse Reactions

>10%:

Cardiovascular: Orthostatic hypotension

Central nervous system: Sleep disorder, excessive dreaming, somnolence, headache

Gastrointestinal: Nausea, diarrhea, anorexia

Neuromuscular & skeletal: Dyskinesia, dystonia, muscle cramps

1% to 10%:

Central nervous system: Hallucinations, fatigue, loss of balance, hyperkinesia

Gastrointestinal: Vomiting, constipation, xerostomia, abdominal pain, flatulence, dyspepsia

Genitourinary: Urine discoloration

Neuromuscular & skeletal: Paresthesia, stiffness

Miscellaneous: Diaphoresis (increased)

Overdosage/Toxicology

Signs and symptoms include nausea, vomiting, and dizziness, particularly in combination with levodopa/carbidopa

Treatment: Hospitalization and general supportive care; hemodialysis is unlikely to be effective

Drug Interactions CYP2A6 and CYP3A4 enzyme substrate

CYP3A3/4 inhibitors: Serum level and/or toxicity of tolcapone may be increased; inhibitors include amiodarone, cimetidine, clarithromycin, erythromycin, delavirdine, diltiazem, dirithromycin, disulfiram, fluoxetine, fluvoxamine, grapefruit juice, indinavir, itraconazole, ketoconazole, nevirapine, propoxyphene, quinupristin-dalfopristin, ritonavir, saquinavir, verapamil, zafirlukast, zileuton; monitor for altered effects

Substrates of COMT: COMT inhibition could slow the metabolism of methyldopa, dobutamine, apomorphine, and isoproterenol

Ethanol/Nutrition/Herb Interactions

Ethanol: Avoid ethanol (may increase CNS depression).

Food: Tolcapone, taken with food within 1 hour before or 2 hours after the dose, decreases bioavailability by 10% to 20%.

Avoid valerian, St John's wort, kava kava, gotu kola (may increase CNS depression).

Mechanism of Action Tolcapone is a selective and reversible inhibitor of catechol-o-methyltransferase (COMT)

Pharmacodynamics/Kinetics

Absorption: Rapid with T_{max} at 2 hours

Distribution: V_d: 9 L

Protein binding: 99.9%

Metabolism: Tolcapone is almost completely metabolized prior to excretion; the main metabolic pathway is glucuronidation; the glucuronide conjugate is inactive. Tolcapone is hydroxylated and subsequently oxidized via CYP3A4 and CYP2A6.

Bioavailability: 65% (empty stomach), 45% to 55% (with food)

Half-life: 2-3 hours

Usual Dosage Adults: Oral: Initial: 100-200 mg 3 times/day; levodopa therapy may need to be decreased upon initiation of tolcapone

Monitoring Parameters Blood pressure, symptoms of Parkinson's disease, liver enzymes at baseline and then every 2 weeks for the first year of therapy, every 4 weeks for the next 6 months, then every 8 weeks thereafter. If the dose is increased to 200 mg 3 times/day, reinitiate LFT monitoring at the previous frequency. Discontinue therapy if the ALT or AST exceeds the upper limit of normal or if the clinical signs and symptoms suggest the onset of liver failure.

Dosage Forms Tablet: 100 mg, 200 mg

- **Tonga** *see Kava on page 186*
- **Topamax®** *see Topiramate on page 403*

Topiramate (toe PYE ra mate)

Related Information
Mood Stabilizers *on page 588*
Patient Information - Miscellaneous Medications *on page 495*

U.S. Brand Names Topamax®

Canadian Brand Names Topamax

Pharmacologic Category Anticonvulsant, Miscellaneous

Generic Available No

Use
In adults and pediatric patients (ages 2-16 years), adjunctive therapy for partial onset seizures and adjunctive therapy of primary generalized tonic-clonic seizures; treatment of seizures associated with Lennox-Gastaut syndrome in patients ≥2 years of age

Unlabeled/Investigational Use
Bipolar disorder, infantile spasms, neuropathic pain

Pregnancy Risk Factor C

Pregnancy/Breast-Feeding Implications
No studies in pregnant women; use only if benefit to the mother outweighs the risk to the fetus. Postmarketing experience includes reports of hypospadias following *in vitro* exposure to topiramate.

Contraindications
Hypersensitivity to topiramate or any component of the formulation

Warnings/Precautions
Avoid abrupt withdrawal of topiramate therapy, it should be withdrawn slowly to minimize the potential of increased seizure frequency. The risk of kidney stones is about 2-4 times that of the untreated population, the risk of this event may be reduced by increasing fluid intake. Use cautiously in patients with hepatic or renal impairment and during pregnancy. May cause paresthesias. Sedation, psychomotor slowing, confusion, and mood disturbances may occur with topiramate use. Has been associated with secondary angle-closure glaucoma in adults and children, typically within 1 month of initiation. Discontinue in patients with acute onset of decreased visual acuity or ocular pain. Safety and efficacy have not been established in children <2 years of age.

Adverse Reactions
>10%:
- Central nervous system: Dizziness, ataxia, somnolence, psychomotor slowing, nervousness, memory difficulties, speech problems, fatigue
- Gastrointestinal: Nausea
- Neuromuscular & skeletal: Paresthesia, tremor
- Ocular: Nystagmus, diplopia, abnormal vision
- Respiratory: Upper respiratory infections

1% to 10%:
- Cardiovascular: Chest pain, edema
- Central nervous system: Language problems, abnormal coordination, confusion, depression, difficulty concentrating, hypoesthesia
- Endocrine & metabolic: Hot flashes
- Gastrointestinal: Dyspepsia, abdominal pain, anorexia, constipation, xerostomia, gingivitis, weight loss
- Neuromuscular & skeletal: Myalgia, weakness, back pain, leg pain, rigors
- Otic: Decreased hearing
- Renal: Nephrolithiasis
- Respiratory: Pharyngitis, sinusitis, epistaxis
- Miscellaneous: Flu-like symptoms

<1%: Apraxia, AV block, bone marrow depression, delirium, dyskinesia, encephalopathy, eosinophilia, granulocytopenia, manic reaction, neuropathy, pancytopenia, paranoid reaction, photosensitivity, psychosis, renal calculus, suicidal behavior, tinnitus

Postmarketing and/or case reports: Hepatic failure, hepatitis, pancreatitis, renal tubular acidosis, syndrome of acute myopia/secondary angle-closure glaucoma

Overdosage/Toxicology
Treatment: Activated charcoal has not been shown to adsorb topiramate and is, therefore, not recommended; hemodialysis can remove

(Continued)

Topiramate *(Continued)*

drug, however, most cases do not require removal and instead is best treated with supportive measures

Drug Interactions CYP2C19 enzyme substrate; CYP2C19 enzyme inhibitor

Carbamazepine: May reduce topiramate levels 40%

Carbonic anhydrase inhibitors: Coadministration with other carbonic anhydrase inhibitors may increase the chance of nephrolithiasis; includes acetazolamide

CNS depressants: Sedative effects may be additive with topiramate; monitor for increased effect; includes barbiturates, benzodiazepines, narcotic analgesics, ethanol, and other sedative agents

CYP2C19 inhibitors: Serum levels of topiramate may be increased; inhibitors include cimetidine, felbamate, fluconazole, fluoxetine, fluvoxamine, omeprazole, teniposide, tolbutamide, and troglitazone

Digoxin: Blood levels of digoxin are decreased when coadministered with topiramate.

Estrogens: Blood levels of estrogens are decreased when coadministered with topiramate, this may lead to a loss of efficacy.

Oral contraceptives: See interaction with Estrogens; use of alternative contraception is recommended.

Phenytoin: May decrease topiramate levels by as much as 48%; topiramate may increase phenytoin concentration by 25%

Valproic acid: May reduce topiramate levels by 14%; topiramate may decrease valproic acid concentration by 11%

Ethanol/Nutrition/Herb Interactions

Ethanol: Avoid ethanol (may increase CNS depression).

Herb/Nutraceutical: Avoid evening primrose (seizure threshold decreased).

Stability Store at room temperature; protect capsules from moisture.

Mechanism of Action Mechanism is not fully understood, it is thought to decrease seizure frequency by blocking sodium channels in neurons, enhancing GABA activity and by blocking glutamate activity

Pharmacodynamics/Kinetics

Absorption: Good; unaffected by food

Protein binding: 13% to 17%

Metabolism: Minimal, less than 5% of metabolites are active

Bioavailability: 80%

Half-life: Mean: 21 hours in adults

Time to peak serum concentration: ~2-4 hours

Elimination: Primarily eliminated unchanged in the urine

Dialyzable: ~30%

Usual Dosage Oral:

Children 2-16 years: Partial seizures (adjunctive therapy), primary generalized tonic-clonic seizures (adjunctive therapy), or seizure associated with Lennox-Gastaut syndrome: Initial dose titration should begin at 25 mg (or less, based on a range of 1-3 mg/kg/day) nightly for the first week; dosage may be increased in increments of 1-3 mg/kg/day (administered in 2 divided doses) at 1- or 2-week intervals to a total daily dose of 5-9 mg/kg/day.

Adults: Partial onset seizures (adjunctive therapy), primary generalized tonic-clonic seizures (adjunctive therapy): Initial: 25-50 mg/day; titrate in increments of 25-50 mg per week until an effective daily dose is reached; the daily dose may be increased by 25 mg at weekly intervals for the first 4 weeks; thereafter, the daily dose may be increased by 25-50 mg weekly to an effective daily dose (usually at least 400 mg); usual maximum dose: 1600 mg/day

Note: A more rapid titration schedule has been previously recommended (ie, 50 mg/week), and may be attempted in some clinical situations; however, this may reduce the patient's ability to tolerate topiramate.

Dosing adjustment in renal impairment: Cl$_{cr}$ <70 mL/minute: Administer 50% dose and titrate more slowly

Hemodialysis: Supplemental dose may be needed during hemodialysis

Dosing adjustment in hepatic impairment: Clearance may be reduced

Administration Oral: May be administered without regard to meals

Capsule sprinkles: May be swallowed whole or opened to sprinkle the contents on soft food (drug/food mixture should not be chewed).

Tablet: Because of bitter taste, tablets should not be broken.

Additional Information May be associated with weight loss in some patients

Dosage Forms

Capsule, sprinkle (Topamax®): 15 mg, 25 mg

Tablet (Topamax®): 25 mg, 100 mg, 200 mg

♦ **Transamine Sulphate** *see* Tranylcypromine *on page 405*

♦ **Tranxene®** *see* Clorazepate *on page 92*

Tranylcypromine (tran il SIP roe meen)

Related Information

Antidepressant Agents Comparison Chart *on page 553*

Patient Information - Antidepressants (MAOIs) *on page 462*

Teratogenic Risks of Psychotropic Medications *on page 594*

Tyramine Content of Foods *on page 595*

U.S. Brand Names Parnate®

Canadian Brand Names Parnate

Synonyms Transamine Sulphate; Tranylcypromine Sulfate

Pharmacologic Category Antidepressant, Monoamine Oxidase Inhibitor

Generic Available No

Use Treatment of major depressive episode without melancholia

Unlabeled/Investigational Use Post-traumatic stress disorder

Pregnancy Risk Factor C

Contraindications Hypersensitivity to tranylcypromine or any component of the formulation; uncontrolled hypertension; pheochromocytoma; hepatic or renal disease; cerebrovascular defect; cardiovascular disease (CHF); concurrent use of sympathomimetics (and related compounds), CNS depressants, ethanol, meperidine, bupropion, buspirone, dexfenfluramine, dextromethorphan, guanethidine, and serotonergic drugs (including SSRIs) - do not use within 5 weeks of fluoxetine discontinuation or 2 weeks of other antidepressant discontinuation; general anesthesia (discontinue 10 days prior to elective surgery); local vasoconstrictors; spinal anesthesia (hypotension may be exaggerated); foods which are high in tyramine, tryptophan, or dopamine, chocolate, or caffeine.

Warnings/Precautions Safety in children <16 years of age has not been established; use with caution in patients who are hyperactive, hyperexcitable, or who have glaucoma, suicidal tendencies, hyperthyroidism, or diabetes; avoid use of meperidine within 2 weeks of tranylcypromine use. Toxic reactions have occurred with dextromethorphan. Hypertensive crisis may occur with tyramine, tryptophan, or dopamine-containing foods. Should not be used in combination with other antidepressants. Hypotensive effects of antihypertensives (beta-blockers, thiazides) may be exaggerated. Use with caution in depressed patients at risk of suicide. May cause orthostatic hypotension (especially at dosages >30 mg/day) - use with caution in patients with hypotension or patients who would not tolerate transient hypotensive episodes - effects may be additive when used with other agents known to cause orthostasis (phenothiazines). Has been associated with activation of hypomania and/or mania in bipolar patients. May worsen psychotic symptoms in some patients. Use with caution in patients at risk of seizures, or in patients receiving other drugs which may lower seizure threshold. Discontinue at least 48 hours prior to myelography. Use with caution in patients receiving disulfiram. Use with caution in patients with renal impairment.

The MAO inhibitors are effective and generally well tolerated by older patients. It is the potential interactions with tyramine or tryptophan-containing foods and other drugs, and their effects on blood pressure that have limited their use.

Adverse Reactions

Cardiovascular: Orthostatic hypotension, edema

(Continued)

Tranylcypromine *(Continued)*

Central nervous system: Dizziness, headache, drowsiness, sleep disturbances, fatigue, hyper-reflexia, twitching, ataxia, mania, akinesia, confusion, disorientation, memory loss

Dermatologic: Rash, pruritus, urticaria, localized scleroderma, cystic acne (flare)

Endocrine & metabolic: Sexual dysfunction (anorgasmia, ejaculatory disturbances, impotence), hypernatremia, hypermetabolic syndrome, SIADH

Gastrointestinal: Xerostomia, constipation, weight gain

Genitourinary: Urinary retention, incontinence

Hematologic: Leukopenia, agranulocytosis

Hepatic: Hepatitis

Neuromuscular & skeletal: Weakness, tremor, myoclonus

Ocular: Blurred vision, glaucoma

Miscellaneous: Diaphoresis

Overdosage/Toxicology

Signs and symptoms: Tachycardia, palpitations, muscle twitching, seizures, insomnia, transient hypotension, hypertension, hyperpyrexia, coma

Treatment: Competent supportive care is the most important treatment for an overdose with a monoamine oxidase (MAO) inhibitor. Both hypertension or hypotension can occur with intoxication. Hypotension may respond to I.V. fluids or vasopressors, and hypertension usually responds to an alpha-adrenergic blocker. While treating the hypertension, care is warranted to avoid sudden drops in blood pressure, since this may worsen the MAO inhibitor toxicity. Muscle irritability and seizures often respond to diazepam, while hyperthermia is best treated antipyretics and cooling blankets. Cardiac arrhythmias are best treated with phenytoin or procainamide.

Drug Interactions CYP2A6 and 2C19 enzyme inhibitor

Amphetamines: MAO inhibitors in combination with amphetamines may result in severe hypertensive reaction; these combinations are best avoided

Anesthetics, general: Discontinue tranylcypromine 10 days prior to elective surgery.

Anorexiants: Concurrent use of anorexiants may result in serotonin syndrome; contraindicated with dexfenfluramine; avoid use with fenfluramine or sibutramine

Barbiturates: MAO inhibitors may inhibit the metabolism of barbiturates and prolong their effect

Bupropion: May cause hypertensive crisis; at least 14 days should elapse before initiating bupropion

Buspirone: May cause hypertensive crisis; at least 10 days should elapse before initiating buspirone

CNS stimulants: MAO inhibitors in combination with stimulants (methylphenidate) may result in severe hypertensive reaction; these combinations are best avoided

Dextromethorphan: Concurrent use of MAO inhibitors may result in serotonin syndrome; concurrent use is contraindicated

Disulfiram: MAO inhibitors may produce delirium in patients receiving disulfiram; monitor

Guanadrel and guanethidine: MAO inhibitors inhibit the antihypertensive response to guanadrel or guanethidine; use an alternative antihypertensive agent

Hypoglycemic agents: MAO inhibitors may produce hypoglycemia in patients with diabetes; monitor

Levodopa: MAO inhibitors in combination with levodopa may result in hypertensive reactions; monitor

Lithium: MAO inhibitors in combination with lithium have resulted in malignant hyperpyrexia; this combination is best avoided

Meperidine: May cause serotonin syndrome when combined with an MAO inhibitor; concurrent use is contraindicated

Nefazodone: Concurrent use of MAO inhibitors may result in serotonin syndrome; these combinations are best avoided

Norepinephrine: MAO inhibitors may increase the pressor response of norepinephrine (effect is generally small); monitor

Reserpine: MAO inhibitors in combination with reserpine may result in hypertensive reactions; monitor

Serotonin agonists: Theoretically may increase the risk of serotonin syndrome; includes sumatriptan, naratriptan, rizatriptan, and zolmitriptan

SSRIs: May cause serotonin syndrome when combined with an MAO inhibitor; avoid this combination

Succinylcholine: MAO inhibitors may prolong the muscle relaxation produced by succinylcholine via decreased plasma pseudocholinesterase

Sympathomimetics (indirect-acting): MAO inhibitors in combination with sympathomimetics such as dopamine, metaraminol, phenylephrine, and decongestants (pseudoephedrine) may result in severe hypertensive reaction; concurrent use is contraindicated

Tramadol: May increase the risk of seizures and serotonin syndrome in patients receiving an MAO inhibitor

Trazodone: Concurrent use of MAO inhibitors may result in serotonin syndrome; these combinations are best avoided

Tricyclic antidepressants: May cause hypertension/seizures when combined with an MAO inhibitor; concurrent use is contraindicated

Tyramine: Foods (eg, cheese) and beverages (eg, ethanol) containing tyramine, should be avoided in patients receiving an MAO inhibitor; hypertensive crisis may result

Venlafaxine: Concurrent use of MAO inhibitors may result in serotonin syndrome; these combinations are best avoided

Ethanol/Nutrition/Herb Interactions

Ethanol: Avoid ethanol (many contain tyramine).

Food: Clinically severe elevated blood pressure may occur if tranylcypromine is taken with tyramine-containing food. Avoid foods containing tryptophan or dopamine, chocolate or caffeine.

Herb/Nutraceutical: Avoid valerian, St John's wort, SAMe, ginseng. Avoid ginkgo (may lead to MAO inhibitor toxicity). Avoid ephedra, yohimbe (can cause hypertension).

Mechanism of Action Thought to act by increasing endogenous concentrations of epinephrine, norepinephrine, dopamine and serotonin through inhibition of the enzyme (monoamine oxidase) responsible for the breakdown of these neurotransmitters

Pharmacodynamics/Kinetics

Onset of action: 2-3 weeks are required of continued dosing to obtain full therapeutic effect

Half-life: 90-190 minutes

Time to peak serum concentration: Within 2 hours

Elimination: In urine

Usual Dosage Adults: Oral: 10 mg twice daily, increase by 10 mg increments at 1- to 3-week intervals; maximum: 60 mg/day

Dosing comments in hepatic impairment: Use with care and monitor plasma levels and patient response closely

Monitoring Parameters Blood pressure, blood glucose

Test Interactions ↓ glucose

Patient Information Tablets may be crushed; avoid alcohol; do not discontinue abruptly; avoid foods high in tyramine (eg, aged cheeses, Chianti wine, raisins, liver, bananas, chocolate, yogurt, sour cream); discuss list of drugs and foods to avoid with pharmacist or physician; arise slowly from prolonged sitting or lying

Nursing Implications Assist with ambulation during initiation of therapy; monitor blood pressure closely, patients should be cautioned against eating foods high in tyramine or tryptophan (cheese, wine, beer, pickled herring, dry sausage)

Additional Information Tranylcypromine has a more rapid onset of therapeutic effect than other MAO inhibitors, but causes more severe hypertensive reactions.

Dosage Forms Tablet, as sulfate: 10 mg

♦ **Tranylcypromine Sulfate** *see* Tranylcypromine *on page 405*

Trazodone (TRAZ oh done)

Related Information

Antidepressant Agents Comparison Chart *on page 553*
Federal OBRA Regulations Recommended Maximum Doses *on page 583*
Patient Information - Antidepressants (Serotonin Blocker) *on page 460*
Teratogenic Risks of Psychotropic Medications *on page 594*

U.S. Brand Names Desyrel®

Canadian Brand Names Desyrel; Trazorel

Synonyms Trazodone Hydrochloride

Pharmacologic Category Antidepressant, Serotonin Reuptake Inhibitor/Antagonist

Generic Available Yes

Use Treatment of depression

Unlabeled/Investigational Use Potential augmenting agent for antidepressants, hypnotic

Pregnancy Risk Factor C

Contraindications Hypersensitivity to trazodone or any component of the formulation

Warnings/Precautions Priapism, including cases resulting in permanent dysfunction, has occurred with the use of trazodone. Not recommended for use in a patient during the acute recovery phase of MI. Trazodone should be initiated with caution in patients who are receiving concurrent or recent therapy with a MAO inhibitor. May cause sedation, resulting in impaired performance of tasks requiring alertness (ie, operating machinery or driving). Sedative effects may be additive with other CNS depressants and ethanol. The degree of sedation is very high relative to other antidepressants. May worsen psychosis in some patients or precipitate a shift to mania or hypomania in patients with bipolar disease. May increase the risks associated with electroconvulsive therapy. This agent should be discontinued, when possible, prior to elective surgery. Therapy should not be abruptly discontinued in patients receiving high doses for prolonged periods.

Use with caution in patients at risk of hypotension or in patients where transient hypotensive episodes would be poorly tolerated (cardiovascular disease or cerebrovascular disease). The risk of postural hypotension is high relative to other antidepressants. Use caution in patients with depression, particularly if suicidal risk may be present. Use caution in patients with a previous seizure disorder or condition predisposing to seizures such as brain damage, alcoholism, or concurrent therapy with other drugs which lower the seizure threshold. Use with caution in patients with hepatic or renal dysfunction and in elderly patients. Use with caution in patients with a history of cardiovascular disease (including previous MI, stroke, tachycardia, or conduction abnormalities). However, the risk of conduction abnormalities with this agent is low relative to other antidepressants.

Adverse Reactions

>10%:
Central nervous system: Dizziness, headache, sedation
Gastrointestinal: Nausea, xerostomia

1% to 10%:
Cardiovascular: Syncope, hypertension, hypotension, edema
Central nervous system: Confusion, decreased concentration, fatigue, incoordination
Gastrointestinal: Diarrhea, constipation, weight gain/loss
Neuromuscular & skeletal: Tremor, myalgia
Ocular: Blurred vision
Respiratory: Nasal congestion

<1%: Agitation, bradycardia, extrapyramidal reactions, hepatitis, priapism, rash, seizures, tachycardia, urinary retention

Overdosage/Toxicology

Signs and symptoms: Drowsiness, vomiting, hypotension, tachycardia, incontinence, coma, priapism

Treatment:

Following initiation of essential overdose management, toxic symptoms should be treated

Ventricular arrhythmias often respond to lidocaine 1.5 mg/kg bolus followed by 2 mg/minute infusion with concurrent systemic alkalinization (sodium bicarbonate 0.5-2 mEq/kg I.V.)

Seizures usually respond to diazepam I.V. boluses (5-10 mg for adults up to 30 mg or 0.25-0.4 mg/kg/dose for children up to 10 mg/dose). If seizures are unresponsive or recur, phenytoin or phenobarbital may be required.

Hypotension is best treated by I.V. fluids and by placing the patient in the Trendelenburg position.

Drug Interactions CYP2D6 and 3A3/4 enzyme substrate

Antipsychotics: Trazodone, in combination with other psychotropics (low potency antipsychotics), may result in additional hypotension (isolated case reports); monitor

Buspirone: Serotonergic effects may be additive (limited documentation); monitor

CNS depressants: Sedative effects may be additive with CNS depressants. Includes ethanol, barbiturates, benzodiazepines, narcotic analgesics, and other sedative agents; monitor for increased effect

CYP2D6 inhibitors: Metabolism of trazodone may be decreased; increasing clinical effect or toxicity; inhibitors include amiodarone, cimetidine, delavirdine, fluoxetine, paroxetine, propafenone, quinidine, and ritonavir; monitor for increased effect/toxicity

CYP3A3/4 inhibitors: Serum level and/or toxicity of trazodone may be increased; inhibitors include amiodarone, cimetidine, clarithromycin, erythromycin, delavirdine, diltiazem, dirithromycin, disulfiram, fluoxetine, fluvoxamine, grapefruit juice, indinavir, itraconazole, ketoconazole, metronidazole, nefazodone, nevirapine, propoxyphene, quinupristin-dalfopristin, ritonavir, saquinavir, verapamil, zafirlukast, zileuton; monitor for altered response

Enzyme inducers: May enhance the hepatic metabolism of trazodone; larger doses may be required; inducers include carbamazepine, rifampin, rifabutin, barbiturates, phenytoin, and cigarette smoking

Linezolid: Due to MAO inhibition (see note on MAO inhibitors), this combination should be avoided

MAO inhibitors: Concurrent use may lead to serotonin syndrome; avoid concurrent use or use within 14 days

Meperidine: Combined use, theoretically, may increase the risk of serotonin syndrome

Serotonin agonists: Theoretically, may increase the risk of serotonin syndrome; includes sumatriptan, naratriptan, rizatriptan, and zolmitriptan

SSRIs: Combined use of trazodone with an SSRI may, theoretically, increase the risk of serotonin syndrome; in addition, some SSRIs may inhibit the metabolism of trazodone resulting in elevated plasma levels and increased sedation; includes fluoxetine and fluvoxamine (see CYP inhibition); low doses of trazodone appear to represent little risk

Venlafaxine: Combined use with trazodone may increase the risk of serotonin syndrome

Ethanol/Nutrition/Herb Interactions

Ethanol: Avoid ethanol (may increase CNS depression).

Food: Time to peak serum levels may be increased if trazodone is taken with food.

Herb/Nutraceutical: Avoid valerian, St John's wort, SAMe, kava kava (may increase risk of serotonin syndrome and/or excessive sedation).

Mechanism of Action Inhibits reuptake of serotonin, causes adrenoreceptor subsensitivity, and induces significant changes in 5-HT presynaptic receptor adrenoreceptors. Trazodone also significantly blocks histamine (H_1) and alpha$_1$-adrenergic receptors.

Pharmacodynamics/Kinetics

Onset of effect: Therapeutic effects take 1-3 weeks to appear

Protein binding: 85% to 95%

(Continued)

Trazodone *(Continued)*

Metabolism: In the liver by hydroxylation, pyridine ring splitting, oxidation, and N-oxidation

Half-life: 7-8 hours, 2 compartment kinetics

Time to peak serum concentration: Within 30-100 minutes, prolonged in the presence of food (up to 2.5 hours)

Elimination: Primarily in urine and secondarily in feces

Usual Dosage Oral: Therapeutic effects may take up to 4 weeks to occur; therapy is normally maintained for several months after optimum response is reached to prevent recurrence of depression

Children 6-12 years: Depression: Initial: 1.5-2 mg/kg/day in divided doses; increase gradually every 3-4 days as needed; maximum: 6 mg/kg/day in 3 divided doses

Adolescents: Depression: Initial: 25-50 mg/day; increase to 100-150 mg/day in divided doses

Adults:

Depression: Initial: 150 mg/day in 3 divided doses (may increase by 50 mg/day every 3-7 days); maximum: 600 mg/day

Sedation/hypnotic (unlabeled use): 25-50 mg at bedtime (often in combination with daytime SSRIs); may increase up to 200 mg at bedtime

Elderly: 25-50 mg at bedtime with 25-50 mg/day dose increase every 3 days for inpatients and weekly for outpatients, if tolerated; usual dose: 75-150 mg/day

Reference Range

Plasma levels do not always correlate with clinical effectiveness

Therapeutic: 0.5-2.5 µg/mL

Potentially toxic: >2.5 µg/mL

Toxic: >4 µg/mL

Patient Information Take shortly after a meal or light snack, can be given as bedtime dose if drowsiness occurs; avoid alcohol; be aware of possible photosensitivity reaction; report any prolonged or painful erection

Nursing Implications Dosing after meals may decrease lightheadedness and postural hypotension; use side rails on bed if administered to the elderly; observe patient's activity and compare with admission level; assist with ambulation; sitting and standing blood pressure and pulse

Additional Information Therapeutic effect for sleep occurs in 1-3 hours

Dosage Forms Tablet, as hydrochloride: 50 mg, 100 mg, 150 mg, 300 mg

- ◆ **Trazodone Hydrochloride** *see* Trazodone *on page 408*
- ◆ **Trazorel (Can)** *see* Trazodone *on page 408*
- ◆ **Tremytoine® (Can)** *see* Phenytoin *on page 308*
- ◆ **Triadapin® (Can)** *see* Doxepin *on page 123*
- ◆ **Triapin®** *see* Butalbital Compound *on page 59*
- ◆ **Triavil®** *see* Amitriptyline and Perphenazine *on page 28*

Triazolam *(trye AY zoe lam)*

Related Information

Anxiolytic/Hypnotic Use in Long-Term Care Facilities *on page 562*

Benzodiazepines Comparison Chart *on page 566*

Federal OBRA Regulations Recommended Maximum Doses *on page 583*

Patient Information - Anxiolytics & Sedative Hypnotics (Benzodiazepines) *on page 483*

U.S. Brand Names Halcion®

Canadian Brand Names Apo®-Triazo; Gen-Triazolam®; Novo-Triolam®; Nu-Triazo®

Pharmacologic Category Benzodiazepine

Generic Available Yes

Use Short-term treatment of insomnia

Restrictions C-IV

Pregnancy Risk Factor X

Contraindications Hypersensitivity to triazolam or any component of the formulation (cross-sensitivity with other benzodiazepines may exist); concurrent therapy with CYP3A3/4 inhibitors (including ketoconazole, itraconazole, and nefazodone); pregnancy

Warnings/Precautions Should be used only after evaluation of potential causes of sleep disturbance. Failure of sleep disturbance to resolve after 7-10 days may indicate psychiatric or medical illness. A worsening of insomnia or the emergence of new abnormalities of thought or behavior may represent unrecognized psychiatric or medical illness and requires immediate and careful evaluation.

An increase in daytime anxiety may occur after as few as 10 days of continuous use, which may be related to withdrawal reaction in some patients. Anterograde amnesia may occur at a higher rate with triazolam than with other benzodiazepines. Use with caution in elderly or debilitated patients, patients with hepatic disease (including alcoholics), or renal impairment. Use with caution in patients with respiratory disease or impaired gag reflex. Avoid use in patients with sleep apnea.

Causes CNS depression (dose-related) resulting in sedation, dizziness, confusion, or ataxia which may impair physical and mental capabilities. Patients must be cautioned about performing tasks which require mental alertness (ie, operating machinery or driving). Use with caution in patients receiving other CNS depressants or psychoactive agents. Effects with other sedative drugs or ethanol may be potentiated. Benzodiazepines have been associated with falls and traumatic injury and should be used with extreme caution in patients who are at risk of these events (especially the elderly).

Use caution in patients with depression, particularly if suicidal risk may be present. Use with caution in patients with a history of drug dependence. Benzodiazepines have been associated with dependence and acute withdrawal symptoms on discontinuation or reduction in dose. Acute withdrawal, including seizures, may be precipitated after administration of flumazenil to patients receiving long-term benzodiazepine therapy.

Paradoxical reactions, including hyperactive or aggressive behavior have been reported with benzodiazepines, particularly in adolescent/pediatric or psychiatric patients. Does not have analgesic, antidepressant, or antipsychotic properties.

Adverse Reactions

>10%: Central nervous system: Drowsiness, anterograde amnesia

1% to 10%:

Central nervous system: Headache, dizziness, nervousness, lightheadedness, ataxia

Gastrointestinal: Nausea, vomiting

<1%: Cramps, confusion, depression, euphoria, fatigue, memory impairment, pain, tachycardia, visual disturbance

Overdosage/Toxicology

Signs and symptoms: Somnolence, confusion, coma, diminished reflexes, dyspnea, and hypotension

Treatment: Supportive; rarely is mechanical ventilation required. Flumazenil has been shown to selectively block the binding of benzodiazepines to CNS receptors, resulting in a reversal of benzodiazepine-induced CNS depression but not always respiratory depression

Drug Interactions CYP3A3/4 and 3A5-7 enzyme substrate

CNS depressants: Sedative effects and/or respiratory depression may be additive with CNS depressants; includes ethanol, barbiturates, narcotic analgesics, and other sedative agents; monitor for increased effect

CYP3A3/4 inhibitors: Serum level and/or toxicity of some benzodiazepines may be increased; inhibitors include amiodarone, cimetidine, clarithromycin, erythromycin, delavirdine, diltiazem, dirithromycin, disulfiram, fluoxetine, fluvoxamine, grapefruit juice, indinavir, itraconazole, ketoconazole, nefazodone, nevirapine, (Continued)

Triazolam *(Continued)*

propoxyphene, quinupristin-dalfopristin, ritonavir, saquinavir, verapamil, zafirlukast, zileuton; monitor for altered benzodiazepine response

Enzyme inducers: Metabolism of some benzodiazepines may be increased, decreasing their therapeutic effect; consider using an alternative sedative/hypnotic agent; potential inducers include phenobarbital, phenytoin, carbamazepine, rifampin, and rifabutin

Levodopa: Therapeutic effects may be diminished in some patients following the addition of a benzodiazepine; limited/inconsistent data

Oral contraceptives: May decrease the clearance of some benzodiazepines (those which undergo oxidative metabolism); monitor for increased benzodiazepine effect

Theophylline: May partially antagonize some of the effects of benzodiazepines; monitor for decreased response; may require higher doses for sedation

Ethanol/Nutrition/Herb Interactions

Ethanol: Avoid ethanol (may increase CNS depression).

Food: Food may decrease the rate of absorption. Triazolam serum concentration may be increased by grapefruit juice; avoid concurrent use.

Herb/Nutraceutical: St John's wort may decrease levels. Avoid valerian, St John's wort, kava kava, gotu kola (may increase CNS depression).

Mechanism of Action Binds to stereospecific benzodiazepine receptors on the postsynaptic GABA neuron at several sites within the central nervous system, including the limbic system, reticular formation. Enhancement of the inhibitory effect of GABA on neuronal excitability results by increased neuronal membrane permeability to chloride ions. This shift in chloride ions results in hyperpolarization (a less excitable state) and stabilization.

Pharmacodynamics/Kinetics

Onset of hypnotic effect: Within 15-30 minutes

Duration: 6-7 hours

Distribution: V_d: 0.8-1.8 L/kg

Protein binding: 89%

Metabolism: Extensively in the liver

Half-life: 1.7-5 hours

Elimination: In urine as unchanged drug and metabolites

Usual Dosage Oral (onset of action is rapid, patient should be in bed when taking medication):

Children <18 years: Dosage not established

Adults:

Hypnotic: 0.125-0.25 mg at bedtime

Preprocedure sedation (dental): 0.25 mg taken the evening before oral surgery; or 0.25 mg 1 hour before procedure

Dosing adjustment/comments in hepatic impairment: Reduce dose or avoid use in cirrhosis

Monitoring Parameters Respiratory and cardiovascular status

Patient Information Avoid alcohol and other CNS depressants; avoid activities needing good psychomotor coordination until CNS effects are known; drug may cause physical or psychological dependence; avoid abrupt discontinuation after prolonged use

Nursing Implications Patients may require assistance with ambulation; lower doses in the elderly are usually effective; institute safety measures

Additional Information Onset of action is rapid, patient should be in bed when taking medication. Prescription should be written for 7-10 days and should not be prescribed in quantities exceeding a 1-month supply. Abrupt discontinuation after sustained use (generally >10 days) may cause withdrawal symptoms.

Dosage Forms Tablet: 0.125 mg, 0.25 mg

- ◆ **Trichloroacetaldehyde Monohydrate** *see* Chloral Hydrate *on page 69*
- ◆ **Tridione®** *see* Trimethadione *on page 420*

Trifluoperazine (trye floo oh PER a zeen)

Related Information

Antipsychotic Agents Comparison Chart *on page 557*
Antipsychotic Medication Guidelines *on page 559*
Discontinuation of Psychotropic Drugs - Withdrawal Symptoms and Recommendations *on page 582*
Federal OBRA Regulations Recommended Maximum Doses *on page 583*
Liquid Compatibility With Antipsychotics and Mood Stabilizers *on page 587*
Patient Information - Antipsychotics (General) *on page 466*

U.S. Brand Names Stelazine®

Canadian Brand Names Novo-Flurazine; Solazine; Stelazine; Terfluzine

Synonyms Trifluoperazine Hydrochloride

Pharmacologic Category Antipsychotic Agent, Phenothiazine, Piperazine

Generic Available Yes

Use Treatment of schizophrenia

Unlabeled/Investigational Use Management of psychotic disorders

Pregnancy Risk Factor C

Contraindications Hypersensitivity to trifluoperazine or any component of the formulation (cross-reactivity between phenothiazines may occur); severe CNS depression; bone marrow suppression; blood dyscrasias; severe hepatic disease; coma

Warnings/Precautions May result in hypotension, particularly after I.M. administration. May be sedating, use with caution in disorders where CNS depression is a feature. Use with caution in Parkinson's disease. Caution in patients with hemodynamic instability; predisposition to seizures; subcortical brain damage; hepatic impairment; severe cardiac, rehal, or respiratory disease. Esophageal dysmotility and aspiration have been associated with antipsychotic use - use with caution in patients at risk of pneumonia (ie, Alzheimer's disease). Caution in breast cancer or other prolactin-dependent tumors (may elevate prolactin levels). May alter temperature regulation or mask toxicity of other drugs due to antiemetic effects. May alter cardiac conduction - life-threatening arrhythmias have occurred with therapeutic doses of phenothiazines. May cause orthostatic hypotension - use with caution in patients at risk of this effect or those who would tolerate transient hypotensive episodes (cerebrovascular disease, cardiovascular disease or other medications which may predispose). Safety in children <6 months of age has not been established.

Phenothiazines may cause anticholinergic effects (confusion, agitation, constipation, dry mouth, blurred vision, urinary retention); therefore, they should be used with caution in patients with decreased gastrointestinal motility, urinary retention, BPH, xerostomia, or visual problems. Conditions which also may be exacerbated by cholinergic blockade include narrow-angle glaucoma (screening is recommended) and worsening of myasthenia gravis. Relative to other antipsychotics, trifluoperazine has a low potency of cholinergic blockade.

May cause extrapyramidal reactions, including pseudoparkinsonism, acute dystonic reactions, akathisia, and tardive dyskinesia (risk of these reactions is high relative to other neuroleptics). May be associated with neuroleptic malignant syndrome (NMS) or pigmentary retinopathy.

Adverse Reactions Frequency not defined.

Cardiovascular: Hypotension, orthostatic hypotension, cardiac arrest

Central nervous system: Extrapyramidal symptoms (pseudoparkinsonism, akathisia, dystonias, tardive dyskinesia), dizziness, headache, neuroleptic malignant syndrome (NMS), impairment of temperature regulation, lowering of seizures threshold

Dermatologic: Increased sensitivity to sun, rash, discoloration of skin (blue-gray)

Endocrine & metabolic: Changes in menstrual cycle, changes in libido, breast pain, hyperglycemia, hypoglycemia, gynecomastia, lactation, galactorrhea

Gastrointestinal: Constipation, weight gain, nausea, vomiting, stomach pain, xerostomia

(Continued)

Trifluoperazine *(Continued)*

Genitourinary: Difficulty in urination, ejaculatory disturbances, urinary retention, priapism

Hematologic: Agranulocytosis, leukopenia, pancytopenia, thrombocytopenic purpura, eosinophilia, hemolytic anemia, aplastic anemia

Hepatic: Cholestatic jaundice, hepatotoxicity

Neuromuscular & skeletal: Tremor

Ocular: Pigmentary retinopathy, cornea and lens changes

Respiratory: Nasal congestion

Overdosage/Toxicology

Signs and symptoms: Deep sleep, coma, extrapyramidal symptoms, abnormal involuntary muscle movements, hypo- or hypertension, cardiac arrhythmias

Treatment:

Following initiation of essential overdose management, toxic symptom treatment and supportive treatment should be initiated

Hypotension usually responds to I.V. fluids or Trendelenburg positioning. If unresponsive to these measures, the use of a parenteral inotrope may be required (eg, norepinephrine 0.1-0.2 mcg/kg/minute titrated to response).

Seizures commonly respond to diazepam (I.V. 5-10 mg bolus in adults every 15 minutes if needed up to a total of 30 mg; I.V. 0.25-0.4 mg/kg/dose up to a total of 10 mg in children) or to phenytoin or phenobarbital

Neuroleptics often cause extrapyramidal symptoms (eg, dystonic reactions) requiring management with diphenhydramine 1-2 mg/kg (adults) up to a maximum of 50 mg I.M. or I.V. slow push followed by a maintenance dose for 48-72 hours or benztropine mesylate I.V. 1-2 mg (adults). These agents are generally effective within 2-5 minutes.

Cardiac arrhythmias are treated with lidocaine 1-2 mg/kg bolus followed by a maintenance infusion

Drug Interactions CYP1A2 enzyme substrate

Aluminum salts: May decrease the absorption of phenothiazines; monitor

Amphetamines: Efficacy may be diminished by antipsychotics; in addition, amphetamines may increase psychotic symptoms; avoid concurrent use

Anticholinergics: May inhibit the therapeutic response to phenothiazines and excess anticholinergic effects may occur; includes benztropine, trihexyphenidyl, biperiden, and drugs with significant anticholinergic activity (TCAs, antihistamines, disopyramide)

Antihypertensives: Concurrent use of phenothiazines with an antihypertensive may produce additive hypotensive effects (particularly orthostasis)

Bromocriptine: Phenothiazines inhibit the ability of bromocriptine to lower serum prolactin concentrations

CNS depressants: Sedative effects may be additive with phenothiazines; monitor for increased effect; includes barbiturates, benzodiazepines, narcotic analgesics, ethanol, and other sedative agents

CYP1A2 inhibitors: Serum concentrations may be increased due to decreased metabolism; includes cimetidine, ciprofloxacin, fluvoxamine, isoniazid, ritonavir, and zileuton.

Enzyme inducers: May enhance the hepatic metabolism of phenothiazines; larger doses may be required; includes rifampin, rifabutin, barbiturates, phenytoin, and cigarette smoking

Epinephrine: Chlorpromazine (and possibly other low potency antipsychotics) may diminish the pressor effects of epinephrine

Guanethidine and guanadrel: Antihypertensive effects may be inhibited by phenothiazines

Levodopa: Phenothiazines may inhibit the antiparkinsonian effect of levodopa; avoid this combination

Lithium: Phenothiazines may produce neurotoxicity with lithium; this is a rare effect

Phenytoin: May reduce serum levels of phenothiazines; phenothiazines may increase phenytoin serum levels

Polypeptide antibiotics: Rare cases of respiratory paralysis have been reported with concurrent use of phenothiazines

Propranolol: Serum concentrations of phenothiazines may be increased; propranolol also increases phenothiazine concentrations

QT_c-prolonging agents: Effects on QT_c interval may be additive with phenothiazines, increasing the risk of malignant arrhythmias; includes type Ia antiarrhythmics, TCAs, and some quinolone antibiotics (sparfloxacin, moxifloxacin, and gatifloxacin)

Sulfadoxine-pyrimethamine: May increase phenothiazine concentrations

Trazodone: Phenothiazines and trazodone may produce additive hypotensive effects

Tricyclic antidepressants: Concurrent use may produce increased toxicity or altered therapeutic response

Valproic acid: Serum levels may be increased by phenothiazines

Ethanol/Nutrition/Herb Interactions

Ethanol: Avoid ethanol (may increase CNS depression).

Herb/Nutraceutical: Avoid kava kava, gotu kola, valerian, St John's wort (may increase CNS depression). Avoid dong quai, St John's wort (may also cause photosensitization).

Stability Store injection at room temperature; protect from heat and from freezing; use only clear or slightly yellow solutions

Mechanism of Action Blocks postsynaptic mesolimbic dopaminergic receptors in the brain; exhibits alpha-adrenergic blocking effect and depresses the release of hypothalamic and hypophyseal hormones

Pharmacodynamics/Kinetics

Metabolism: Extensive in the liver

Half-life: >24 hours with chronic use

Usual Dosage

Children 6-12 years: Schizophrenia/psychoses:

Oral: Hospitalized or well-supervised patients: Initial: 1 mg 1-2 times/day, gradually increase until symptoms are controlled or adverse effects become troublesome; maximum: 15 mg/day

I.M.: 1 mg twice daily

Adults:

Schizophrenia/psychoses:

Outpatients: Oral: 1-2 mg twice daily

Hospitalized or well-supervised patients: Initial: 2-5 mg twice daily with optimum response in the 15-20 mg/day range; do not exceed 40 mg/day

I.M.: 1-2 mg every 4-6 hours as needed up to 10 mg/24 hours maximum

Nonpsychotic anxiety: Oral: 1-2 mg twice daily; maximum: 6 mg/day; therapy for anxiety should not exceed 12 weeks; do not exceed 6 mg/day for longer than 12 weeks when treating anxiety; agitation, jitteriness, or insomnia may be confused with original neurotic or psychotic symptoms

Elderly:

Schizophrenia/psychoses:

Oral: Refer to adult dosing. Dose selection should start at the low end of the dosage range and titration must be gradual.

I.M.: Initial: 1 mg every 4-6 hours; increase at 1 mg increments; do not exceed 6 mg/day

Behavioral symptoms associated with dementia behavior: Oral: Initial: 0.5-1 mg 1-2 times/day; increase dose at 4- to 7-day intervals by 0.5-1 mg/day; increase dosing intervals (bid, tid, etc) as necessary to control response or side effects. Maximum daily dose: 40 mg. Gradual increases (titration) may prevent some side effects or decrease their severity.

Hemodialysis: Not dialyzable (0% to 5%)

Dietary Considerations May be administered with food to decrease GI distress.

Administration Administer I.M. injection deep in upper outer quadrant of buttock

Monitoring Parameters Mental status, blood pressure

(Continued)

Trifluoperazine *(Continued)*

Reference Range Therapeutic response and blood levels have not been established

Test Interactions False-positive for phenylketonuria; ↑ cholesterol (S), ↑ glucose; ↓ uric acid (S)

Patient Information This drug usually requires up to 6 weeks for a full therapeutic response to be seen. Avoid excessive exposure to sunlight or tanning lamps; concentrate must be diluted in 2-4 oz of liquid (water, carbonated drinks, fruit juices, tomato juice, milk, or pudding); wash hands if undiluted concentrate is spilled on skin to prevent contact dermatosis.

Nursing Implications Watch for hypotension when administering I.M. or I.V.; observe for extrapyramidal effects

Additional Information Do not exceed 6 mg/day for longer than 12 weeks when treating anxiety. Agitation, jitteriness, or insomnia may be confused with original neurotic or psychotic symptoms.

Dosage Forms
Injection, as hydrochloride: 2 mg/mL (10 mL)
Solution, oral concentrate, as hydrochloride: 10 mg/mL (60 mL)
Tablet, as hydrochloride: 1 mg, 2 mg, 5 mg, 10 mg

♦ **Trifluoperazine Hydrochloride** *see Trifluoperazine on page 413*

Triflupromazine *(trye floo PROE ma zeen)*

Related Information
Federal OBRA Regulations Recommended Maximum Doses *on page 583*
Patient Information - Antipsychotics (General) *on page 466*

U.S. Brand Names Vesprin®

Synonyms Triflupromazine Hydrochloride

Pharmacologic Category Antipsychotic Agent, Phenothiazine, Aliphatic

Generic Available No

Use Treatment of psychoses; severe nausea and vomiting

Unlabeled/Investigational Use Pain; hiccups

Pregnancy Risk Factor C

Contraindications Hypersensitivity to triflupromazine or any component of the formulation (cross-sensitivity with other phenothiazines may exist); angle-closure glaucoma; bone marrow depression; severe liver or cardiac disease; subcortical brain damage

Warnings/Precautions Safety and efficacy have not been established in children <2.5 years of age. Highly sedating, use with caution in disorders where CNS depression is a feature. Use with caution in Parkinson's disease. Caution in patients with hemodynamic instability; bone marrow suppression; predisposition to seizures; subcortical brain damage; severe cardiac, hepatic, renal, or respiratory disease. Esophageal dysmotility and aspiration have been associated with antipsychotic use; use with caution in patients at risk of pneumonia (ie, Alzheimer's disease).

Caution in breast cancer or other prolactin-dependent tumors (may elevate prolactin levels). May alter temperature regulation or mask toxicity of other drugs due to antiemetic effects. May alter cardiac conduction; life-threatening arrhythmias have occurred with therapeutic doses of phenothiazines. May cause orthostatic hypotension - use with caution in patients at risk of this effect or those who would tolerate transient hypotensive episodes (cerebrovascular disease, cardiovascular disease, or other medications which may predispose).

Phenothiazines may cause anticholinergic effects (confusion, agitation, constipation, dry mouth, blurred vision, urinary retention). Therefore, they should be used with caution in patients with decreased gastrointestinal motility, urinary retention, BPH, xerostomia, or visual problems. Conditions which also may be exacerbated by cholinergic blockade include narrow-angle glaucoma (screening is recommended) and worsening of myasthenia gravis. Relative to other antipsychotics, triflupromazine has a moderate potency of cholinergic blockade.

May cause extrapyramidal reactions, including pseudoparkinsonism, acute dystonic reactions, akathisia, and tardive dyskinesia (risk of these reactions is moderate relative to other neuroleptics). May be associated with neuroleptic malignant syndrome (NMS) or pigmentary retinopathy.

Adverse Reactions

Cardiovascular: Hypotension, tachycardia, syncope, peripheral edema, QT prolongation

Central nervous system: Neuroleptic malignant syndrome, extrapyramidal symptoms (dystonia, akathisia, pseudoparkinsonism, tardive dyskinesia), sedation, dizziness, drowsiness, insomnia, anxiety, depression, headache, seizures, NMS hyperpyrexia

Dermatologic: Photosensitivity, dermatitis, urticaria

Endocrine & metabolic: Syndrome of inappropriate antidiuretic hormone, galactorrhea, gynecomastia, hyperglycemia, hypoglycemia, breast engorgement, lactation, mastalgia

Gastrointestinal: Xerostomia, weight gain

Hematologic: Agranulocytosis, leukopenia, eosinophilia, thrombocytopenia, aplastic anemia, hemolytic anemia

Hepatic: Jaundice

Neuromuscular & skeletal: Weakness

Ocular: Nystagmus, blurred vision, keratopathy, lacrimation, pigment deposition

Drug Interactions

Aluminum salts: May decrease the absorption of phenothiazines; monitor

Amphetamines: Efficacy may be diminished by antipsychotics; in addition, amphetamines may increase psychotic symptoms; avoid concurrent use

Anticholinergics: May inhibit the therapeutic response to phenothiazines and excess anticholinergic effects may occur; includes benztropine, trihexyphenidyl, biperiden, and drugs with significant anticholinergic activity (TCAs, antihistamines, disopyramide)

Antihypertensives: Concurrent use of phenothiazines with an antihypertensive may produce additive hypotensive effects (particularly orthostasis)

Bromocriptine: Phenothiazines inhibit the ability of bromocriptine to lower serum prolactin concentrations

CNS depressants: Sedative effects may be additive with phenothiazines; monitor for increased effect; includes barbiturates, benzodiazepines, narcotic analgesics, ethanol, and other sedative agents

CYP inhibitors: Metabolism of phenothiazines may be decreased, increasing clinical effect or toxicity; monitor for increased effect/toxicity

Enzyme inducers: May enhance the hepatic metabolism of phenothiazines; larger doses may be required; includes rifampin, rifabutin, barbiturates, phenytoin, and cigarette smoking

Epinephrine: Chlorpromazine (and possibly other low potency antipsychotics) may diminish the pressor effects of epinephrine

Guanethidine and guanadrel: Antihypertensive effects may be inhibited by phenothiazines

Levodopa: Phenothiazines may inhibit the antiparkinsonian effect of levodopa; avoid this combination

Lithium: Phenothiazines may produce neurotoxicity with lithium; this is a rare effect

Phenytoin: May reduce serum levels of phenothiazines; phenothiazines may increase phenytoin serum levels

Polypeptide antibiotics: Rare cases of respiratory paralysis have been reported with concurrent use of phenothiazines

Propranolol: Serum concentrations of phenothiazines may be increased; propranolol also increases phenothiazine concentrations

(Continued)

Triflupromazine (Continued)

QT$_c$-prolonging agents: Effects on QT$_c$ interval may be additive with phenothiazines, increasing the risk of malignant arrhythmias; includes type Ia antiarrhythmics, TCAs, and some quinolone antibiotics (sparfloxacin, moxifloxacin, and gatifloxacin)

Sulfadoxine-pyrimethamine: May increase phenothiazine concentrations

Trazodone: Phenothiazines and trazodone may produce additive hypotensive effects

Tricyclic antidepressants: Concurrent use may produce increased toxicity or altered therapeutic response

Valproic acid: Serum levels may be increased by phenothiazines

Ethanol/Nutrition/Herb Interactions

Ethanol: Avoid ethanol (may increase CNS depression).

Herb/Nutraceutical: Avoid valerian, St John's wort, kava kava, gotu kola (may increase CNS depression).

Mechanism of Action The sites of action appear to be the reticular activity system of the midbrain, limbic system, hypothalamus, globus pallidus, and corpus striatum. Postsynaptic, adrenergic, dopaminergic, and serotonergic receptors are blocked.

Usual Dosage Safety and efficacy have not been established for children <2.5 years of age

Psychosis:

Children ≥2.5 years: I.M.: 0.2-0.25 mg/kg, up to a maximum total daily dose of 10 mg

Adults:

I.M.: 5-15 mg every 4 hours; initial dose: 60 mg, up to a maximum total daily dose of 150 mg

I.V.: 1 mg, may be repeated every 4 hours, up to a maximum total daily dose of 3 mg

Nausea and vomiting:

Children ≥2.5 years:

I.M.: 0.2-0.25 mg/kg, up to a maximum total daily dose of 10 mg

I.V.: Not recommended for use in children

Adults:

I.M.: 5-15 mg, may be repeated every 4 hours, up to a maximum total daily dose of 60 mg

I.V.: 1 mg, may be repeated every 4 hours, up to a maximum total daily dose of 3 mg

Elderly: I.M.: 2.5 mg, up to a maximum total daily dose of 15 mg

Dietary Considerations Should be administered with food, milk, or water.

Monitoring Parameters Monitor EKG for 24 hours

Test Interactions May cause false positive results in pregnancy tests

Dosage Forms Injection, as hydrochloride: 10 mg/mL (10 mL) [multidose vial]; 20 mg/mL (1 mL)

♦ **Triflupromazine Hydrochloride** *see* Triflupromazine *on page 416*

♦ **Trihexyphen® (Can)** *see* Trihexyphenidyl *on page 418*

Trihexyphenidyl (trye heks ee FEN i dil)

Related Information

Antiparkinsonian Agents Comparison Chart *on page 556*

Discontinuation of Psychotropic Drugs - Withdrawal Symptoms and Recommendations *on page 582*

Patient Information - Agents for Treatment of Extrapyramidal Symptoms *on page 493*

U.S. Brand Names Artane®

Canadian Brand Names Apo®-Trihex; Novo-Hexidyl®; PMS-Trihexyphenidyl; Trihexyphen®

Synonyms Benzhexol Hydrochloride; Trihexyphenidyl Hydrochloride

Pharmacologic Category Anticholinergic Agent; Anti-Parkinson's Agent (Anticholinergic)

Generic Available Yes

Use Adjunctive treatment of Parkinson's disease; treatment of drug-induced extrapyramidal effects

Pregnancy Risk Factor C

Contraindications Hypersensitivity to trihexyphenidyl or any component of the formulation; narrow-angle glaucoma; pyloric or duodenal obstruction; stenosing peptic ulcers; bladder neck obstructions; achalasia; myasthenia gravis

Warnings/Precautions Use with caution in hot weather or during exercise. Elderly patients require strict dosage regulation. Use with caution in patients with tachycardia, cardiac arrhythmias, hypertension, hypotension, prostatic hypertrophy or any tendency toward urinary retention, liver or kidney disorders, and obstructive disease of the GI or GU tract. May exacerbate mental symptoms when used to treat extrapyramidal reactions. When given in large doses or to susceptible patients, may cause weakness. Does not improve symptoms of tardive dyskinesias.

Adverse Reactions

Cardiovascular: Tachycardia

Central nervous system: Confusion, agitation, euphoria, drowsiness, headache, dizziness, nervousness, delusions, hallucinations, paranoia

Dermatologic: Dry skin, increased sensitivity to light, rash

Gastrointestinal: Constipation, xerostomia, dry throat, ileus, nausea, vomiting, parotitis

Genitourinary: Urinary retention

Neuromuscular & skeletal: Weakness

Ocular: Blurred vision, mydriasis, increase in intraocular pressure, glaucoma

Respiratory: Dry nose

Miscellaneous: Diaphoresis (decreased)

Overdosage/Toxicology

Signs and symptoms: Blurred vision, urinary retention, tachycardia; anticholinergic toxicity is caused by strong binding of the drug to cholinergic receptors; anticholinesterase inhibitors reduce acetylcholinesterase

Treatment: For anticholinergic overdose with severe life-threatening symptoms, physostigmine 1-2 mg (0.5 or 0.02 mg/kg for children) S.C. or I.V., slowly may be given to reverse these effects

Drug Interactions

Amantadine, rimantadine: Central and/or peripheral anticholinergic syndrome can occur when administered with amantadine or rimantadine

Anticholinergic agents: Central and/or peripheral anticholinergic syndrome can occur when administered with narcotic analgesics, phenothiazines and other antipsychotics (especially with high anticholinergic activity), tricyclic antidepressants, quinidine and some other antiarrhythmics, and antihistamines

Atenolol: Anticholinergics may increase the bioavailability of atenolol (and possibly other beta-blockers); monitor for increased effect

Cholinergic agents: Anticholinergics may antagonize the therapeutic effect of cholinergic agents: Includes tacrine and donepezil

Digoxin: Anticholinergics may decrease gastric degradation and increase the amount of digoxin absorbed by delaying gastric emptying

Levodopa: Anticholinergics may increase gastric degradation and decrease the amount of levodopa absorbed by delaying gastric emptying

Neuroleptics: Anticholinergics may antagonize the therapeutic effects of neuroleptics

Ethanol/Nutrition/Herb Interactions Ethanol: Avoid ethanol (may increase CNS depression).

Mechanism of Action Exerts a direct inhibitory effect on the parasympathetic nervous system. It also has a relaxing effect on smooth musculature; exerted both directly on the muscle itself and indirectly through parasympathetic nervous system (inhibitory effect)

(Continued)

Trihexyphenidyl *(Continued)*

Pharmacodynamics/Kinetics
Peak effect: Within 1 hour
Half-life: 3.3-4.1 hours
Time to peak serum concentration: Within 1-1.5 hours
Elimination: Primarily in urine

Usual Dosage Adults: Oral: Initial: 1-2 mg/day, increase by 2 mg increments at intervals of 3-5 days; usual dose: 5-15 mg/day in 3-4 divided doses

Monitoring Parameters IOP monitoring and gonioscopic evaluations should be performed periodically

Patient Information Take after meals or with food if GI upset occurs; do not discontinue drug abruptly; notify physician if adverse GI effects, rapid or pounding heartbeat, confusion, eye pain, rash, fever or heat intolerance occurs. Observe caution when performing hazardous tasks or those that require alertness such as driving, as may cause drowsiness. Avoid alcohol and other CNS depressants. May cause dry mouth - adequate fluid intake or hard sugar free candy may relieve. Difficult urination or constipation may occur - notify physician if effects persist; may increase susceptibility to heat stroke.

Nursing Implications Tolerated best if given in 3 daily doses and with food; high doses may be divided into 4 doses, at meal times and at bedtime

Additional Information Incidence and severity of side effects are dose related. Patients may be switched to sustained-action capsules when stabilized on conventional dosage forms.

Dosage Forms
Elixir, as hydrochloride: 2 mg/5 mL (480 mL)
Tablet, as hydrochloride: 2 mg, 5 mg

+ **Trihexyphenidyl Hydrochloride** *see Trihexyphenidyl on page 418*
+ **Trilafon®** *see Perphenazine on page 295*
+ **Trileptal®** *see Oxcarbazepine on page 278*

Trimethadione *(trye meth a DYE one)*

U.S. Brand Names Tridione®

Synonyms Troxidone

Pharmacologic Category Anticonvulsant, Oxazolidinedione

Generic Available No

Use Control absence (petit mal) seizures refractory to other drugs

Pregnancy Risk Factor D

Contraindications Hypersensitivity to trimethadione or any component of the formulation

Warnings/Precautions May cause severe blood dyscrasias; use with caution in patients with renal and hepatic impairment, SLE, myasthenia gravis, or intermittent porphyria; do not abruptly discontinue medication

Adverse Reactions
Central nervous system: Drowsiness, hiccups
Dermatologic: Alopecia, exfoliative dermatitis, rash
Endocrine & metabolic: Porphyria
Gastrointestinal: Anorexia, vomiting, stomach upset, abdominal pain, weight loss
Hematologic: Aplastic anemia, agranulocytosis, thrombocytopenia,
Hepatic: Hepatitis, jaundice
Neuromuscular & skeletal: Myasthenia gravis-like syndrome
Ocular: Diplopia, photophobia, hemeralopia, nystagmus, scotomata
Renal: Nephrosis, proteinuria
Miscellaneous: Lupus

Overdosage/Toxicology
Signs and symptoms: Nausea, drowsiness, ataxia, coma
Treatment: General supportive care is required; urine alkalinization can increase elimination of active metabolites

Drug Interactions

Acetylcholinesterase inhibitors: May reduce the antimyasthenic effects of these agents (limited documentation); monitor

CNS depressants: Sedative effects may be additive with other CNS depressants; monitor for increased effect; includes ethanol, sedatives, antidepressants, narcotic analgesics, other anticonvulsants, and benzodiazepines

Mechanism of Action An oxazolidinedione with anticonvulsant sedative properties; elevates the cortical and basal seizure thresholds, and reduces the synaptic response to low frequency impulses

Pharmacodynamics/Kinetics

Metabolism: Metabolized in the liver by microsomal enzymes to dimethadione (active)

Half-life:

Parent drug: 12-24 hours

Dimethadione: 6-13 days

Time to peak serum concentration: Within 30-120 minutes

Elimination: In the urine (3% as unchanged drug)

Usual Dosage Oral:

Children: Seizure disorders: Initial: 25-50 mg/kg/24 hours in 3-4 equally divided doses every 6-8 hours

Adults: Seizure disorders: Initial: 900 mg/day in 3-4 equally divided doses, increase by 300 mg/day at weekly intervals until therapeutic results or toxic symptoms appear

Dosing interval in renal impairment:

Cl_{cr} 10-50 mL/minute: Administer every 8-12 hours

Cl_{cr} <10 mL/minute: Administer every 12-24 hours

Patient Information Blood test monitoring must be performed periodically, notify physician of persistent or severe fatigue, sore throat, fever, rash, unusual bleeding or bruising; may take with food, may cause drowsiness, impair judgment and coordination, and blurred vision; visual disturbances are normally controlled by reduction of dose

Nursing Implications Caution patient that even minor skin rash and signs of infection or bleeding must be reported to the physician

Dosage Forms

Capsule: 300 mg

Solution: 40 mg/mL (473 mL)

Tablet, chewable: 150 mg

Trimipramine (trye MI pra meen)

Related Information

Antidepressant Agents Comparison Chart *on page 553*

Discontinuation of Psychotropic Drugs - Withdrawal Symptoms and Recommendations *on page 582*

Federal OBRA Regulations Recommended Maximum Doses *on page 583*

Patient Information - Antidepressants (TCAs) *on page 454*

Teratogenic Risks of Psychotropic Medications *on page 594*

U.S. Brand Names Surmontil®

Canadian Brand Names Apo®-Trimip; Novo-Tripramine®; Nu-Trimipramine®; Rhotrimine®

Synonyms Trimipramine Maleate

Pharmacologic Category Antidepressant, Tricyclic (Tertiary Amine)

Generic Available No

Use Treatment of depression

Pregnancy Risk Factor C

Contraindications Hypersensitivity to trimipramine, any component of the formulation, or other dibenzodiazepines; use of MAO inhibitors within 14 days; use in a patient during the acute recovery phase of MI

Warnings/Precautions Often causes sedation, resulting in impaired performance of tasks requiring alertness (ie, operating machinery or driving). Sedative effects (Continued)

Trimipramine *(Continued)*

may be additive with other CNS depressants and/or ethanol. The degree of sedation is very high relative to other antidepressants. May worsen psychosis in some patients or precipitate a shift to mania or hypomania in patients with bipolar disease. May increase the risks associated with electroconvulsive therapy. This agent should be discontinued, when possible, prior to elective surgery. Therapy should not be abruptly discontinued in patients receiving high doses for prolonged periods. Use with caution in patients with hepatic or renal dysfunction and in elderly patients.

May cause orthostatic hypotension (risk is high relative to other antidepressants) - use with caution in patients at risk of hypotension or in patients where transient hypotensive episodes would be poorly tolerated (cardiovascular disease or cerebrovascular disease). The degree of anticholinergic blockade produced by this agent is very high relative to other cyclic antidepressants - use caution in patients with urinary retention, benign prostatic hypertrophy, narrow-angle glaucoma, xerostomia, visual problems, constipation, or history of bowel obstruction. May cause alteration in glucose regulation - use with caution in patients with diabetes.

Use caution in patients with depression, particularly if suicidal risk may be present. Use with caution in patients with a history of cardiovascular disease (including previous MI, stroke, tachycardia, or conduction abnormalities). The risk conduction abnormalities with this agent is high relative to other antidepressants. Use caution in patients with a previous seizure disorder or condition predisposing to seizures such as brain damage, alcoholism, or concurrent therapy with other drugs which lower the seizure threshold. Use with caution in hyperthyroid patients or those receiving thyroid supplementation.

Adverse Reactions

Cardiovascular: Arrhythmias, hypotension, hypertension, tachycardia, palpitations, heart block, stroke, myocardial infarction

Central nervous system: Headache, exacerbation of psychosis, confusion, delirium, hallucinations, nervousness, restlessness, delusions, agitation, insomnia, nightmares, anxiety, seizures

Dermatologic: Photosensitivity, rash, petechiae, itching

Endocrine & metabolic: Sexual dysfunction, breast enlargement, galactorrhea, SIADH

Gastrointestinal: Xerostomia, constipation, increased appetite, nausea, unpleasant taste, weight gain, diarrhea, heartburn, vomiting, anorexia, trouble with gums, decreased lower esophageal sphincter tone may cause GE reflux

Genitourinary: Difficult urination, urinary retention, testicular edema

Hematologic: Agranulocytosis, eosinophilia, purpura, thrombocytopenia

Hepatic: Cholestatic jaundice, increased liver enzymes

Neuromuscular & skeletal: Tremors, numbness, tingling, paresthesia, incoordination, ataxia, peripheral neuropathy, extrapyramidal symptoms

Ocular: Blurred vision, eye pain, disturbances in accommodation, mydriasis, increased intraocular pressure

Otic: Tinnitus

Miscellaneous: Allergic reactions

Overdosage/Toxicology

Signs and symptoms: Agitation, confusion, hallucinations, urinary retention, hypothermia, hypotension, tachycardia, cardiac arrhythmias

Treatment:

Following initiation of essential overdose management, toxic symptoms should be treated

Ventricular arrhythmias often respond to systemic alkalinization (sodium bicarbonate 0.5-2 mEq/kg I.V.). Arrhythmias unresponsive to this therapy may respond to lidocaine 1 mg/kg I.V. followed by a titrated infusion. Physostigmine (1-2 mg I.V. slowly for adults or 0.5 mg I.V. slowly for children) may be indicated in reversing cardiac arrhythmias that are life-threatening.

Seizures usually respond to diazepam I.V. boluses (5-10 mg for adults up to 30 mg or 0.25-0.4 mg/kg/dose for children up to 10 mg/dose). If seizures are unresponsive or recur, phenytoin or phenobarbital may be required.

Drug Interactions CYP2D6 enzyme substrate

Altretamine: Concurrent use may cause orthostatic hypertension

Amphetamines: TCAs may enhance the effect of amphetamines; monitor for adverse CV effects

Anticholinergics: Combined use with TCAs may produce additive anticholinergic effects

Antihypertensives: TCAs may inhibit the antihypertensive response to bethanidine, clonidine, debrisoquin, guanadrel, guanethidine, guanabenz, guanfacine; monitor BP; consider alternate antihypertensive agent

Beta-agonists: When combined with TCAs may predispose patients to cardiac arrhythmias

Bupropion: May increase the levels of tricyclic antidepressants; based on limited information; monitor response

Carbamazepine: Tricyclic antidepressants may increase carbamazepine levels; monitor

Cholestyramine and colestipol: May bind TCAs and reduce their absorption; monitor for altered response

Clonidine: Abrupt discontinuation of clonidine may cause hypertensive crisis, amitriptyline may enhance the response (also see note on antihypertensives)

CNS depressants: Sedative effects may be additive with TCAs; monitor for increased effect; includes benzodiazepines, barbiturates, antipsychotics, ethanol, and other sedative medications

CYP2D6 inhibitors: Serum levels and/or toxicity of some tricyclic antidepressants may be increased; inhibitors include amiodarone, cimetidine, delavirdine, fluoxetine, paroxetine, propafenone, quinidine, and ritonavir; monitor for increased effect/toxicity

Enzyme inducers: May increase the metabolism of TCAs resulting in decreased effect; includes carbamazepine, phenobarbital, phenytoin, and rifampin; monitor for decreased response

Epinephrine (and other direct alpha-agonists): Pressor response to I.V. epinephrine, norepinephrine, and phenylephrine may be enhanced in patients receiving TCAs (**Note:** Effect is unlikely with epinephrine or levonordefrin dosages typically administered as infiltration in combination with local anesthetics).

Fenfluramine: May increase tricyclic antidepressant levels/effects

Hypoglycemic agents (including insulin): TCAs may enhance the hypoglycemic effects of tolazamide, chlorpropamide, or insulin; monitor for changes in blood glucose levels; reported with chlorpropamide, tolazamide, and insulin

Levodopa: Tricyclic antidepressants may decrease the absorption (bioavailability) of levodopa; rare hypertensive episodes have also been attributed to this combination

Linezolid: Hyperpyrexia, hypertension, tachycardia, confusion, seizures, and **deaths have been reported** with agents which inhibit MAO (serotonin syndrome); this combination should be avoided

Lithium: Concurrent use with a TCA may increase the risk for neurotoxicity

MAO Inhibitors: Hyperpyrexia, hypertension, tachycardia, confusion, seizures, and **deaths have been reported** (serotonin syndrome); this combination should be avoided

Methylphenidate: Metabolism of TCAs may be decreased

Phenothiazines: Serum concentrations of some TCAs may be increased; in addition, TCAs may increase concentration of phenothiazines; monitor for altered clinical response

QT_c-prolonging agents: Concurrent use of tricyclic agents with other drugs which may prolong QT_c interval may increase the risk of potentially fatal arrhythmias; includes type Ia and type III antiarrhythmics agents, selected quinolones (sparfloxacin, gatifloxacin, moxifloxacin, grepafloxacin), cisapride, and other agents

Sucralfate: Absorption of tricyclic antidepressants may be reduced with coadministration

(Continued)

Trimipramine *(Continued)*

Sympathomimetics, indirect-acting: Tricyclic antidepressants may result in a decreased sensitivity to indirect-acting sympathomimetics; includes dopamine and ephedrine; also see interaction with epinephrine (and direct-acting sympathomimetics)

Valproic acid: May increase serum concentrations/adverse effects of some tricyclic antidepressants

Warfarin (and other oral anticoagulants): TCAs may increase the anticoagulant effect in patients stabilized on warfarin; monitor INR

Ethanol/Nutrition/Herb Interactions

Ethanol: Avoid ethanol (may increase CNS depression).

Food: Grapefruit juice may inhibit the metabolism of some TCAs and clinical toxicity may result.

Herb/Nutraceutical: Avoid valerian, St John's wort, SAMe, kava kava (may increase risk of serotonin syndrome and/or excessive sedation).

Stability Solutions stable at a pH of 4-5; turns yellowish or reddish on exposure to light. Slight discoloration does not affect potency; marked discoloration is associated with loss of potency. Capsules stable for 3 years following date of manufacture.

Mechanism of Action Increases the synaptic concentration of serotonin and/or norepinephrine in the central nervous system by inhibition of their reuptake by the presynaptic neuronal membrane

Pharmacodynamics/Kinetics

Therapeutic plasma levels: Oral: Occurs within 6 hours

Protein binding: 95%

Metabolism: Undergoes significant first-pass metabolism; metabolized in the liver

Half-life: 20-26 hours

Elimination: In urine

Usual Dosage Oral:

Adults: 50-150 mg/day as a single bedtime dose up to a maximum of 200 mg/day outpatient and 300 mg/day inpatient

Elderly: Adequate studies have not been done in the elderly. In general, dosing should be cautious, starting at the lower end of dosing range.

Monitoring Parameters Blood pressure and pulse rate prior to and during initial therapy; evaluate mental status; monitor weight; EKG in older adults

Test Interactions ↑ glucose

Patient Information Avoid unnecessary exposure to sunlight; avoid alcohol ingestion; do not discontinue medication abruptly; may cause urine to turn blue-green; may cause drowsiness; can use sugarless gum or hard candy for dry mouth; full effect may not occur for 4-6 weeks

Nursing Implications May increase appetite; may cause drowsiness, raise bed rails, institute safety precautions

Additional Information May cause alterations in bleeding time.

Dosage Forms Capsule, as maleate: 25 mg, 50 mg, 100 mg

♦ **Unithroid**™ *see Levothyroxine on page 198*

Valerian
Synonyms Radix; Red Valerian; *Valeriana edulis*; *Valeriana wallichi*
Pharmacologic Category Herb
Use Herbal medicine use as a sleep-promoting agent and minor tranquilizer (similar to benzodiazepines); used in anxiety, panic attacks, intestinal cramps, headaches
Per Commission E: Restlessness, sleep disorders based on nervous conditions
Adverse Reactions
Cardiovascular: Cardiac disturbances (unspecified)
Central nervous system: Lightheadedness, restlessness, fatigue
Gastrointestinal: Nausea
Neuromuscular & skeletal: Tremor
Ocular: Blurred vision
Overdosage/Toxicology
Signs and symptoms: Headache, blurred vision, fine tremor, fatigue, mydriasis, abdominal cramping; intravenous exposure can cause hypotension, lethargy, hypophosphatemia, hypocalcemia, hypokalemia, and piloerection. Contact with the plant can cause contact dermatitis. Hepatotoxicity (probably due to an idiosyncratic hypersensitivity) has been noted.
Decontamination: Lavage (within 1 hour)/activated charcoal with cathartic
Treatment: Supportive therapy; hypotension can be treated with I.V. crystalloid therapy
Drug Interactions CNS depressants: Potentiation of effect by valerian is possible; no effect noted in some studies with ethanol
Usual Dosage Adults:
Sedative: 1-3 g (1-3 mL of tincture)
Sleep aid: 1-3 mL of tincture at bedtime
Dried root: 0.3-1 g
Additional Information *Valeriana officinalis* is a perennial plant that can reach 5 feet in height with tiny white or pink flowers. It is found in Europe, Canada, and Northern U.S. Preparations may contain multiple components.

♦ ***Valeriana edulis*** *see Valerian on page 425*
♦ ***Valeriana wallichi*** *see Valerian on page 425*
♦ **Valium**® *see Diazepam on page 110*
♦ **Valproate Semisodium** *see Valproic Acid and Derivatives on page 425*
♦ **Valproate Sodium** *see Valproic Acid and Derivatives on page 425*
♦ **Valproic Acid** *see Valproic Acid and Derivatives on page 425*

Valproic Acid and Derivatives
(val PROE ik AS id & dah RIV ah tives)
Related Information
Clozapine-Induced Side Effects *on page 568*
Liquid Compatibility With Antipsychotics and Mood Stabilizers *on page 587*
Mood Stabilizers *on page 588*
Patient Information - Mood Stabilizers (Valproic Acid) *on page 473*
U.S. Brand Names Depacon™; Depakene®; Depakote® Delayed Release; Depakote® ER; Depakote® Sprinkle®
Canadian Brand Names Epival®
Synonyms Dipropylacetic Acid; Divalproex Sodium; DPA; 2-Propylpentanoic Acid; 2-Propylvaleric Acid; Valproate Semisodium; Valproate Sodium; Valproic Acid
Pharmacologic Category Anticonvulsant, Miscellaneous
Generic Available Yes
Use
Mania associated with bipolar disorder (Depakote®)
Migraine prophylaxis (Depakote®, Depakote® ER)
(Continued)

Valproic Acid and Derivatives *(Continued)*

Monotherapy and adjunctive therapy in the treatment of patients with complex partial seizures that occur either in isolation or in association with other types of seizures (Depacon™, Depakote®)

Sole and adjunctive therapy of simple and complex absence seizures (Depacon™, Depakene®, Depakote®)

Adjunctively in patients with multiple seizure types that include absence seizures (Depacon™, Depakene®)

Unlabeled/Investigational Use Behavior disorders in Alzheimer's disease

Pregnancy Risk Factor D

Pregnancy/Breast-Feeding Implications

Clinical effects on the fetus: Crosses the placenta. Neural tube, cardiac, facial (characteristic pattern of dysmorphic facial features), skeletal, multiple other defects reported. Epilepsy itself, number of medications, genetic factors, or a combination of these probably influence the teratogenicity of anticonvulsant therapy. Risk of neural tube defects with use during first 30 days of pregnancy warrants discontinuation prior to pregnancy and through this period of possible.

Breast-feeding/lactation: Crosses into breast milk. AAP considers **compatible** with breast-feeding.

Contraindications Hypersensitivity to valproic acid, derivatives, or any component of the formulation; hepatic dysfunction; pregnancy

Warnings/Precautions Hepatic failure resulting in fatalities has occurred in patients; children <2 years of age are at considerable risk; other risk factors include organic brain disease, mental retardation with severe seizure disorders, congenital metabolic disorders, and patients on multiple anticonvulsants. Hepatotoxicity has been reported after 3 days to 6 months of therapy. Monitor patients closely for appearance of malaise, weakness, facial edema, anorexia, jaundice, and vomiting; may cause severe thrombocytopenia, inhibition of platelet aggregation and bleeding; tremors may indicate overdosage; use with caution in patients receiving other anticonvulsants.

Cases of life-threatening pancreatitis, occurring at the start of therapy or following years of use, have been reported in adults and children. Some cases have been hemorrhagic with rapid progression of initial symptoms to death.

In vitro studies have suggested valproate stimulates the replication of HIV and CMV viruses under experimental conditions. The clinical consequence of this is unknown, but should be considered when monitoring affected patients.

Anticonvulsants should not be discontinued abruptly because of the possibility of increasing seizure frequency; valproate should be withdrawn gradually to minimize the potential of increased seizure frequency, unless safety concerns require a more rapid withdrawal. Concomitant use with clonazepam may induce absence status.

Hyperammonemia may occur, even in the absence of overt liver function abnormalities. Asymptomatic elevations require continued surveillance; symptomatic elevations should prompt modification or discontinuation of valproate therapy. CNS depression may occur with valproate use. Patients must be cautioned about performing tasks which require mental alertness (operating machinery or driving). Effects with other sedative drugs or ethanol may be potentiated.

Adverse Reactions

Adverse reactions reported when used as monotherapy for complex partial seizures:

>10%:

Central nervous system: Somnolence (18% to 30%), dizziness (13% to 18%), insomnia (9% to 15%), nervousness (7% to 11%)

Dermatologic: Alopecia (13% to 24%)

Gastrointestinal: Nausea (26% to 34%), diarrhea (19% to 23%), vomiting (15% to 23%), abdominal pain (9% to 12%), dyspepsia (10% to 11%), anorexia (4% to 11%)

Hematologic: Thrombocytopenia (1% to 24%)

Neuromuscular & skeletal: Tremor (19% to 57%), weakness (10% to 21%)

Respiratory: Respiratory tract infection (13% to 20%), pharyngitis (2% to 8%), dyspnea (1% to 5%)

1% to 10%

Cardiovascular: Hypertension, palpitation, peripheral edema (3% to 8%), tachycardia, chest pain

Central nervous system: Amnesia (4% to 7%), abnormal dreams, anxiety, confusion, depression (4% to 5%), malaise, personality disorder

Dermatologic: Bruising (4% to 5%), dry skin, petechia, pruritus, rash

Endocrine & metabolic: Amenorrhea, dysmenorrhea

Gastrointestinal: Eructation, flatulence, hematemesis, increased appetite, pancreatitis, periodontal abscess, taste perversion, weight gain (4% to 9%)

Genitourinary: Urinary frequency, urinary incontinence, vaginitis

Hepatic: Increased AST and ALT

Neuromuscular & skeletal: Abnormal gait, arthralgia, back pain, hypertonia, incoordination, leg cramps, myalgia, myasthenia, paresthesia, twitching

Ocular: Amblyopia/blurred vision (4% to 8%), abnormal vision, nystagmus (1% to 7%)

Otic: Deafness, otitis media, tinnitus (1% to 7%)

Respiratory: Epistaxis, increased cough, pneumonia, sinusitis

Additional adverse effects:

Cardiovascular: Bradycardia

Central nervous system: Aggression, ataxia, behavioral deterioration, cerebral atrophy (reversible), dementia, emotional upset, encephalopathy (rare), fever, hallucinations, headache, hostility, hyperactivity, hypesthesia, incoordination, Parkinsonism, psychosis, vertigo

Dermatologic: Cutaneous vasculitis, erythema multiforme, photosensitivity, Stevens-Johnson syndrome, toxic epidermal necrolysis (rare)

Endocrine & metabolic: Breast enlargement, galactorrhea, hyperammonemia, hyponatremia, inappropriate ADH secretion, irregular menses, parotid gland swelling, polycystic ovary disease (rare), abnormal thyroid function tests

Genitourinary: Enuresis, urinary tract infection

Hematologic: Anemia, aplastic anemia, bone marrow suppression, eosinophilia, hematoma formation, hemorrhage, hypofibrinogenemia, intermittent porphyria, leukopenia, lymphocytosis, macrocytosis, pancytopenia

Hepatic: Increased bilirubin

Neuromuscular & skeletal: Asterixis, bone pain, dysarthria

Ocular: Diplopia, "spots before the eyes"

Renal: Fanconi-like syndrome (rare, in children)

Miscellaneous: Anaphylaxis, decreased carnitine, hyperglycinemia, lupus

Case reports: Life-threatening pancreatitis (2 cases out of 2416 patients), occurring at the start of therapy or following years of use, has been reported in adults and children. Some cases have been hemorrhagic with rapid progression of initial symptoms to death. Cases have also been reported upon rechallenge.

Overdosage/Toxicology

Signs and symptoms: Coma, deep sleep, motor restlessness, visual hallucinations

Treatment: Supportive treatment is necessary; naloxone has been used to reverse CNS depressant effects, but may block action of other anticonvulsants

In an overdose situation, the fraction of unbound valproate is high and hemodialysis or tandem hemodialysis plus hemoperfusion may lead to significant removal of the drug.

Drug Interactions CYP2C19 enzyme substrate; CYP2C9 and 2D6 enzyme inhibitor; CYP3A3/4 enzyme inhibitor (weak)

Acyclovir: Serum levels of valproate may be reduced; monitor

Carbamazepine: Valproic acid may increase, decrease, or have no effect on carbamazepine levels; valproic acid may increase serum concentrations of carbamazepine - epoxide (active metabolite); carbamazepine may induce the metabolism of carbamazepine; monitor

(Continued)

Valproic Acid and Derivatives *(Continued)*

Cholestyramine: Cholestyramine (and possibly colestipol) may bind valproic acid in GI tract; monitor

Clonazepam: Absence seizures have been reported in patients receiving valproic acid and clonazepam

Clozapine: Valproic acid may displace clozapine from protein-binding site resulting in decreased clozapine serum concentrations

CYP2C18/19 inhibitors: May increase serum concentrations of valproic acid; inhibitors include cimetidine, felbamate, fluoxetine, fluvoxamine, monitor

Diazepam: Valproic acid may increase serum concentrations; monitor

Enzyme inducers: Carbamazepine, lamotrigine, and phenytoin may induce the metabolism of valproic acid; monitor

Isoniazid: May decrease valproic acid metabolism (limited documentation)

Lamotrigine: Valproic acid inhibits the metabolism of lamotrigine; combination therapy has been proposed to increase the risk of toxic epidermal necrolysis; monitor

Macrolide antibiotics: May decrease valproic acid metabolism (limited documentation); includes clarithromycin, erythromycin, troleandomycin; monitor

Nimodipine: Valproic acid appears to inhibit the metabolism of nimodipine; monitor for increased effect

Phenobarbital: Valproic acid appears to inhibit the metabolism of phenobarbital; monitor for increased effect

Phenothiazines: Chlorpromazine may increase valproic acid concentrations. Other phenothiazines may share this effect; monitor

Phenytoin: Valproic acid may increase, decrease, or have no effect on phenytoin levels

Risperidone: A case report of generalized edema occurred during combination therapy

Salicylates: May displace valproic acid from plasma proteins, leading to acute toxicity

Tricyclic antidepressants: Valproate may increase serum concentrations and/or toxicity of tricyclic antidepressants

Ethanol/Nutrition/Herb Interactions

Ethanol: Avoid ethanol (may increase CNS depression).

Food: Food may delay but does not affect the extent of absorption. Valproic acid serum concentrations may be decreased if taken with food. Milk has no effect on absorption.

Herb/Nutraceutical: Avoid evening primrose (seizure threshold decreased)

Stability Injection is physically compatible and chemically stable in D_5W, NS, and LR for at least 24 hours when stored in glass or PVC; store vials at room temperature 15°C to 30°C (59°F to 86°F)

Mechanism of Action Causes increased availability of gamma-aminobutyric acid (GABA), an inhibitory neurotransmitter, to brain neurons or may enhance the action of GABA or mimic its action at postsynaptic receptor sites

Pharmacodynamics/Kinetics

Distribution: Total valproate: 11 L/1.73 m²; free valproate 92 L/1.73 m²

Protein binding: 80% to 90% (dose dependent)

Metabolism: Extensively in the liver; glucuronide conjugation and mitochondrial beta-oxidation

Bioavailability: Extended release: 90% of I.V. dose, 81% to 90% of delayed release dose

Half-life (increased in neonates and patients with liver disease): Children: 4-14 hours; Adults: 8-17 hours

Time to peak serum concentration: Within 1-4 hours; 3-5 hours after divalproex (enteric coated)

Elimination: Urine (30% to 50% as glucuronide conjugate, 3% unchanged)

Usual Dosage

Seizures:

Children >10 years and Adults:

Oral: Initial: 10-15 mg/kg/day in 1-3 divided doses; increase by 5-10 mg/kg/day at weekly intervals until therapeutic levels are achieved; maintenance: 30-60 mg/kg/day in 2-3 divided doses. Adult usual dose: 1000-2500 mg/day

Children receiving more than one anticonvulsant (ie, polytherapy) may require doses up to 100 mg/kg/day in 3-4 divided doses

I.V.: Administer as a 60-minute infusion (≤20 mg/minute) with the same frequency as oral products; switch patient to oral products as soon as possible

Rectal: Dilute syrup 1:1 with water for use as a retention enema; loading dose: 17-20 mg/kg one time; maintenance: 10-15 mg/kg/dose every 8 hours

Mania: Adults: Oral: 750 mg/day in divided doses; dose should be adjusted as rapidly as possible to desired clinical effect; a loading dose of 20 mg/kg may be used; maximum recommended dosage: 60 mg/kg/day

Migraine prophylaxis: Adults: Oral:

Extended release tablets: 500 mg once daily for 7 days, then increase to 1000 mg once daily; adjust dose based on patient response; usual dosage range 500-1000 mg/day

Delayed release tablets: 250 mg twice daily; adjust dose based on patient response, up to 1000 mg/day

Elderly: Elimination is decreased in the elderly. Studies of elderly patients with dementia show a high incidence of somnolence. In some patients, this was associated with weight loss. Starting doses should be lower and increases should be slow, with careful monitoring of nutritional intake and dehydration. Safety and efficacy for use in patients >65 years have not been studied for migraine prophylaxis.

Dosing adjustment in renal impairment: A 27% reduction in clearance of unbound valproate is seen in patients with Cl_{cr} <10 mL/minute. Hemodialysis reduces valproate concentrations by 20%, therefore no dose adjustment is needed in patients with renal failure. Protein binding is reduced, monitoring only total valproate concentrations may be misleading.

Dosing adjustment/comments in hepatic impairment: Reduce dose. Clearance is decreased with liver impairment. Hepatic disease is also associated with increased albumin concentrations and 2- to 2.6-fold increase in the unbound fraction. Free concentrations of valproate may be elevated while total concentrations appear normal.

Dietary Considerations Valproic acid may cause GI upset; take with large amount of water or food to decrease GI upset. May need to split doses to avoid GI upset.

Coated particles of divalproex sodium may be mixed with semisolid food (eg, applesauce or pudding) in patients having difficulty swallowing; particles should be swallowed and not chewed

Valproate sodium oral solution will generate valproic acid in carbonated beverages and may cause mouth and throat irritation; do not mix valproate sodium oral solution with carbonated beverages

Administration Depakote® ER: Swallow whole, do not crush or chew. Patients who need dose adjustments smaller than 500 mg/day for migraine prophylaxis should be changed to Depakote® delayed release tablets. Sprinkle capsules may be swallowed whole or open cap and sprinkle on small amount (1 teaspoonful) of soft food and use immediately (do not store or chew).

Monitoring Parameters Liver enzymes, CBC with platelets

Reference Range

Therapeutic: 50-100 µg/mL (SI: 350-690 µmol/L)

Toxic: >200 µg/mL (SI: >1390 µmol/L)

Seizure control: May improve at levels >100 µg/mL (SI: 690 µmol/L), but toxicity may occur at levels of 100-150 µg/mL (SI: 690-1040 µmol/L)

(Continued)

Valproic Acid and Derivatives *(Continued)*

Mania: Clinical response seen with trough levels between 50-125 μg/mL; risk of toxicity increases at levels >125 μg/mL

Test Interactions False-positive result for urine ketones

Patient Information When used to treat generalized seizures, patient instructions are determined by patient's condition and ability to understand.

Oral: Take as directed; do not alter dose or timing of medication. Do not increase dose or take more than recommended. Do not crush or chew capsule or enteric-coated pill. While using this medication, do not use alcohol and other prescription or OTC medications (especially pain medications, sedatives, antihistamines, or hypnotics) without consulting prescriber. Maintain adequate hydration (2-3 L/day of fluids unless instructed to restrict fluid intake). Diabetics should monitor serum glucose closely (valproic acid will alter results of urine ketones). Report alterations in menstrual cycle; abdominal cramps, unresolved diarrhea, vomiting, or constipation; skin rash; unusual bruising or bleeding; blood in urine, stool or vomitus; malaise; weakness; facial swelling; yellowing of skin or eyes; excessive sedation; or restlessness.

Do not get pregnant while taking this medication; use appropriate contraceptive measures

Nursing Implications Do not crush enteric coated drug product or capsule; do not crush or chew gelatin capsules or tablet formulations

Additional Information

Sodium content of valproate sodium syrup (5 mL): 23 mg (1 mEq)

Extended release tablets have 10% to 20% less fluctuation in serum concentration than delayed release tablets. Extended release tablets are not bioequivalent to delayed release tablets.

Dosage Forms

Capsule, as valproic acid (Depakene®): 250 mg

Capsule, sprinkles, as divalproex sodium (Depakote® Sprinkle®): 125 mg

Injection, as sodium valproate (Depacon™): 100 mg/mL (5 mL)

Syrup, as sodium valproate (Depakene®): 250 mg/5 mL (5 mL, 50 mL, 480 mL)

Tablet, delayed release, as divalproex sodium (Depakote®): 125 mg, 250 mg, 500 mg

Tablet, extended release, as divalproex sodium (Depakote® ER): 500 mg

♦ **Vanatrip®** *see Amitriptyline on page 22*

Venlafaxine *(VEN la faks een)*

Related Information

Antidepressant Agents Comparison Chart *on page 553*

Patient Information - Antidepressants (Venlafaxine) *on page 458*

U.S. Brand Names Effexor®; Effexor® XR

Canadian Brand Names Effexor

Pharmacologic Category Antidepressant, Serotonin/Norepinephrine Reuptake Inhibitor

Generic Available No

Use Treatment of depression, generalized anxiety disorder (GAD)

Unlabeled/Investigational Use Obsessive-compulsive disorder (OCD), chronic fatigue syndrome; attention-deficit/hyperactivity disorder (ADHD) and autism in children

Pregnancy Risk Factor C

Pregnancy/Breast-Feeding Implications There are no adequate or well-controlled studies in pregnant women. Use only in pregnancy if clearly needed. Venlafaxine is excreted in human milk; breast-feeding is not recommended.

Contraindications Hypersensitivity to venlafaxine or any component of the formulation; use of MAO inhibitors within 14 days; should not initiate MAO inhibitor within 7 days of discontinuing venlafaxine

Warnings/Precautions May cause sustained increase in blood pressure; may cause increase in anxiety, nervousness, insomnia; may cause weight loss (use with caution in patients where weight loss is undesirable). May worsen psychosis in some patients or precipitate a shift to mania or hypomania in patients with bipolar disease. May increase the risks associated with electroconvulsive therapy. Use caution in patients with depression, particularly if suicidal risk may be present. The risks of cognitive or motor impairment, as well as the potential for anticholinergic effects are very low. May cause or exacerbate sexual dysfunction. Abrupt discontinuation or dosage reduction after extended (>6 weeks) therapy may lead to agitation, dysphoria, nervousness, anxiety, and other symptoms. When discontinuing therapy, dosage should be tapered gradually over at least a 2-week period. Use caution in patients with increased intraocular pressure or at risk of acute narrow-angle glaucoma.

Adverse Reactions

≥10%:

Central nervous system: Headache (25%), somnolence (23%), dizziness (19%), insomnia (18%), nervousness (13%)

Gastrointestinal: Nausea (37%), xerostomia (22%), constipation (15%), anorexia (11%)

Genitourinary: Abnormal ejaculation/orgasm (12%)

Neuromuscular & skeletal: Weakness (12%)

Miscellaneous: Diaphoresis (12%)

1% to 10%:

Cardiovascular: Vasodilation (4%), hypertension (dose-related; 3% in patients receiving <100 mg/day, up to 13% in patients receiving >300 mg/day), tachycardia (2%), chest pain (2%), postural hypotension (1%)

Central nervous system: Anxiety (6%), abnormal dreams (4%), yawning (3%), agitation (2%), confusion (2%), abnormal thinking (2%), depersonalization (1%), depression (1%)

Dermatologic: Rash (3%), pruritus (1%)

Endocrine & metabolic: Decreased libido

Gastrointestinal: Diarrhea (8%), vomiting (6%), dyspepsia (5%), flatulence (3%), taste perversion (2%), weight loss (1%)

Genitourinary: Impotence (6%), urinary frequency (3%), impaired urination (2%), orgasm disturbance (2%), urinary retention (1%)

Neuromuscular & skeletal: Tremor (5%), hypertonia (3%), twitching (1%)

Ocular: Blurred vision (6%), mydriasis (2%)

Otic: Tinnitus (2%)

Miscellaneous: Infection (6%), chills (3%), trauma (2%)

<1%, postmarketing reports and/or case reports: Abnormal vision, agranulocytosis, akathisia, anaphylaxis, aplastic anemia, asthma, bronchitis, catatonia, delirium, dyspnea, emotional lability, epidermal necrolysis, erythema multiforme, erythema nodosum, exfoliative dermatitis, extrapyramidal symptoms, hallucinations, hepatic necrosis, hirsutism, increased transaminases/GGT, manic reaction (0.5%), metrorrhagia, paresthesia, prostatitis, psychosis, rash (maculopapular, pustular, or vesiculobullous), seizure, Stevens-Johnson syndrome, tardive dyskinesia, torticollis, vaginitis, vertigo

Overdosage/Toxicology

Symptoms of overdose include somnolence and occasionally EKG changes (Q-T prolongation, QRS prolongation, bundle branch block), tachycardia, bradycardia, seizures, vertigo, (rare coma); deaths have been reported

Most overdoses resolve with only supportive treatment. Use of activated charcoal, inductions of emesis, or gastric lavage should be considered for acute ingestion; forced diuresis, dialysis, and hemoperfusion not effective due to large volume of distribution

Drug Interactions CYP2D6, 2E1, and 3A3/4 enzyme substrate; CYP2D6 enzyme inhibitor (weak)

Buspirone: Concurrent use may result in serotonin syndrome; these combinations are best avoided

(Continued)

Venlafaxine *(Continued)*

Clozapine: Addition of venlafaxine has been associated with case reports of increased clozapine serum concentrations and seizures.

CYP2D6 inhibitors: Serum levels and/or toxicity venlafaxine may be increased; inhibitors include amiodarone, cimetidine, delavirdine, fluoxetine, paroxetine, propafenone, quinidine, and ritonavir; monitor for increased effect/toxicity

CYP2E1 inhibitors: Serum levels and/or toxicity venlafaxine may be increased; inhibitors include disulfiram, metronidazole, and ritonavir

CYP3A3/4 inhibitors: Serum level and/or toxicity of venlafaxine may be increased; inhibitors include amiodarone, cimetidine, clarithromycin, erythromycin, delavirdine, diltiazem, dirithromycin, disulfiram, fluoxetine, fluvoxamine, grapefruit juice, indinavir, itraconazole, ketoconazole, metronidazole, nefazodone, nevirapine, propoxyphene, quinupristin-dalfopristin, ritonavir, saquinavir, verapamil, zafirlukast, zileuton; monitor for altered response

Enzyme inducers: May increase the metabolism of venlafaxine, reducing its effectiveness; inducers include phenytoin, carbamazepine, phenobarbital, and rifampin

Haloperidol: Serum levels may be increased during concurrent administration; AUC may be increased by as much as 70%

Indinavir: Serum levels may be reduced by venlafaxine (AUC reduced by 28%); clinical significance unknown

MAO inhibitors: Serotonin syndrome may result when venlafaxine is used in combination or within 2 weeks of an MAO inhibitor; these combinations should be avoided

Meperidine: Concurrent use may increase risk of serotonin syndrome

Methylphenidate: Neuroleptic malignant syndrome (NMS) has been reported in a patient receiving methylphenidate and venlafaxine

Mirtazapine: Concurrent use may increase risk of serotonin syndrome

Nefazodone: Concurrent use may increase risk of serotonin syndrome; in addition, nefazodone may inhibit the metabolism of venlafaxine

Selegiline: Concurrent use may predispose to serotonin syndrome

Serotonin agonists: Theoretically, may increase the risk of serotonin syndrome; includes sumatriptan, naratriptan, rizatriptan, and zolmitriptan

Sibutramine: Concurrent use may increase risk of serotonin syndrome

SSRIs: Concurrent use may increase risk of serotonin syndrome

Trazodone: Concurrent use may increase risk of serotonin syndrome

Tricyclic antidepressants: Concurrent use may increase risk of serotonin syndrome

Warfarin: Case reports of increased INR when venlafaxine was added to therapy.

Ethanol/Nutrition/Herb Interactions

Ethanol: Avoid ethanol (may increase CNS effects).

Herb/Nutraceutical: Avoid valerian, St John's wort, SAMe, kava kava (may increase risk of serotonin syndrome and/or excessive sedation).

Mechanism of Action Venlafaxine and its active metabolite o-desmethylvenlafaxine (ODV) are potent inhibitors of neuronal serotonin and norepinephrine reuptake and weak inhibitors of dopamine reuptake; causes beta-receptor down regulation and reduces adenylcyclase coupled beta-adrenergic systems in the brain

Pharmacodynamics/Kinetics

Absorption: Oral: 92% to 100%

Protein binding: Bound to human plasma 27% to 30%; steady-state achieved within 3 days of multiple dose therapy

Metabolism: In the liver by cytochrome P450 enzyme system to active metabolite, O-desmethyl-venlafaxine (ODV)

Half-life: 3-7 hours (venlafaxine) and 11-13 hours (ODV)

Time to peak: 1-2 hours

Elimination: Primarily by renal route

Usual Dosage Oral:

Children and Adolescents:

ADHD (unlabeled use): 60 mg or 1.4 mg/kg administered in 2-3 divided doses

Autism (unlabeled use): Initial: 12.5 mg/day; adjust to 6.25-50 mg/day

Adults:

Immediate-release tablets: 75 mg/day, administered in 2 or 3 divided doses, taken with food; dose may be increased in 75 mg/day increments at intervals of at least 4 days, up to 225-375 mg/day

Extended-release capsules: 75 mg once daily taken with food; for some new patients, it may be desirable to start at 37.5 mg/day for 4-7 days before increasing to 75 mg once daily; dose may be increased by up to 75 mg/day increments every 4 days as tolerated, up to a maximum of 225 mg/day

Note: When discontinuing this medication, it is imperative to taper the dose. If venlafaxine is used >6 weeks, the dose should be tapered over 2 weeks when discontinuing its use.

Dosing adjustment in renal impairment: Cl_{cr} 10-70 mL/minute: Decrease dose by 25%; decrease total daily dose by 50% if dialysis patients; dialysis patients should receive dosing after completion of dialysis

Dosing adjustment in moderate hepatic impairment: Reduce total daily dosage by 50%

Child/Adolescent Considerations Sixteen children and adolescents (mean age: 11.6 years) with attention-deficit/hyperactivity disorder (ADHD) received a mean daily dose of 60 mg (1.4 mg/kg) administered in 2-3 divided doses (Olvera, 1996). Thirty-three children 8-17 years of age with major depression participated in a 6-week trial (Mandoki, 1997). Ten children with autism spectrum disorder were initiated at 12.5 mg/day and adjusted on a flexible basis (mean: 24.4 mg/day; range 6.25-50 mg/day) (Hollander, 2000).

Dietary Considerations May be taken without regard to food.

Monitoring Parameters Blood pressure should be regularly monitored, especially in patients with a high baseline blood pressure

Reference Range Peak serum level of 163 ng/mL (325 ng/mL of ODV metabolite) obtained after a 150 mg oral dose

Test Interactions Elevations in thyroid, uric acid, glucose, potassium, AST, and cholesterol (S)

Patient Information Avoid use of alcohol; use caution when operating hazardous machinery

Nursing Implications Causes mean increase in heart rate of 4 beats/minute; tapering to minimize symptoms of discontinuation is recommended when the drug is discontinued; tapering should be over a 2-week period if the patient has received it longer than 6 weeks

Dosage Forms

Capsule, extended release: 37.5 mg, 75 mg, 150 mg

Tablet: 25 mg, 37.5 mg, 50 mg, 75 mg, 100 mg

Vitamin E (VYE ta min ee)

U.S. Brand Names Amino-Opti-E® [OTC]; Aquasol E® [OTC]; E-Complex-600® [OTC]; E-Vitamin® [OTC]; Vita-Plus® E Softgels® [OTC]; Vitec® [OTC]; Vite E® Creme [OTC]

Canadian Brand Names Aquasol E; Novo E; Nutrol E; Organex; Vita-E

Synonyms d-Alpha Tocopherol; dl-Alpha Tocopherol

Pharmacologic Category Vitamin, Fat Soluble

Generic Available Yes

Use Prevention and treatment hemolytic anemia secondary to vitamin E deficiency, dietary supplement

(Continued)

Vitamin E (Continued)

Unlabeled/Investigational Use To reduce the risk of bronchopulmonary dysplasia or retrolental fibroplasia in infants exposed to high concentrations of oxygen; prevention and treatment of tardive dyskinesia and Alzheimer's disease

Pregnancy Risk Factor A/C (dose exceeding RDA recommendation)

Contraindications Hypersensitivity to vitamin E or any component of the formulation; I.V. route

Warnings/Precautions May induce vitamin K deficiency; necrotizing enterocolitis has been associated with oral administration of large dosages (eg, >200 units/day) of a hyperosmolar vitamin E preparation in low birth weight infants

Adverse Reactions <1%: Blurred vision, contact dermatitis with topical preparation, diarrhea, fatigue, gonadal dysfunction, headache, intestinal cramps, nausea, weakness

Drug Interactions

Cholestyramine (and colestipol): May reduce absorption of vitamin E

Iron: Vitamin E may impair the hematologic response to iron in children with iron-deficiency anemia; monitor

Orlistat: May reduce absorption of vitamin E

Warfarin: Vitamin E may alter the effect of vitamin K actions on clotting factors resulting in an increase hypoprothrombinemic response to warfarin; monitor

Stability Protect from light

Mechanism of Action Prevents oxidation of vitamin A and C; protects polyunsaturated fatty acids in membranes from attack by free radicals and protects red blood cells against hemolysis

Pharmacodynamics/Kinetics

Absorption: Oral: Depends upon the presence of bile; absorption is reduced in conditions of malabsorption, in low birth weight premature infants, and as dosage increases; water miscible preparations are better absorbed than oil preparations

Distribution: Distributes to all body tissues, especially adipose tissue, where it is stored

Metabolism: In the liver to glucuronides

Elimination: In feces and bile

Usual Dosage One unit of vitamin E = 1 mg *dl*-alpha-tocopherol acetate. Oral:

Recommended daily allowance (RDA):

Premature infants ≤3 months: 17 mg (25 units)

Infants:

≤6 months: 3 mg (4.5 units)

7-12 months: 4 mg (6 units)

Children:

1-3 years: 6 mg (9 units); upper limit of intake should not exceed 200 mg/day

4-8 years: 7 mg (10.5 units); upper limit of intake should not exceed 300 mg/day

9-13 years: 11 mg (16.5 units); upper limit of intake should not exceed 600 mg/day

14-18 years: 15 mg (22.5 units); upper limit of intake should not exceed 800 mg/day

Adults: 15 mg (22.5 units); upper limit of intake should not exceed 1000 mg/day

Pregnant female:

≤18 years: 15 mg (22.5 units); upper level of intake should not exceed 800 mg/day

19-50 years: 15 mg (22.5 units); upper level of intake should not exceed 1000 mg/day

Lactating female:

≤18 years: 19 mg (28.5 units); upper level of intake should not exceed 800 mg/day

19-50 years: 19 mg (28.5 units); upper level of intake should not exceed 1000 mg/day

Vitamin E deficiency:
Children (with malabsorption syndrome): 1 unit/kg/day of water miscible vitamin E (to raise plasma tocopherol concentrations to the normal range within 2 months and to maintain normal plasma concentrations)
Adults: 60-75 units/day
Prevention of vitamin E deficiency: Adults: 30 units/day
Prevention of retinopathy of prematurity or BPD secondary to O_2 therapy (AAP considers this use investigational and routine use is not recommended):
Retinopathy prophylaxis: 15-30 units/kg/day to maintain plasma levels between 1.5-2 µg/mL (may need as high as 100 units/kg/day)
Cystic fibrosis, beta-thalassemia, sickle cell anemia may require higher daily maintenance doses:
Children:
Cystic fibrosis: 100-400 units/day
Beta-thalassemia: 750 units/day
Adults:
Sickle cell: 450 units/day
Alzheimer's disease: 1000 units twice daily
Tardive dyskinesia: 1600 units/day
Reference Range Therapeutic: 0.8-1.5 mg/dL (SI: 19-35 µmol/L), some method variation
Patient Information Drops can be placed directly in the mouth or mixed with cereal, fruit juice, or other food; take only the prescribed dose. Vitamin E toxicity appears as blurred vision, diarrhea, dizziness, flu-like symptoms, nausea, headache; swallow capsules whole, do not crush or chew
Nursing Implications Monitor plasma tocopherol concentrations (normal range: 6-14 mcg/mL)
Additional Information 1 mg dl-alpha tocopheryl acetate = 1 int. unit
Dosage Forms
Capsule: 100 units, 200 units, 400 units, 500 units, 600 units, 1000 units
Capsule, water miscible: 73.5 mg, 147 mg, 165 mg, 330 mg, 400 units
Cream: 50 mg/g (15 g, 30 g, 60 g, 75 g, 120 g, 454 g)
Liquid, oral [drops]: 50 mg/mL (12 mL, 30 mL)
Liquid, topical: 10 mL, 15 mL, 30 mL, 60 mL
Lotion: 120 mL
Oil: 15 mL, 30 mL, 60 mL
Ointment, topical: 30 mg/g (45 g, 60 g)
Tablet: 200 units, 400 units

Wormwood

Synonyms Absinthe; Artemisia absinthium; Green Ginger
Pharmacologic Category Herb
Use Homeopathic medicine, used as an anthelmintic, bitter tonic, hair tonic, sedative, flavoring agent (in vermouth)
Per Commission E: Loss of appetite, dyspepsia, biliary dyskinesia
(Continued)

Wormwood *(Continued)*

Adverse Reactions Vomiting, stomach cramps, intestinal cramps, dizziness, CNS disturbances, headache

Overdosage/Toxicology

Signs and symptoms: Headache, vertigo, thirst, vomiting, giddiness, paranoia, tremors, diarrhea, diaphoresis, color vision disturbance, psychosis, seizures (>15 g ingestion), visual hallucinations, euphoria, coma, respiratory depression, contact dermatitis (from flowers), dysphoria, delirium, mania, anorexia, memory impairment

Decontamination: Lavage (within 1 hour)/activated charcoal with cathartic

Treatment: Supportive therapy; seizures can be managed with a benzodiazepine or barbiturate; psychiatric abnormalities can be managed with a benzodiazepine or neuroleptic agent

Usual Dosage Tea: 2-3 g/day

Patient Information Considered unsafe; avoid long-term use

Additional Information Not popular in the U.S.; taste threshold (Absinthin): 1 part in 70,000: A shrub with small green-yellow flowers from July through September. Grows naturally in Europe but found in Northeastern and North Central U.S. Wormwood extract has been used in absinth, an emerald green bitter liquor banned in Europe and U.S. Absinth has been thought to cause Vincent van Gogh's psychosis. The tea uses dried leaves and flowering tops.

Per Commission E: In toxic doses, thujone, the active component of the oil, acts as a convulsant poison. Thus, essential oil must not be used except in combinations.

+ **Xanax®** see Alprazolam on page 16
+ **Xenical®** see Orlistat on page 274
+ **X-Prep® Liquid [OTC]** see Senna on page 373
+ **Yellow Indian Paint** see Golden Seal on page 169
+ **Yellow Root** see Golden Seal on page 169
+ **Yocon®** see Yohimbine on page 436

Yohimbine *(yo HIM bine)*

U.S. Brand Names Aphrodyne™; Dayto Himbin®; Yocon®; Yohimex™

Canadian Brand Names Yocon

Synonyms Yohimbine Hydrochloride

Pharmacologic Category Miscellaneous Product

Generic Available Yes

Unlabeled/Investigational Use Treatment of SSRI-induced sexual dysfunction; weight loss; impotence; sympatholytic and mydriatic; may have activity as an aphrodisiac

Contraindications Hypersensitivity to yohimbine or any component of the formulation; renal disease

Warnings/Precautions Do not use in pregnancy; do not use in children; not for use in geriatric, psychiatric, or cardio-renal patients with a history of gastric or duodenal ulcer; generally not for use in females. Should not be used in kidney disease or psychiatric disorders; can cause high blood pressure and anxiety, tachycardia, nausea, or vomiting.

Adverse Reactions

Cardiovascular: Tachycardia, hypertension, hypotension (orthostatic), flushing

Central nervous system: Anxiety, mania, hallucinations, irritability, dizziness, psychosis, insomnia, headache, panic attacks

Gastrointestinal: Nausea, vomiting, anorexia, salivation

Neuromuscular & skeletal: Tremors

Miscellaneous: Antidiuretic action, diaphoresis

Drug Interactions CYP2D6 and 3A3/4 enzyme substrate; CYP2D6 enzyme inhibitor

Antihypertensives: Effect of antihypertensives may be reduced by yohimbine

CNS active agents: Caution with other CNS acting drugs

CYP3A3/4 inhibitors: Serum level and/or toxicity of yohimbine may be increased; inhibitors include amiodarone, cimetidine, clarithromycin, erythromycin, delavirdine, diltiazem, dirithromycin, disulfiram, fluoxetine, fluvoxamine, grape-fruit juice, indinavir, itraconazole, ketoconazole, metronidazole, nefazodone, nevirapine, propoxyphene, quinupristin-dalfopristin, ritonavir, saquinavir, verapamil, zafirlukast, zileuton; monitor for altered response

Linezolid: Due to MAO inhibition (see note on MAO inhibitors), combinations with this agent should generally be avoided

MAO inhibitors: Theoretically may increase toxicity or adverse effects

Mechanism of Action Derived from the bark of the yohimbe tree (*Corynanthe yohimbe*), this indole alkaloid produces a presynaptic alpha$_2$-adrenergic blockade. Peripheral autonomic effect is to increase cholinergic and decrease adrenergic activity; yohimbine exerts a stimulating effect on the mood and a mild antidiuretic effect.

Pharmacodynamics/Kinetics

Duration of action: Usually 3-4 hours, but may last 36 hours

Absorption: Oral: 33%

Distribution: V_d: 0.3-3 L/kg

Half-life: 0.6 hours

Usual Dosage Adults: Oral:

Male erectile impotence: 5.4 mg tablet 3 times/day have been used. If side effects occur, reduce to $1/2$ tablet (2.7 mg) 3 times/day followed by gradual increases to 1 tablet 3 times/day. Results of therapy >10 weeks are not known.

Orthostatic hypotension: Doses of 12.5 mg/day have been utilized; however, more research is necessary

Patient Information Considered unsafe

Additional Information Also a street drug of abuse that can be smoked; has a bitter taste. Dissociative state may resemble phencyclidine intoxication.

Dosage Forms Tablet, as hydrochloride: 5.4 mg

♦ **Yohimbine Hydrochloride** *see* Yohimbine *on page 436*

♦ **Yohimex**™ *see* Yohimbine *on page 436*

Zaleplon (ZAL e plon)

Related Information

Anxiolytic/Hypnotic Use in Long-Term Care Facilities *on page 562*

Nonbenzodiazepine Anxiolytics and Hypnotics *on page 589*

Patient Information - Anxiolytics & Sedative Hypnotics (Nonbenzodiazepine Hypnotics) *on page 489*

U.S. Brand Names Sonata®

Pharmacologic Category Hypnotic, Nonbenzodiazepine

Generic Available No

Use Short-term (7-10 days) treatment of insomnia (has been demonstrated to be effective for up to 5 weeks in controlled trial)

Restrictions C-IV

Pregnancy Risk Factor C

Pregnancy/Breast-Feeding Implications Not recommended for use during pregnancy

Contraindications Hypersensitivity to zaleplon or any component of the formulation

Warnings/Precautions Symptomatic treatment of insomnia should be initiated only after careful evaluation of potential causes of sleep disturbance. Failure of sleep disturbance to resolve after 7-10 days may indicate psychiatric and/or medical illness.

Use with caution in patients with depression, particularly if suicidal risk may be present. Use with caution in patients with a history of drug dependence. Abrupt discontinuance may lead to withdrawal symptoms. May impair physical and mental capabilities. Patients must be cautioned about performing tasks which require (Continued)

Zaleplon *(Continued)*

mental alertness (operating machinery or driving). Use with caution in patients receiving other CNS depressants or psychoactive medications. Effects with other sedative drugs or ethanol may be potentiated.

Use with caution in the elderly, those with compromised respiratory function, or renal and hepatic impairment. Because of the rapid onset of action, zaleplon should be administered immediately prior to bedtime or after the patient has gone to bed and is having difficulty falling asleep.

Adverse Reactions

1% to 10%:

Cardiovascular: Peripheral edema, chest pain

Central nervous system: Amnesia, anxiety, depersonalization, dizziness, hallucinations, hypesthesia, somnolence, vertigo, malaise, depression, lightheadedness, impaired coordination, fever, migraine

Dermatologic: Photosensitivity reaction, rash, pruritus

Gastrointestinal: Abdominal pain, anorexia, colitis, dyspepsia, nausea, constipation, xerostomia

Genitourinary: Dysmenorrhea

Neuromuscular & skeletal: Paresthesia, tremor, myalgia, weakness, back pain, arthralgia

Ocular: Abnormal vision, eye pain

Otic: Hyperacusis

Miscellaneous: Parosmia

1% (Limited to important or life-threatening symptoms): Alopecia, angina, ataxia, bundle branch block, dysarthria, dystonia, eosinophilia, facial paralysis, glaucoma, intestinal obstruction, paresthesia, pericardial effusion, ptosis, pulmonary embolus, syncope, urinary retention, ventricular tachycardia

Overdosage/Toxicology Symptoms include CNS depression, ranging from drowsiness to coma. Mild overdose is associated with drowsiness, confusion, and lethargy. Serious case may result in ataxia, respiratory depression, hypotension, hypotonia, coma, and rarely death. Treatment is supportive.

Drug Interactions CYP3A3/4 substrate (minor metabolic pathway)

Antipsychotics: Zaleplon potentiates the CNS effects of thioridazine (and potentially other antipsychotics)

Cimetidine: May increase zaleplon levels by decreasing its metabolism; cimetidine inhibits both aldehyde oxidase and CYP3A4 leading to an 85% increase in C_{max} and AUC of zaleplon; use 5 mg zaleplon as starting dose in patients receiving cimetidine

CNS depressants: Sedative effects may be additive with phenothiazines; monitor for increased effect; includes barbiturates, benzodiazepines, narcotic analgesics, ethanol, and other sedative agents

CYP3A3/4 inhibitors: Serum level and/or toxicity of zaleplon may be increased; inhibitors include amiodarone, cimetidine, clarithromycin, erythromycin, delavirdine, diltiazem, dirithromycin, disulfiram, fluoxetine, fluvoxamine, grapefruit juice, indinavir, itraconazole, ketoconazole, metronidazole, nefazodone, nevirapine, propoxyphene, quinupristin-dalfopristin, ritonavir, saquinavir, verapamil, zafirlukast, zileuton; monitor for altered response

CYP3A3/4 inducers: May increase the metabolism of zaleplon, reducing its effectiveness; inducers include phenytoin, carbamazepine, phenobarbital, and rifampin; rifampin decreased AUC by 80%; consider an alternative hypnotic

Tricyclic antidepressants: Zaleplon potentiates the CNS effects of imipramine (and potentially other TCAs)

Ethanol/Nutrition/Herb Interactions

Ethanol: Avoid ethanol (may increase CNS depression).

Food: High fat meal prolonged absorption; delayed t_{max} by 2 hours, and reduced C_{max} by 35%.

Herb/Nutraceutical: St John's wort may decrease zaleplon levels. Avoid valerian, St John's wort, kava kava, gotu kola (may increase CNS depression).

Stability Store at controlled room temperature of 20°C to 25°C (68°F to 77°F); protect from light

Mechanism of Action Zaleplon is unrelated to benzodiazepines, barbiturates, or other hypnotics. However, it interacts with the benzodiazepine GABA receptor complex. Nonclinical studies have shown that it binds selectively to the brain omega-1 receptor situated on the alpha subunit of the GABA-A receptor complex.

Pharmacodynamics/Kinetics

Onset: Rapid

Peak effect: Within 1 hour

Duration: 6-8 hours

Absorption: Rapid and almost complete

Distribution: V_d: 1.4 L/kg

Protein binding: 60% ± 15%

Metabolism: Extensively metabolized with <1% of dose excreted unchanged in urine. Primarily metabolized by aldehyde oxidase to form 5-oxo-zaleplon and to a lesser extent by CYP3A4 to desethylzaleplon. All metabolites are pharmacologically inactive. Oral dose plasma clearance: 3 L/hour/kg

Bioavailability: 30%

Half-life: 1 hour

Time to peak serum concentration: 1 hour

Elimination: In urine as metabolites

Usual Dosage Oral:

Adults: 10 mg at bedtime (range: 5-20 mg); has been used for up to 5 weeks of treatment in controlled trial setting

Elderly: 5 mg at bedtime

Dosage adjustment in renal impairment: No adjustment for mild to moderate renal impairment; use in severe renal impairment has not been adequately studied

Dosage adjustment in hepatic impairment: Mild to moderate impairment: 5 mg; not recommended for use in patients with severe hepatic impairment

Administration Immediately before bedtime or when the patient is in bed and cannot fall asleep

Patient Information May cause drowsiness, dizziness, or lightheadedness. Avoid alcohol and other CNS depressants. Consult prescriber before taking any prescription or OTC medication. Do not operate machinery or drive while taking this medication. Dose should be taken immediately before bedtime or when you are in bed and cannot fall asleep.

Additional Information Prescription quantities should not exceed a 1-month supply.

Dosage Forms Capsule: 5 mg, 10 mg

♦ **Zantryl**® *see* Phentermine *on page 307*

♦ **Zapex**® **(Can)** *see* Oxazepam *on page 276*

♦ **Zarontin**® *see* Ethosuximide *on page 138*

♦ **Zeldox** *see* Ziprasidone *on page 439*

♦ **Zingiber officinale** *see* Ginger *on page 167*

Ziprasidone (zi PRAY si done)

Related Information

Atypical Antipsychotics *on page 565*

Patient Information - Antipsychotics (General) *on page 466*

U.S. Brand Names Geodon®

Synonyms Zeldox; Ziprasidone Hydrochloride

Pharmacologic Category Antipsychotic Agent, Benzothiazolylpiperazine

Generic Available No

Use Treatment of schizophrenia

Unlabeled/Investigational Use Tourette's syndrome

Pregnancy Risk Factor C

(Continued)

Ziprasidone *(Continued)*

Pregnancy/Breast-Feeding Implications Developmental toxicity demonstrated in animals. There are no adequate and well-controlled studies in pregnant women. Use only if potential benefit justifies risk to the fetus. Excretion in breast milk is unknown; breast-feeding is not recommended.

Contraindications Hypersensitivity to ziprasidone or any component of the formulation; history (or current) prolonged QT; congenital long QT syndrome; recent myocardial infarction; uncompensated heart failure; concurrent use of other QT_c-prolonging agents, including amiodarone, dofetilide, class Ia antiarrhythmics (quinidine, procainamide), cisapride, pimozide, some quinolone antibiotics (moxifloxacin, sparfloxacin, gatifloxacin), sotalol, mesoridazine, and thioridazine.

Warnings/Precautions May result in QT_c prolongation (dose-related), which has been associated with the development of malignant ventricular arrhythmias (torsade de pointes) and sudden death. Observed prolongation was greater than with other atypical antipsychotic agents (risperidone, olanzapine, quetiapine), but less than with thioridazine. Avoid hypokalemia, hypomagnesemia. Use caution in patients with bradycardia. Discontinue in patients found to have persistent QT_c intervals >500 msec. Patients with symptoms of dizziness, palpitations, or syncope should receive further cardiac evaluation.

May cause extrapyramidal reactions, including pseudoparkinsonism, acute dystonic reactions, akathisia, and tardive dyskinesia. Disturbances of temperature regulation have been reported with antipsychotics (not reported in premarketing trials of ziprasidone). Antipsychotic use may also be associated with neuroleptic malignant syndrome (NMS). Use with caution in patients at risk of seizures, including those with a history of seizures, head trauma, brain damage, alcoholism, or concurrent therapy with medications which may lower seizure threshold. Elderly patients may be at increased risk of seizures due to an increased prevalence of predisposing factors.

May cause orthostatic hypotension; use with caution in patients at risk of this effect or in those who would tolerate transient hypotensive episodes (cerebrovascular disease, cardiovascular disease, hypovolemia, or other medications which may predispose).

Cognitive and/or motor impairment (sedation) is common with ziprasidone, resulting in impaired performance of tasks requiring alertness (ie, operating machinery or driving). Use with caution in disorders where CNS depression is a feature. Use with caution in Parkinson's disease. Esophageal dysmotility and aspiration have been associated with antipsychotic use; use with caution in patients at risk of aspiration pneumonia (ie, Alzheimer's disease). Caution in breast cancer or other prolactin-dependent tumors (may elevate prolactin levels). Ziprasidone has been associated with a fairly high incidence of rash (5%); discontinue if alternative etiology is not identified. Safety and efficacy have not been established in pediatric patients.

Adverse Reactions Note: Although minor QT_c prolongation (mean 10 msec at 160 mg/day) may occur more frequently (incidence not specified), clinically relevant prolongation (>500 msec) was rare (0.06%).

>10%: Central nervous system: Somnolence (14%)

1% to 10%:
Cardiovascular: Tachycardia (2%), postural hypotension (1%)
Central nervous system: Akathisia (8%), dizziness (8%), extrapyramidal symptoms (5%), dystonia (4%), hypertonia (3%)
Dermatologic: Rash (with urticaria, 4% to 5%), fungal dermatitis (2%)
Gastrointestinal: Nausea (10%), constipation (9%), dyspepsia (8%), diarrhea (5%), xerostomia (4%), anorexia (2%), weight gain (10%)
Neuromuscular & skeletal: Weakness (5%), myalgia (1%)
Ocular: Abnormal vision (3%)
Respiratory: Respiratory disorder (8%, primarily cold symptoms, upper respiratory infection), rhinitis (4%), increased cough (3%)
Miscellaneous: Accidental injury (4%)

<1%: Abdominal pain, abnormal ejaculation, abnormal gait, accidental fall, agitation, akinesia, albuminuria, alopecia, amenorrhea, amnesia, anemia, angina, anorgasmia, atrial fibrillation, ataxia, AV block (first degree), basophilia, blepharitis, buccoglossal syndrome, bundle branch block, bradycardia, cardiomegaly, cataract, cerebral infarction, chills, cholestatic jaundice, choreoathetosis, circumoral paresthesia, cogwheel rigidity, confusion, conjunctivitis, contact dermatitis, dehydration, delirium, diplopia, dry eyes, dysarthria, dyskinesia, dysphagia, dyspnea, ecchymosis, eczema, eosinophilia, epistaxis, exfoliative dermatitis, facial edema, fecal impaction, fatty liver, fever, flank pain, flu syndrome, gingival bleeding, gout, gynecomastia, hematemesis, hemoptysis, hematuria, hepatitis, hepatomegaly, hostility, hypercholesterolemia, hyperglycemia, hyperkalemia, hyperlipemia, hypertension, hyperthyroidism, hyperuricemia, hypesthesia, hypocalcemia, hypoglycemia, hypokalemia, hypokinesia, hypomagnesemia, hyponatremia, hypoproteinemia, hypothyroidism, hypotonia, impotence, incoordination, increased alkaline phosphatase, increased BUN, increased creatinine (serum), increased CPK, increased GGT, increased LDH, increased transaminases, jaundice, keratitis, keratoconjunctivitis, ketosis, lactation (female), laryngismus, leukocytosis, leukoplakia (mouth), lymphadenopathy, lymphedema, lymphocytosis, maculopapular rash, melena, menorrhagia, metrorrhagia, monocytosis, motor vehicle accident, myoclonus, myopathy, nocturia, nystagmus, ocular hemorrhage, phlebitis, polycythemia, myocarditis, neuropathy, oculogyric crisis, oliguria, opisthotonos, paresthesia, peripheral edema, photophobia, photosensitivity reaction, pneumonia, polyuria, pulmonary embolism, priapism (1 case reported), QT_c prolongation >500 msec (0.06%), rectal hemorrhage, respiratory alkalosis, seizures (0.4%), sexual dysfunction (male and female), stroke, syncope (0.6%), tenosynovitis, thirst, thrombocytopenia, thrombocythemia, thrombophlebitis, thyroiditis, tinnitus, tongue edema, torticollis, tremor, trismus, urinary retention, urticaria, uterine hemorrhage, vaginal hemorrhage, vertigo, vesiculobullous rash, visual field defect, vomiting, withdrawal syndrome

Overdosage/Toxicology Reported symptoms include somnolence, slurring of speech, and hypertension. Acute extrapyramidal reactions may also occur. Treatment is symptom-directed and supportive. Not removed by dialysis.

Drug Interactions CYP3A3/4 substrate (limited), CYP1A2 substrate (minor)

Amphetamines: Efficacy may be diminished by antipsychotics; in addition, amphetamines may increase psychotic symptoms; avoid concurrent use

Antihypertensives: Concurrent use of ziprasidone with an antihypertensive may produce additive hypotensive effects (particularly orthostasis)

Carbamazepine: May decrease serum concentrations of ziprasidone (AUC is decreased by 35%); other enzyme-inducing agents may share this potential

CNS depressants: Sedative effects may be additive with ziprasidone; monitor for increased effect; includes barbiturates, benzodiazepines, narcotic analgesics, ethanol, and other sedative agents

CYP3A3/4 inhibitors: Serum level and/or toxicity may be increased; inhibitors include amiodarone, clarithromycin, erythromycin, delavirdine, diltiazem, dirithromycin, disulfiram, fluoxetine, fluvoxamine, grapefruit juice, indinavir, itraconazole, ketoconazole, nefazodone, nevirapine, propoxyphene, quinupristin-dalfopristin, ritonavir, saquinavir, verapamil, zafirlukast, zileuton; monitor for altered response

Enzyme inducers: May enhance the hepatic metabolism of ziprasidone; larger doses may be required; includes rifampin, rifabutin, barbiturates, phenytoin, and cigarette smoking

Ketoconazole: May increase serum concentrations of ziprasidone (AUC is increased by 35% to 40%); other CYP3A3/4 inhibitors may share this potential. QT_c prolongation was not demonstrated.

Levodopa: Ziprasidone may inhibit the antiparkinsonian effect of levodopa; avoid this combination

(Continued)

Ziprasidone *(Continued)*

Potassium- or magnesium-depleting agents: May increase the risk of serious arrhythmias with ziprasidone; includes many diuretics, aminoglycosides, cyclosporine, and amphotericin; monitor serum potassium and magnesium levels closely

QT_c-prolonging agents: May result in additive effects on cardiac conduction, potentially resulting in malignant or lethal arrhythmias; concurrent use is contraindicated. Includes dofetilide, class Ia antiarrhythmics (quinidine, procainamide), pimozide, some quinolones antibiotics (moxifloxacin, sparfloxacin, gatifloxacin), sotalol, mesoridazine, and thioridazine.

Ethanol/Nutrition/Herb Interactions

Ethanol: Avoid ethanol (may increase CNS depression).

Food: Administration with food increases serum levels twofold. Grapefruit juice may increase serum concentration of ziprasidone.

Herb/Nutraceutical: St John's wort may decrease serum levels of ziprasidone, due to a potential effect on CYP3A3/4. This has not been specifically studied. Avoid kava kava, chamomile (may increase CNS depression).

Stability Store at controlled room temperature of 15°C to 30°C (59°F to 86°F)

Mechanism of Action The exact mechanism of action is unknown. However, *in vitro* radioligand studies show that ziprasidone has high affinity for D_2, 5-HT_{2a}, 5-HT_{1A}, 5-HT_{2c} and 5-HT_{1d}, moderate affinity for alpha$_1$ adrenergic and histamine H_1 receptors, and low affinity for alpha$_2$ adrenergic, beta adrenergic, 5-HT_3, 5-HT_4, cholinergic, mu, sigma, or benzodiazepine receptors. Ziprasidone moderately inhibits the reuptake of serotonin and norepinephrine.

Pharmacodynamics/Kinetics

Absorption: Well absorbed after oral administration

Distribution: V_d: 1.5 L/kg

Protein binding: 99%; primarily to albumin and alpha-1-acid glycoprotein

Metabolism: Hepatic (extensive), primarily via aldehyde oxidase; less than $\frac{1}{3}$ of total metabolism via cytochrome P450 isoenzymes: CYP3A3/4 and CYP1A2 (minor)

Bioavailability: Oral: 60% when administered with food (food increases up to twofold)

Half-life: 7 hours

Time to peak: Oral: 6-8 hours

Excretion: In feces 66% and urine 20%, as metabolites; little elimination of unchanged drug (1% in urine and 4% in feces)

Usual Dosage Oral:

Children and adolescents: Tourette's syndrome (unlabeled use): 5-40 mg/day

Adults: Psychosis: Initial: 20 mg twice daily (with food)

Adjustment: Increases (if indicated) should be made no more frequently than every 2 days; ordinarily patients should be observed for improvement over several weeks before adjusting the dose

Maintenance: Range 20-100 mg twice daily; however, dosages >80 mg twice daily are generally not recommended

Elderly: No dosage adjustment is recommended; consider initiating at a low end of the dosage range, with slower titration

Dosage adjustment in renal impairment: No dosage adjustment is recommended

Dosage adjustment in hepatic impairment: No dosage adjustment is recommended

Child/Adolescent Considerations Twenty-eight children 7-17 years of age with Tourette's syndrome and chronic tic disorder were randomly assigned to ziprasidone or placebo for 56 days. Ziprasidone was initiated at 5 mg/day and titrated to a maximum of 40 mg/day (Sallee, 2000).

Administration Administer with food

Monitoring Parameters Serum potassium, magnesium, improvements in symptomatology. The value of routine ECG screening or monitoring has not been established. Potential for extrapyramidal effects. Fever, confusion, and/or stiffness should prompt evaluation of possible NMS.

Test Interactions Increased cholesterol, triglycerides, and eosinophils

Additional Information The increased potential to prolong QT_c, as compared to other available antipsychotic agents, should be considered in the evaluation of available alternatives.

Dosage Forms Capsule, as hydrochloride: 20 mg, 40 mg, 60 mg, 80 mg

♦ **Ziprasidone Hydrochloride** *see* Ziprasidone *on page 439*

Zolmitriptan (zohl mi TRIP tan)

Related Information
Patient Information - Miscellaneous Medications - Antimigraine Medications *on page 521*

U.S. Brand Names Zomig®; Zomig-ZMT™

Canadian Brand Names Zomig

Synonyms 311C90

Pharmacologic Category Serotonin 5-HT$_{1D}$ Receptor Agonist

Generic Available No

Use Acute treatment of migraine with or without auras

Pregnancy Risk Factor C

Pregnancy/Breast-Feeding Implications In pregnant animals, zolmitriptan caused embryolethality and fetal abnormalities at doses ≥11 times the equivalent human dose.

Contraindications Hypersensitivity to zolmitriptan or any component of the formulation; ischemic heart disease or Prinzmetal's angina; signs or symptoms of ischemic heart disease; uncontrolled hypertension; symptomatic Wolff-Parkinson-White syndrome or arrhythmias associated with other cardiac accessory conduction pathway disorders; use with ergotamine derivatives (within 24 hours of); use within 24 hours of another 5-HT$_1$ agonist; concurrent administration or within 2 weeks of discontinuing an MAO inhibitor; management of hemiplegic or basilar migraine

Warnings/Precautions Zolmitriptan is indicated only in patient populations with a clear diagnosis of migraine. Not for prophylactic treatment of migraine headaches. Cardiac events (coronary artery vasospasm, transient ischemia, myocardial infarction, ventricular tachycardia/fibrillation, cardiac arrest, and death) have been reported with 5-HT$_1$ agonist administration. Should not be given to patients who have risk factors for CAD (eg, hypertension, hypercholesterolemia, smoker, obesity, diabetes, strong family history of CAD, menopause, male >40 years of age) without adequate cardiac evaluation. Patients with suspected CAD should have cardiovascular evaluation to rule out CAD before considering zolmitriptan's use; if cardiovascular evaluation negative, first dose would be safest if given in the healthcare provider's office. Periodic evaluation of those without cardiovascular disease, but with continued risk factors should be done. Significant elevation in blood pressure, including hypertensive crisis, has also been reported on rare occasions in patients with and without a history of hypertension. Vasospasm-related reactions have been reported other than coronary artery vasospasm. Peripheral vascular ischemia and colonic ischemia with abdominal pain and bloody diarrhea have occurred. Use with caution in patients with hepatic impairment. Zomig-ZMT™ 2.5 mg tablet contains 2.81 mg phenylalanine. Safety and efficacy not established in pediatric patients.

Adverse Reactions

1% to 10%:

Cardiovascular: Chest pain (2% to 4%), palpitations (up to 2%)

Central nervous system: Dizziness (6% to 10%), somnolence (5% to 8%), pain (2% to 3%), vertigo (≤2%)

Gastrointestinal: Nausea (4% to 9%), xerostomia (3% to 5%), dyspepsia (1% to 3%), dysphagia (≤2%)

(Continued)

Zolmitriptan *(Continued)*

Neuromuscular & skeletal: Paresthesia (5% to 9%), weakness (3% to 9%), warm/cold sensation (5% to 7%), hypesthesia (1% to 2%), myalgia (1% to 2%), myasthenia (up to 2%)

Miscellaneous: Neck/throat/jaw pain (4% to 10%), diaphoresis (up to 3%), allergic reaction (up to 1%)

<1% Agitation, akathisia, alkaline phosphatase increase, amnesia, anorexia, anxiety, apathy, apnea, appetite increased, arrhythmia, arthritis, ataxia, back pain, bradycardia, bronchitis, bronchospasm, bruising, cerebral ischemia, chills, constipation, cyanosis, cystitis, depression, diplopia, dry eyes, dysmenorrhea, dystonia, ear pain, edema, emotional lability, eosinophilia, epistaxis, esophagitis, extrasystole, euphoria, eye pain, facial edema, fever, gastritis, gastroenteritis, hallucinations, hematemesis, hematuria, hiccups, hyperacusis, hyperesthesia, hyperglycemia, hyperkinesias, hypertension, hypertensive crisis, hypertonia, hypotonia, insomnia, irritability, lacrimation, laryngitis, leg cramps, leukopenia, liver function abnormality, malaise, melena, miscarriage, pancreatitis, parosmia, photosensitivity, polyuria, postural hypotension, pruritus, QT prolongation, rash, syncope, tachycardia, tenosynovitis, tetany, thirst, thrombocytopenia, thrombophlebitis, tinnitus, tongue edema, twitching, ulcer, urinary frequency, urinary urgency, urticaria, voice alteration, yawning

Postmarketing and/or case reports: Angina pectoris, coronary artery vasospasm, myocardial infarction, myocardial ischemia

Events related to related to other serotonin 5-HT$_{1D}$ receptor agonists: Cerebral hemorrhage, stroke, subarachnoid hemorrhage, peripheral vascular ischemia, colonic ischemia

Drug Interactions

Cimetidine: Zolmitriptan serum levels increased; avoid concurrent use

Ergot-containing drugs (dihydroergotamine, methysergide): Concurrent use may lead to vasospastic reactions; separate by at least 24 hours.

MAO inhibitors: Increases systemic exposure to zolmitriptan. Avoid concurrent use and use within 2 weeks of discontinuing a MAO inhibitor.

Oral contraceptives: Zolmitriptan serum levels increased with concurrent use.

Propranolol: Increased zolmitriptan toxicity

Selective serotonin reuptake inhibitors (SSRIs): Concurrent use may lead to serotonin syndrome.

Sibutramine: Concurrent use may lead to serotonin syndrome.

Stability Store at 20°C to 25°C (68°F to 77°F); protect from light and moisture

Mechanism of Action Selective agonist for serotonin (5-HT$_{1B}$ and 5-HT$_{1D}$ receptors) in cranial arteries to cause vasoconstriction and reduce sterile inflammation associated with antidromic neuronal transmission correlating with relief of migraine

Usual Dosage Oral:

Children: Safety and efficacy have not been established

Adults: Migraine:

Tablet: Initial: ≤2.5 mg at the onset of migraine headache; may break 2.5 mg tablet in half

Orally-disintegrating tablet: Initial: 2.5 mg at the onset of migraine headache

Note: Use the lowest possible dose to minimize adverse events. If the headache returns, the dose may be repeated after 2 hours; do not exceed 10 mg within a 24-hour period. Controlled trials have not established the effectiveness of a second dose if the initial one was ineffective

Elderly: No dosage adjustment needed but elderly patients are more likely to have underlying cardiovascular disease and should have careful evaluation of cardiovascular system before prescribing.

Dosage adjustment in renal impairment: No dosage adjustment recommended. There is a 25% reduction in zolmitriptan's clearance in patients with severe renal impairment (Cl$_{cr}$ 5-25 mL/minute)

Dosage adjustment in hepatic impairment: Administer with caution in patients with liver disease, generally using doses <2.5 mg. Patients with moderate-to-severe hepatic impairment may have decreased clearance of zolmitriptan, and significant elevation in blood pressure was observed in some patients.

Administration Administer as soon as migraine headache starts. Tablets may be broken. Orally-disintegrating tablets must be taken whole; do not break, crush or chew; place on tongue and allow to dissolve.

Patient Information This drug is to be used to reduce your migraine, not to prevent or reduce number of attacks. If first dose brings relief, second dose may be taken anytime after 2 hours if migraine returns. If you have no relief with first dose, do not take a second dose without consulting prescriber. Do not exceed 10 mg in 24 hours. You may experience some dizziness or drowsiness; use caution when driving or engaging in tasks requiring alertness until response to drug is known. Frequent mouth care and sucking on lozenges may relieve dry mouth. Report immediately any chest pain, heart throbbing or tightness in throat; swelling of eyelids, face, or lips; skin rash or hives; easy bruising; blood in urine, stool, or vomitus; pain or itching with urination; or pain, warmth, or numbness in extremities.

Nursing Implications Ethanol: Limit use (may have additive CNS toxicity)

Additional Information Not recommended if the patient has risk factors for heart disease (high blood pressure, high cholesterol, obesity, diabetes, smoking, strong family history of heart disease, postmenopausal woman, or a male >40 years of age).

This agent is intended to relieve migraine, but not to prevent or reduce the number of attacks. Use only to treat an actual migraine attack.

Dosage Forms
Tablet (Zomig®): 2.5 mg, 5 mg
Tablet, orally-disintegrating (Zomig-ZMT™): 2.5 mg [contains 2.81 mg phenylalanine]

♦ **Zoloft®** see Sertraline on page 374

Zolpidem (zole PI dem)

Related Information
Anxiolytic/Hypnotic Use in Long-Term Care Facilities on page 562
Nonbenzodiazepine Anxiolytics and Hypnotics on page 589
Patient Information - Anxiolytics & Sedative Hypnotics (Nonbenzodiazepine Hypnotics) on page 489

U.S. Brand Names Ambien™

Synonyms Zolpidem Tartrate

Pharmacologic Category Hypnotic, Nonbenzodiazepine

Generic Available No

Use Short-term treatment of insomnia

Restrictions C-IV

Pregnancy Risk Factor B

Contraindications Hypersensitivity to zolpidem or any component of the formulation

Warnings/Precautions Should be used only after evaluation of potential causes of sleep disturbance. Failure of sleep disturbance to resolve after 7-10 days may indicate psychiatric or medical illness. Use with caution in patients with depression. Behavioral changes have been associated with sedative-hypnotics. Causes CNS depression, which may impair physical and mental capabilities. Effects with other sedative drugs or ethanol may be potentiated. Closely monitor elderly or debilitated patients for impaired cognitive or motor performance; not recommended for use in children <18 years of age. Avoid use in patients with sleep apnea or a history of sedative-hypnotic abuse.

Adverse Reactions 1% to 10%:
Cardiovascular: Palpitations
Central nervous system: Headache, drowsiness, dizziness, lethargy, lightheadedness, depression, abnormal dreams, amnesia
Dermatologic: Rash
Gastrointestinal: Nausea, diarrhea, xerostomia, constipation
Respiratory: Sinusitis, pharyngitis
(Continued)

Zolpidem *(Continued)*

Overdosage/Toxicology
Signs and symptoms: Coma

Treatment: Supportive; rarely is mechanical ventilation required. Flumazenil has been shown to selectively block the binding of benzodiazepines to CNS receptors, resulting in a reversal of benzodiazepine-induced CNS depression but not always respiratory depression

Drug Interactions CYP3A3/4 enzyme substrate
Antipsychotics: Sedative effects may be additive with antipsychotics, including phenothiazines; monitor for increased effect

CNS depressants: Sedative effects may be additive with other CNS depressants; monitor for increased effect; includes barbiturates, benzodiazepines, narcotic analgesics, ethanol, and other sedative agents

CYP3A3/4 inhibitors: Serum level and/or toxicity of zolpidem may be increased; inhibitors include amiodarone, cimetidine, clarithromycin, erythromycin, delavirdine, diltiazem, dirithromycin, disulfiram, fluoxetine, fluvoxamine, grapefruit juice, indinavir, itraconazole, ketoconazole, metronidazole, nefazodone, nevirapine, propoxyphene, quinupristin-dalfopristin, ritonavir, saquinavir, verapamil, zafirlukast, zileuton; monitor for increased response

Enzyme inducers: May increase the metabolism of zolpidem, reducing its effectiveness; inducers include phenytoin, carbamazepine, phenobarbital, and rifampin

SSRIs: Sertraline and fluoxetine (to a lesser extent) have been demonstrated to increase zaleplon levels; pharmacodynamic effects were not significantly changed; monitor

Ethanol/Nutrition/Herb Interactions
Ethanol: Avoid ethanol (may increase CNS depression).

Herb/Nutraceutical: St John's wort may decrease zolpidem levels. Avoid valerian, St John's wort, kava kava, gotu kola (may increase CNS depression).

Mechanism of Action
Structurally dissimilar to benzodiazepine, however, has much or all of its actions explained by its effects on benzodiazepine (BZD) receptors, especially the omega-1 receptor (with a high affinity ratio of the alpha 1/alpha 5 subunits); retains hypnotic and much of the anxiolytic properties of the BZD, but has reduced effects on skeletal muscle and seizure threshold.

Pharmacodynamics/Kinetics
Onset of action: 30 minutes

Duration: 6-8 hours

Absorption: Rapid

Distribution: Very low amounts secreted into breast milk

Protein binding: 92%

Metabolism: Hepatic to inactive metabolites

Half-life: 2-2.6 hours, in cirrhosis increased to 9.9 hours

Usual Dosage
Duration of therapy should be limited to 7-10 days

Adults: Oral: 10 mg immediately before bedtime; maximum dose: 10 mg

Elderly: 5 mg immediately before bedtime

Hemodialysis: Not dialyzable

Dosing adjustment in hepatic impairment: Decrease dose to 5 mg

Administration
Ingest immediately before bedtime due to rapid onset of action

Monitoring Parameters
Daytime alertness; respiratory and cardiac status

Reference Range
80-150 ng/mL

Patient Information
Avoid alcohol and other CNS depressants while taking this medication

Nursing Implications
Patients may require assistance with ambulation; lower doses in the elderly are usually effective; institute safety measures

Additional Information
Causes less disturbances in sleep stages as compared to benzodiazepines. Time spent in sleep stages 3 and 4 are maintained; decreases sleep latency. Should not be prescribed in quantities exceeding a 1-month supply.

Dosage Forms
Tablet, as tartrate: 5 mg, 10 mg

Zonisamide (zoe NIS a mide)

U.S. Brand Names Zonegran™

Pharmacologic Category Anticonvulsant, Miscellaneous

Generic Available No

Use Adjunct treatment of partial seizures in children >16 years of age and adults with epilepsy

Pregnancy Risk Factor C

Pregnancy/Breast-Feeding Implications Fetal abnormalities and death have been reported in animals, however, there are no studies in pregnant women. It is not known if zonisamide is excreted in human milk. Use during pregnancy/lactation only if the potential benefits outweigh the potential risks.

Contraindications Hypersensitivity to zonisamide, sulfonamides, or any component of the formulation

Warnings/Precautions Rare, but potentially fatal sulfonamide reactions have occurred following the use of zonisamide. These reactions include Stevens-Johnson syndrome and toxic epidermal necrolysis, usually appearing within 2-16 weeks of drug initiation. Discontinue zonisamide if rash develops. Chemical similarities are present among sulfonamides, sulfonylureas, carbonic anhydrase inhibitors, thiazides, and loop diuretics (except ethacrynic acid). Use in patients with sulfonamide allergy is specifically contraindicated in product labeling, however a risk of cross-reaction exists in patients with allergy to any of these compounds; avoid use when previous reaction has been severe. Decreased sweating and hyperthermia requiring hospitalization have been reported in children. The safety and efficacy in children <16 years of age has not been established.

Discontinue zonisamide in patients who develop acute renal failure or a significant sustained increase in creatinine/BUN concentration. Kidney stones have been reported. Use cautiously in patients with renal and hepatic dysfunction. Do not use if estimated Cl_{cr} <50 mL/minute. Significant CNS effects include psychiatric symptoms, psychomotor slowing, and fatigue or somnolence. Fatigue and somnolence occur within the first month of treatment, most commonly at doses of 300-500 mg/day. Abrupt withdrawal may precipitate seizures; discontinue or reduce doses gradually.

Adverse Reactions Adjunctive Therapy: Frequencies noted in patients receiving other anticonvulsants:

>10%:
  Central nervous system: Somnolence (17%), dizziness (13%)
  Gastrointestinal: Anorexia (13%)

1% to 10%:
  Central nervous system: Headache (10%), agitation/irritability (9%), fatigue (8%), tiredness (7%), ataxia (6%), confusion (6%), decreased concentration (6%), memory impairment (6%), depression (6%), insomnia (6%), speech disorders (5%), mental slowing (4%), anxiety (3%), nervousness (2%), schizophrenic/schizophreniform behavior (2%), difficulty in verbal expression (2%), status epilepticus (1%), tremor (1%), convulsion (1%), hyperesthesia (1%), incoordination (1%)
  Dermatologic: Rash (3%), bruising (2%), pruritus (1%)
  Gastrointestinal: Nausea (9%), abdominal pain (6%), diarrhea (5%), dyspepsia (3%), weight loss (3%), constipation (2%), dry mouth (2%), taste perversion (2%), vomiting (1%)
  Neuromuscular & skeletal: Paresthesia (4%), weakness (1%), abnormal gait (1%)
  Ocular: Diplopia (6%), nystagmus (4%), amblyopia (1%)

(Continued)

Zonisamide *(Continued)*

Otic: Tinnitus (1%)

Respiratory: Rhinitis (2%), pharyngitis (1%), increased cough (1%)

Miscellaneous: Flu-like syndrome (4%) accidental injury (1%)

<1%: Flank pain, malaise, abnormal dreams, vertigo, movement disorder, hypotonia, euphoria, chest pain, facial edema, palpitations, tachycardia, vascular insufficiency, hypotension, hypertension, syncope, bradycardia, peripheral edema, edema, cerebrovascular accident, maculopapular rash, acne, alopecia, dry skin, eczema, urticaria, hirsutism, pustular rash, vesiculobullous rash, dehydration, decreased libido, amenorrhea, flatulence, gingivitis, gum hyperplasia, gastritis, gastroenteritis, stomatitis, glossitis, ulcerative stomatitis, gastroduodenal ulcer, dysphagia, weight gain, urinary frequency, dysuria, urinary incontinence, impotence, urinary retention, urinary urgency, polyuria, nocturia, rectal hemorrhage, gum hemorrhage, leukopenia, anemia, cholelithiasis, thrombophlebitis, neck rigidity, leg cramps, myalgia, myasthenia, arthralgia, arthritis, hypertonia, neuropathy, twitching, hyperkinesia, dysarthria, peripheral neuritis, paresthesia, increased reflexes, allergic reaction, lymphadenopathy, immunodeficiency, thirst, diaphoresis, parosmia, conjunctivitis, visual field defect, glaucoma, deafness, hematuria, dyspnea, dystonia, encephalopathy, atrial fibrillation, heart failure, ventricular extrasystoles, petechia, hypoglycemia, hyponatremia, gynecomastia, mastitis, menorrhagia, cholangitis, hematemesis, colitis, duodenitis, esophagitis, fecal incontinence, mouth ulceration, enuresis, bladder pain, bladder calculus, thrombocytopenia, microcytic anemia, cholecystitis, cholestatic jaundice, increased AST (SGOT), increased ALT (SGPT), circumoral paresthesia, dyskinesia, facial paralysis, hypokinesia, myoclonus, lupus erythematosus, increased lactic dehydrogenase, oculogyric crisis, photophobia, iritis, albuminuria, pulmonary embolus, apnea, hemoptysis

Postmarketing and/or case reports: Stevens-Johnson syndrome, toxic epidermal necrolysis, aplastic anemia, agranulocytosis, kidney stones, increased BUN, increased serum creatinine, increased serum alkaline phosphatase

Overdosage/Toxicology No specific antidotes are available; experience with doses >800 mg/day is limited. Emesis or gastric lavage, with airway protection, should be done following a recent overdose. General supportive care and close observation are indicated. Renal dialysis may not be effective due to low protein binding (40%).

Drug Interactions CYP3A3/4 enzyme substrate

Note: Zonisamide did NOT affect steady state levels of carbamazepine, phenytoin, or valproate; zonisamide half-life is decreased by carbamazepine, phenytoin, phenobarbital, and valproate

Cimetidine: Single dose zonisamide levels were not altered by cimetidine

CNS depressants: Sedative effects may be additive with other CNS depressants; monitor for increased effect; includes barbiturates, benzodiazepines, narcotic analgesics, ethanol, and other sedative agents

CYP3A3/4 inhibitors: Serum level and/or toxicity of zonisamide may be increased; inhibitors include amiodarone, cimetidine, clarithromycin, erythromycin, delavirdine, diltiazem, dirithromycin, disulfiram, fluoxetine, fluvoxamine, grapefruit juice, indinavir, itraconazole, ketoconazole, metronidazole, nefazodone, nevirapine, propoxyphene, quinupristin-dalfopristin, ritonavir, saquinavir, verapamil, zafirlukast, zileuton; monitor for increased response

Enzyme inducers: May increase the metabolism of zonisamide, reducing its effectiveness; inducers include phenytoin, carbamazepine, phenobarbital, and rifampin

Ethanol/Nutrition/Herb Interactions

Ethanol: Avoid ethanol (may increase CNS depression).

Food: Food delays time to maximum concentration, but does not affect bioavailability.

Stability Store at controlled room temperature 25°C (77°F). Protect from moisture and light.

Mechanism of Action The exact mechanism of action is not known. May stabilize neuronal membranes and suppress neuronal hypersynchronization through action at sodium and calcium channels. Does not affect GABA activity.

Pharmacodynamics/Kinetics

Distribution: V_d: 1.45 L/kg

Protein binding: 40%

Metabolism: Hepatic (CYP3A4), forms N-acetyl zonisamide and 2-sulfamoylacetyl phenol (SMAP)

Half-life: 63 hours

Time to peak: 2-6 hours

Elimination: Urine, 62% (35% as parent drug, 65% as metabolites); feces, 3%

Usual Dosage Oral:

Children >16 years and Adults: Adjunctive treatment of partial seizures: Initial: 100 mg/day; dose may be increased to 200 mg/day after 2 weeks. Further dosage increases to 300 mg/day and 400 mg/day can then be made with a minimum of 2 weeks between adjustments, in order to reach steady state at each dosage level. Doses of up to 600 mg/day have been studied, however, there is no evidence of increased response with doses above 400 mg/day.

Elderly: Data from clinical trials is insufficient for patients >65 years; begin dosing at the low end of the dosing range.

Dosage adjustment in renal/hepatic impairment: Slower titration and frequent monitoring are indicated in patients with renal or hepatic disease. Do not use if Cl_{cr} <50 mL/minute.

Dietary Considerations May be taken with or without food.

Administration Capsules should be swallowed whole. Dose may be given once or twice daily. Doses of 300 mg/day and higher are associated with increased side effects. Steady-state levels are reached in 14 days.

Monitoring Parameters Monitor BUN and serum creatinine

Patient Information May cause drowsiness, especially at higher doses. Do not drive a car or operate other complex machinery until effects on performance can be determined. Avoid alcohol and other CNS depressants. Contact healthcare provider immediately if seizures worsen or for any of the following symptoms: skin rash; sudden back pain, abdominal pain, blood in the urine; fever, sore throat, oral ulcers, or easy bruising. Contact healthcare provider before becoming pregnant or breast-feeding. Swallow capsules whole, do not bite or break. It is important to drink 6-8 glasses of water each day while using this medication. Do not stop taking this or other seizure medications without talking to your healthcare professional first.

Nursing Implications See Contraindications and Warning/Precautions for use.

Dosage Forms Capsule: 100 mg

♦ **Zyban**™ *see* Bupropion *on page 52*

♦ **Zyprexa®** *see* Olanzapine *on page 272*

♦ **Zyprexa® Zydis®** *see* Olanzapine *on page 272*

SPECIAL TOPICS/ISSUES

TABLE OF CONTENTS

ANTIDEPRESSANT MEDICATIONS

SELECTIVE SEROTONIN REUPTAKE INHIBITORS (SSRIs)

TYPE OF MEDICATION:

Antidepressant medication, selective serotonin reuptake inhibitor (SSRI)

MEDICATIONS IN THIS GROUP

Citalopram (Celexa™) *on page 79*
Fluoxetine (Prozac® - depression;
    Sarafem™ - premenstrual disorder) *on page 146*
Fluvoxamine (Luvox®) *on page 157*
Paroxetine (Paxil™) *on page 283*
Sertraline (Zoloft®) *on page 374*

THIS MEDICATION IS USED FOR:

Treatment of depression; may also be used for obsessive-compulsive disorder and other anxiety disorders (eg, post-traumatic stress disorder, panic disorder, or social phobia), eating disorders, premenstrual dysphoric disorder, and addiction disorders. Usual duration of treatment is at least 1 year; may be used indefinitely for severe or relapsing depressive or related conditions.

DIRECTIONS BEFORE TAKING THIS MEDICATION

Tell your healthcare provider (HCP) if any of the following circumstances apply to you:

1. You are pregnant, intending to become pregnant, or are breast-feeding.
2. You have any medication allergies.
3. You are using any prescription medications or over-the-counter medications; remember to include any medications prescribed by your dentist and any herbal or natural products.
4. You have any medical problems.
5. You have had any problems with this medication in the past.

INSTRUCTIONS ON APPROPRIATE USE OF THIS MEDICATION

*   Take this medication exactly as recommended by your HCP. Do not take more or less than recommended dosage. Talk with your HCP concerning what you ought to do about missed doses of medication should this occur.
*   Know the name, spelling, and milligram dosage amount of your medication. This may be written down on a card kept in your wallet or purse. This information is extremely important should you become suddenly ill or are involved in an emergency situation.
*   Always try to take this medication at the same time of day. SSRIs are usually taken 1-2 times daily. Fluoxetine (Prozac®) is available in a formulation that may be taken once weekly.
*   SSRI antidepressants are generally best tolerated if taken with or shortly after food. This may minimize any potential digestive system upset.
*   Store medication in a clean, dry place at room temperature, away from children.

PRECAUTIONS

- Improvement in energy level and sleep/appetite may occur during the first week, while depressive symptoms may take up to 4-6 weeks to improve. Do not abruptly stop medication as there may be a drug withdrawal reaction.

- This medication may add to the effects of alcohol or other drugs.

- Do not use alcohol or street drugs while on this medication.

- If this medication makes you sleepy or drowsy, do not operate a machine or motor vehicle as this may be dangerous.

- Tell your HCP immediately if you become pregnant while on this medication.

- Do not take any new or additional prescription or over-the-counter medications without discussing them with your HCP. This includes herbal and natural products.

- Do not take SSRI antidepressant medications if you have taken a monoamine oxidase inhibitor (MAOI) within the past 2 weeks. This may be associated with potentially life-threatening high blood pressure.

- Prozac® and Sarafem™ are the same medication (fluoxetine) sold under different brand names for different disorders. Discuss all your medications with your healthcare provider to ensure that you are only taking one prescription of fluoxetine at a time.

COMMON SIDE EFFECTS

All drugs are associated with side effects. Most side effects are mild, and often may improve over time. Discuss side effects of this medication with your HCP prior to starting therapy, including how you should contact your HCP if side effects occur. The following side effects are more common and should be discussed with your HCP.

- Drowsiness
- Decreased appetite/weight loss/weight gain
- Decrease in sexual function
- Nausea or digestive system upset
- Dry mouth

More rare side effects include agitation, anxiety, or other physical symptoms such as rash, itching, or muscle twitching. Report these symptoms immediately to your HCP. Other side effects not listed may occur in some individuals. If these occur, report them to your HCP.

ANTIDEPRESSANT MEDICATIONS *(Continued)*

TRICYCLIC ANTIDEPRESSANTS (TCA) AND RELATED MEDICATIONS

TYPE OF MEDICATION:

Antidepressant medication, cyclic/tricyclic class

MEDICATIONS IN THIS GROUP

Amitriptyline (Elavil®, Enovil®) *on page 22*
Amoxapine (Asendin®) *on page 36*
Clomipramine (Anafranil®) *on page 82*
Desipramine (Norpramin®) *on page 101*
Doxepin (Adapin®, Sinequan®) *on page 123*
Imipramine (Janamine®, Tofranil®) *on page 180*
Maprotiline (Ludiomil®) *on page 216*
Nortriptyline (Aventyl®, Pamelor®) *on page 267*
Protriptyline (Vivactil®) *on page 344*
Trimipramine (Surmontil®) *on page 421*

THIS MEDICATION IS USED FOR:

Treatment of depression; may also be used for some anxiety disorders such as obsessive-compulsive disorder, panic disorder, and post-traumatic stress disorder as well as eating disorders, chronic pain conditions, and enuresis (bedwetting) in children. Usual duration of the treatment for depression and anxiety disorders is at least 1 year, although may be used indefinitely for severe or relapsing depressive or related conditions.

DIRECTIONS BEFORE TAKING THIS MEDICATION

Tell your healthcare provider (HCP) if any of the following circumstances apply to you:

1. You are pregnant, intending to become pregnant, or are breast-feeding.
2. You have any medication allergies.
3. You are using any prescription medications or over-the-counter medications; remember to include any medications prescribed by your dentist and any herbal or natural products.
4. You have any medical problems.
5. You have had any problems with this medication in the past.

INSTRUCTIONS ON APPROPRIATE USE OF THIS MEDICATION

- Take this medication exactly as recommended by your HCP. Do not take more or less than recommended dosage. Talk with your HCP concerning what you ought to do about missed doses of medication should this occur.
- Know the name, spelling, and milligram dosage amount of your medication. This may be written down on a card kept in your wallet or purse. This information is extremely important should you become suddenly ill or are involved in an emergency situation.
- Always try to take this medication at the same time of day. TCAs are usually taken 1-2 times daily, frequently with a larger proportion of medication at bedtime.
- Store medication in a clean, dry place at room temperature, away from children.

PRECAUTIONS

- Improvement in energy level and sleep/appetite may occur during the first week, while depressive symptoms may take up to 4-6 weeks to improve. Do not abruptly stop medication as there may be a drug withdrawal reaction.

- TCAs may cause drowsiness or sleepiness. If this medication makes you sleepy or drowsy, do not operate a dangerous machine or motor vehicle as this may be hazardous.

- Dizziness or light-headedness may occur, particularly when getting up quickly from a seated or lying down position. Getting up slowly may help.

- Dry mouth may occur; sucking on sugarless candy or chewing gum may help.

- This medication may add to the effects of alcohol or "street" drugs.

- Do not use alcohol or "street" drugs while on this medication.

- Tell your HCP immediately if you become pregnant while on this medication.

- Do not take any new or additional prescription or over-the-counter medications without discussing them with your HCP. This includes herbal and natural products.

COMMON SIDE EFFECTS

All drugs are associated with side effects. Most side effects are mild, and often may improve over time. Discuss side effects of this medication with your HCP prior to starting therapy, including how you should contact your HCP if side effects occur. The following side effects are more common with TCAs and should be discussed with your HCP.

- Drowsiness/sleepiness/fatigue
- Dizziness
- Dry mouth
- Constipation
- Increased appetite/weight gain
- Headache
- Blurred vision
- Unpleasant metallic taste in mouth

More rare side effects include irregular heart beat or fainting, confusion, twitching, seizures, problems in urination, skin rash, or yellowing of eyes or skin. Report these symptoms immediately to your HCP. Other side effects not listed may occur in some individuals. If these occur, report them to your HCP.

ANTIDEPRESSANT MEDICATIONS *(Continued)*

BUPROPION

TYPE OF MEDICATION:

Antidepressant medication, dopamine-reuptake inhibitor

MEDICATIONS IN THIS GROUP

Bupropion (Wellbutrin® -depression; Zyban™ - smoking cessation) *on page 52* is the only medication in this group available in the U.S.

THIS MEDICATION IS USED FOR:

Treatment of depression and to help in stopping smoking.

DIRECTIONS BEFORE TAKING THIS MEDICATION

Tell your healthcare provider (HCP) if any of the following circumstances apply to you:

1. You are pregnant, intending to become pregnant, or are breast-feeding.

2. You have any medication allergies.

3. You are using any prescription medications or over-the-counter medications; remember to include any medications prescribed by your dentist and any herbal or natural products.

4. You have any medical problems.

5. You have had any problems with this medication in the past.

6. You have or have had an eating disorder such as bulimia or anorexia.

7. You have a seizure disorder or have ever had a seizure disorder (convulsion).

INSTRUCTIONS ON APPROPRIATE USE OF THIS MEDICATION

- Take this medication exactly as recommended by your HCP. Do not take more or less than recommended dosage. Talk with your HCP concerning what you ought to do about missed doses of medication should this occur.

- Know the name, spelling, and milligram dosage amount of your medication. This may be written down on a card kept in your wallet or purse. This information is extremely important should you become suddenly ill or are involved in an emergency situation.

- Always try to take this medication at the same time of day. Bupropion is generally prescribed 2-3 times/day. A slow-release (SR) form is also available to be taken 1-2 times/day.

- Store medication in a clean, dry place at room temperature, away from children.

PRECAUTIONS

- Improvement in energy level and sleep/appetite may occur during the first week, while depressive symptoms may take up to 4-6 weeks to improve. Do not abruptly stop medication as there may be a drug withdrawal reaction.

- This medication may add to the effects of alcohol or other drugs.

- Do not use alcohol or "street" drugs while on this medication.

- If this medication makes you sleepy or drowsy, do not operate heavy machinery or a motor vehicle as this may be hazardous.

- Tell your HCP immediately if you become pregnant while on this medication.

- Do not take any new or additional prescription or over-the-counter medications without discussing them with your HCP. This includes herbal and natural products.

- Dizziness or light-headedness may occur, particularly when getting up quickly from a seated or lying down position. Getting up slowly may help.

- Do not take bupropion if you have taken a monoamine oxidase inhibitor (MAOI) within the past 2 weeks; this may be associated with potentially life-threatening high blood pressure.

- Bupropion is sold under different brand names for different uses. Discuss all your medications with your HCP so that you only take one prescription of bupropion at a time.

COMMON SIDE EFFECTS

All drugs are associated with side effects. Most side effects are mild, and often may improve over time. Discuss side effects of this medication with your HCP prior to starting therapy, including how you should contact your HCP if side effects occur. The following side effects are more common with bupropion and should be discussed with your HCP.

- Agitation/anxiety
- Nausea, constipation, loss of appetite
- Trembling/shaking
- Dizziness
- Sleepiness
- Transient weight loss

More rare side effects include seizures, confusion, headache, or skin rash. Report these symptoms immediately to your HCP. Other side effects not listed may occur in some individuals. If these occur, report them to your HCP.

ANTIDEPRESSANT MEDICATIONS *(Continued)*

VENLAFAXINE

TYPE OF MEDICATION:

Antidepressant, selective serotonin-norepinephrine reuptake inhibitor

MEDICATIONS IN THIS GROUP

Venlafaxine (Effexor®) *on page 430* is the only medication in this group available in the U.S.

THIS MEDICATION IS USED FOR:

Treatment of depression and anxiety

DIRECTIONS BEFORE TAKING THIS MEDICATION

Tell your healthcare provider (HCP) if any of the following circumstances apply to you:

1. You are pregnant, intending to become pregnant, or are breast-feeding.
2. You have any medication allergies.
3. You are using any prescription medications or over-the-counter medications; remember to include any medications prescribed by your dentist and any herbal or natural products.
4. You have any medical problem.
5. You have had any problems with this medication in the past.

INSTRUCTIONS ON APPROPRIATE USE OF THIS MEDICATION

- Take this medication exactly as recommended by your HCP. Do not take more or less than recommended dosage. Talk with your HCP concerning what you ought to do about missed doses of medication should this occur.
- Know the name, spelling, and milligram dosage amount of your medication. This may be written down on a card kept in your wallet or purse. This information is extremely important should you become suddenly ill or are involved in an emergency situation.
- Always try to take this medication at the same time of day. Venlafaxine is generally prescribed 1-3 times/day. A slow-acting formulation is available which is prescribed once daily.
- Store medication in a clean, dry place at room temperature, away from children.

PRECAUTIONS

- Improvement in energy level and sleep/appetite may occur during the first week, while depressive symptoms may take up to 4-6 weeks to improve. Do not abruptly stop medication as there may be a drug withdrawal reaction.
- This medication may add to the effects of alcohol or other drugs.
- Do not use alcohol or "street" drugs while on this medication.
- If this medication makes you sleepy or drowsy, do not operate heavy machinery or a motor vehicle as this may be hazardous.
- Tell your HCP immediately if you become pregnant while on this medication.
- Do not take any new or additional prescription or over-the-counter medications without discussing them with your HCP. This includes herbal and natural products.
- Dizziness or light-headedness may occur, particularly when getting up quickly from a seated or lying down position. Getting up slowly may help.
- Venlafaxine may be associated with increases in blood pressure, even in individuals who do not have high blood pressure to begin with. Your blood pressure should be monitored during the initial period when you begin to take venlafaxine.

COMMON SIDE EFFECTS

All drugs are associated with side effects. Most side effects are mild, and often may improve over time. Discuss side effects of this medication with your HCP prior to starting therapy, including how you should contact your HCP if side effects occur. The following side effects are more common with venlafaxine and should be discussed with your HCP.

- Nausea
- Dizziness
- Dry mouth
- Anxiety or difficulty sleeping
- Headache
- Sleepiness
- Constipation
- Abnormal ejaculation or abnormal orgasm
- Blurred vision

More rare side effects include irregular heart beat, confusion, difficulty urinating, skin rash, seizures. Report these symptoms immediately to your HCP. Other side effects not listed may occur in some individuals. If these occur, report them to your HCP.

ANTIDEPRESSANT MEDICATIONS *(Continued)*

SEROTONIN BLOCKER

TYPE OF MEDICATION:

Antidepressant medication, serotonin antagonist

MEDICATIONS IN THIS GROUP

Nefazodone (Serzone®) *on page 259*

Trazodone (Desyrel®) *on page 408*

THIS MEDICATION IS USED FOR:

Treatment of depression; also used in anxiety disorders such as post-traumatic stress disorder. Trazodone is sometimes used as a sleep inducer.

DIRECTIONS BEFORE TAKING THIS MEDICATION

Tell your healthcare provider (HCP) if any of the following circumstances apply to you:

1.   You are pregnant, intending to become pregnant, or are breast-feeding.

2.   You have any medication allergies.

3.   You are using any prescription medications or over-the-counter medications; remember to include any medications prescribed by your dentist and any herbal or natural products.

4.   You have any medical problems.

5.   You have had any problems with this medication in the past.

INSTRUCTIONS ON APPROPRIATE USE OF THIS MEDICATION

*   Take this medication exactly as recommended by your HCP. Do not take more or less than recommended dosage. Talk with your HCP concerning what you ought to do about missed doses of medication should this occur.

*   Know the name, spelling, and milligram dosage amount of your medication. This may be written down on a card kept in your wallet or purse. This information is extremely important should you become suddenly ill or are involved in an emergency situation.

*   Always try to take this medication at the same time of day. Serotonin blockers are generally prescribed 2-3 times/day.

*   Store medication in a clean, dry place at room temperature, away from children.

PRECAUTIONS

- Improvement in energy level and sleep/appetite may occur during the first week, while depressive symptoms may take up to 4-6 weeks to improve. Do not abruptly stop medication as there may be a drug withdrawal reaction.

- This medication may add to the effects of alcohol or other drugs.

- Do not use alcohol or "street" drugs while on this medication.

- If this medication makes you sleepy or drowsy, do not operate heavy machinery or a motor vehicle as this may be hazardous.

- Tell your HCP immediately if you become pregnant while on this medication.

- Do not take any new or additional prescription or over-the-counter medications without discussing them with your HCP. This includes herbal and natural products.

- Dizziness or light-headedness may occur, particularly when getting up quickly from a seated or lying down position. Getting up slowly may help.

- Do not take nefazodone if you have taken a monoamine oxidase inhibitor (MAOI) within the past 2 weeks; this may be associated with potentially life-threatening high blood pressure.

- Nefazodone should not be taken if you are on the following medications:

  - Cisapride (Propulsid®) for gastrointestinal problems
  - Pimozide (Orap™) *on page 316* for psychological problems of tics in children/adolescents

COMMON SIDE EFFECTS

All drugs are associated with side effects. Most side effects are mild, and often may improve over time. Discuss side effects of this medication with your HCP prior to starting therapy, including how you should contact your HCP if side effects occur. The following side effects are more common with this group of antidepressants and should be discussed with your HCP:

- Sleepiness
- Dry mouth
- Blurred vision
- Dizziness
- Constipation
- Nausea

More rare side effects include irregular heartbeat (with trazodone), painful, prolonged erection (with trazodone), confusion, or headache. Report these symptoms immediately to your HCP. Other side effects not listed may occur in some individuals. If these occur, report them to your HCP.

ANTIDEPRESSANT MEDICATIONS *(Continued)*

MONOAMINE OXIDASE INHIBITORS (MAOIs)

TYPE OF MEDICATION:

Antidepressant medication, monoamine oxidase inhibitor

MEDICATIONS IN THIS GROUP

Isocarboxazid (Marplan®) *on page 184*
Phenelzine (Nardil®) *on page 300*
Selegiline (Eldepryl®) *on page 370*
Tranylcypromine (Parnate®) *on page 405*

THIS MEDICATION IS USED FOR:

Treatment of depression; also used in the treatment of anxiety disorders (eg, obsessive-compulsive disorders), and sometimes used to treat severe sleep disorders

DIRECTIONS BEFORE TAKING THIS MEDICATION

Tell your healthcare provider (HCP) if any of the following circumstances apply to you:

1. You are pregnant, intending to become pregnant, or are breast-feeding.
2. You have any medication allergies.
3. You are using any prescription medications or over-the-counter medications; remember to include any medications prescribed by your dentist and any herbal or natural products.
4. You have any medical problems.
5. You have had any problems with this medication in the past.

INSTRUCTIONS ON APPROPRIATE USE OF THIS MEDICATION

- Take this medication exactly as recommended by your HCP. Do not take more or less than recommended dosage. Talk with your HCP concerning what you ought to do about missed doses of medication should this occur.
- Know the name, spelling, and milligram dosage amount of your medication. This may be written down on a card kept in your wallet or purse. This information is extremely important should you become suddenly ill or are involved in an emergency situation.
- Always try to take this medication at the same time of day. MAOIs are generally prescribed twice daily.
- Store medication in a clean, dry place at room temperature, away from children.

PRECAUTIONS

- Improvement in energy level and sleep/appetite may occur during the first week, while depressive symptoms may take up to 4-6 weeks to improve. Do not abruptly stop medication as there may be a drug withdrawal reaction.
- If this medication makes you sleepy or drowsy, do not operate heavy machinery or a motor vehicle as this may be hazardous.
- Tell your HCP immediately if you become pregnant while on this medication.

- Do not take any new or additional prescription or over-the-counter medications without discussing them with your HCP. This includes herbal and natural products.

- Dizziness or light-headedness may occur, particularly when getting up quickly from a seated or lying down position. Getting up slowly may help.

- MAOIs can cause very dangerous reactions (life-threatening high blood pressure) with certain foods, drinks, or medications. These include:

  - Foods that are fermented or aged (eg, smoked or pickled meats, sauerkraut or other pickled fruits or vegetables)
  - Aged cheeses, yogurt, sour cream, tofu
  - Meat tenderizers or soy sauce
  - Some types of red wine, beer (including nonalcoholic), champagne
  - Tea, coffee, cola
  - Chocolate
  - Nuts
  - Narcotics (eg, codeine or other painkillers)
  - Cold preparations (eg, antihistamines, cough syrups, nasal spray)
  - Medications to induce sleep
  - Stimulant medications (eg, some diet pills)
  - Yeast or dietary supplements

- If you need to have any surgery or dental procedure, notify your HCP or dentist that you are taking an MAOI or have taken an MAOI within the past 2 weeks.

- After stopping an MAOI, you must adhere to all the above precautions and instructions for at least 2 weeks, as there may be enough MAOI in your body to interact with certain foods, drinks, or medications.

COMMON SIDE EFFECTS

All drugs are associated with side effects. Most side effects are mild, and often may improve over time. Discuss side effects of this medication with your HCP prior to starting therapy, including how you should contact your HCP if side effects occur. The following side effects are more common with MAOIs and should be discussed with your HCP.

- Drowsiness
- Mild/moderate headache
- Mild/moderate agitation
- Dry mouth
- Dizziness
- Blurred vision
- Gastrointestinal problems (eg, nausea, constipation)
- Shakiness or trembling

More rare side effects include severe headache, skin rash, fever, or sore throat. Symptoms of potentially life-threatening high blood pressure (hypertensive crisis) include chest pain, increased sweating, enlarged pupils, eye sensitivity to light, severe headache and sore neck. Report any of these symptoms immediately to your HCP. Other side effects not listed may occur in some individuals. If these occur, report them to your HCP.

ANTIDEPRESSANT MEDICATIONS *(Continued)*

MIRTAZAPINE

TYPE OF MEDICATION:

Antidepressant medication, alpha-adrenoceptor antagonist

MEDICATIONS IN THIS GROUP

Mirtazapine (Remeron®) *on page 244* is the only medication in this group available in the U.S.

THIS MEDICATION IS USED FOR:

Treatment of depression

DIRECTIONS BEFORE TAKING THIS MEDICATION

Tell your healthcare provider (HCP) if any of the following circumstances apply to you:

1. You are pregnant, intending to become pregnant, or are breast-feeding.

2. You have any medication allergies.

3. You are using any prescription medications or over-the-counter medications; remember to include any medications prescribed by your dentist and any herbal or natural products.

4. You have any medical problems.

5. You have had any problems with this medication in the past.

6. You have ever had a disorder of low red blood cell count (anemia) or low white blood cell count (neutropenia).

INSTRUCTIONS ON APPROPRIATE USE OF THIS MEDICATION

- Take this medication exactly as recommended by your HCP. Do not take more or less than recommended dosage. Talk with your HCP concerning what you ought to do about missed doses of medication should this occur.

- Know the name, spelling, and milligram dosage amount of your medication. This may be written down on a card kept in your wallet or purse. This information is extremely important should you become suddenly ill or are involved in an emergency situation.

- Always try to take this medication at the same time of day. Mirtazapine is generally prescribed once daily.

- Store medication in a clean, dry place at room temperature, away from children.

464

PRECAUTIONS

- Improvement in energy level and sleep/appetite may occur during the first week, while depressive symptoms may take up to 4-6 weeks to improve. Do not abruptly stop medication as there may be a drug withdrawal reaction.
- This medication may add to the effects of alcohol or other drugs.
- Do not use alcohol or "street" drugs while on this medication.
- If this medication makes you sleepy or drowsy, do not operate heavy machinery or a motor vehicle as this may be hazardous.
- Tell your HCP immediately if you become pregnant while on this medication.
- Do not take any new or additional prescription or over-the-counter medications without discussing them with your HCP. This includes herbal and natural products.
- Dizziness or light-headedness may occur, particularly when getting up quickly from a seated or lying down position. Getting up slowly may help.
- Do not take mirtazapine if you have taken a monoamine oxidase inhibitor (MAOI) within the past 2 weeks; this may be associated with potentially life-threatening high blood pressure.

COMMON SIDE EFFECTS

All drugs are associated with side effects. Most side effects are mild, and often may improve over time. Discuss side effects of this medication with your HCP prior to starting therapy, including how you should contact your HCP if side effects occur. The following side effects are more common with mirtazapine and should be discussed with your HCP.

- Dry mouth
- Constipation
- Dizziness
- Tiredness
- Increased appetite/weight gain

More rare side effects include seizures, confusion, headache, or fever. Report these symptoms immediately to your HCP. Other side effects not listed may occur in some individuals. If these occur, report them to your HCP.

ANTIPSYCHOTIC MEDICATIONS

GENERAL

TYPE OF MEDICATION:

Antipsychotic medication, typical group and atypical group

MEDICATIONS IN THIS GROUP

Typical medications in this group include:

THIS MEDICATION IS USED FOR:

Treatment of psychosis which may be seen in a variety of mental disorders such as schizophrenia, manic-depressive disorder, and dementia. Other uses of antipsychotic medications include tic disorders (Tourette's disorder) or severe aggressive or impulsive conditions. Olanzapine (Zyprexa™) is approved by the FDA for the treatment of manic symptoms of bipolar disorder.

DIRECTIONS BEFORE TAKING THIS MEDICATION

Tell your healthcare provider (HCP) if any of the following circumstances apply to you:

1. You are pregnant, intending to become pregnant, or are breast-feeding.
2. You have any medication allergies.
3. You are using any prescription medications or over-the-counter medications; remember to include any medications prescribed by your dentist and any herbal or natural products.
4. You have any medical problems.
5. You have had any problems with this medication in the past.
6. You have ever had neuroleptic malignant syndrome in the past with antipsychotic medications.

INSTRUCTIONS ON APPROPRIATE USE OF THIS MEDICATION

- Take this medication exactly as recommended by your HCP. Do not take more or less than recommended dosage. Talk with your HCP concerning what you ought to do about missed doses of medication should this occur.
- Know the name, spelling, and milligram dosage amount of your medication. This may be written down on a card kept in your wallet or purse. This information is extremely important should you become suddenly ill or are involved in an emergency situation.
- Always try to take this medication at the same time of day. Antipsychotic medications are usually taken as tablets, 1-2 times/day. Alternatively, your HCP may prescribe antipsychotic medications in other forms which include:
  1. Short-acting injectable medications to treat symptoms quickly
  2. Liquid form for ease of swallowing
  3. Long-acting injectable medications usually given once or twice monthly to minimize missed doses. Currently no atypical antipsychotic medications are available in either short- or long-acting injectable forms.
- Store medication in a clean, dry place at room temperature, away from children.

PRECAUTIONS

- Full effect of antipsychotic medication may take 6 weeks or longer to occur. Do not abruptly stop medication as there may be a drug withdrawal reaction.
- This medication may add to the effects of alcohol or other drugs.
- Do not use alcohol or "street" drugs while on this medication.
- If this medication makes you sleepy or drowsy, do not operate heavy machinery or a motor vehicle as this may be hazardous.
- Tell your HCP immediately if you become pregnant while on this medication.
- Do not take any new or additional prescription or over-the-counter medications without discussing them with your HCP. This includes natural and herbal products.
- Dizziness or light-headedness may occur, particularly when getting up quickly from a seated or lying down position. Getting up slowly may help.
- Avoid extreme heat (eg, saunas) or activities that may lead to becoming overheated as some antipsychotic medications disturb the body's ability to self-regulate body temperature.
- Avoid direct, prolonged sun exposure and take appropriate sun precautions (eg, sun screen, protective clothing/headgear) as antipsychotic medications may increase risk of severe sunburn/reactivity to the sun.
- Minimize cigarette smoking, as this may alter blood levels of antipsychotic medication in the body.

COMMON SIDE EFFECTS

All drugs are associated with side effects. Most side effects are mild, and often may improve over time. Discuss side effects of this medication with your HCP prior to starting therapy, including how you should contact your HCP if side effects occur. The following side effects are more common with antipsychotic medications and should be discussed with your HCP.

- Muscle spasm, shaking, muscle stiffness, or restlessness (extrapyramidal symptoms). These are more common with typical antipsychotic medications and may be improved or resolved with the use of agents to treat extrapyramidal symptoms. Risk of extrapyramidal symptoms are greater with typical antipsychotic medications and less with atypical antipsychotic medications.
- Tiredness

ANTIPSYCHOTIC MEDICATIONS *(Continued)*

- Dizziness
- Dry mouth
- Blurred vision
- Weight gain (generally more common with atypical antipsychotic medications)
- Breast enlargement, menstrual irregularities (generally more common with typical antipsychotic medications)
- Constipation
- Involuntary body movements (tardive dyskinesia), usually of the lips, tongue, and face. May also involve arms, legs, or trunk. These usually only occur after long-term use of antipsychotic medication (months to years). Risk of tardive dyskinesia appears to be greater with typical antipsychotic medications and less with atypical antipsychotic medications.

More rare side effects include seizures, confusion, skin rash, changes in the eyes/decreased vision, fast or irregular heartbeat, liver damage, or yellowing of skin or eyes. If you experience fever, sweating, muscle stiffness, you may have a very serious medical condition called neuroleptic malignant syndrome. Report any of these symptoms to your HCP immediately. Other side effects not listed may occur in some individuals. If these occur, report them to your HCP.

CLOZAPINE

TYPE OF MEDICATION:

Antipsychotic medication, atypical group

MEDICATIONS IN THIS GROUP

Clozapine (Clozaril® and others) *on page 94* is the only medication approved by the FDA for treatment-resistant schizophrenia

THIS MEDICATION IS USED FOR:

Treatment-resistant schizophrenia; also used sometimes for severe manic-depressive illness, other severe psychotic conditions, and severe aggressive behavior. Due to the need for regular blood tests (every 1-2 weeks) and potential for serious side effects, clozapine therapy is generally reserved for situations where other medications have been ineffective.

DIRECTIONS BEFORE TAKING THIS MEDICATION

Tell your healthcare provider (HCP) if any of the following circumstances apply to you:

1. You are pregnant, intending to become pregnant, or are breast-feeding.
2. You have any medication allergies.
3. You are using any prescription medications or over-the-counter medications; remember to include any medications prescribed by your dentist and any herbal or natural products.
4. You have any medical problems.
5. You have had any problems with this medication in the past.
6. You have ever had a disorder of low blood cell count (anemia) or low white blood cell count (neutropenia)
7. You have ever had a seizure or a seizure disorder.

INSTRUCTIONS ON APPROPRIATE USE OF THIS MEDICATION

- Take this medication exactly as recommended by your HCP. Do not take more or less than recommended dosage. Talk with your HCP concerning what you ought to do about missed doses of medication should this occur.
- Know the name, spelling, and milligram dosage amount of your medication. This may be written down on a card kept in your wallet or purse. This information is extremely important should you become suddenly ill or are involved in an emergency situation.
- Always try to take this medication at the same time of day. Clozapine is generally prescribed twice daily.
- Store medication in a clean, dry place at room temperature, away from children.

ANTIPSYCHOTIC MEDICATIONS *(Continued)*

PRECAUTIONS

- Full effect of antipsychotic medications may take 6 weeks or longer to occur. Do not abruptly stop medication as there may be a drug withdrawal reaction.
- This medication may add to the effects of alcohol or other drugs.
- Do not use alcohol or "street" drugs while on this medication.
- If this medication makes you sleepy or drowsy, do not operate heavy machinery or a motor vehicle as this may be hazardous.
- Tell your HCP immediately if you become pregnant while on this medication.
- Do not take any new or additional prescription or over-the-counter medications without discussing them with your HCP. This includes natural and herbal products.
- Dizziness or light-headedness may occur, particularly when getting up quickly from a seated or lying down position. Getting up slowly may help.
- In rare cases (less than 1% of patients) clozapine has been associated with a decrease in white blood cells, which are used by the body to fight infection. In order to closely follow white blood cell levels, your HCP will order a blood test once weekly during the first 6 months of clozapine therapy. If there are no blood count abnormalities after 6 months, blood checks are reduced to once every 2 weeks. These will continue indefinitely, as long as you are on clozapine. After stopping clozapine, the blood checks should continue for 4 additional weeks.

COMMON SIDE EFFECTS

All drugs are associated with side effects. Most side effects are mild, and often may improve over time. Discuss side effects of this medication with your HCP prior to starting therapy, including how you should contact your HCP if side effects occur. The following side effects are common with clozapine and should be discussed with your HCP.

- Tiredness
- Dizziness
- Dry mouth or drooling
- Constipation
- Weight gain
- Blurred vision

More rare side effects include seizures, confusion, fast or irregular heartbeat, skin rash, or liver damage. If you experience fever, sweating, muscle stiffness, you may have a serious medical condition called neuroleptic malignant syndrome. Report any of these symptoms immediately to your HCP. Other side effects not listed may occur in some individuals. If these occur, report them to your HCP.

MEDICATIONS TO STABILIZE MOOD

LITHIUM

TYPE OF MEDICATION:

Mood stabilizer

MEDICATIONS IN THIS GROUP

Typical medications in this group include:

Lithium (Lithobid®, generic formulations) *on page 205*

THIS MEDICATION IS USED FOR:

Treatment of manic-depressive (bipolar) disorder; also used sometimes in the treatment of depression, post-traumatic stress disorder, severe aggressive behaviors, and personality disorders.

DIRECTIONS BEFORE TAKING THIS MEDICATION

Tell your healthcare provider (HCP) if any of the following circumstances apply to you:

1. You are pregnant, intending to become pregnant, or are breast-feeding

2. You have any medication allergies

3. You are using any prescription medications or over-the-counter medications; remember to include any medications prescribed by your dentist and any herbal or natural products.

4. You have any medical problems

5. You have had any problems with this medication in the past

INSTRUCTIONS ON APPROPRIATE USE OF THIS MEDICATION

- Improvement in mood stability (mood "leveling out") may require 1-3 weeks. Do not abruptly stop medication as there may be a drug withdrawal reaction.

- Know the name, spelling, and milligram dosage amount of your medication. This may be written down on a card kept in your wallet or purse. This information is extremely important should you become suddenly ill or are involved in an emergency situation.

- Always try to take this medication at the same time of day. Lithium is generally prescribed twice daily. Your HCP will check blood level of lithium to determine the most appropriate dosage for you. Lithium blood levels are usually done in the morning. On the morning of your lithium blood level test, wait to take your morning dose of lithium until **after** the blood test.

- Store medication in a clean, dry place at room temperature, away from children.

PRECAUTIONS

- Improvement in mood stability (mood "leveling out") may require 1-3 weeks. Do not abruptly stop medication as there may be a drug withdrawal reaction.

- This medication may add to the effects of alcohol or other drugs.

MEDICATIONS TO STABILIZE MOOD (Continued)

- Do not use alcohol or "street" drugs while on this medication.

- If this medication makes you sleepy or drowsy, do not operate heavy machinery or a motor vehicle as this may be hazardous.

- Tell your HCP immediately if you become pregnant while on this medication.

- Do not take any new or additional prescription or over-the-counter medications without discussing them with your HCP. This includes herbal or natural products.

- Dizziness or light-headedness may occur, particularly when getting up quickly from a seated or lying down position. Getting up slowly may help.

- Excessive heat or exercise in hot weather may cause extreme sweating and dehydration. This, in the presence of taking lithium may cause serious problems with blood pressure or heart functioning. Avoid circumstances of extreme heat or physical activity that can lead to dehydration/body fluid imbalance.

- Do not take diuretic medications ("water pills") while on lithium without consulting your HCP.

- Avoid excessive amount of caffeine-containing drinks such as coffee and cola.

COMMON SIDE EFFECTS

All drugs are associated with side effects. Most side effects are mild, and often may improve over time. Discuss side effects of this medication with your HCP prior to starting therapy, including how you should contact your HCP if side effects occur. The following side effects are more common with lithium and should be discussed with your HCP.

- Increased thirst

- Frequent urination

- Tiredness

- Muscle tremor or shakiness

- Weight gain

- Skin changes (eg, rashes)

- Nausea

More rare side effects include problems in coordination or balance, severe muscle tremor, diarrhea, confusion, slurred speech, rapid heart rate or irregular pulse, blurred vision, severe weakness, severe rash, and neck swelling (goiter). Report these symptoms immediately to your HCP. Your HCP may use a blood test to check for lithium overdose (lithium toxicity) as well as any physical or neurological examinations. Other side effects not listed may occur in some individuals. If these occur, report them to your HCP.

VALPROIC ACID (valproate, divalproex)

TYPE OF MEDICATION:
Mood stabilizer, anticonvulsant type

MEDICATIONS IN THIS GROUP

Valproate (Depakote®, and others) *on page 425* is the only mood stabilizer in the anticonvulsant group which is FDA approved as an agent to treat mania in bipolar disorder

THIS MEDICATION IS USED FOR:
Treatment of bipolar disorder; also FDA approved to treat seizures

DIRECTIONS BEFORE TAKING THIS MEDICATION
Tell your healthcare provider (HCP) if any of the following circumstances apply to you:
1. You are pregnant, intending to become pregnant, or are breast-feeding
2. You have any medication allergies
3. You are using any prescription medications or over-the-counter medications; remember to include any medications prescribed by your dentist and any herbal or natural products
4. You have any medical problems
5. You have had any problems with this medication in the past

INSTRUCTIONS ON APPROPRIATE USE OF THIS MEDICATION
- Take this medication exactly as recommended by your HCP. Do not take more or less than recommended dosage. Talk with your HCP concerning what you ought to do about missed doses of medication should this occur.
- Know the name, spelling, and milligram dosage amount of your medication. This may be written down on a card kept in your wallet or purse. This information is extremely important should you become suddenly ill or are involved in an emergency situation.
- Always try to take this medication at the same time of day. Valproate is usually taken 2-3 times/day. Your HCP will determine the appropriate dosage of valproate for you by checking valproate blood levels periodically.
- Store medication in a clean, dry place at room temperature, away from children.

PRECAUTIONS
- Improvement in mood stability (mood "leveling out") may require 1-3 weeks. Do not abruptly stop medication as there may be a drug withdrawal reaction.
- This medication may add to the effects of alcohol or other drugs.
- Do not use alcohol or "street" drugs while on this medication.
- If this medication makes you sleepy or drowsy, do not operate heavy machinery or a motor vehicle as this may be hazardous.
- Tell your HCP immediately if you become pregnant while on this medication.
- Do not take any new or additional prescription or over-the-counter medications without discussing them with your HCP. This includes herbal or natural products.
- Dizziness or light-headedness may occur, particularly when getting up quickly from a seated or lying down position. Getting up slowly may help.

MEDICATIONS TO STABILIZE MOOD *(Continued)*

COMMON SIDE EFFECTS

All drugs are associated with side effects. Most side effects are mild, and often may improve over time. Discuss side effects of this medication with your HCP prior to starting therapy, including how you should contact your HCP if side effects occur. The following side effects are common with valproate and should be discussed with your HCP.

- Tiredness
- Nausea, abdominal cramping (mild)
- Hand/arm trembling
- Weight change (usually gain)
- Menstrual period changes
- Blurred vision
- Unsteadiness

More rare side effects include severe nausea/abdominal cramping, severe fatigue, easy bruising/bleeding, severe dizziness, soreness of mouth or gums, eye rolling/abnormal movements. Report these symptoms immediately to your HCP. Your HCP may use a blood test to check for valproate overdose (toxicity) as well as any physical or neurological examinations. Other side effects not listed may occur in some individuals. If these occur, report them to your HCP.

CARBAMAZEPINE

TYPE OF MEDICATION:
Anticonvulsant; used in psychiatry as a mood stabilizer

MEDICATIONS IN THIS GROUP

Carbamazepine (Tegretol®, generic formulations) *on page 61* is not approved by the FDA as a mood stabilizer but has been widely used in this capacity by physicians for many years.

THIS MEDICATION IS USED FOR:

Treatment of manic-depressive (bipolar) disorder, seizure disorder, post-traumatic stress disorder, chronic pain, and severe aggressive behavior.

DIRECTIONS BEFORE TAKING THIS MEDICATION

Tell your healthcare provider (HCP) if any of the following circumstances apply to you:

1. You are pregnant, intending to become pregnant, or are breast-feeding

2. You have any medication allergies

3. You are using any prescription medications or over-the-counter medications; remember to include any medications prescribed by your dentist and any herbal or natural products

4. You have any medical problems

5. You have had any problems with this medication in the past

6. You have ever had a disorder of low red blood cell count (anemia) or low white blood cell count (neutropenia)

INSTRUCTIONS ON APPROPRIATE USE OF THIS MEDICATION

- Take this medication exactly as recommended by your HCP. Do not take more or less than recommended dosage. Talk with your HCP concerning what you ought to do about missed doses of medication should this occur.

- Know the name, spelling, and milligram dosage amount of your medication. This may be written down on a card kept in your wallet or purse. This information is extremely important should you become suddenly ill or are involved in an emergency situation.

- Always try to take this medication at the same time of day. Carbamazepine is usually taken 2-3 times/day. Your HCP will determine the appropriate dosage of carbamazepine for you by checking carbamazepine blood levels periodically.

- Store medication in a clean, dry place at room temperature, away from children.

PRECAUTIONS

- Improvement in mood stability (mood "leveling out") may require 1-3 weeks. Do not abruptly stop medication as there may be a drug withdrawal reaction.

- This medication may add to the effects of alcohol or other drugs.

- Do not use alcohol or "street" drugs while on this medication.

MEDICATIONS TO STABILIZE MOOD *(Continued)*

- If this medication makes you sleepy or drowsy, do not operate heavy machinery or a motor vehicle as this may be hazardous.

- Tell your HCP immediately if you become pregnant while on this medication.

- Do not take any new or additional prescription or over-the-counter medications without discussing them with your HCP. This includes herbal or natural products.

- Dizziness or light-headedness may occur, particularly when getting up quickly from a seated or lying down position. Getting up slowly may help.

- In rare cases, carbamazepine may be associated with a decrease in white blood cells, the cells in a person's blood which fight infection. For this reason, your HCP may decide to order a blood test periodically to screen for blood abnormalities.

COMMON SIDE EFFECTS

All drugs are associated with side effects. Most side effects are mild, and often may improve over time. Discuss side effects of this medication with your HCP prior to starting therapy, including how you should contact your HCP if side effects occur. The following side effects are common with carbamazepine and should be discussed with your HCP.

- Tiredness
- Dizziness
- Blurred vision
- Muscle incoordination
- Dry mouth
- Weight gain
- Nausea

More rare side effects include confusion, severe nausea, severe fatigue, easy bruising or bleeding, gum or mouth soreness, skin rash. Report these symptoms immediately to your HCP. Your HCP may use a blood test to check for carbamazepine overdose (toxicity) as well as any physical or neurological examinations. Other side effects not listed may occur in some individuals. If these occur, report them to your HCP.

GABAPENTIN

TYPE OF MEDICATION:

Anticonvulsant; used in psychiatry as a mood stabilizer

MEDICATIONS IN THIS GROUP

Gabapentin (Neurontin®) *on page 161* is not approved by the FDA as a mood stabilizer but has been used in this capacity by physicians.

THIS MEDICATION IS USED FOR:

Prevention or reduction of the number of seizures a person has; also used to treat painful neuropathies and as a mood stabilizer in bipolar disorder.

DIRECTIONS BEFORE TAKING THIS MEDICATION

Tell your healthcare provider (HCP) if any of the following circumstances apply to you:

1. You are pregnant, intending to become pregnant, or are breast-feeding.
2. You have any medication allergies.
3. You are using any prescription medications or over-the-counter medications; remember to include any medications prescribed by your dentist and any herbal or natural products.
4. You have any medical problem.
5. You have had any problems with this medication in the past.

INSTRUCTIONS ON APPROPRIATE USE OF THIS MEDICATION

- Take this medication exactly as recommended by your HCP. Do not take more or less than recommended dosage. Talk with your HCP concerning what you ought to do about missed doses of medication should this occur.
  - Take a missed dose as soon as possible. If it is almost time for the next dose, skip the missed one and return to your regular schedule. Do not take a double dose or extra doses.
- Know the name, spelling, and milligram dosage amount of your medication. This may be written down on a card kept in your wallet or purse. This information is extremely important should you become suddenly ill or are involved in an emergency situation. Give this list to your HCP.
- Do not share your medication with others and do not take anyone else's medication.
- Take with or without food; take with food if medication causes stomach upset.
- Do not suddenly stop taking this medication if you have been taking it for a long time (dose should be slowly decreased).
- Store medication in a tight, light-resistant container at room temperature, away from children and pets.

MEDICATIONS TO STABILIZE MOOD *(Continued)*

PRECAUTIONS

- Avoid alcohol and other depressant medications (sedatives, tranquilizers, mood stabilizers, and pain medication) that slow your actions and reactions. Talk with your HCP.

- Wear disease medical alert identification if for seizure disorder.

- If this medication makes you sleepy or drowsy, do not operate heavy machinery or a motor vehicle as this may be hazardous.

- Tell your HCP immediately if you become pregnant while on this medication.

- Do not take any new or additional prescription or over-the-counter medications without discussing them with your HCP. This includes herbal and natural products.

COMMON SIDE EFFECTS

All drugs are associated with side effects. Most side effects are mild, and often may improve over time. Discuss side effects of this medication with your HCP prior to starting therapy, including how you should contact your HCP if side effects occur. The following side effects are more common and should be discussed with your HCP.

- Drowsiness

- Dizziness

- Fatigue

- Impaired judgment

- Changes in balance (staggering or feeling drunk)

- Weight gain

- Muscle jerks

More rare side effects include signs or symptoms of life-threatening reactions (eg, wheezing, tightness in the chest, fever, itching, severe cough, blue color to skin, convulsions), persistent sedation or drowsiness, passing out, fainting, dizziness, light-headedness, or any rash. Report these symptoms immediately to your HCP. Other side effects not listed may occur in some individuals. If these occur, report them to your HCP.

LAMOTRIGINE

TYPE OF MEDICATION:
Anticonvulsant; used in psychiatry as a mood stabilizer

MEDICATIONS IN THIS GROUP

Lamotrigine (Lamictal®) *on page 187* is not approved by the FDA as a mood stabilizer but has been used in this capacity by physicians.

THIS MEDICATION IS USED FOR:
Prevention or reduction of the number of seizures a person has; also used to treat painful neuropathies and as a mood stabilizer in bipolar disorder.

DIRECTIONS BEFORE TAKING THIS MEDICATION
Tell your healthcare provider (HCP) if any of the following circumstances apply to you:

1. You are pregnant, intending to become pregnant, or are breast-feeding.
2. Notify HCP if you are currently taking valproic acid (Depacon®, Depakene®, Depakote®) or carbamazepine (Tegretol® Epitol®) as dosing modifications are necessary.
3. You have any medication allergies.
4. You are using any prescription medications or over-the-counter medications; remember to include any medications prescribed by your dentist and any herbal or natural products.
5. You have any medical problem.
6. You have had any problems with this medication in the past.

INSTRUCTIONS ON APPROPRIATE USE OF THIS MEDICATION

- Take this medication exactly as recommended by your HCP. Do not take more or less than recommended dosage. Talk with your HCP concerning what you ought to do about missed doses of medication should this occur.

  - Take a missed dose as soon as possible. If it is almost time for the next dose, skip the missed one and return to your regular schedule. Do not take a double dose or extra doses.

- Know the name, spelling, and milligram dosage amount of your medication. This may be written down on a card kept in your wallet or purse. This information is extremely important should you become suddenly ill or are involved in an emergency situation. Give this list to your HCP.

- Do not share your medication with others and do not take anyone else's medication.

- Take with or without food; take with food if medication causes stomach upset.

- Do not suddenly stop taking this medication if you have been taking it for a long time (dose should be slowly decreased).

- Store medication in a tight, light-resistant container protected from moisture at room temperature, away from children and pets.

MEDICATIONS TO STABILIZE MOOD *(Continued)*

PRECAUTIONS

- Avoid alcohol and other depressant medications (sedatives, tranquilizers, mood stabilizers, and pain medication) that slow your actions and reactions. Talk with your HCP.
- There may be an interaction with valproic acid (Depakote®, Depakene®, Depacon®) or carbamazepine (Epitol®, Tegretol®); notify HCP; dosing adjustment is necessary.
- Wear disease medical alert identification if for seizure disorder.
- If this medication makes you sleepy or drowsy, do not operate heavy machinery or a motor vehicle as this may be hazardous.
- Tell your HCP immediately if you become pregnant while on this medication.
- Do not take any new or additional prescription or over-the-counter medications without discussing them with your HCP. This includes herbal and natural products.

COMMON SIDE EFFECTS

All drugs are associated with side effects. Most side effects are mild, and often may improve over time. Discuss side effects of this medication with your HCP prior to starting therapy, including how you should contact your HCP if side effects occur. The following side effects are more common and should be discussed with your HCP.

- Drowsiness
- Dizziness
- Fatigue
- Impaired judgment
- Nausea
- Vomiting
- Headache
- Changes in balance
- Blurred or double vision
- Rash (call your HCP immediately if this occurs)

More rare side effects include signs or symptoms of life-threatening reactions (eg, wheezing, tightness in the chest, fever, itching, severe cough, blue color to skin, convulsions), persistent sedation or drowsiness, passing out, fainting, dizziness, light-headedness, or any rash. Report these symptoms immediately to your HCP. Other side effects not listed may occur in some individuals. If these occur, report them to your HCP.

STIMULANTS

TYPE OF MEDICATION:

Stimulant

MEDICATIONS IN THIS GROUP

Typical medications in this group include:

Dextroamphetamine (Dexedrine®, Oxydess®, Spancap®) *on page 105*

Methylphenidate (Ritalin®) *on page 236*

Modafinil (Provigil®) *on page 247*

Pemoline (Cylert®) *on page 287*

THIS MEDICATION IS USED FOR:

Pemoline and amphetamine compounds: Treatment of attention deficit hyperactivity disorder (ADHD), primarily in children, for some types of depressive illness, for some sleep disorders, and in Parkinson's disease

Modafinil (Provigil®): Treatment of daytime sleepiness due to narcolepsy

DIRECTIONS BEFORE TAKING THIS MEDICATION

Tell your healthcare provider (HCP) if any of the following circumstances apply to you:

1. You are pregnant, intending to become pregnant, or are breast-feeding

2. You have any medication allergies

3. You are using any prescription medications or over-the-counter medications; remember to include any medications prescribed by your dentist and any herbal or natural products

4. You have any medical problems

5. You have had any problems with this medication in the past

INSTRUCTIONS ON APPROPRIATE USE OF THIS MEDICATION

- Know the name, spelling, and milligram dosage amount of your medication. This may be written down on a card kept in your wallet or purse. This information is extremely important should you become suddenly ill or are involved in an emergency situation.

- Always try to take this medication at the same time of day. Stimulants are generally given 1-2 times daily. Some stimulants are available in short-acting and slow-release (SR) forms.

- Store medication in a clean, dry place at room temperature, away from children.

STIMULANTS *(Continued)*

PRECAUTIONS

- Improvement in attention span and restless in ADHD may require up to 3 weeks to improve.

- This medication may add to the effects of alcohol or other drugs.

- Do not use alcohol or "street" drugs while on this medication.

- If this medication makes you sleepy or drowsy, do not operate heavy machinery or a motor vehicle as this may be hazardous.

- Tell your HCP immediately if you become pregnant while on this medication.

- Do not take any new or additional prescription or over-the-counter medications without discussing them with your HCP. This includes any herbal or natural products.

- Dizziness or light-headedness may occur, particularly when getting up quickly from a seated or lying down position. Getting up slowly may help.

- All stimulant drugs have potential for addiction. Pemoline is generally less likely to become a drug of abuse compared to methylphenidate and dextroamphetamine. All medications should be used responsibly and exactly as prescribed. Care should be taken that they are not used by anyone except the individual for whom they are prescribed.

- Liver damage has been reported in rare cases with pemoline. Tell your HCP if you have ever had liver disease before beginning to take pemoline.

COMMON SIDE EFFECTS

All drugs are associated with side effects. Most side effects are mild, and often may improve over time. Discuss side effects of this medication with your HCP prior to starting therapy, including how you should contact your HCP if side effects occur. The following side effects are more common with stimulants and should be discussed with your HCP.

- Decreased sleep
- Decreased appetite and weight
- Anxiousness
- Increased pulse rate and blood pressure
- Headache
- Nausea
- Blurred vision

More rare side effects include muscle twitching, severe headache, extreme increase in pulse rate, severe agitation, elevated mood, or skin rash. Report these symptoms immediately to your HCP. Other side effects not listed may occur in some individuals. If these occur, report them to your HCP.

ANXIOLYTICS & SEDATIVE/HYPNOTICS

BENZODIAZEPINES

TYPE OF MEDICATION:

Anxiolytic, sedative/hypnotic

MEDICATIONS IN THIS GROUP

Typical medications in this group include:

THIS MEDICATION IS USED FOR:

Treatment of insomnia, anxiety/agitation, panic disorder, and alcohol withdrawal. Frequently prescribed with other psychiatric medications, such as antidepressants.

DIRECTIONS BEFORE TAKING THIS MEDICATION

Tell your healthcare provider (HCP) if any of the following circumstances apply to you:

1. You are pregnant, intending to become pregnant, or are breast-feeding.

2. You have any medication allergies.

3. You are using any prescription medications or over-the-counter medications; remember to include any medications prescribed by your dentist and any herbal or natural products.

4. You have any medical problems.

5. You have had any problems with this medication in the past.

6. You have ever been addicted to or abused alcohol or any other drugs, especially benzodiazepines.

ANXIOLYTICS & SEDATIVE/HYPNOTICS *(Continued)*

INSTRUCTIONS ON APPROPRIATE USE OF THIS MEDICATION

- Take this medication exactly as recommended by your HCP. Do not take more or less than recommended dosage. Talk with your HCP concerning what you ought to do about missed doses of medication should this occur.

- Know the name, spelling, and milligram dosage amount of your medication. This may be written down on a card kept in your wallet or purse. This information is extremely important should you become suddenly ill or are involved in an emergency situation.

- Benzodiazepines may be prescribed to be taken on a regular basis, either at bedtime or several times daily. In some cases, benzodiazepines are prescribed to be taken on as "as needed" basis.

- Store medication in a clean, dry place at room temperature, away from children.

PRECAUTIONS

- Benzodiazepines may be habit-forming. Do not exceed prescribed dosage, or take medication for a longer period than is prescribed. Do not abruptly stop medication as there may be a drug withdrawal reaction

- This medication may add to the effects of alcohol or other drugs.

- Do not use alcohol or "street" drugs while on this medication.

- If this medication makes you sleepy or drowsy, do not operate heavy machinery or a motor vehicle as this may be hazardous.

- Tell your HCP immediately if you become pregnant while on this medication.

- Do not take any new or additional prescription or over-the-counter medications without discussing them with your HCP. This includes natural and herbal products.

- Dizziness or light-headedness may occur, particularly when getting up quickly from a seated or lying down position. Getting up slowly may help.

- Coffee or other caffeine-containing beverages may counteract the effects of benzodiazepines. Limiting the amount of caffeine-containing beverages consumed will avoid this problem.

COMMON SIDE EFFECTS

All drugs are associated with side effects. Most side effects are mild, and often may improve over time. Discuss side effects of this medication with your HCP prior to starting therapy, including how you should contact your HCP if side effects occur. The following side effects are more common with benzodiazepine medications and should be discussed with your HCP.

- Drowsiness

- Muscle weakness or problems with muscle coordination

- Forgetfulness or difficulty concentrating

- Slurred speech

- Dizziness

More rare side effects include severe drowsiness or clumsiness, confusion, agitation or excitement, severe dizziness, skin rash, slowed heart rate. Report these symptoms immediately to your HCP. Other side effects not listed may occur in some individuals. If these occur, report them to your HCP.

BARBITURATES

TYPE OF MEDICATION:

Anxiolytic, sedative/hypnotic

MEDICATIONS IN THIS GROUP

Typical medications in this group include:

Amobarbital (Amytal®) *on page 31*
Amobarbital and Secobarbital (Tuinal®) *on page 34*
Butabarbital Sodium (Butalan®, Buticaps®, Butisol®) *on page 57*
Hexobarbital (Pre-Sed®) *on page 176*
Mephobarbital (Mebaral®)
Pentobarbital (Nembutal®) *on page 289*
Phenobarbital (Barbita®, Luminal®, Solfoton®) *on page 302*
Primidone (Mysoline®) *on page 325*
Secobarbital (Seconal™) *on page 367*
Thiopental (Pentothal®) *on page 390*

THIS MEDICATION IS USED FOR:

Treatment of insomnia, anxiety/agitation. Generally reserved for situations where other medications have been ineffective.

DIRECTIONS BEFORE TAKING THIS MEDICATION

Tell your healthcare provider (HCP) if any of the following circumstances apply to you:

1. You are pregnant, intending to become pregnant, or are breast-feeding.

2. You have any medication allergies.

3. You are using any prescription medications or over-the-counter medications; remember to include any medications prescribed by your dentist and any herbal or natural products.

4. You have any medical problems.

5. You have had any problems with this medication in the past.

6. You have ever been addicted to or abused alcohol or any other drugs, especially barbiturates.

INSTRUCTIONS ON APPROPRIATE USE OF THIS MEDICATION

*   Take this medication exactly as recommended by your HCP. Do not take more or less than recommended dosage. Talk with your HCP concerning what you ought to do about missed doses of medication should this occur.

*   Know the name, spelling, and milligram dosage amount of your medication. This may be written down on a card kept in your wallet or purse. This information is extremely important should you become suddenly ill or are involved in an emergency situation.

*   Barbiturates may be prescribed to be taken on a regular basis, either at bedtime or several times daily. In some cases, barbiturates are prescribed to be taken on as "as needed" basis.

*   Store medication in a clean, dry place at room temperature, away from children.

ANXIOLYTICS & SEDATIVE/HYPNOTICS *(Continued)*

PRECAUTIONS

- Barbiturates may be habit-forming. Do not exceed prescribed dosage, or take medication for a longer period than is prescribed. Do not abruptly stop medication as there may be a drug withdrawal reaction

- This medication may add to the effects of alcohol or other drugs.

- Do not use alcohol or "street" drugs while on this medication.

- If this medication makes you sleepy or drowsy, do not operate heavy machinery or a motor vehicle as this may be hazardous.

- Tell your HCP immediately if you become pregnant while on this medication.

- Do not take any new or additional prescription or over-the-counter medications without discussing them with your HCP. This includes natural and herbal products.

- Dizziness or light-headedness may occur, particularly when getting up quickly from a seated or lying down position. Getting up slowly may help.

- Coffee or other caffeine-containing beverages may counteract the effects of barbiturates. Limiting the amount of caffeine-containing beverages consumed will avoid this problem.

COMMON SIDE EFFECTS

All drugs are associated with side effects. Most side effects are mild, and often may improve over time. Discuss side effects of this medication with your HCP prior to starting therapy, including how you should contact your HCP if side effects occur. The following side effects are more common with barbiturate medications and should be discussed with your HCP.

- Drowsiness

- Muscle weakness or problems with muscle coordination

- Forgetfulness or difficulty concentrating

- Slurred speech

- Dizziness

More rare side effects include severe drowsiness or clumsiness, confusion, agitation or excitement, severe dizziness, skin rash, slowed heart rate. Report these symptoms immediately to your HCP. Other side effects not listed may occur in some individuals. If these occur, report them to your HCP.

BUSPIRONE

TYPE OF MEDICATION:

Anxiolytic (antianxiety medication)

MEDICATIONS IN THIS GROUP

Buspirone (BuSpar®) *on page 55* is the only medication in this group available in the U.S.

THIS MEDICATION IS USED FOR:

Treatment of generalized anxiety. Also used sometimes to treat premenstrual syndrome and to treat agitation, especially in older people.

DIRECTIONS BEFORE TAKING THIS MEDICATION

Tell your healthcare provider (HCP) if any of the following circumstances apply to you:

1. You are pregnant, intending to become pregnant, or are breast-feeding.

2. You have any medication allergies.

3. You are using any prescription medications or over-the-counter medications; remember to include any medications prescribed by your dentist and any herbal or natural products.

4. You have any medical problems.

5. You have had any problems with this medication in the past.

INSTRUCTIONS ON APPROPRIATE USE OF THIS MEDICATION

• Take this medication exactly as recommended by your HCP. Do not take more or less than recommended dosage. Talk with your HCP concerning what you ought to do about missed doses of medication should this occur.

• Know the name, spelling, and milligram dosage amount of your medication. This may be written down on a card kept in your wallet or purse. This information is extremely important should you become suddenly ill or are involved in an emergency situation.

• Always try to take this medication at the same time of day. Buspirone is generally prescribed twice daily.

• Store medication in a clean, dry place at room temperature, away from children.

PRECAUTIONS

• This medication may add to the effects of alcohol or other drugs.

• Do not use alcohol or "street" drugs while on this medication.

• If this medication makes you sleepy or drowsy, do not operate heavy machinery or a motor vehicle as this may be hazardous.

• Tell your HCP immediately if you become pregnant while on this medication.

• Do not take any new or additional prescription or over-the-counter medications without discussing them with your HCP. This includes natural and herbal products.

• Dizziness or light-headedness may occur, particularly when getting up quickly from a seated or lying down position. Getting up slowly may help.

ANXIOLYTICS & SEDATIVE/HYPNOTICS *(Continued)*

COMMON SIDE EFFECTS

All drugs are associated with side effects. Most side effects are mild, and often may improve over time. Discuss side effects of this medication with your HCP prior to starting therapy, including how you should contact your HCP if side effects occur. The following side effects are more common with buspirone and should be discussed with your HCP.

- Dizziness

- Headache

- Nausea

- Drowsiness

More rare side effects include severe drowsiness or dizziness, confusion, chest pain, fast heart rate, fever, weakness, or skin rash. Report these symptoms immediately to your HCP. Other side effects not listed may occur in some individuals. If these occur, report them to your HCP.

NONBENZODIAZEPINE HYPNOTICS

TYPE OF MEDICATION:

Sedative/hypnotic

MEDICATIONS IN THIS GROUP

Zaleplon (Sonata®) *on page 437*

Zolpidem (Ambien™) *on page 445*

THIS MEDICATION IS USED FOR:

Treatment of insomnia

DIRECTIONS BEFORE TAKING THIS MEDICATION

Tell your healthcare provider (HCP) if any of the following circumstances apply to you:

1. You are pregnant, intending to become pregnant, or are breast-feeding.

2. You have any medication allergies.

3. You are using any prescription medications or over-the-counter medications; remember to include any medications prescribed by your dentist and any herbal or natural products.

4. You have any medical problems.

5. You have had any problems with this medication in the past.

INSTRUCTIONS ON APPROPRIATE USE OF THIS MEDICATION

- Take this medication exactly as recommended by your HCP. Do not take more or less than recommended dosage. Talk with your HCP concerning what you ought to do about missed doses of medication should this occur.

- Know the name, spelling, and milligram dosage amount of your medication. This may be written down on a card kept in your wallet or purse. This information is extremely important should you become suddenly ill or are involved in an emergency situation.

- Always try to take this medication at the same time of day. Zolpidem and zaleplon are generally prescribed at bedtime. Zaleplon may be taken after going to bed and experiencing difficulty falling asleep.

- Store medication in a clean, dry place at room temperature, away from children.

PRECAUTIONS

- This medication may add to the effects of alcohol or other drugs.

- Do not use alcohol or "street" drugs while on this medication.

- If this medication makes you sleepy or drowsy, do not operate heavy machinery or a motor vehicle as this may be hazardous.

- Tell your HCP immediately if you become pregnant while on this medication.

- Do not take any new or additional prescription or over-the-counter medications without discussing them with your HCP. This includes natural and herbal products.

- Dizziness or light-headedness may occur, particularly when getting up quickly from a seated or lying down position. Getting up slowly may help.

ANXIOLYTICS & SEDATIVE/HYPNOTICS *(Continued)*

COMMON SIDE EFFECTS

All drugs are associated with side effects. Most side effects are mild, and often may improve over time. Discuss side effects of this medication with your HCP prior to starting therapy, including how you should contact your HCP if side effects occur. The following side effects are more common with zaleplon and zolpidem and should be discussed with your HCP.

- Drowsiness
- Dizziness
- Lightheadedness
- Difficulty with coordination

More rare side effects include severe dizziness or drowsiness, confusion, vomiting, shakiness, and memory loss. Report these symptoms immediately to your HCP. Other side effects not listed may occur in some individuals. If these occur, report them to your HCP.

AGENTS FOR THE TREATMENT OF ALZHEIMER'S DISEASE

ACETYLCHOLINESTERASE INHIBITOR

TYPE OF MEDICATION:
Alzheimer drug, acetylcholinesterase inhibitor

MEDICATIONS IN THIS GROUP

Donepezil (Aricept®) *on page 121*
Galantamine (Reminyl®) *on page 163*
Rivastigmine (Exelon®) *on page 357*
Tacrine (Cognex®) *on page 386*

THIS MEDICATION IS USED FOR:
Treatment of mild to moderate dementia of the Alzheimer's patient.

DIRECTIONS BEFORE TAKING THIS MEDICATION
Tell your healthcare provider (HCP) if any of the following circumstances apply to you:

1. You are pregnant, intending to become pregnant, or are breast-feeding.
2. You have any medication allergies.
3. You are using any prescription medications or over-the-counter medications; remember to include any medications prescribed by your dentist and any herbal or natural products.
4. You have any medical problems.
5. You have had any problems with this medication in the past.

INSTRUCTIONS ON APPROPRIATE USE OF THIS MEDICATION

- Take this medication exactly as recommended by your HCP. Do not take more or less than recommended dosage. Talk with your HCP concerning what you ought to do about missed doses of medication should this occur.
  - Take a missed dose as soon as possible. If it is almost time for the next dose, skip the missed dose and return to your regular schedule. Do not take a double dose or extra doses. Do not change dose or stop medicine. Talk with your HCP.
- Know the name, spelling, and milligram dosage amount of your medication. This may be written down on a card kept in your wallet or purse. This information is extremely important should you become suddenly ill or are involved in an emergency situation. Give this list to your HCP.
- Do not share your medication with others and do not take anyone else's medication.
- Take with food.
- Store medication in a tight container at room temperature, away from children and pets.

AGENTS FOR THE TREATMENT OF ALZHEIMER'S
DISEASE *(Continued)*

PRECAUTIONS

- Wear disease medical alert identification for Alzheimer's disease.
- Tell your HCP immediately if you become pregnant while on this medication.
- Do not take any new or additional prescription or over-the-counter medications without discussing them with your HCP. This includes herbal and natural products.
- Cautious use in liver disease; talk with your HCP.

COMMON SIDE EFFECTS

All drugs are associated with side effects. Most side effects are mild, and often may improve over time. Discuss side effects of this medication with your HCP prior to starting therapy, including how you should contact your HCP if side effects occur. The following side effects are more common and should be discussed with your HCP.

- Nausea
- Vomiting
- Diarrhea

More rare side effects include signs or symptoms of life-threatening reactions (eg, wheezing, tightness in the chest, fever, itching, severe cough, blue color to skin, convulsions), insomnia, muscle cramps, feeling tired, lack of appetite, belly pain, gas, or any rash. Report these symptoms immediately to your HCP. Other side effects not listed may occur in some individuals. If these occur, report them to your HCP.

AGENTS FOR TREATMENT OF EXTRAPYRAMIDAL SYMPTOMS

(Anti-EPS Medications)

TYPE OF MEDICATION:

Agent for the treatment of extrapyramidal symptoms

MEDICATIONS IN THIS GROUP

Typical medications in this group include:

THIS MEDICATION IS USED FOR:

Treatment of abnormal body movements caused by antipsychotic medications; also used to treat the symptoms of Parkinson's disease.

DIRECTIONS BEFORE TAKING THIS MEDICATION

Tell your healthcare provider (HCP) if any of the following circumstances apply to you:

1. You are pregnant, intending to become pregnant, or are breast-feeding

2. You have any medication allergies

3. You are using any prescription medications or over-the-counter medications; remember to include any medications prescribed by your dentist and any herbal or natural products

4. You have any medical problems

5. You have had any problems with this medication in the past

INSTRUCTIONS ON APPROPRIATE USE OF THIS MEDICATION

- Know the name, spelling, and milligram dosage amount of your medication. This may be written down on a card kept in your wallet or purse. This information is extremely important should you become suddenly ill or are involved in an emergency situation.

- Always try to take this medication at the same time of day. Anti-EPS medications are generally prescribed 2-3 times/day. Medications may be given in rapidly acting injectable forms, or as a tablet or liquid. In some cases, your HCP may recommend that you take this medication only "as needed."

- Store medication in a clean, dry place at room temperature, away from children.

AGENTS FOR TREATMENT OF EXTRAPYRAMIDAL
SYMPTOMS *(Continued)*

PRECAUTIONS

- Anti-EPS agents may work within a few minutes for injectable forms, and oral tablets may take up to several hours for full effectiveness. Your HCP may prescribe anti-EPS medications to be taken on a regular basis if abnormal body movements related to antipsychotic medication are a continuing problem for you.

- This medication may add to the effects of alcohol or other drugs.

- Do not use alcohol or "street" drugs while on this medication.

- If this medication makes you sleepy or drowsy, do not operate heavy machinery or a motor vehicle as this may be hazardous.

- Tell your HCP immediately if you become pregnant while on this medication.

- Do not take any new or additional prescription or over-the-counter medications without discussing them with your HCP.

- Dizziness or light-headedness may occur, particularly when getting up quickly from a seated or lying down position. Getting up slowly may help.

- Avoid extreme heat (eg, saunas) or activities that may lead to becoming overheated. Some individuals experience decreased ability for their body to tolerate high temperatures while on anti-EPS medications.

COMMON SIDE EFFECTS

All drugs are associated with side effects. Most side effects are mild, and often may improve over time. Discuss side effects of this medication with your HCP prior to starting therapy, including how you should contact your HCP if side effects occur. The following side effects are more common with EPS medications and should be discussed with your HCP.

- Tiredness
- Dizziness
- Blurred vision
- Dry mouth
- Constipation
- Nausea

More rare side effects include rapid heart rate, confusion, severe dizziness or fatigue, inability to urinate, small pupils of the eyes, or muscle cramping. Report these symptoms immediately to your HCP. Other side effects not listed may occur in some individuals. If these occur, report them to your HCP.

MISCELLANEOUS MEDICATIONS

CLONIDINE

TYPE OF MEDICATION:

Antihypertensive, alpha-adrenergic agonist, second-line agent for heroin or nicotine withdrawal.

MEDICATIONS IN THIS GROUP

Clonidine (Catapres®; Duraclon®) *on page 88*

THIS MEDICATION IS USED FOR:

Management of high blood pressure and to help with symptoms from heroin or nicotine withdrawal.

DIRECTIONS BEFORE TAKING THIS MEDICATION

Tell your healthcare provider (HCP) if any of the following circumstances apply to you:

1. You are pregnant, intending to become pregnant, or are breast-feeding.
2. You have any medication allergies.
3. You are using any prescription medications or over-the-counter medications; remember to include any medications prescribed by your dentist and any herbal or natural products.
4. You have any medical problems.
5. You have had any problems with this medication in the past.

INSTRUCTIONS ON APPROPRIATE USE OF THIS MEDICATION

- Take this medication exactly as recommended by your HCP. Do not take more or less than recommended dosage. Do not stop taking this medication abruptly. Talk with your HCP concerning what you ought to do about missed doses of medication should this occur.
  - For the tablet: Take a missed dose as soon as possible. If it is almost time for the next dose, skip the missed dose and return to your regular schedule.
  - For the skin patch: Apply the missed patch as soon as possible after removing the old one. If it is almost time for the next patch, then place the new patch immediately and keep on for 7 days. Start new schedule from the time the patch is replaced. Do not take a double dose or extra doses. Do not change dose or stop without talking with your HCP.
- Know the name, spelling, and milligram dosage amount of your medication. This may be written down on a card kept in your wallet or purse. This information is extremely important should you become suddenly ill or are involved in an emergency situation. Give this list to your HCP.
- Do not share your medication with others and do not take anyone else's medication.
- Store tablets in tight, light-resistant container at room temperature; store skin patch at room temperature away from children and pets.

MISCELLANEOUS MEDICATIONS (Continued)

PRECAUTIONS

- Avoid alcohol and other depressant medications (sedatives, tranquilizers, mood stabilizers, and pain medication) that slow your actions and reactions. Talk with your HCP.

- Wear disease medical alert identification if for high blood pressure.

- Do not take any new or additional prescription or over-the-counter medications without discussing them with your HCP. This includes herbal and natural products.

- If this medication makes you sleepy or drowsy, do not operate a machine or motor vehicle, as this may be dangerous.

- Tell your HCP immediately if you become pregnant while on this medication.

- If you are 65 or older, you may be more sensitive to side effects (drowsiness).

COMMON SIDE EFFECTS

All drugs are associated with side effects. Most side effects are mild, and often may improve over time. Discuss side effects of this medication with your HCP prior to starting therapy, including how you should contact your HCP if side effects occur. The following side effects are more common and should be discussed with your HCP.

- Drowsiness

- Dizziness (rise slowly over several minutes from sitting or lying position); be cautious when climbing

- Fatigue

- Impaired judgment

- Dry mouth

- Constipation

More rare side effects include life-threatening reactions (eg, wheezing, tightness in the chest, fever, itching, severe cough, blue color to skin, convulsions), persistent sedation or drowsiness, passing out, fainting, dizziness, or light-headedness, or any rash. Report these symptoms immediately to your HCP. Other side effects not listed may occur in some individuals. If these occur, report them to your HCP.

DISULFIRAM

TYPE OF MEDICATION:

Alcohol deterrent

MEDICATIONS IN THIS GROUP

Disulfiram (Antabuse®) *on page 119*

THIS MEDICATION IS USED FOR:

Treatment of chronic alcoholism; to prevent drinking alcohol.

DIRECTIONS BEFORE TAKING THIS MEDICATION

Tell your healthcare provider (HCP) if any of the following circumstances apply to you:

1.   You are pregnant, intending to become pregnant, or are breast-feeding.
2.   You have any medication allergies.
3.   You are using any prescription medications or over-the-counter medications; remember to include any medications prescribed by your dentist and any herbal or natural products.
4.   You have any medical problems.
5.   You have had any problems with this medication in the past.

INSTRUCTIONS ON APPROPRIATE USE OF THIS MEDICATION

•   Take this medication exactly as recommended by your HCP. Do not take more or less than recommended dosage. Talk with your HCP concerning what you ought to do about missed doses of medication should this occur.

   •   Take a missed dose as soon as possible. If it is almost time for the next dose, skip the missed dose and return to your regular schedule. Do not take a double dose or extra doses.

•   Know the name, spelling, and milligram dosage amount of your medication. This may be written down on a card kept in your wallet or purse. This information is extremely important should you become suddenly ill or are involved in an emergency situation. Give this list to your HCP.

•   Do not share your medication with others and do not take anyone else's medication.

•   Tablet may be crushed and mixed with nonalcoholic beverages.

•   Store in tight, light-resistant container at room temperature, away from children and pets.

MISCELLANEOUS MEDICATIONS *(Continued)*

PRECAUTIONS

- No alcohol intake (includes wine, beer, liquor, cough syrups, elixirs, and foods with alcohol) as it can cause a reaction that includes rapid heartbeats, sweating, chest pain, flushing, headache, nausea, shortness of breath, and low blood pressure.
- Do not use with other medications like chlorpropamide or metronidazole.
- Do not take any new or additional prescription or over-the-counter medications without discussing them with your HCP. This includes herbal and natural products.
- Limit caffeine (teas, coffee, colas) and chocolate intake.
- If this medication makes you sleepy or drowsy, do not operate a machine or motor vehicle, as this may be dangerous.
- Tell your HCP immediately if you become pregnant while on this medication.
- Inform your HCP if you are taking phenytoin.

COMMON SIDE EFFECTS

All drugs are associated with side effects. Most side effects are mild, and often may improve over time. Discuss side effects of this medication with your HCP prior to starting therapy, including how you should contact your HCP if side effects occur. The following side effects are more common and should be discussed with your HCP.

- Drowsiness
- Headache (mild pain medicine may help)

More rare side effects include life-threatening reactions (eg, wheezing, tightness in chest, fever, itching, severe cough, blue color to skin, convulsions), or any rash. Report these symptoms immediately to your HCP. Other side effects not listed may occur in some individuals. If these occur, report them to your HCP.

LEVODOPA AND CARBIDOPA

TYPE OF MEDICATION:

Anti-Parkinson's agent

MEDICATIONS IN THIS GROUP

Levodopa and Carbidopa (Sinemet®) *on page 193*

THIS MEDICATION IS USED FOR:

Treatment of symptoms of Parkinson's syndrome.

DIRECTIONS BEFORE TAKING THIS MEDICATION

Tell your healthcare provider (HCP) if any of the following circumstances apply to you:

1. You are pregnant, intending to become pregnant, or are breast-feeding.
2. You have any medication allergies.
3. You are using any prescription medications or over-the-counter medications; remember to include any medications prescribed by your dentist and any herbal or natural products.
4. You have any medical problems.
5. You have had any problems with this medication in the past.

INSTRUCTIONS ON APPROPRIATE USE OF THIS MEDICATION

- Take this medication exactly as recommended by your HCP. Do not take more or less than recommended dosage. Talk with your HCP concerning what you ought to do about missed doses of medication should this occur.
  - Take a missed dose as soon as possible. If it is almost time for the next dose, skip the missed dose and return to your regular schedule. Do not take a double dose or extra doses. Do not change dose or stop medicine. Talk with your HCP.
- Know the name, spelling, and milligram dosage amount of your medication. This may be written down on a card kept in your wallet or purse. This information is extremely important should you become suddenly ill or are involved in an emergency situation. Give this list to your HCP.
- Do not share your medication with others and do not take anyone else's medication.
- Take with or without food; take with food if medication causes stomach upset.
- Do not take high protein foods with this medication.
- May break sustained release tablet in half, but do not chew or crush.
- Store medication in a tight, light-resistant container at room temperature, away from children and pets.

PRECAUTIONS

- Tell your HCP immediately if you become pregnant while on this medication.
- Do not take any new or additional prescription or over-the-counter medications without discussing them with your HCP. This includes herbal and natural products.

MISCELLANEOUS MEDICATIONS *(Continued)*

COMMON SIDE EFFECTS

All drugs are associated with side effects. Most side effects are mild, and often may improve over time. Discuss side effects of this medication with your HCP prior to starting therapy, including how you should contact your HCP if side effects occur. The following side effects are more common and should be discussed with your HCP.

- Nausea
- Vomiting
- Stomach pain and cramps
- Constipation
- Involuntary movements

More rare side effects include signs or symptoms of life-threatening reactions (eg, wheezing, tightness in the chest, fever, itching, severe cough, blue color to skin, convulsions), or any rash. Report these symptoms immediately to your HCP. Other side effects not listed may occur in some individuals. If these occur, report them to your HCP.

LEVOMETHADYL ACETATE HYDROCHLORIDE

TYPE OF MEDICATION:
Narcotic, analgesic

MEDICATIONS IN THIS GROUP
Levomethadyl Acetate Hydrochloride (ORLAAM®) *on page 196*

THIS MEDICATION IS USED FOR:
Treatment of narcotic dependence; prevents drug-seeking behavior and blocks the high from heroin.

DIRECTIONS BEFORE TAKING THIS MEDICATION
Tell your healthcare provider (HCP) if any of the following circumstances apply to you:

1. You are pregnant, intending to become pregnant, or are breast-feeding.
2. You have any medication allergies.
3. You are using any prescription medications or over-the-counter medications; remember to include any medications prescribed by your dentist and any herbal or natural products.
4. You have any medical problems.
5. You have had any problems with this medication in the past.

INSTRUCTIONS ON APPROPRIATE USE OF THIS MEDICATION
- Take this medication exactly as recommended by your HCP. Do not take more or less than recommended dosage. Talk with your HCP concerning what you ought to do about missed doses of medication should this occur.
- Know the name, spelling, and milligram dosage amount of your medication. This may be written down on a card kept in your wallet or purse. This information is extremely important should you become suddenly ill or are involved in an emergency situation. Give this list to your HCP.
- Do not share your medication with others and do not take anyone else's medication.
- This medication must always be diluted before taking and should be mixed before administration; it is usually given 3 times/week.
- Store medication in original container, protected from light, at room temperature, away from children and pets.

PRECAUTIONS
- No alcohol intake (includes wine, beer, and liquor) or illicit drug use as it could result in death or serious injury.
- You may not be alert; use care when driving, doing other tasks, or hobbies.
- If you have lung disease tell your HCP; you may be more sensitive to this medication and your breathing may worsen.
- Tell your HCP immediately if you become pregnant while on this medication.
- Do not take any new or additional prescription or over-the-counter medications without discussing them with your HCP. This includes herbal and natural products.

MISCELLANEOUS MEDICATIONS *(Continued)*

COMMON SIDE EFFECTS

All drugs are associated with side effects. Most side effects are mild, and often may improve over time. Discuss side effects of this medication with your HCP prior to starting therapy, including how you should contact your HCP if side effects occur. The following side effects are more common and should be discussed with your HCP:

- Feeling tired and worn out
- Stomach pain and cramps
- Constipation
- Inability to sleep
- Nervousness
- Sweating
- Change in sexual ability or desire

More rare side effects include signs or symptoms of life-threatening reactions (eg, wheezing, tightness in the chest, fever, itching, severe cough, blue color to skin, convulsions), hot flashes, abnormal dreams, headache, or any rash. Report these symptoms immediately to your HCP. Other side effects not listed may occur in some individuals. If these occur, report them to your HCP.

METHADONE

TYPE OF MEDICATION:
Narcotic; analgesic

MEDICATIONS IN THIS GROUP
Methadone (Dolophine®) *on page 228*

THIS MEDICATION IS USED FOR:
Treatment of narcotic dependence; prevents drug-seeking behavior and blocks the high from heroin.

DIRECTIONS BEFORE TAKING THIS MEDICATION
Tell your healthcare provider (HCP) if any of the following circumstances apply to you:
1. You are pregnant, intending to become pregnant, or are breast-feeding.
2. You have any medication allergies.
3. You are using any prescription medications or over-the-counter medications; remember to include any medications prescribed by your dentist and any herbal or natural products.
4. You have any medical problems.
5. You have had any problems with this medication in the past.

INSTRUCTIONS ON APPROPRIATE USE OF THIS MEDICATION
- Take this medication exactly as recommended by your HCP. Do not take more or less than recommended dosage. Talk with your HCP concerning what you ought to do about missed doses of medication should this occur.
- Know the name, spelling, and milligram dosage amount of your medication. This may be written down on a card kept in your wallet or purse. This information is extremely important should you become suddenly ill or are involved in an emergency situation. Give this list to your HCP.
- Do not share your medication with others and do not take anyone else's medicine.
- Dissolve dispersible tablet in fruit juice or water. Dilute liquid concentrate with half a glass of water.
- Store medication in a tight container at room temperature, away from children and pets.

PRECAUTIONS
- No alcohol intake (includes wine, beer, and liquor) or illicit drug use as it could result in death or serious injury.
- You may not be alert; use care when driving, doing other tasks, or hobbies.
- Tell your HCP immediately if you become pregnant while on this medication.
- Do not take any new or additional prescription or over-the-counter medications without discussing them with your HCP. This includes herbal and natural products.
- If you have lung disease tell your HCP; you may be more sensitive to this medication and your breathing may worsen.

MISCELLANEOUS MEDICATIONS *(Continued)*

COMMON SIDE EFFECTS

All drugs are associated with side effects. Most side effects are mild, and often may improve over time. Discuss side effects of this medication with your HCP prior to starting therapy, including how you should contact your HCP if side effects occur. The following side effects are more common and should be discussed with your HCP.

- Light-headedness
- Feeling tired and worn out
- Nausea
- Vomiting
- Constipation

More rare side effects include signs or symptoms of life-threatening reactions (eg, wheezing, tightness in the chest, fever, itching, severe cough, blue color to skin, convulsions), or any rash. Report any of these symptoms immediately to your HCP. Other side effects not listed may occur in some individuals. If these occur, report them to your HCP.

NALTREXONE

TYPE OF MEDICATION:
Antidote

MEDICATIONS IN THIS GROUP
Naltrexone (ReVia®) *on page 256*

THIS MEDICATION IS USED FOR:
Maintaining a narcotic-free state; can also be used in recovering alcoholics to maintain an alcohol-free state.

DIRECTIONS BEFORE TAKING THIS MEDICATION
Tell your healthcare provider (HCP) if any of the following circumstances apply to you:

1. You are pregnant, intending to become pregnant, or are breast-feeding.
2. You have any medication allergies.
3. You are using any prescription medications or over-the-counter medications; remember to include any medications prescribed by your dentist and any herbal or natural products.
4. You have any medical problems.
5. You have had any problems with this medication in the past.

INSTRUCTIONS ON APPROPRIATE USE OF THIS MEDICATION

- Take this medication exactly as recommended by your HCP. Do not take more or less than recommended dosage. Talk with your HCP concerning what you ought to do about missed doses of medication should this occur.
- Know the name, spelling, and milligram dosage amount of your medication. This may be written down on a card kept in your wallet or purse. This information is extremely important should you become suddenly ill or are involved in an emergency situation. Give this list to your HCP.
- Do not share your medication with others and do not take anyone else's medication.
- Take with or without food; take with food if medication causes stomach upset.
- Store medication in a tight container at room temperature, away from children and pets.

PRECAUTIONS

- You may not be alert; use care when driving, doing other tasks, or hobbies.
- Tell your HCP immediately if you become pregnant while on this medication.
- Do not take any new or additional prescription or over-the-counter medications without discussing them with your HCP. This includes herbal and natural products.
- No alcohol intake (includes wine, beer, and liquor) or illicit drug use as it could result in death or serious injury.
- If you have lung disease tell your HCP; you may be more sensitive to this medication and your breathing may worsen.

MISCELLANEOUS MEDICATIONS *(Continued)*

COMMON SIDE EFFECTS

All drugs are associated with side effects. Most side effects are mild, and often may improve over time. Discuss side effects of this medication with your HCP prior to starting therapy, including how you should contact your HCP if side effects occur. The following side effects are more common and should be discussed with your HCP.

- Light-headedness
- Dizziness
- Feeling tired and worn out
- Nausea
- Vomiting
- Headache
- Inability to sleep
- Nervousness

More rare side effects include signs or symptoms of life-threatening reactions (eg, wheezing, tightness in the chest, fever, itching, severe cough, blue color to skin, convulsions), or any rash. Report these symptoms immediately to your HCP. Other side effects not listed may occur in some individuals. If these occur, report them to your HCP.

NICOTINE

TYPE OF MEDICATION:
Antidote

MEDICATIONS IN THIS GROUP
Nicotine (various products) *on page 264*

THIS MEDICATION IS USED FOR:
Treatment of symptoms of nicotine withdrawal when you stop smoking.

DIRECTIONS BEFORE TAKING THIS MEDICATION
Tell your healthcare provider (HCP) if any of the following circumstances apply to you:

1. You are pregnant, intending to become pregnant, or are breast-feeding.
2. You have any medication allergies.
3. You are using any prescription medications or over-the-counter medications; remember to include any medications prescribed by your dentist and any herbal or natural products.
4. You have any medical problems.
5. You have had any problems with this medication in the past.

INSTRUCTIONS ON APPROPRIATE USE OF THIS MEDICATION
- Take this medication exactly as recommended by your HCP. Do not take more or less than recommended dosage. Talk with your HCP concerning what you ought to do about missed doses of medication should this occur.
- Know the name, spelling, and milligram dosage amount of your medication. This may be written down on a card kept in your wallet or purse. This information is extremely important should you become suddenly ill or are involved in an emergency situation. Give this list to your HCP.
- Do not share your medication with others and do not take anyone else's medication.
- If using gum, chew slowly over 30 minutes; do not swallow gum. Do not eat or drink within 15 minutes of using gum. Gum chewing can cause problems with dental work.
- If using patch, use on clean, dry skin. Move site for each patch; use on trunk of body or upper arm (this includes chest, back, and belly).
- Store at room temperature, away from children and pets.

PRECAUTIONS
- Tell your HCP immediately if you become pregnant while on this medication.
- Do not take any new or additional prescription or over-the-counter medications without discussing them with your HCP. This includes herbal and natural products.
- Gum chewing can cause problems with dental work.
- When you stop smoking, other medications may be affected; talk with your HCP.

MISCELLANEOUS MEDICATIONS *(Continued)*

COMMON SIDE EFFECTS

All drugs are associated with side effects. Most side effects are mild, and often may improve over time. Discuss side effects of this medication with your HCP prior to starting therapy, including how you should contact your HCP if side effects occur. The following side effects are more common and should be discussed with your HCP.

- Light-headedness
- Dizziness
- Feeling tired and worn out
- Nausea
- Vomiting
- Headache
- Inability to sleep
- Nervousness
- Jaw ache when using gum
- Redness, itching, and burning at site when using patch

More rare side effects include signs or symptoms of life-threatening reactions (eg, wheezing, tightness in the chest, fever, itching, severe cough, blue color to skin, convulsions), or any rash. Report these symptoms immediately to your HCP. Other side effects not listed may occur in some individuals. If these occur, report them to your HCP.

ORLISTAT

TYPE OF MEDICATION:

Antiobesity

MEDICATIONS IN THIS GROUP

Orlistat (Xenical®) *on page 274*

THIS MEDICATION IS USED FOR:

Treatment of obesity.

DIRECTIONS BEFORE TAKING THIS MEDICATION

Tell your healthcare provider (HCP) if any of the following circumstances apply to you:

1. You are pregnant, intending to become pregnant, or are breast-feeding.
2. You have any medication allergies.
3. You are using any prescription medications or over-the-counter medications; remember to include any medications prescribed by your dentist and any herbal or natural products.
4. You have any medical problems.
5. You have had any problems with this medication in the past.

INSTRUCTIONS ON APPROPRIATE USE OF THIS MEDICATION

- Take this medication exactly as recommended by your HCP. Do not take more or less than recommended dosage. Talk with your HCP concerning what you ought to do about missed doses of medication should this occur.
  - Take a missed dose as soon as possible. If it is almost time for the next dose, skip the missed one and return to your regular schedule. Do not take a double dose or extra doses. Do not change dose or stop medicine. Talk with your HCP.
- Know the name, spelling, and milligram dosage amount of your medication. This may be written down on a card kept in your wallet or purse. This information is extremely important should you become suddenly ill or are involved in an emergency situation. Give this list to your HCP.
- Do not share your medication with others and do not take anyone else's medication.
- Take 3 times/day with each main meal containing fat.
- Store medication in a tight, light-resistant container at room temperature, away from children and pets.

PRECAUTIONS

- Tell your HCP immediately if you become pregnant while on this medication.
- Do not take any new or additional prescription or over-the-counter medications without discussing them with your HCP. This includes herbal and natural products.
- Vitamins should be taken 2 hours before or 2 hours after this medication.

MISCELLANEOUS MEDICATIONS *(Continued)*

COMMON SIDE EFFECTS

All drugs are associated with side effects. Most side effects are mild, and often may improve over time. Discuss side effects of this medication with your HCP prior to starting therapy, including how you should contact your HCP if side effects occur. The following side effects are more common and should be discussed with your HCP.

- Gas with discharge and/or oil spotting
- Feeling like you have to go to the bathroom

More rare side effects include signs or symptoms of life-threatening reactions (eg, wheezing, tightness in the chest, fever, itching, severe cough, blue color to skin, convulsions), or any rash. Report these symptoms immediately to your HCP. Other side effects not listed may occur in some individuals. If these occur, report them to your HCP.

PRAMIPEXOLE

TYPE OF MEDICATION:
Anti-Parkinson's agent

MEDICATIONS IN THIS GROUP

Pramipexole (Mirapex®) *on page 321*

THIS MEDICATION IS USED FOR:
Treatment of Parkinson's syndrome.

DIRECTIONS BEFORE TAKING THIS MEDICATION
Tell your healthcare provider (HCP) if any of the following circumstances apply to you:

1. You are pregnant, intending to become pregnant, or are breast-feeding.
2. You have any medication allergies.
3. You are using any prescription medications or over-the-counter medications; remember to include any medications prescribed by your dentist and any herbal or natural products.
4. You have any medical problems.
5. You have had any problems with this medication in the past.

INSTRUCTIONS ON APPROPRIATE USE OF THIS MEDICATION

- Take this medication exactly as recommended by your HCP. Do not take more or less than recommended dosage. Talk with your HCP concerning what you ought to do about missed doses of medication should this occur.

  - Take a missed dose as soon as possible. If it is almost time for the next dose, skip the missed dose and return to your regular schedule. Do not take a double dose or extra doses. Do not change dose or stop medicine. Talk with your HCP.

- Know the name, spelling, and milligram dosage amount of your medication. This may be written down on a card kept in your wallet or purse. This information is extremely important should you become suddenly ill or are involved in an emergency situation. Give this list to your HCP.

- Do not share your medication with others and do not take anyone else's medication.

- Take with or without food; take with food if medication causes stomach upset.

- Store medication in a tight, light-resistant container at room temperature, away from children and pets.

PRECAUTIONS

- Tell your HCP immediately if you become pregnant while on this medication.

- Do not take any new or additional prescription or over-the-counter medications without discussing them with your HCP. This includes herbal and natural products.

- Avoid alcohol (includes wine, beer, and liquor) and other medications that slow your actions and reactions. This includes sedatives, tranquilizers, mood stabilizers, and pain medication; talk with your HCP.

MISCELLANEOUS MEDICATIONS *(Continued)*

COMMON SIDE EFFECTS

All drugs are associated with side effects. Most side effects are mild, and often may improve over time. Discuss side effects of this medication with your HCP prior to starting therapy, including how you should contact your HCP if side effects occur. The following side effects are more common and should be discussed with your HCP.

- Tiredness, sleepiness
- Dizziness (rise slowly over several minutes form sitting or lying position); use caution when climbing
- Inability to sleep
- Nausea
- Vomiting
- Constipation
- Hallucinations

More rare side effects include signs or symptoms of life-threatening reactions (eg, wheezing, tightness in the chest, fever, itching, severe cough, blue color to skin, convulsions), or any rash. Report these symptoms immediately to your HCP. Other side effects not listed may occur in some individuals. If these occur, report them to your HCP.

ROPINIROLE

TYPE OF MEDICATION:
Anti-Parkinson's agent

MEDICATIONS IN THIS GROUP
Ropinirole (Requip™) *on page 361*

THIS MEDICATION IS USED FOR:
Treatment and symptoms of Parkinson's syndrome.

DIRECTIONS BEFORE TAKING THIS MEDICATION
Tell your healthcare provider (HCP) if any of the following circumstances apply to you:

1.   You are pregnant, intending to become pregnant, or are breast-feeding.
2.   You have any medication allergies.
3.   You are using any prescription medications or over-the-counter medications; remember to include any medications prescribed by your dentist and any herbal or natural products.
4.   You have any medical problems.
5.   You have had any problems with this medication in the past.

INSTRUCTIONS ON APPROPRIATE USE OF THIS MEDICATION
*   Take this medication exactly as recommended by your HCP. Do not take more or less than recommended dosage. Talk with your HCP concerning what you ought to do about missed doses of medication should this occur.
    *   Take a missed dose as soon as possible. If it is almost time for the next dose, skip the missed dose and return to your regular schedule. Do not take a double dose or extra doses.
*   Know the name, spelling, and milligram dosage amount of your medication. This may be written down on a card kept in your wallet or purse. This information is extremely important should you become suddenly ill or are involved in an emergency situation. Give this list to your HCP.
*   Do not share your medication with others and do not take anyone else's medication.
*   Take with or without food; take with food if medication causes stomach upset.
*   Store medication in a tight, light-resistant container at room temperature, away from children and pets.

PRECAUTIONS
*   Tell your HCP immediately if you become pregnant while on this medication.
*   You may not be alert; use care when driving, doing other tasks, or hobbies.
*   If you are 65 or older, you may have more side effects; you could feel dizzy and confused.
*   Do not take any new or additional prescription or over-the-counter medications without discussing them with your HCP. This includes herbal and natural products.
*   Avoid alcohol (includes wine, beer, and liquor) and other medications that slow your actions and reactions. This includes sedatives, tranquilizers, mood stabilizers, and pain medication; talk with your HCP.

MISCELLANEOUS MEDICATIONS *(Continued)*

COMMON SIDE EFFECTS

All drugs are associated with side effects. Most side effects are mild, and often may improve over time. Discuss side effects of this medication with your HCP prior to starting therapy, including how you should contact your HCP if side effects occur. The following side effects are more common and should be discussed with your HCP.

- Light-headedness
- Dizziness (rise slowly over several minutes form sitting or lying position); use caution when climbing
- Sleepiness/feeling tired
- Nausea
- Vomiting

More rare side effects include signs or symptoms of life-threatening reactions (eg, wheezing, tightness in the chest, fever, itching, severe cough, blue color to skin, convulsions), confusion, hallucinations, feeling faint, or any rash. Report these symptoms immediately to your HCP. Other side effects not listed may occur in some individuals. If these occur, report them to your HCP.

SELEGILINE

TYPE OF MEDICATION:
Anti-Parkinson's agent

MEDICATIONS IN THIS GROUP
Selegiline (Eldepryl®) *on page 370*

THIS MEDICATION IS USED FOR:
Treatment of early symptoms of Parkinson's disease.

DIRECTIONS BEFORE TAKING THIS MEDICATION
Tell your healthcare provider (HCP) if any of the following circumstances apply to you:

1. You are pregnant, intending to become pregnant, or are breast-feeding.
2. You have any medication allergies.
3. You are using any prescription medications or over-the-counter medications; remember to include any medications prescribed by your dentist and any herbal or natural products.
4. You have any medical problems.
5. You have had any problems with this medication in the past.

INSTRUCTIONS ON APPROPRIATE USE OF THIS MEDICATION
- Take this medication exactly as recommended by your HCP. Do not take more or less than recommended dosage. Talk with your HCP concerning what you ought to do about missed doses of medication should this occur.
  - Take a missed dose as soon as possible. If it is almost time for the next dose, skip the missed dose and return to your regular schedule. Do not take a double dose or extra doses. Do not change dose or stop medicine. Talk with your HCP.
- Know the name, spelling, and milligram dosage amount of your medication. This may be written down on a card kept in your wallet or purse. This information is extremely important should you become suddenly ill or are involved in an emergency situation. Give this list to your HCP.
- Do not share your medication with others and do not take anyone else's medication.
- Take with breakfast and lunch. Take early in the day to avoid sleep problems.
- Store medication in a tight, light-resistant container at room temperature, away from children and pets.

PRECAUTIONS
- Avoid alcohol (includes wine, beer, and liquor) as it can worsen side effects.
- Do not use this medicine with monoamine oxidase inhibitors. These include isocarboxazid, phenelzine, and tranylcypromine. Separate use by 2 weeks.
- Use caution if you have high blood pressure. Talk with HCP.
- Do not use over-the-counter products that may affect blood pressure. These include cough or cold remedies, diet pills, stimulants, ibuprofen or like products, certain herbs or supplements. Talk with HCP.

MISCELLANEOUS MEDICATIONS *(Continued)*

COMMON SIDE EFFECTS

All drugs are associated with side effects. Most side effects are mild, and often may improve over time. Discuss side effects of this medication with your HCP prior to starting therapy, including how you should contact your HCP if side effects occur. The following side effects are more common and should be discussed with your HCP.

- Feeling lightheaded or faint
- Nausea or vomiting
- Dizziness

More rare side effects include signs or symptoms of life-threatening reactions (eg, wheezing, tightness in the chest, fever, itching, severe cough, blue color to skin, convulsions), or any rash. Report these symptoms immediately to your HCP. Other side effects not listed may occur in some individuals. If these occur, report them to your HCP.

SIBUTRAMINE

TYPE OF MEDICATION:
Anorexiant

MEDICATIONS IN THIS GROUP
Sibutramine (Meridia®) *on page 378*

THIS MEDICATION IS USED FOR:
Treatment of obesity.

DIRECTIONS BEFORE TAKING THIS MEDICATION
Tell your healthcare provider (HCP) if any of the following circumstances apply to you:
1. You are pregnant, intending to become pregnant, or are breast-feeding.
2. You have any medication allergies.
3. You are using any prescription medications or over-the-counter medications; remember to include any medications prescribed by your dentist and any herbal or natural products.
4. You have any medical problems.
5. You have had any problems with this medication in the past.

INSTRUCTIONS ON APPROPRIATE USE OF THIS MEDICATION
*   Take this medication exactly as recommended by your HCP. Do not take more or less than recommended dosage. Talk with your HCP concerning what you ought to do about missed doses of medication should occur.
    *   Take a missed dose as soon as possible. If it is almost time for the next dose, skip the missed dose and return to your regular schedule. Do not take a double dose or extra doses.
*   Know the name, spelling, and milligram dosage amount of your medication. This may be written down on a card kept in your wallet or purse. This information is extremely important should you become suddenly ill or are involved in an emergency situation. Give this list to your HCP.
*   Do not share your medication with others and do not take anyone else's medication.
*   Follow diet as directed by your HCP. Take with or without food; take with food if medication causes stomach upset.
*   Store medication in a tight, light-resistant container at room temperature, away from children and pets.

PRECAUTIONS
*   Tell your HCP immediately if you become pregnant while on this medication.
*   Do not take any new or additional prescription or over-the-counter medications without discussing them with your HCP. This includes herbal and natural products.
*   Do not use if taking monoamine oxidase inhibitors (MAOIs).
*   Cautious use with high blood pressure; talk with your HCP.
*   Do not use over-the-counter products that may affect blood pressure (eg, cough/cold remedies, diet pills, stimulants, ibuprofen or like products, certain herbs/supplements); talk with your HCP.

MISCELLANEOUS MEDICATIONS *(Continued)*

COMMON SIDE EFFECTS

All drugs are associated with side effects. Most side effects are mild, and often may improve over time. Discuss side effects of this medication with your HCP prior to starting therapy, including how you should contact your HCP if side effects occur. The following side effects are more common and should be discussed with your HCP.

- Headache
- Loss of appetite
- Constipation
- Dry mouth
- Inability to sleep
- Light-headedness

More rare side effects include signs or symptoms of life-threatening reactions (eg, wheezing, tightness in the chest, fever, itching, severe cough, blue color to skin, convulsions), or any rash. Report these symptoms immediately to your HCP. Other side effects not listed may occur in some individuals. If these occur, report them to your HCP.

TOPIRAMATE

TYPE OF MEDICATION:
Anticonvulsant

MEDICATIONS IN THIS GROUP

Topiramate (Topamax®) *on page 403*

THIS MEDICATION IS USED FOR:
Treatment of partial onset seizures in adults along with other medication.

DIRECTIONS BEFORE TAKING THIS MEDICATION
Tell your healthcare provider (HCP) if any of the following circumstances apply to you:

1. You are pregnant, intending to become pregnant, or are breast-feeding.
2. You have any medication allergies.
3. You are using any prescription medications or over-the-counter medications; remember to include any medications prescribed by your dentist and any herbal or natural products.
4. You have any medical problems.
5. You have had any problems with this medication in the past.

INSTRUCTIONS ON APPROPRIATE USE OF THIS MEDICATION

- Take this medication exactly as recommended by your HCP. Do not take more or less than recommended dosage. Talk with your HCP concerning what you ought to do about missed doses of medication should this occur.
  - Take a missed dose as soon as possible. If it is almost time for the next dose, skip the missed dose and return to your regular schedule. Do not take a double dose or extra doses.
- Know the name, spelling, and milligram dosage amount of your medication. This may be written down on a card kept in your wallet or purse. This information is extremely important should you become suddenly ill or are involved in an emergency situation. Give this list to your HCP.
- Do not share your medication with others and do not take anyone else's medication.
- Take with or without food; take with food if medicine causes stomach upset.
- Swallow tablet whole; do not break (bitter taste).
- Take plenty of liquid everyday unless told to drink less liquid. Rarely causes kidney stones.
- Store medication in a tight container protected from moisture at room temperature, away from children and pets.

PRECAUTIONS

- Tell your HCP immediately if you become pregnant while on this medication.
- Do not take any new or additional prescription or over-the-counter medications without discussing them with your HCP. This includes herbal and natural products.
- Avoid alcohol (includes wine, beer, and liquor) and other medicines that slow your actions and reactions. This includes sedatives, tranquilizers, mood stabilizers, pain medication; talk with your HCP.
- You may not be alert; use care when driving, doing other tasks, or hobbies.

MISCELLANEOUS MEDICATIONS *(Continued)*

COMMON SIDE EFFECTS

All drugs are associated with side effects. Most side effects are mild, and often may improve over time. Discuss side effects of this medication with your HCP prior to starting therapy, including how you should contact your HCP if side effects occur. The following side effects are more common and should be discussed with your HCP.

- Light-headedness
- Dizziness
- Tired feeling
- Slowing of reactions
- Changes in balance
- Feeling shaky or unsteady
- Problems speaking
- Numbness and tingling of hands and feet

More rare side effects include signs or symptoms of life-threatening reactions (eg, wheezing, tightness in the chest, fever, itching, severe cough, blue color to skin, convulsions), nausea, depression, difficulty concentrating, kidney stones, and any rash. Report these symptoms immediately to your HCP. Other side effects not listed may occur in some individuals. If these occur, report them to your HCP.

ANTIMIGRAINE MEDICATIONS

ALMOTRIPTAN

TYPE OF MEDICATION:

Antimigraine, Serotonin 5-HT$_{1D}$ Receptor Agonist

MEDICATIONS IN THIS GROUP

Almotriptan (Axert™) *on page 14*

THIS MEDICATION IS USED FOR:

This medicine is used to get rid of, or decrease the pain and symptoms of, a migraine headache. It is **not** used to prevent future attacks. It may take 1-3 hours to feel the full benefits of this medicine.

DIRECTIONS BEFORE TAKING THIS MEDICATION

Tell your healthcare provider (HCP) if any of the following circumstances apply to you:

1. You are pregnant, intending to become pregnant, or are breast-feeding

2. You have any medication allergies

3. You are using any prescription medications or over-the-counter medications; remember to include any medications prescribed by your dentist and any herbal or natural products

4. You have any medical problems

5. You have had any problems with this medication in the past

INSTRUCTIONS ON APPROPRIATE USE OF THIS MEDICATION

*   Take with or without food. Take with food if this medicine causes an upset stomach.

*   If your headache comes back, take a second dose at least 2 hours after the first dose.

*   Do not take more than 2 doses in a 24-hour period.

*   Do not take within 24 hours of other migraine medication without consulting healthcare provider.

*   If you do not get any headache relief after the first dose call healthcare provider. Do not take a second dose.

MISCELLANEOUS MEDICATIONS (Continued)

PRECAUTIONS

- Avoid alcohol (includes wine, beer, and liquor). Can worsen headache.

- Do not take if you have a history of angina (chest pain from the heart), heart spasms, heart attack, or uncontrolled high blood pressure.

- Do not take within 24 hours of other headache medicines, like monoamine oxidase inhibitors. These include isocarboxazid, phenelzine, and tranylcypromine. Certain medicines do not mix well with this medicine. Talk with healthcare provider.

- Use caution if you have risk factors for heart disease (high blood pressure, high cholesterol, overweight, diabetes, cigarette smoking, a male >40 years of age, other family members with heart disease, postmenopausal women). Talk with healthcare provider.

- Tell healthcare provider if you are allergic to any medicine. Make sure to tell about the allergy and how it affected you. This includes telling about rash; hives; itching; shortness of breath; wheezing; cough; swelling of face, lips, tongue, throat; or any other symptoms involved.

COMMON SIDE EFFECTS

All drugs are associated with side effects. Most side effects are mild, and often may improve over time. Discuss side effects of this medication with your HCP prior to starting therapy, including how you should contact your HCP if side effects occur. The following side effects are more common and should be discussed with your HCP.

- Feeling sleepy or tired. Avoid driving, doing other tasks or activities that require you to be alert until you see how this medicine affects you.

- Nausea.

- Dry mouth.

- Numbness and tingling of feet, legs, hands, or arms.

More rare side effects include signs or symptoms of life-threatening reactions (eg, wheezing, chest pains, tightness in the chest, fever, itching, bad cough, blue skin color, fits, swelling of face, lips, tongue, or throat); no relief of headache after treatment, throat pain or tightness, fast heartbeats or shortness of breath, fainting, dizziness, light-headedness, and any rash. Report these symptoms immediately to your HCP. Other side effects not listed may occur in some individuals. If these occur, report them to your HCP.

NARATRIPTAN

TYPE OF MEDICATION:

Antimigraine, Serotonin 5-HT$_{1D}$ Receptor Agonist

MEDICATIONS IN THIS GROUP

Naratriptan (Amerge®) *on page 257*

THIS MEDICATION IS USED FOR:

This medicine is used to get rid of, or decrease the pain and symptoms of, a migraine headache. It is **not** used to prevent future attacks. It may take 1-3 hours to feel the full benefits of this medicine.

DIRECTIONS BEFORE TAKING THIS MEDICATION

Tell your healthcare provider (HCP) if any of the following circumstances apply to you:

1. You are pregnant, intending to become pregnant, or are breast-feeding

2. You have any medication allergies

3. You are using any prescription medications or over-the-counter medications; remember to include any medications prescribed by your dentist and any herbal or natural products

4. You have any medical problems

5. You have had any problems with this medication in the past

INSTRUCTIONS ON APPROPRIATE USE OF THIS MEDICATION

- Swallow tablet whole. Do not chew, break, or crush.

- Take with liquids as early as possible after the attack has started.

- If no headache relief by 4 hours after the first dose, then take another dose.

- Do not take more than 5 mg as a total daily dose.

- Do not take within 24 hours of other migraine medication without consulting healthcare provider.

MISCELLANEOUS MEDICATIONS *(Continued)*

PRECAUTIONS

- Avoid alcohol (includes wine, beer, and liquor). Can worsen headache.

- Do not take if you have a history of angina (chest pain from the heart), heart spasms, heart attack, or uncontrolled high blood pressure.

- Do not take within 24 hours of other headache medicines, like monoamine oxidase inhibitors. These include isocarboxazid, phenelzine, and tranylcypromine. Certain medicines do not mix well with this medicine. Talk with healthcare provider.

- Use caution if you have risk factors for heart disease (high blood pressure, high cholesterol, overweight, diabetes, cigarette smoking, a male >40 years of age, other family members with heart disease, postmenopausal women). Talk with healthcare provider.

- Tell healthcare provider if you are allergic to any medicine. Make sure to tell about the allergy and how it affected you. This includes telling about rash; hives; itching; shortness of breath; wheezing; cough; swelling of face, lips, tongue, throat; or any other symptoms involved.

COMMON SIDE EFFECTS

All drugs are associated with side effects. Most side effects are mild, and often may improve over time. Discuss side effects of this medication with your HCP prior to starting therapy, including how you should contact your HCP if side effects occur. The following side effects are more common and should be discussed with your HCP.

- Feeling sleepy, light-headed, or dizzy. Avoid driving, doing other tasks or hobbies that require you to be alert until you see how this medicine affects you.

- Nausea or vomiting. Small frequent meals, frequent mouth care, sucking hard candy, or chewing gum may help.

- Numbness or tingling of hands or feet.

More rare side effects include signs or symptoms of life-threatening reactions (eg, wheezing, chest pains, tightness in the chest, fever, itching, bad cough, blue skin color, fits, swelling of face, lips, tongue, or throat); no relief of headache after treatment, throat pain or tightness, fast heartbeats or shortness of breath, fainting, dizziness, light-headedness, and any rash. Report these symptoms immediately to your HCP. Other side effects not listed may occur in some individuals. If these occur, report them to your HCP.

RIZATRIPTAN

TYPE OF MEDICATION:
Antimigraine, Serotonin 5-HT$_{1D}$ Receptor Agonist

MEDICATIONS IN THIS GROUP
Rizatriptan (Maxalt®, Maxalt-MLT™) *on page 360*

THIS MEDICATION IS USED FOR:
This medicine is used to get rid of, or decrease the pain and symptoms of, a migraine headache. It is **not** used to prevent future attacks.

DIRECTIONS BEFORE TAKING THIS MEDICATION
Tell your healthcare provider (HCP) if any of the following circumstances apply to you:
1. You are pregnant, intending to become pregnant, or are breast-feeding
2. You have any medication allergies
3. You are using any prescription medications or over-the-counter medications; remember to include any medications prescribed by your dentist and any herbal or natural products
4. You have any medical problems
5. You have had any problems with this medication in the past

INSTRUCTIONS ON APPROPRIATE USE OF THIS MEDICATION
- Swallow Maxalt® tablet whole. Do not chew, break, or crush.
- Take with liquids as early as possible after the attack has started.
- Leave the Maxalt-MLT™ orally disintegrating tablet in the package until ready to use. When ready to use put tablet on tongue. This tablet will dissolve quickly.
- If no headache relief within 2 hours after first dose, do not take another dose. Talk with HCP.
- If your headache comes back after your first dose, another dose may be taken anytime 2 hours after the first dose.
- Do not take more than 30 mg in a 24-hour period.
- If you are taking propranolol, do not take more than 15 mg in a 24-hour period.

PRECAUTIONS
- Do not take if you have a history of angina (chest pain from the heart), heart spasms, heart attack, or uncontrolled high blood pressure.
- Do not take within 24 hours of other headache medicines. Talk with health-care provider.
- Tell healthcare provider if you are taking any medicines for depression. Certain medicines do not mix well with this medicine.
- Tell healthcare provider if you have had any history of seizures or are on seizure medicine.
- Use caution if you have risk factors for heart disease (high blood pressure, high cholesterol, overweight, diabetes, cigarette smoking, a male >40 years of age, other family members with heart disease, postmenopausal women). Talk with healthcare provider.
- Tell healthcare provider if you are allergic to any medicine. Make sure to tell about the allergy and how it affected you. This includes telling about rash; hives; itching; shortness of breath; wheezing; cough; swelling of face, lips, tongue, throat; or any other symptoms involved.

MISCELLANEOUS MEDICATIONS *(Continued)*

COMMON SIDE EFFECTS

All drugs are associated with side effects. Most side effects are mild, and often may improve over time. Discuss side effects of this medication with your HCP prior to starting therapy, including how you should contact your HCP if side effects occur. The following side effects are more common and should be discussed with your HCP.

- Feeling sleepy, light-headed, or dizzy. Avoid driving, doing other tasks or hobbies that require you to be alert until you see how this medicine affects you.

- Nausea or vomiting. Small frequent meals, frequent mouth care, sucking hard candy, or chewing gum may help.

- For the intranasal spray, a bad or unusual taste, nausea and vomiting, nasal cavity discomfort are common.

- For the oral tablet and shot, tingling, warm sensation, flushing, and chest tightness, pressure, or heaviness are common. The shot also causes pain at the site of injection.

More rare side effects include signs or symptoms of life-threatening reactions (eg, wheezing, chest pains, tightness in the chest, fever, itching, bad cough, blue skin color, fits, swelling of face, lips, tongue, or throat); no relief of headache after treatment, throat pain or tightness, fast heartbeats or shortness of breath, fainting, dizziness, light-headedness, and any rash. Report these symptoms immediately to your HCP. Other side effects not listed may occur in some individuals. If these occur, report them to your HCP.

SUMATRIPTAN

TYPE OF MEDICATION:
Antimigraine, Serotonin 5-HT$_{1D}$ Receptor Agonist

MEDICATIONS IN THIS GROUP

Sumatriptan (Imitrex®) *on page 383*

THIS MEDICATION IS USED FOR:
This medicine is used to get rid of, or decrease the pain and symptoms of, a migraine headache or cluster headache attacks (injection only). It is **not** used to prevent future attacks.

DIRECTIONS BEFORE TAKING THIS MEDICATION
Tell your healthcare provider (HCP) if any of the following circumstances apply to you:

1. You are pregnant, intending to become pregnant, or are breast-feeding
2. You have any medication allergies
3. You are using any prescription medications or over-the-counter medications; remember to include any medications prescribed by your dentist and any herbal or natural products
4. You have any medical problems
5. You have had any problems with this medication in the past

INSTRUCTIONS ON APPROPRIATE USE OF THIS MEDICATION
- Oral:
    - Swallow tablet whole. Do not chew, break, or crush.
    - Take with liquids as early as possible after the attack has started.
    - If no headache relief 2 hours after first dose, take another dose up to 100 mg. There may be additional doses given at 2-hour intervals.
    - Do not take more than 200 mg as a total daily dose; 100 mg as a total daily dose after an injection.
- Intranasal spray:
    - Give as a single dose in one nostril as early as possible after the attack has started.
    - If the dose is 10 mg, a single 5 mg spray can be given into each nostril.
    - If the headache returns, the dose may be repeated once after 2 hours.
    - Do not take more than 40 mg as a total daily dose.
- Injectable:
    - The shot is given under the skin as early as possible after the attack has started.
    - Do not give more than two 6 mg shots (must be separated by 1 hour) in a day.
    - Follow instructions given by nurse on how to give shot. Throw away needles in red box and return box to healthcare provider when full.

MISCELLANEOUS MEDICATIONS *(Continued)*

PRECAUTIONS

- Avoid alcohol (includes wine, beer, and liquor). Can worsen headache.

- Do not take if you have a history of angina (chest pain from the heart), heart spasms, heart attack, or uncontrolled high blood pressure.

- Do not take within 24 hours of other headache medicines. Talk with health-care provider.

- Tell healthcare provider if you are taking any medicines for depression. Certain medicines do not mix well with this medicine.

- Tell healthcare provider if you have had any history of seizures or are on seizure medicine.

- Use caution if you have risk factors for heart disease (high blood pressure, high cholesterol, overweight, diabetes, cigarette smoking, a male >40 years of age, other family members with heart disease, postmenopausal women). Talk with healthcare provider.

- Tell healthcare provider if you are allergic to any medicine. Make sure to tell about the allergy and how it affected you. This includes telling about rash; hives; itching; shortness of breath; wheezing; cough; swelling of face, lips, tongue, throat; or any other symptoms involved.

COMMON SIDE EFFECTS

All drugs are associated with side effects. Most side effects are mild, and often may improve over time. Discuss side effects of this medication with your HCP prior to starting therapy, including how you should contact your HCP if side effects occur. The following side effects are more common and should be discussed with your HCP.

- Feeling sleepy, light-headed, or dizzy. Avoid driving, doing other tasks or hobbies that require you to be alert until you see how this medicine affects you.

- Nausea or vomiting. Small frequent meals, frequent mouth care, sucking hard candy, or chewing gum may help.

- For the intranasal spray, a bad or unusual taste, nausea and vomiting, nasal cavity discomfort are common.

- For the oral tablet and shot, tingling, warm sensation, flushing, and chest tightness, pressure, or heaviness are common. The shot also causes pain at the site of injection.

More rare side effects include signs or symptoms of life-threatening reactions (eg, wheezing, chest pains, tightness in the chest, fever, itching, bad cough, blue skin color, fits, swelling of face, lips, tongue, or throat); no relief of headache after treatment, throat pain or tightness, fast heartbeats or shortness of breath, fainting, dizziness, light-headedness, and any rash. Report these symptoms immediately to your HCP. Other side effects not listed may occur in some individuals. If these occur, report them to your HCP.

ZOLMITRIPTAN

TYPE OF MEDICATION:

Antimigraine, Serotonin 5-HT$_{1D}$ Receptor Agonist

MEDICATIONS IN THIS GROUP

Zolmitriptan (Zomig®) *on page 443*

THIS MEDICATION IS USED FOR:

This medicine is used to get rid of, or decrease the pain and symptoms of, a migraine headache. It is **not** used to prevent future attacks.

DIRECTIONS BEFORE TAKING THIS MEDICATION

Tell your healthcare provider (HCP) if any of the following circumstances apply to you:

1. You are pregnant, intending to become pregnant, or are breast-feeding
2. You have any medication allergies
3. You are using any prescription medications or over-the-counter medications; remember to include any medications prescribed by your dentist and any herbal or natural products
4. You have any medical problems
5. You have had any problems with this medication in the past

INSTRUCTIONS ON APPROPRIATE USE OF THIS MEDICATION

- Swallow tablet whole. Do not chew, break, or crush.
- Take with liquids as early as possible after the attack has started.
- If no headache relief 2 hours after first dose, take another dose up to 10 mg. There may be additional doses given at 2-hour intervals.
- Do not take more than 5 mg as a total daily dose.

PRECAUTIONS

- Avoid alcohol (includes wine, beer, and liquor). Can worsen headache.
- Do not take it if you have a history of angina (chest pain from the heart), heart spasms, heart attack, or uncontrolled high blood pressure.
- Do not take within 24 hours of other headache medicines. Talk with health-care provider.
- Tell healthcare provider if you are taking any medicines for depression. Certain medicines do not mix well with this medicine.
- Tell healthcare provider if you have had any history of seizures or are on seizure medicine.
- Use caution if you have risk factors for heart disease (high blood pressure, high cholesterol, overweight, diabetes, cigarette smoking, a male >40 years of age, other family members with heart disease, postmenopausal women). Talk with healthcare provider.
- Tell healthcare provider if you are allergic to any medicine. Make sure to tell about the allergy and how it affected you. This includes telling about rash; hives; itching; shortness of breath; wheezing; cough; swelling of face, lips, tongue, throat; or any other symptoms involved.

MISCELLANEOUS MEDICATIONS *(Continued)*

COMMON SIDE EFFECTS

All drugs are associated with side effects. Most side effects are mild, and often may improve over time. Discuss side effects of this medication with your HCP prior to starting therapy, including how you should contact your HCP if side effects occur. The following side effects are more common and should be discussed with your HCP.

- Feeling sleepy, light-headed, or dizzy. Avoid driving, doing other tasks or hobbies that require you to be alert until you see how this medicine affects you.
- Nausea or vomiting. Small frequent meals, frequent mouth care, sucking hard candy, or chewing gum may help.
- Dry mouth
- Warm-cold feelings

More rare side effects include signs or symptoms of life-threatening reactions (eg, wheezing, chest pains, tightness in the chest, fever, itching, bad cough, blue skin color, fits, swelling of face, lips, tongue, or throat); no relief of headache after treatment, throat pain or tightness, fast heartbeats or shortness of breath, fainting, dizziness, light-headedness, and any rash. Report these symptoms immediately to your HCP. Other side effects not listed may occur in some individuals. If these occur, report them to your HCP.

DSM-IV CLASSIFICATION

Used with permission from the American Psychiatric Association, *Diagnostic and Statistical Manual of Mental Disorders*, 4th ed, Washington, DC: American Psychiatric Association, 1994, 13-24,6,7.

AXIS I AND II CATEGORIES AND CODES

An ellipsis (...) is used in the names of certain disorders to indicate that the name of a specific mental disorder or general medical condition should be inserted when recording the name.

An "x" appearing in a diagnostic code indicates that a specific code number is required.

If criteria are currently met, one of the following severity specifiers may be noted after the diagnosis:

- Mild
- Moderate
- Severe

If criteria are no longer met, one of the following specifiers may be noted:

- In partial remission
- In full remission
- Prior history
- NOS = Not otherwise specified

AXIS I: CLINICAL DISORDERS; OTHER CONDITIONS THAT MAY BE A FOCUS OF CLINICAL ATTENTION

Axis I is for reporting all the various disorders or conditions in the Classification except for the Personality Disorders and Mental Retardation (which are reported on Axis II). The major groups of disorders to be reported on Axis I are listed in the box. Also reported on Axis I are Other Conditions That May Be a Focus of Clinical Attention.

AXIS I
Clinical Disorders
Other Conditions That May Be a Focus of Clinical Attention

Disorders Usually First Diagnosed in Infancy, Childhood, or Adolescence (excluding Mental Retardation, which is diagnosed on Axis II)
Delirium, Dementia, and Amnestic and Other Cognitive Disorders
Mental Disorders Due to a General Medical Condition
Substance-Related Disorders
Schizophrenia and Other Psychotic Disorders
Mood Disorders
Anxiety Disorders
Somatoform Disorders
Factitious Disorders
Dissociative Disorders
Sexual and Gender Identity Disorders
Eating Disorders
Sleep Disorders
Impulse-Control Disorders Not Elsewhere Classified
Adjustment Disorders
Other Conditions That May Be a Focus of Clinical Attention

AXIS II: PERSONALITY DISORDERS; MENTAL RETARDATION

Axis II is for reporting Personality Disorders and Mental Retardation. It may also be used for noting prominent maladaptive personality features and defense mechanisms. The listing of Personality Disorders and Mental Retardation on a separate axis ensures that consideration

DSM-IV CLASSIFICATION *(Continued)*

will be given to the possible presence of Personality Disorders and Mental Retardation that might otherwise be overlooked when attention is directed to the usually more florid Axis I disorders. The coding of Personality Disorders on Axis II should not be taken to imply that their pathogenesis or range of appropriate treatment is fundamentally different from that for the disorders coded on Axis I. The disorders to be reported on Axis II are listed in the box.

AXIS II
Personality Disorders
Mental Retardation

Paranoid Personality Disorder

Schizoid Personality Disorder

Schizotypal Personality Disorder

Antisocial Personality Disorder

Borderline Personality Disorder

Histrionic Personality Disorder

Narcissistic Personality Disorder

Avoidant Personality Disorder

Dependent Personality Disorder

Obsessive-Compulsive Personality Disorder

Personality Disorder Not Otherwise Specified

Mental Retardation

DISORDERS USUALLY FIRST DIAGNOSED IN INFANCY, CHILDHOOD, OR ADOLESCENCE

MENTAL RETARDATION

Note: These are coded on Axis II.

317	Mild Mental Retardation
318.0	Moderate Mental Retardation
318.1	Severe Mental Retardation
318.2	Profound Mental Retardation
319	Mental Retardation, Severity Unspecified

LEARNING DISORDERS

315.00	Reading Disorder
315.1	Mathematics Disorder
315.2	Disorder of Written Expression
315.9	Learning Disorder NOS

MOTOR SKILLS DISORDER

315.4	Development Coordination Disorder

COMMUNICATION DISORDERS

315.31	Expressive Language Disorder
315.32	Mixed Receptive-Expressive Language Disorder
315.39	Phonological Disorder
307.0	Stuttering
307.9	Communication Disorder NOS

PERVASIVE DEVELOPMENTAL DISORDERS

299.00	Autistic Disorder
299.80	Rett's Disorder
299.10	Childhood Disintegrative Disorder
299.80	Asperger's Disorder
299.80	Pervasive Developmental Disorder NOS

ATTENTION-DEFICIT AND DISRUPTIVE BEHAVIOR DISORDERS

314.xx	Attention-Deficit/Hyperactivity Disorder
.01	Combined Type
.00	Predominantly Inattentive Type
.01	Predominantly Hyperactive-Impulsive Type
314.9	Attention-Deficit/Hyperactivity Disorder NOS
312.xx	Conduct Disorder
.81	Childhood-Onset Type
.82	Adolescent-Onset Type
.89	Unspecified Onset
313.81	Oppositional Defiant Disorder
312.9	Disruptive Behavior Disorder NOS

FEEDING AND EATING DISORDERS OF INFANCY OR EARLY CHILDHOOD

307.52	Pica
307.53	Rumination Disorder
307.59	Feeding Disorder of Infancy or Early Childhood

TIC DISORDERS

307.23	Tourette's Disorder
307.22	Chronic Motor or Vocal Tic Disorder
307.21	Transient Tic Disorder
	Specify if: Single Episode/Recurrent
307.20	Tic Disorder NOS

ELIMINATION DISORDERS

__.__	Encopresis
787.6	With Constipation and Overflow Incontinence
307.7	Without Constipation and Overflow Incontinence
307.6	Enuresis (Not Due to a General Medical Condition)
	Specify type: Nocturnal Only/Diurnal Only/Nocturnal and Diurnal

DSM-IV CLASSIFICATION *(Continued)*

OTHER DISORDERS OF INFANCY, CHILDHOOD, OR ADOLESCENCE

309.21	Separation Anxiety Disorder	

Specify if: Early Onset

313.23	Selective Mutism	
313.89	Reactive Attachment Disorder of Infancy or Early Childhood	

Specify type: Inhibited Type/Disinhibited Type

307.3	Stereotypic Movement Disorder	

Specify if: With Self-Injurious Behavior

313.9	Disorder of Infancy, Childhood, or Adolescence NOS	

DELIRIUM, DEMENTIA, AND AMNESTIC AND OTHER COGNITIVE DISORDERS

DELIRIUM

293.0	Delirium Due to ... [Indicate the General Medical Condition]
___.__	Substance Intoxication Delirium (refer to Substance-Related Disorders for substance-specific codes)
___.__	Substance Withdrawal Delirium (refer to Substance-Related Disorders for substance-specific codes)
___.__	Delirium Due to Multiple Etiologies (code each of the specific etiologies)
780.09	Delirium NOS

DEMENTIA

290.xx	Dementia of the Alzheimer's Type, With Early Onset (also code 331.0 Alzheimer's disease on Axis III)]
.10	Uncomplicated
.11	With Delirium
.12	With Delusions
.13	With Depressed Mood

Specify if: With Behavioral Disturbance

290.xx	Dementia of the Alzheimer's Type, With Late Onset (also code 331.0 Alzheimer's disease on Axis III)
.0	Uncomplicated
.3	With Delirium
.20	With Delusions
.21	With Depressed Mood

Specify if: With Behavioral Disturbance

290.xx	Vascular Dementia
.40	Uncomplicated
.41	With Delirium
.42	With Delusions
.43	With Depressed Mood

Specify if: With Behavioral Disturbance

294.1	Dementia Due to HIV Disease (also code 042 HIV infection on Axis III)
294.1	Dementia Due to Head Trauma (also code 854.00 head injury on Axis III)
294.1	Dementia Due to Parkinson's Disease (also code 332.0 Parkinson's disease on Axis III)
294.1	Dementia Due to Huntington's Disease (also code 333.4 Huntington's disease on Axis III)

290.10	Dementia Due to Pick's Disease (also code 331.1 Pick's disease on Axis III)
290.10	Dementia Due to Creutzfeldt-Jakob Disease (also code 046.1 Creutzfeldt-Jakob disease on Axis III)
294.1	Dementia Due to ... [Indicate the General Medical Condition not listed above] (also code the general medical condition on Axis III)
___.__	Substance-Induced Persisting Dementia (refer to Substance-Related Disorders for substance-specific codes)
___.__	Dementia Due to Multiple Etiologies (code each of the specific etiologies)
294.8	Dementia NOS

AMNESTIC DISORDERS

| 294.0 | Amnestic Disorder Due to ... [Indicate the General Medical Condition] |

Specify if: Transient/Chronic

| ___.__ | Substance-Induced Persisting Amnestic Disorder (refer to Substance-Related Disorders for substance-specific codes) |
| 294.8 | Amnestic Disorder NOS |

OTHER COGNITIVE DISORDERS

| 294.9 | Cognitive Disorder NOS |

MENTAL DISORDERS DUE TO A GENERAL MEDICAL CONDITION NOT ELSEWHERE CLASSIFIED

| 293.89 | Catatonic Disorder Due to ... [Indicate the General Medical Condition] |
| 310.1 | Personality Change Due to ... [Indicate the General Medical Condition] |

Specify type: Labile Type/Disinhibited Type/Aggressive Type/Apathetic Type/Paranoid Type/Other Type/Combined Type/Unspecified Type

| 293.9 | Mental Disorder NOS Due to ... [Indicate the General Medical Condition] |

SUBSTANCE-RELATED DISORDERS

[a]The following specifiers may be applied to Substance Dependence:

With Physiological Dependence/Without Physiological Dependence

Early Full Remission/Early Partial Remission

Sustained Full Remission/ Sustained Partial Remission

On Agonist Therapy/In a Controlled Environment

The following specifiers apply to Substance-Induced Disorders as noted:

[I]With Onset During Intoxication/[W]With Onset During Withdrawal

ALCOHOL-RELATED DISORDERS

___ Alcohol Use Disorders

| 303.90 | Alcohol Dependence[a] |
| 305.00 | Alcohol Abuse |

___ Alcohol-Induced Disorders

| 303.00 | Alcohol Intoxication |
| 291.81 | Alcohol Withdrawal |

Specify if: With Perceptual Disturbances

DSM-IV CLASSIFICATION *(Continued)*

291.0	Alcohol Intoxication Delirium
291.0	Alcohol Withdrawal Delirium
291.2	Alcohol-Induced Persisting Dementia
291.1	Alcohol-Induced Persisting Amnestic Disorder
291.x	Alcohol-Induced Psychotic Disorder
.5	With Delusions[I,W]
.3	With Hallucinations[I,W]
291.89	Alcohol-Induced Mood Disorder[I,W]
291.89	Alcohol-Induced Anxiety Disorder[I,W]
291.89	Alcohol-Induced Sexual Dysfunction[I]
291.89	Alcohol-Induced Sleep Disorder[I,W]
291.9	Alcohol-Related Disorder NOS

AMPHETAMINE (or Amphetamine-Like) - Related Disorders

___ Amphetamine Use Disorders

304.40	Amphetamine Dependence[a]]
305.70	Amphetamine Abuse

___ Amphetamine-Induced Disorders

292.89	Amphetamine Intoxication

Specify if: With Perceptual Disturbances

292.0	Amphetamine Withdrawal
292.81	Amphetamine Intoxication Delirium
292.xx	Amphetamine-Induced Psychotic Disorder
.11	With Delusions[I]
.12	With Hallucinations[I]
292.84	Amphetamine-Induced Mood Disorder[I,W]
292.89	Amphetamine-Induced Anxiety Disorder[I]
292.89	Amphetamine-Induced Sexual Dysfunction[I]
292.89	Amphetamine-Induced Sleep Disorder[I,W]
292.9	Amphetamine-Related Disorder NOS

CAFFEINE-RELATED DISORDERS

___ Caffeine-Induced Disorders

305.90	Caffeine Intoxication
292.89	Caffeine-Induced Anxiety Disorder[I]
292.89	Caffeine-Induced Sleep Disorder[I]
292.9	Caffeine-Related Disorder NOS

CANNABIS-RELATED DISORDERS

___ Cannabis Use Disorders

304.30	Cannabis Dependence[a]
305.20	Cannabis Abuse

___ Cannabis-Induced Disorders

292.89	Cannabis Intoxication

Specify if: With Perceptual Disturbance

292.81	Cannabis Intoxication Delirium

292.xx	Cannabis-Induced Psychotic Disorder
.11	With Delusions[I]
.12	With Hallucinations[I]
292.89	Cannabis-Induced Anxiety Disorder[I]
292.9	Cannabis-Related Disorder NOS

COCAINE-RELATED DISORDERS

___ Cocaine Use Disorders

| 304.20 | Cocaine Dependence[a] |
| 305.60 | Cocaine Abuse |

___ Cocaine-Induced Disorders

| 292.89 | Cocaine Intoxication |

Specify if: With Perceptual Disturbance

292.0	Cocaine Withdrawal
292.81	Cocaine Intoxication Delirium
292.xx	Cocaine-Induced Psychotic Disorder
.11	With Delusions[I]
.12	With Hallucinations[I]
292.84	Cocaine-Induced Mood Disorder[I,W]
292.89	Cocaine-Induced Anxiety Disorder[I,W]
292.89	Cocaine-Induced Sexual Dysfunction[I]
292.89	Cocaine-Induced Sleep Disorder[I,W]
292.9	Cocaine-Related Disorder NOS

HALLUCINOGEN-RELATED DISORDERS

___ Hallucinogen Use Disorders

| 304.50 | Hallucinogen Dependence[a] |
| 305.30 | Hallucinogen Abuse |

___ Hallucinogen-Induced Disorders

292.89	Hallucinogen Intoxication
292.89	Hallucinogen Persisting Perception Disorder (Flashbacks)
292.81	Hallucinogen Intoxication Delirium
292.xx	Hallucinogen-Induced Psychotic Disorder
.11	With Delusions[I]
.12	With Hallucinations[I]
292.84	Hallucinogen-Induced Mood Disorder[I]
292.89	Hallucinogen-Induced Anxiety Disorder[I]
292.9	Hallucinogen-Related Disorder NOS

INHALANT-RELATED DISORDERS

___ Inhalant Use Disorders

| 304.60 | Inhalant Dependence[a] |
| 305.90 | Inhalant Abuse |

DSM-IV CLASSIFICATION *(Continued)*

___ **Inhalant-Induced Disorders**

292.89	Inhalant Intoxication
292.81	Inhalant Intoxication Delirium
292.82	Inhalant-Induced Persisting Dementia
292.xx	Inhalant-Induced Psychotic Disorder
.11	With Delusions[I]
.12	With Hallucinations[I]
292.84	Inhalant-Induced Mood Disorder[I]
292.89	Inhalant-Induced Anxiety Disorder[I]
292.9	Inhalant-Related Disorder NOS

NICOTINE-RELATED DISORDERS

___ **Nicotine Use Disorders**

305.10	Nicotine Dependence[a]

___ **Nicotine-Induced Disorders**

292.0	Nicotine Withdrawal
292.9	Nicotine-Related Disorder NOS

OPIOID-RELATED DISORDERS

___ **Opioid Use Disorders**

304.00	Opioid Dependence[a]
305.50	Opioid Abuse

___ **Opioid-Induced Disorders**

292.89	Opioid Intoxication

Specify if: With Perceptual Disturbances

292.0	Opioid Withdrawal
292.81	Opioid Intoxication Delirium
292.xx	Opioid-Induced Psychotic Disorder
.11	With Delusions[I]
.12	With Hallucinations[I]
292.84	Opioid-Induced Mood Disorder[I]
292.89	Opioid-Induced Sexual Dysfunction[I]
292.89	Opioid-Induced Sleep Disorder[I,W]
292.9	Opioid-Related Disorder NOS

PHENCYCLIDINE (or Phencyclidine-Like)-RELATED DISORDERS

___ **Phencyclidine Use Disorders**

304.60	Phencyclidine Dependence[a]
305.90	Phencyclidine Abuse

___ **Phencyclidine-Induced Disorders**

292.89	Phencyclidine Intoxication

Specify if: With Perceptual Disturbances

292.81	Phencyclidine Intoxication Delirium
292.xx	Phencyclidine-Induced Psychotic Disorder
.11	With Delusions[I]

.12	With Hallucinations[I]
292.84	Phencyclidine-Induced Mood Disorder[I]
292.89	Phencyclidine-Induced Anxiety Disorder[I]
292.9	Phencyclidine-Related Disorder NOS

SEDATIVE-, HYPNOTIC-, OR ANXIOLYTIC-RELATED DISORDERS

___ **Sedative, Hypnotic, or Anxiolytic Use Disorders**

304.10	Sedative, Hypnotic, or Anxiolytic Dependence[a]
305.40	Sedative, Hypnotic, or Anxiolytic Abuse

___ **Sedative-, Hypnotic-, or Anxiolytic-Induced Disorders**

292.89	Sedative, Hypnotic, or Anxiolytic Intoxication
292.0	Sedative, Hypnotic, or Anxiolytic Withdrawal

Specify if: With Perceptual Disturbances

292.81	Sedative, Hypnotic, or Anxiolytic Intoxication Delirium
292.81	Sedative, Hypnotic, or Anxiolytic Withdrawal Delirium
292.82	Sedative-, Hypnotic-, or Anxiolytic-Induced Persisting Dementia
292.83	Sedative-, Hypnotic-, or Anxiolytic-Induced Persisting Amnestic Disorder
292.xx	Sedative-, Hypnotic-, or Anxiolytic-Induced Psychotic Disorder
.11	With Delusions[I,W]
.12	With Hallucinations[I,W]
292.84	Sedative-, Hypnotic-, or Anxiolytic-Induced Mood Disorder[I,W]
292.89	Sedative-, Hypnotic-, or Anxiolytic-Induced Anxiety Disorder[W]
292.89	Sedative-, Hypnotic-, or Anxiolytic-Induced Sexual Dysfunction[I]
292.89	Sedative-, Hypnotic-, or Anxiolytic-Induced Sleep Disorder[I,W]
292.9	Sedative-, Hypnotic-, or Anxiolytic-Related Disorder NOS

POLYSUBSTANCE-RELATED DISORDER

304.80	Polysubstance Dependence[a]

OTHER (or Unknown) SUBSTANCE-RELATED DISORDERS

___ **Other (or Unknown) Substance Use Disorders**

304.90	Other (or Unknown) Substance Dependence[a]
305.90	Other (or Unknown) Substance Abuse

___ **Other (or Unknown) Substance-Induced Disorders**

292.89	Other (or Unknown) Substance Intoxication

Specify if: With Perceptual Disturbances

292.0	Other (or Unknown) Substance Withdrawal

Specify if: With Perceptual Disturbances

292.81	Other (or Unknown) Substance-Induced Delirium
292.82	Other (or Unknown) Substance-Induced Persisting Dementia
292.83	Other (or Unknown) Substance-Induced Persisting Amnestic Disorder
292.xx	Other (or Unknown) Substance-Induced Psychotic Disorder
.11	With Delusions[I,W]
.12	With Hallucinations[I,W]
292.84	Other (or Unknown) Substance-Induced Mood Disorder[I,W]

DSM-IV CLASSIFICATION *(Continued)*

292.89	Other (or Unknown) Substance-Induced Anxiety Disorder[I,W]
292.89	Other (or Unknown) Substance-Induced Sexual Dysfunction[I]
292.89	Other (or Unknown) Substance-Induced Sleep Disorder[I,W]
292.9	Other (or Unknown) Substance-Related Disorder NOS

SCHIZOPHRENIA AND OTHER PSYCHOTIC DISORDERS

295.xx   Schizophrenia

The following Classification of Longitudinal Course applies to all subtypes of Schizophrenia:

Episodic With Interepisode Residual Symptoms

(specify if: With Prominent Negative Symptoms)/Episodic With No Interepisode Residual Symptoms/Continuous (specify if: With Prominent Negative Symptoms)

Single Episode In Partial Remission

(specify if: With Prominent Negative Symptoms)/Single Episode In Full Remission

Other or Unspecified Pattern

.30	Paranoid Type
.10	Disorganized Type
.20	Catatonic Type
.90	Undifferentiated Type
.60	Residual Type
295.40	Schizophreniform Disorder

Specify if: Without Good Prognostic Features/With Good Prognostic Features

295.70   Schizoaffective Disorder

Specify type: Bipolar Type/Depressive Type

297.1   Delusional Disorder

Specify type: Erotomanic Type/Grandiose Type/Jealous Type/Persecutory Type/Somatic Type/Mixed Type/Unspecified Type

298.8   Brief Psychotic Disorder

Specify if: With Marked Stressor(s)/Without Marked Stressor(s)/With Postpartum Onset

297.3   Shared Psychotic Disorder

293.xx   Psychotic Disorder Due to ... [Indicate the General Medical Condition]

.81	With Delusions
.82	With Hallucinations
___.__	Substance-Induced Psychotic Disorder

(Refer to Substance-Related Disorders for substance-specific codes)

Specify if: With Onset During Intoxication/With Onset During Withdrawal

298.9   Psychotic Disorder NOS

MOOD DISORDERS

Code current state of Major Depressive Disorder or Bipolar I Disorder in fifth digit:

1 = Mild

2 = Moderate

3 = Severe Without Psychotic Features

4 = Severe With Psychotic Features

Specify: Mood-Congruent Psychotic Features/Mood-Incongruent Psychotic Features

5 = In Partial Remission

6 = In Full Remission

0 = Unspecified

The following specifiers apply (for current or most recent episode) to Mood Disorders as noted:

[a]Severity/Psychotic/Remission Specifiers
[b]Chronic
[c]With Catatonic Features
[d]With Melancholic Features
[e]With Atypical Features
[f]With Postpartum Onset

The following specifiers apply to Mood Disorders as noted:

[g]With or Without Full Interepisode Recovery
[h]With Seasonal Pattern
[i]With Rapid Cycling

DEPRESSIVE DISORDERS

296.xx	Major Depressive Disorder,	
.2x	Single Episode[a,b,c,d,e,f]	
.3x	Recurrent[a,b,c,d,e,f,g,h]	
300.4	Dysthymic Disorder	

Specify if: Early Onset/Late Onset

Specify: With Atypical Features

311	Depressive Disorder NOS

BIPOLAR DISORDERS

296.xx	Bipolar I Disorder,	
.0x	Single Manic Episode[a,c,f]	

Specify if: Mixed

.40	Most Recent Episode Hypomanic[g,h,i]
.4x	Most Recent Episode Manic[a,c,f,g,h,i]
.6x	Most Recent Episode Mixed[a,c,f,g,h,i]
.5x	Most Recent Episode Depressed[a,b,c,d,e,f,g,h,i]
.7	Most Recent Episode Unspecified[g,h,i]
296.89	Bipolar II Disorder[a,b,c,d,e,f,g,h,i]

Specify (current or most recent episode):

Hypomanic/Depressed

301.13	Cyclothymic Disorder
296.80	Bipolar Disorder NOS
293.83	Mood Disorder Due to ... [Indicate the General Medical Condition]

Specify type: With Depressive Features/With Major Depressive-Like Episode/With Manic Features/With Mixed Features

___.__	Substance-Induced Mood Disorder (refer to Substance-Related Disorders for substance-specific codes)

Specify type: With Depressive Features/With Manic Features/With Mixed Features

Specify if: With Onset During Intoxication/With Onset During Withdrawal

296.90	Mood Disorder NOS

ANXIETY DISORDERS

300.01	Panic Disorder Without Agoraphobia
300.21	Panic Disorder With Agoraphobia
300.22	Agoraphobia Without History of Panic Disorder
300.29	Specific Phobia

Specify type: Animal Type/Natural Environment Type/Blood-Injection-Injury Type/Situational Type/Other Type

DSM-IV CLASSIFICATION *(Continued)*

300.23   Social Phobia
Specify if: Generalized
300.3   Obsessive-Compulsive Disorder
Specify if: With Poor Insight
309.81   Post-traumatic Stress Disorder
Specify if: Acute/Chronic
Specify if: With Delayed Onset
308.3   Acute Stress Disorder
300.02   Generalized Anxiety Disorder
293.84   Anxiety Disorder Due to ... [Indicate the General Medical Condition]
Specify if: With Generalized Anxiety/With Panic Attacks/With Obsessive-Compulsive Symptoms
___.___   Substance-Induced Anxiety Disorder (refer to Substance-Related Disorders for substance-specific codes)
Specify if: With Generalized Anxiety/With Panic Attacks/With Obsessive-Compulsive Symptoms/With Phobic Symptoms
Specify if: With Onset During Intoxication/With Onset During Withdrawal
300.00   Anxiety Disorder NOS

SOMATOFORM DISORDERS

300.81   Somatization Disorder
300.82   Undifferentiated Somatoform Disorder
300.11   Conversion Disorder
Specify type: With Motor Symptom or Deficit/With Sensory Symptom or Deficit/With Seizures or Convulsions/With Mixed Presentation
307.xx   Pain Disorder
   .80   Associated With Psychological Factors
   .89   Associated With Both Psychological Factors and a General Medical Condition
Specify if: Acute/Chronic
300.7   Hyperchondriasis
Specify if: With Poor Insight
300.7   Body Dysmorphic Disorder
300.82   Somatoform Disorder NOS

FACTITIOUS DISORDERS

300.xx   Factitious Disorder
   .16   With Predominantly Psychological Signs and Symptoms
   .19   With Predominantly Physical Signs and Symptoms
   .19   With Combined Psychological and Physical Signs and Symptoms
300.19   Factitious Disorder NOS

DISSOCIATIVE DISORDERS

300.12   Dissociative Amnesia
300.13   Dissociative Fugue
300.14   Dissociative Identity Disorder
300.6   Depersonalization Disorder
300.15   Dissociative Disorder NOS

SEXUAL AND GENDER IDENTITY DISORDERS

SEXUAL DYSFUNCTION

The following specifiers apply to all primary Sexual Dysfunctions:
Lifelong Type/Acquired Type
Generalized Type/Situational Type
Due to Psychological Factors/Due to Combined Factors

___ Sexual Desire Disorders

302.71	Hypoactive Sexual Desire Disorder
302.79	Sexual Aversion Disorder

___ Sexual Arousal Disorders

302.72	Female Sexual Arousal Disorder
302.72	Male Erectile Disorder

___ Orgasmic Disorders

302.73	Female Orgasmic Disorder
302.74	Male Orgasmic Disorder
302.75	Premature Ejaculation

___ Sexual Pain Disorders

302.76	Dyspareunia (Not Due to a General Medical Condition)
306.51	Vaginismus (Not Due to a General Medical Condition)

___ Sexual Dysfunction Due to a General Medical Condition

625.8	Female Hypoactive Sexual Desire Disorder Due to ... [Indicate the General Medical Condition]
608.89	Male Hypoactive Sexual Desire Disorder Due to ... [Indicate the General Medical Condition]
607.84	Male Erectile Disorder Due to ... [Indicate the General Medial Condition]
625.0	Female Dyspareunia Due to ... [Indicate the General Medial Condition]
608.89	Male Dyspareunia Due to ... [Indicate the General Medial Condition]
625.8	Other Female Sexual Dysfunction Due to ... [Indicate the General Medial Condition]
608.89	Other Male Sexual Dysfunction Due to ... [Indicate the General Medial Condition]
___.__	Substance-Induced Sexual Dysfunction (refer to Substance-Related Disorders for substance-specific codes)

Specify if: With Impaired Desire/With Impaired Arousal/With Impaired Orgasm/With Sexual Pain

Specify if: With Onset During Intoxication

302.70	Sexual Dysfunction NOS

PARAPHILIAS

302.4	Exhibitionism
302.81	Fetishism
302.89	Frotteurism
302.2	Pedophilia

Specify if: Sexually Attracted to Males/Sexually Attracted to Females/Sexually Attracted to Both

Specify if: Limited to Incest

Specify type: Exclusive Type/Nonexclusive Type

302.83	Sexual Masochism
302.84	Sexual Sadism

DSM-IV CLASSIFICATION *(Continued)*

302.3   Transvestic Fetishism
Specify if: With Gender Dysphoria
302.82   Voyeurism
302.9   Paraphilia NOS

GENDER IDENTITY DISORDERS

302.xx   Gender Identity Disorder
.6   in Children
.85   in Adolescents or Adults
Specify if: Sexually Attracted to Males/Sexually Attracted to Females/Sexually Attracted to Both/Sexually Attracted to Neither
302.6   Gender Identity Disorder NOS
302.9   Sexual Disorder NOS

EATING DISORDERS

307.1   Anorexia Nervosa
Specify type: Restricting Type; Binge-Eating/Purging Type
307.51   Bulimia Nervosa
Specify type: Purging Type/Nonpurging Type
307.50   Eating Disorder NOS

SLEEP DISORDERS

PRIMARY SLEEP DISORDERS

___ **Dyssomnias**
307.42   Primary Insomnia
307.44   Primary Hypersomnia
Specify if: Recurrent
347   Narcolepsy
780.59   Breathing-Related Sleep Disorder
307.45   Circadian Rhythm Sleep Disorder
Specify type: Delayed Sleep Phase Type/Jet Lag Type/Shift Work Type/Unspecified Type
307.47   Dyssomnia NOS
___ **Parasomnias**
307.47   Nightmare Disorder
307.46   Sleep Terror Disorder
307.46   Sleepwalking Disorder
307.47   Parasomnia NOS

SLEEP DISORDERS RELATED TO ANOTHER MENTAL DISORDER

307.42   Insomnia Related to ... [Indicate the Axis I or Axis II Disorder]
307.44   Hypersomnia Related to ... [Indicate the Axis I or Axis II Disorder]

OTHER SLEEP DISORDERS

780.xx   Sleep Disorder Due to ... [Indicate the Axis I or Axis II Disorder]

.52	Insomnia Type
.54	Hypersomnia Type
.59	Parasomnia Type
.59	Mixed Type
__.__	Substance-Induced Sleep Disorder (refer to Substance-Related Disorders for substance-specific codes)

Specify type: Insomnia Type/Hypersomnia Type/Parasomnia Type/Mixed Type
Specify if: With Onset During Intoxication/With Onset During Withdrawal

IMPULSE-CONTROL DISORDERS NOT ELSEWHERE CLASSIFIED

312.34	Intermittent Explosive Disorder
312.32	Kleptomania
312.33	Pyromania
312.31	Pathological Gambling
312.39	Trichotillomania
312.30	Impulse-Control Disorder NOS

ADJUSTMENT DISORDERS

309.xx	Adjustment Disorder
.0	With Depressed Mood
.24	With Anxiety
.28	With Mixed Anxiety and Depressed Mood
.3	With Disturbance of Conduct
.4	With Mixed Disturbance of Emotions and Conduct
.9	Unspecified

Specify if: Acute/Chronic

PERSONALITY DISORDERS

Note: These are coded on Axis II.

301.0	Paranoid Personality Disorder
301.20	Schizoid Personality Disorder
301.22	Schizotypal Personality Disorder
301.7	Antisocial Personality Disorder
301.83	Borderline Personality Disorder
301.50	Histrionic Personality Disorder
301.81	Narcissistic Personality Disorder
301.82	Avoidant Personality Disorder
301.6	Dependent Personality Disorder
301.4	Obsessive-Compulsive Personality Disorder
301.9	Personality Disorder NOS

DSM-IV CLASSIFICATION *(Continued)*

OTHER CONDITIONS THAT MAY BE A FOCUS OF CLINICAL ATTENTION

PSYCHOLOGICAL FACTORS AFFECTING MEDICAL CONDITION

316	... [Specified Psychological Factor] Affecting
	... [Indicate the General Medical Condition]
	Choose name based on nature of factors:
	Mental Disorder Affecting Medical Condition
	Psychological Symptoms Affecting Medical Condition
	Personality Traits or Coping Style Affecting Medical Condition
	Maladaptive Health Behaviors Affecting Medical Condition
	Stress-Related Physiological Response Affecting Medical Condition
	Other or Unspecified Psychological Factors Affecting Medical Condition

MEDICATION-INDUCED MOVEMENT DISORDERS

332.1	Neuroleptic-Induced Parkinsonism
333.92	Neuroleptic Malignant Syndrome
333.7	Neuroleptic-Induced Acute Dystonia
333.99	Neuroleptic-Induced Acute Akathisia
333.82	Neuroleptic-Induced Tardive Dyskinesia
333.1	Medication-Induced Postural Tremor
333.90	Medication-Induced Movement Disorder NOS

OTHER MEDICATION-INDUCED DISORDER

995.2	Adverse Effects of Medication NOS

RELATIONAL PROBLEMS

V61.9	Relational Problem Related to a Mental Disorder or General Medical Condition
V61.20	Parent-Child Relational Problem
V61.10	Partner Relational Problem
V61.8	Sibling Relational Problem
V62.81	Relational Problem NOS

PROBLEMS RELATED TO ABUSE OR NEGLECT

V61.21	Physical Abuse of Child (code 99.54 if focus of attention is on victim)
V61.21	Sexual Abuse of Child (code 995.53 if focus of attention is on victim)
V61.21	Neglect of Child (code 995.52 if focus of attention is on victim)
___.___	Physical Abuse of Adult (682)
V61.12	(if by partner)
V62.83	(if by person other than partner) (code 995.81 if focus of attention is on victim)
___.___	Sexual Abuse of Adult (682)
V61.12	(if by partner)
V62.83	(if by person other than partner) (code 995.83 if focus of attention is on victim)

ADDITIONAL CONDITIONS THAT MAY BE A FOCUS OF CLINICAL ATTENTION

V15.81	Noncompliance With Treatment
V65.2	Malingering
V71.01	Adult Antisocial Behavior
V71.02	Child or Adolescent Antisocial Behavior
V62.89	Borderline Intellectual Functioning

Note: This is coded on Axis II

780.9	Age-Related Cognitive Decline
V62.82	Bereavement
V62.3	Academic Problem
V62.2	Occupational Problem
313.82	Identity Problem
V62.89	Religious or Spiritual Problem
V62.4	Acculturation Problem
V62.89	Phase of Life Problem

ADDITIONAL CODES

300.9	Unspecified Mental Disorder (nonpsychotic)
V71.09	No Diagnosis or Condition on Axis I
799.9	Diagnosis or Condition Deferred on Axis I
V71.09	No Diagnosis on Axis II
799.9	Diagnosis Deferred on Axis II

MULTIAXIAL SYSTEM

Axis I	Clinical Disorders
	Other Conditions That May Be a Focus of Clinical Attention
Axis II	Personality Disorders
	Mental Retardation
Axis III	General Medical Conditions
Axis IV	Psychosocial and Environmental Problems
Axis V	Global Assessment of Functioning

APPENDIX
TABLE OF CONTENTS

ADDICTION TREATMENTS

Bupropion SR (Zyban®)	Smoking cessation: Initiate at 150 mg every morning for 3 days. If tolerated, increase to 150 mg twice daily on day 4 of dosing. Should be an interval of at least 8 hours between successive doses. Target quit date after at least 1 week of treatment. Trial may be up to 12 weeks. Contraindicated in patients with seizures, anorexia, or bulimia.
Clonidine (Catapres®)	Alcohol, nicotine, opioid withdrawal: Initiate 0.1 mg 2-3 times/day
Disulfiram (Antabuse®)	Sobriety: 125-500 mg/day; patients must be free of alcohol for at least 12 hours prior to initiation. Contraindicated with metronidazole and alcohol (including cough syrups).
Levomethadyl (Orlaam®)	Narcotic dependence: Initiate at 20-40 mg 3 times/week
Methadone (Dolophine®)	Narcotic dependence: 15-60 mg every 6-8 hours; can only be initiated in approved treatment programs
Naltrexone (ReVia®)	Alcohol and narcotic dependence: Initiate 25-50 mg/day; patient should be free of opioid for 7-10 days prior to initiation
Nicotine gum	Smoking cessation: 1-2 pieces/hour; maximum: 30 pieces/day (2 mg/piece). If high tobacco use, give DS (4 mg/piece); maximum: 20/day
Nicotine nasal spray	Smoking cessation: 1 spray in each nostril once or twice per hour; maximum: 80 sprays
Nicotine patches	Smoking cessation: One patch daily for 8 weeks

ANTICHOLINERGIC EFFECTS OF COMMON PSYCHOTROPICS

Drug	Atropine Equivalence Factor*	Common Daily Dose (mg)	Atropine Equivalent (mg/dose)
ANTICHOLINERGICS			
Benztropine	0.849	2	1.70
Diphenhydramine	0.011	50	0.55
Trihexyphenidyl	0.828	5	4.14
NEUROLEPTICS			
Chlorpromazine	0.030	500	15.00
Clozapine	0.125	500	62.50
Fluphenazine	0.001	25	0.03
Haloperidol	0.000	20	0.00
Loxapine	0.005	150	0.75
Mesoridazine	0.025	150	3.75
Molindone	0.000	150	0.00
Perphenazine	0.001	32	0.03
Thioridazine	0.104	300	31.20
Thiothixene	0.001	40	0.04
Trifluoperazine	0.003	25	0.08
ANTIDEPRESSANTS			
Amitriptyline	0.121	150	18.15
Amoxapine	0.002	150	0.30
Desipramine	0.011	150	1.65
Doxepin	0.026	150	3.90
Fluoxetine	0.001	20	0.02
Imipramine	0.024	150	3.60
Maprotiline	0.004	150	0.60
Nortriptyline	0.015	75	1.13
Trazodone	0.000	100	0.00

*Anticholinergic effects of 1 mg of drug in equivalent mg of atropine.

ANTICHOLINERGIC EFFECTS OF COMMON
PSYCHOTROPICS (Continued)

FREQUENTLY PRESCRIBED DRUGS FOR THE ELDERLY

Drug*	Atropine Equivalent	Common Dose	Anticholinergic Drug Level (ng/mL of atropine equivalents)
Captopril	1.5	75	0.02
Cimetidine	344	400	0.86
Codeine	9.9	90	0.11
Digoxin	0.03	0.125	0.25
Dipyridamole	24.8	225	0.11
Dyazide	2	25/37.5	0.08
Furosemide	8.8	40	0.22
Isosorbide dinitrate	9	60	0.15
Nifedipine	6.6	30	0.22
Prednisolone	11	20	0.55
Ranitidine	33	150	0.22
Theophylline	176	400	0.44
Warfarin	0.6	5	0.12

*At a 10^{-8} M concentration.

Adapted from Tune L, Carr S, Hoag E, et al, "Anticholinergic Effects of Drugs Commonly Prescribed for the Elderly: Potential Means for Assessing Risk of Delirium," *Am J Psychiatry*, 1992, 149(10):1393-4.

ANTIDEPRESSANT AGENTS

Comparison of Usual Dosage, Mechanism of Action, and Adverse Effects of Antidepressants

Drug	Initial Dose	Usual Dosage (mg/d)	Dosage Forms	Adverse Effects						Comments
				ACH	Drowsiness	Orthostatic Hypotension	Cardiac Arrhythmias**	GI Distress	Weight Gain	
TRICYCLIC ANTIDEPRESSANTS & RELATED COMPOUNDS**										
Amitriptyline (Elavil®, Enovil®)	25-75 mg qhs	100-300	T, I	4+	4+	4+	3+	1	4+	Also used in chronic pain, migraine, and as a hypnotic
Amoxapine (Asendin®)	50 mg bid	100-400	T	2+	2+	2+	2+	0	2+	May cause EPS
Clomipramine* (Anafranil®)	25-75 mg qhs	100-250	C	4+	4+	2+	3+	1+	4+	Approved for OCD
Desipramine (Norpramin®)	25-75 mg qhs	100-300	T	1+	2+	2+	2+	0	1+	Blood levels useful for therapeutic monitoring
Doxepin (Adapin®, Sinequan®)	25-75 mg qhs	100-300	C, L	3+	4+	2+	2+	0	4+	
Imipramine (Janimine®, Tofranil®)	25-75 mg qhs	100-300	T, C, I	3+	3+	4+	3+	1+	4+	Blood levels useful for therapeutic monitoring
Maprotiline (Ludiomil®)	25-75 mg qhs	100-225	T	2+	3+	2+	2+	0	2+	
Nortriptyline (Aventyl®, Pamelor®)	25-50 mg qhs	50-150	C, L	2+	2+	1+	2+	0	1+	Blood levels useful for therapeutic monitoring
Protriptyline (Vivactil®)	15 mg qAM	15-60	T	2+	1+	2+	3+	0	0	
Trimipramine (Surmontil®)	25-75 mg qhs	100-300	C	4+	4+	3+	3+	0	4+	

ANTIDEPRESSANT AGENTS (Continued)

Comparison of Usual Dosage, Mechanism of Action, and Adverse Effects of Antidepressants (continued)

Drug	Initial Dose	Usual Dosage (mg/d)	Dosage Forms	ACH	Drowsiness	Orthostatic Hypotension	Cardiac Arrhythmias	GI Distress	Weight Gain	Comments
						Adverse Effects				
SELECTIVE SEROTONIN REUPTAKE INHIBITORS††										
Citalopram (Celexa™)	20 mg qAM	20-60	T	0	0	0	0	3+§	1+	CYP2D6 inhibitor (weak)
Fluoxetine (Prozac®, Sarafem™)	10-20 mg qAM	20-80	C, L, T	0	0	0	0	3+§	1+	CYP2D6, 2C19, and 3A3/4 inhibitor
Fluvoxamine (Luvox®)*	50 mg qhs	100-300	T	0	0	0	0	3+§	1+	Contraindicated with astemizole, cisapride, terfenadine; CYP1A2, 2C19, and 3A3/4 inhibitors
Paroxetine (Paxil™)	10-20 mg qAM	20-50	T, L	1+	1+	0	0	3+§	1+	CYP2D6 inhibitor
Sertraline (Zoloft™)	25-50 mg qAM	50-150	T	0	0	0	0	3+§	1+	CYP2D6 inhibitor (weak)
DOPAMINE-REUPTAKE BLOCKING COMPOUNDS										
Bupropion (Wellbutrin®, Wellbutrin SR®, Zyban®)	100 mg tid IR 150 mg for 3-7 days, then 150 mg bid SR	300-450†	T	0	0	0	1+	1+	0	Contraindicated with seizures, bulimia, and anorexia; low incidence of sexual dysfunction
SEROTONIN/NOREPINEPHRINE REUPTAKE INHIBITORS***										
Venlafaxine (Effexor®, Effexor-XR®)	25 mg bid-tid IR 37.5 mg qd XR	75-375	T	1+	1+	0	1+	3+§	0	High-dose is useful to treat refractory depression

Comparison of Usual Dosage, Mechanism of Action, and Adverse Effects of Antidepressants (continued)

Drug	Initial Dose	Usual Dosage (mg/d)	Dosage Forms	Adverse Effects							Comments
				ACH	Drowsiness	Orthostatic Hypotension	Cardiac Arrhythmias	GI Distress	Weight Gain		
5HT2 RECEPTOR ANTAGONIST PROPERTIES											
Nefazodone (Serzone®)	100 mg bid	300–600	T	1+	1+	0	0	1+	0		Contraindicated with astemizole, cisapride, and terfenadine; caution with triazolam and alprazolam; low incidence of sexual dysfunction
Trazodone (Desyrel®)	50 mg tid	150–600	T	0	4+	3+	1+	1+	2+		
NORADRENERGIC ANTAGONIST											
Mirtazapine (Remeron®)	15 mg qhs	15–45	T	1+	3+	0	0	0	3+		Dose >15 mg/d less sedating, low incidence of sexual dysfunction
MONOAMINE OXIDASE INHIBITORS											
Phenelzine (Nardil®)	15 mg tid	15–90	T	2+	2+	2+	1+	1+	3+		Diet must be low in tyramine; avoid concurrent sympathomimetics and other antidepressants
Tranylcypromine (Parnate®)	10 mg bid	10–60	T	2+	1+	2+	1+	1+	2+		

**IMPORTANT NOTE: A 1-week supply taken all at once in a patient receiving the maximum dose can be fatal.

*** Do not use with sibutramine; relatively safe in overdose.

Key: N = norepinephrine; S = serotonin; ACH = anticholinergic effects (dry mouth, blurred vision, urinary retention, constipation); 0 - 4+ = absent or rare - relatively common. T= Tablet, L = Liquid, I = Injectable, C = Capsule

*Not approved by FDA for depression. Approved for OCD.

†Not to exceed 150 mg/dose to minimize seizure risk for IR and 200 mg/dose for SR.

††Flat dose response curve, headache, nausea, and sexual dysfunction are common side effects for SSRIs

§Nausea is usually mild and transient.

ANTIPARKINSONIAN AGENTS

Generic Name	Brand Name	Formulation	Dosage Range (mg/day)	Relative Oral Potency
ANTICHOLINERGIC				
Benztropine	Cogentin®*	Tablet: 0.5 mg, 1 mg, 2 mg Injection: 1 mg/mL (2 mL ampul)	1-6	2
Biperiden	Akineton®	Tablet: 2 mg Injection: 5 mg/mL (1 mL ampul)	2-8	2
Orphenadrine	Norflex®	Tablet: 100 mg Tablet, sustained release: 100 mg Injection: 30 mg/mL (2 mL, 10 mL)	50-400	50
ANTIHISTAMINIC				
Diphenhydramine	Benadryl®*	Capsule: 25 mg, 50 mg Elixir: 12.5 mg/5 mL (4 oz, 8 oz, 16 oz bottle) Injection: 10 mg/mL (10 mL, 30 mL); 50 mg/mL (1 mL, 10 mL) Syrup: 12.5 mg/5 mL Tablet: 25 mg, 50 mg	25-300	25
Ethopropazine	Parsidol®	Tablet: 10 mg, 50 mg	100-400	50
Procyclidine	Kemadrin®	Tablet: 5 mg	7.5-20	5
Trihexyphenidyl	Artane®*	Capsule: 5 mg Tablet: 2 mg, 5 mg Elixir: 2 mg/5 mL	2-15	5
DOPAMINERGIC				
Amantadine	Symmetrel®*, Symadine®	Tablet: 100 mg Syrup: 50 mg/5 mL (16 oz bottle)	100-400	N/A

*Available in generic form.

ANTIPSYCHOTIC AGENTS

Antipsychotic Agent	Dosage Forms	I.M./P.O. Potency	Equiv. Dosages (approx) (mg)	Usual Adult Daily Maint. Dose (mg)	Sedation (Incidence)	Extrapyramidal Side Effects	Anticholinergic Side Effects	Cardiovascular Side Effects	Comments
Chlorpromazine (Thorazine®)	Cap, Conc, Inj, Supp, Syr, Tab	4:1	100	200-1000	High	Moderate	Moderate	Moderate/High	
Chlorprothixene* (Taractan®)			100	75-600	High	Moderate	Moderate	Moderate	
Clozapine (Clozaril®)	Tab		50	75-900	High	Very Low	High	High	~1% incidence of agranulocytosis; weekly-biweekly CBC required
Fluphenazine (Prolixin®, Permitil®)	Conc, Elix, Inj, Tab	2:1	2	0.5-40	Low	High	Low	Low	
Haloperidol (Haldol®)	Conc, Inj, Tab	2:1	2	1-15	Low	High	Low	Low	
Loxapine (Loxitane®)	Cap, Conc, Inj		10	25-250	Moderate	Moderate	Low	Low	
Mesoridazine (Serentil®)	Inj, Liq, Tab	3:1	50	30-400	High	Low	High	Moderate	Prolongs QTc; use only in treatment of refractory illness
Molindone (Moban®)	Conc, Tab		15	15-225	Low	Moderate	Low	Low	May cause less weight gain
Olanzapine (Zyprexa™)	Tab		4	5-20	Moderate/ High	Low	Moderate	Moderate	Potential for weight gain, lipid abnormalities, diabetes
Perphenazine (Trilafon®)	Conc, Inj, Tab		10	16-64	Low	Moderate	Low	Low	
Pimozide (Orap®)	Tab		2	1-20	Moderate	High	Moderate	Low	Contraindicated with CYP3A inhibitors
Promazine (Sparine®)	Inj, Tab		200	40-1000	Moderate	Moderate	High	Moderate	
Quetiapine (Seroquel®)	Tab		80	75-750	Moderate	Very Low	Moderate	Moderate	Low weight gain

ANTIPSYCHOTIC AGENTS (Continued)

Antipsychotic Agent	Dosage Forms	I.M./P.O. Potency	Equiv. Dosages (approx) (mg)	Usual Adult Daily Maint. Dose (mg)	Sedation (Incidence)	Extrapyramidal Side Effects	Anticholinergic Side Effects	Cardiovascular Side Effects	Comments
Risperidone (Risperdal®)	Sol, Tab		1	0.5-6	Low/ Moderate	Low	Low	Low/Moderate	Target dose: ≤6 mg/d; low weight gain
Thioridazine (Mellaril®)	Conc, Susp, Tab		100	200-800	High	Low	High	Moderate/High	May cause irreversible retinitis pigmentosa at doses >800 mg/d; prolongs QTc; use only in treatment of refractory illness
Thiothixene (Navane®)	Cap, Conc, Inj, Powder for inj	4:1	4	5-40	Low	High	Low	Low/Moderate	
Trifluoperazine (Stelazine®)	Conc, Inj, Tab		5	2-40	Low	High	Low	Low	
Ziprasidone (Geodon®)	Cap	2:1	40	40-160	Low/ Moderate	Low	Low	Low/Moderate	Low weight gain; contraindicated with QTc-prolonging agents

NA = not available
*Withdrawn from market

ANTIPSYCHOTIC MEDICATION GUIDELINES

Appropriate indications for use of antipsychotic medications are outlined in the Health Care Finance Administration's Omnibus Reconciliation Act (OBRA) of 1987. These regulations require that antipsychotics be used to treat specific conditions (listed below) and not solely for behavior control.

Approved indications include:

- acute psychotic episode
- atypical psychosis
- brief reactive psychosis
- delusional disorder
- Huntington's disease
- psychotic mood disorder (including manic depression and depression with psychotic features)
- schizo-affective disorder
- schizophrenia
- schizophrenic form disorder
- Tourette's disease
- short-term (7 days) for hiccups, nausea, vomiting, or pruritus
- organic mental syndrome with psychotic or agitated features:
    - behaviors are quantitatively and objectively documented
    - behaviors must be **persistent**
    - behaviors are not caused by preventable reasons
    - patient presents a danger to self or others
    - continuous crying or screaming if this impairs functional status
    - psychotic symptoms (hallucinations, paranoia, delusions) which cause resident distress or impaired functional capacity

"Clinically contraindicated" means that a resident with a "specific condition" who has had a history of recurrence of psychotic symptoms (eg, delusions, hallucinations) which have been stabilized with a maintenance dose of an antipsychotic drug without incurring significant side effects (eg, tardive dyskinesia) **should not receive gradual dose reductions**. In residents with organic mental syndromes (eg, dementia, delirium), "clinically contraindicated" means that a gradual dose reduction has been attempted **twice** in 1 year and that attempt resulted in the return of symptoms for which the drug was prescribed to a degree that a cessation in the gradual dose reduction, or a return to previous dose levels was necessary.

If the medication is being used outside the guidelines, the physician must provide justification why the continued use of the drug and the dose of the drug is clinically appropriate.

Antipsychotics should not be used if one or more of the following is/are the **only** indication:

- wandering
- poor self care
- restlessness
- impaired memory
- anxiety
- depression (without psychotic features)
- insomnia
- unsociability
- indifference to surroundings
- fidgeting
- nervousness

ANTIPSYCHOTIC MEDICATION GUIDELINES *(Continued)*

- uncooperativeness
- agitated behaviors which do **not** represent danger to the resident or others

Selection of an antipsychotic agent should be based on the side effect profile since all antipsychotic agents are equally effective at equivalent doses. Coadministration of two or more antipsychotics does not have any pharmacological basis or clinical advantage and increases the potential for side effects. See Antipsychotic Agents table in Comparison Charts.

DOSING GUIDELINES

1. Daily dosages should be equal to or less than those listed below, unless documentation exists to support the need for higher doses to maintain or improve functional status.

Generic	Brand	Daily Dose for Patients With Organic Mental Syndrome
Chlorpromazine	Thorazine®	75 mg
Clozapine	Clozaril®	50 mg
Fluphenazine	Prolixin®	4 mg
Haloperidol	Haldol®	4 mg
Loxapine	Loxitane®	10 mg
Mesoridazine	Serentil®	25 mg
Molindone	Moban®	10 mg
Olanzapine	Zyprexa®	5 mg
Perphenazine	Trilafon®	8 mg
Pimozide	Orap™	4 mg
Prochlorperazine	Compazine®	10 mg
Promazine	Sparine®	150 mg
Quetiapine	Seroquel®	100 mg
Risperidone	Risperdal®	2 mg
Thioridazine	Mellaril®	75 mg
Thiothixene	Navane®	7 mg
Trifluoperazine	Stelazine®	8 mg

2. The dose of prochlorperazine may be exceeded for short-term (up to 7 days) for treatment of nausea and vomiting. Residents with nausea and vomiting secondary to cancer or cancer chemotherapy can also be treated with higher doses for longer periods of time.

3. The residents must receive adequate monitoring for significant side effects such as tardive dyskinesia, postural hypotension, cognitive-behavioral impairment, akathisia, and parkinsonism.

4. Gradual dosage reductions are to be attempted twice in 1 year if prescribed for OMS. If symptoms for which the drug has been prescribed return and both reduction attempts have proven unsuccessful, the physician may indicate further reductions are clinically contraindicated.

5. "Clinically contraindicated" means that a resident **need not undergo** a "gradual dose reduction" or "behavioral interventions" if:

- The resident has a "specific condition" and has a history of recurrence of psychotic symptoms (eg, delusions, hallucinations), which have been stabilized with a maintenance dose of an antipsychotic drug without incurring significant side effects.

- The resident has organic mental syndrome (now called "delirium, dementia, and amnestic and other cognitive disorders" by DSM IV) and has had a gradual dose reduction attempted **twice** in 1 year and that attempt resulted in the return of symptoms for which the drug was prescribed to a degree that a cessation in the gradual dose reduction, or a return to previous dose reduction was necessary.

- The resident's physician provides a justification why the continued use of the drug and the dose of the drug is clinically appropriate. This justification should include: a) a diagnosis, but not simply a diagnostic label or code, but the description of symptoms, b) a discussion of the differential psychiatric and medical diagnosis (eg, why the resident's behavioral symptom is thought to be a result of a dementia with associated psychosis and/or agitated behaviors, and not the result of an unrecognized painful medical condition or a psychosocial or environmental stressor), c) a description of the justification for the choice of a particular treatment, or treatments, and d) a discussion of why the present dose is necessary to manage the symptoms of the resident. This information need not necessarily be in the physician's progress notes, but must be a part of the resident's clinical record.

Examples of evidence that would support a justification of why a drug is being used outside these guidelines but in the best interests of the resident may include, but are not limited to the following.

1. A physician's note indicating for example, that the dosage, duration, indication, and monitoring are clinically appropriate, **and the reasons why they are clinically appropriate**; this note should demonstrate that the physician has carefully considered the risk/benefit to the resident in using drugs outside the guidelines.

2. A medical or psychiatric consultation or evaluation (eg, Geriatric Depression Scale) that confirms the physician's judgment that use of a drug outside the guidelines is in the best interest of the resident.

3. Physician, nursing, or other health professional documentation indicating that the resident is being monitored for adverse consequences or complications of the drug therapy.

4. Documentation confirming that previous attempts at dosage reduction have been unsuccessful.

5. Documentation (including MDS documentation) showing resident's subjective or objective improvement, or maintenance of function while taking the medication.

6. Documentation showing that a resident's decline or deterioration is evaluated by the interdisciplinary team to determine whether a particular drug, or a particular dose, or duration of therapy, may be the cause.

7. Documentation showing why the resident's age, weight, or other factors would require a unique drug dose or drug duration, indication, or monitoring.

8. Other evidence you may deem appropriate.

ANXIOLYTIC/HYPNOTIC USE IN LONG-TERM CARE FACILITIES

One of the regulations regarding medication use in long-term care facilities concerns "unnecessary drugs." The regulation states, "Each resident's drug regimen must be free from unnecessary drugs." Recently, the Health Care Financing Administration (HCFA) issued the final interpretive guidelines on this regulation. The following is a summary of these guidelines as they pertain to anxiolytic/hypnotic agents.

A. **Long-Acting Benzodiazepines**

Long-acting benzodiazepine drugs should not be used in residents unless an attempt with a shorter-acting drug has failed. If they are used, the doses must be no higher than the listed dose, unless higher doses are necessary for maintenance or improvement in the resident's functional status. Daily use should be less then 4 continuous months unless an attempt at a gradual dose reduction is unsuccessful. Residents on diazepam for seizure disorders or for the treatment of tardive dyskinesia are exempt from this restriction. Residents on clonazepam for bipolar disorder, tardive dyskinesia, nocturnal myoclonus, or seizure disorder are also exempt. Residents on long-acting benzodiazepines should have a gradual dose reduction at least twice within 1 year before it can be concluded that the gradual dose reduction is "clinically contraindicated."

Generic	Brand	Maximum Daily Geriatric Dose (mg)
Chlordiazepoxide	Librium®	20
Clonazepam	Klonopin™	1.5
Clorazepate	Tranxene®	15
Diazepam	Valium®	5
Flurazepam	Dalmane®	15
Halazepam	Paxipam®	40
Quazepam	Doral®	7.5

B. **Benzodiazepines or Other Anxiolytic/Sedative Drugs**

Anxiolytic/sedative drugs should be used for purposes other than sleep induction only when other possible causes of the resident's distress have been ruled out and the use results in maintenance or improvement in the resident's functional status. Daily use should not exceed 4 continuous months unless an attempt at gradual dose reduction has failed. Anxiolytics should only be used for generalized anxiety disorder, dementia with agitated states that either endangers the resident or others, or is a source of distress or dysfunction; panic disorder or symptomatic anxiety associated with other psychiatric disorders. The dose should not exceed those listed below unless a higher dose is needed as evidenced by the resident's response. Gradual dosage reductions should be attempted at least twice within 1 year before it can be concluded that a gradual dose reduction is "clinically contraindicated."

Short-Acting Benzodiazepines

Generic	Brand	Maximum Daily Geriatric Dose (mg)
Alprazolam	Xanax®	0.75
Estazolam*	ProSom®	0.5
Lorazepam	Ativan®	2
Oxazepam	Serax®	30

*Primarily used as a hypnotic agent.

Other Anxiolytic and Sedative Drugs

Generic	Brand	Maximum Daily Geriatric Dose (mg)
Chloral hydrate	Noctec®, etc	750
Diphenhydramine	Benadryl®	50
Hydroxyzine	Atarax®, Vistaril®	50

Note: Chloral hydrate, diphenhydramine, and hydroxyzine are not necessarily drugs of choice for treatment of anxiety disorders. HCFA lists them only in the event of their possible use.

C. **Drugs Used for Sleep Induction**

Drugs for sleep induction should only be used when all possible reasons for insomnia have been ruled out (ie, pain, noise, caffeine). The use of the drug must result in the maintenance or improvement of the resident's functional status. Daily use of a hypnotic should not exceed 10 consecutive days unless an attempt at a gradual dose reduction is unsuccessful. The dose should not exceed those listed below unless a higher dose has been deemed necessary. Gradual dose reductions should be attempted at least three times within 6 months before it can be concluded that a gradual dose reduction is "clinically contraindicated."

Hypnotic Drugs

Generic	Brand	Daily Geriatric Dose (mg)
Alprazolam*	Xanax®	0.25
Chloral hydrate	Noctec®	500
Diphenhydramine	Benadryl®	25
Estazolam	ProSom™	0.5
Hydroxyzine	Atarax®, Vistaril®	50
Lorazepam*	Ativan®	1
Oxazepam*	Serax®	15
Temazepam	Restoril®	7.5
Triazolam	Halcion®	0.125
Zaleplon	Sonata®	5
Zolpidem	Ambien®	5

*Not officially indicated as a hypnotic agent.

Note: Chloral hydrate, diphenhydramine, and hydroxyzine are not necessarily drugs of choice for sleep disorders. HCFA lists them only in the event of their possible use.

ANXIOLYTIC/HYPNOTIC USE IN
LONG-TERM CARE FACILITIES *(Continued)*

D. **Miscellaneous Hypnotic/Sedative/Anxiolytic Drugs**

The initiation of the following medications should not occur in any dose in any resident. Residents currently using these drugs or residents admitted to the facility while using these drugs should receive gradual dose reductions. Newly admitted residents should have a period of adjustment before attempting reduction. Dose reductions should be attempted at least twice within 1 year before it can be concluded that it is "clinically contraindicated."

Examples of Barbiturates

Generic	Brand
Amobarbital	Amytal®
Amobarbital/Secobarbital	Tuinal®
Butabarbital	Butisol Sodium®
Combinations	Fiorinal®, etc
Pentobarbital	Nembutal®
Secobarbital	Seconal™

Miscellaneous Hypnotic/Sedative/Anxiolytic Agents

Generic	Brand
Ethchlorvynol	Placidyl®
Glutethimide	Doriden®
Meprobamate	Equanil®, Miltown®
Methyprylon	Noludar®
Paraldehyde	Paral®

ATYPICAL ANTIPSYCHOTICS*

Drug	DR EPS	PROL	TD	ACH	SZ	OH	LFTs	SED	WT GAIN	NMS	AGRAN	TX REFR	Lipid	DM	QTc
Clozapine (Clozaril®)	No	No	No	High	DD	High	Low	High	High	Yes	Yes	Yes	High	High	Low
Risperidone (Risperdal®)	Yes	Yes	Yes	Very low	Low	Low	Very low	Low	Low	Yes	Yes**	Maybe	Low	Low	Low
Olanzapine (Zyprexa®)	Yes	No	Yes	Moderate	Low	Low/Moderate	Low	Moderate	High	Yes	Yes**	Maybe	High	Moderate	Low
Quetiapine (Seroquel®)	No	No	Yes	Moderate	Low	Moderate	Low	Moderate	Low/Moderate	Yes	Yes**	No	Moderate	Low	Low
Ziprasidone (Geodon®)	Yes	Yes	?	Low	Low	Low/Moderate	Low	Low	Mild	?	?	No	Low	Low	Moderate†

*Defined as 1) decrease or no EPS at doses producing antipsychotic effect; 2) minimum or no increase in prolactin; 3) decrease in both positive and negative symptoms of schizophrenia.

**Case reports

†Dose related within 40-160 mg dosage range

DR EPS = dose related extrapyramidal symptoms

PROL = sustained prolactin elevation (may cause amenorrhea, galactorrhea, gynecomastia, impotence)

TD = tardive dyskinesia

ACH = anticholinergic side effects (dry mouth, blurred vision, constipation, urinary hesitancy)

SZ = seizures

OH = orthostatic hypotension (blood pressure drops upon standing)

LFTs = increased liver function test results

SED = sedation

WT GAIN = weight gain

NMS = neuroleptic malignant syndrome

AGRAN = agranulocytosis (without white blood cells to fight infection)

TX REFR = efficacy in treatment refractory schizophrenia

DD = dose dependent

Lipid = lipid abnormalities; cholesterol and/or triglyceride elevations

DM = diabetes (based on case reports)

QTc = QTc prolongation

BENZODIAZEPINES

Agent	Dosage Forms	Relative Potency	Peak Blood Levels (oral) (h)	Protein Binding (%)	Volume of Distribution (L/kg)	Major Active Metabolite	Half-Life (parent) (h)	Half-Life* (metabolite) (h)	Usual Initial Dose	Adult Oral Dosage Range
ANXIOLYTIC										
Alprazolam (Xanax®)	Tab	0.5	1-2	80	0.9-1.2	No	12-15	—	0.25-0.5 tid	0.75-4 mg/d
Chlordiazepoxide (Librium®)	Cap, Powd for Inj, Tab	10	2-4	90-98	0.3	Yes	5-30	24-96	5-25 mg tid-qid	15-100 mg/d
Diazepam (Valium®)	Gel, Inj, Sol, Tab	5	0.5-2	98	1.1	Yes	20-80	50-100	2-10 mg bid-qid	4-40 mg/d
Halazepam (Paxipam®)	Tab	20			1.3	Yes	14	50-100	20-40 mg tid-qid	80-160 mg/d
Lorazepam (Ativan®)**	Inj, Sol, Tab	1	1-6	88-92		No	10-20	—	0.5-2 mg tid-qid	2-4 mg/d
Oxazepam (Serax®)	Cap, Tab	15-30	2-4	86-99	0.6-2	No	5-20	—	10-30 mg tid-qid	30-120 mg/d
Prazepam (Centrax®)	Cap, Tab	10				Yes	1.2	30-100	10 mg tid	30 mg/d
SEDATIVE/HYPNOTIC										
Estazolam (ProSom™)	Tab	0.3	2	93	—	No	10-24	—	1 mg qhs	1-2 mg
Flurazepam (Dalmane®)	Cap	5	0.5-2	97	—	Yes	Not significant	40-114	15 mg qhs	15-60 mg
Quazepam (Doral®)	Tab	5	2	95	5	Yes	25-41	28-114	15 mg qhs	7.5-15 mg
Temazepam (Restoril®)	Cap	5	2-3	96	1.4	No	10-40	—	15-30 mg qhs	15-30 mg
Triazolam (Halcion®)	Tab	0.1	1	89-94	0.8-1.3	No	2.3	—	0.125-0.25 qhs	0.125-0.25 mg

Agent	Dosage Forms	Relative Potency	Peak Blood Levels (oral) (h)	Protein Binding (%)	Volume of Distribution (L/kg)	Major Active Metabolite	Half-Life (parent) (h)	Half-Life* (metabolite) (h)	Usual Initial Dose	Adult Oral Dosage Range
					MISCELLANEOUS					
Clonazepam (Klonopin™)	Tab	0.25-0.5	1-2	86	1.8-4	No	18-50 h	—	0.5 mg tid	1.5-20 mg/d
Clorazepate (Tranxene®)	Cap, Tab	7.5	1-2	80-95	—	Yes	Not significant	50-100 h	7.5-15 mg bid-qid	15-60 mg
Midazolam (Versed®)	Inj		0.4-0.7†	95	0.8-6.6	No	2-5 h	—	NA	

* = significant metabolite.

**Reliable bioavailability when given I.M.

† = I.V. only.

NA = not available.

567

CLOZAPINE-INDUCED SIDE EFFECTS

INCIDENCE AND MANAGEMENT

Effect	Incidence	Management
Sedation & fatigue	35%	Initiate split dosing with long-term goal to administer twice daily with larger portion at bedtime (appears to be dose-dependent). For chronic sedation, consider an empiric trial of methylphenidate 5-20 mg/day.
Sialorrhea	25%	Clozapine may affect the swallowing mechanism; behavioral approach may be best. Consider lowering the dose. Pharmacological management consists of clonidine 0.1-0.9 mg/day (monitor blood pressure) or benztropine 0.5-2 mg/day (monitor for increased anticholinergic side effects).
Weight gain	35%	Diet and exercise best. No pharmacological agent shown to be consistently useful; one study showed the addition of quetiapine to clozapine minimized weight gain; consider lowering dose.
Urinary incontinence	25%	If patient receiving co-pharmacy with typical antipsychotic, consider discontinuing; pharmacological management consists of ephedrine 25-150 mg/d, oxybutynin 5 mg tid, or desmopressin.
Tachycardia	25%	Dose dependent. Beta-blocker; atenolol 50 mg/d or propranolol 10 mg tid (adjust for rate)
Constipation	20%	Discontinue other medications with anticholinergic activity, if possible. May need chronic psyllium and/or docusate.
Seizures	4%	Dose dependent. Valproic acid/valproate; initiate at 250 mg tid or 500 mg bid and titrate to serum level of at least 50 mcg/mL
Agranulocytosis	1%	Stop drug. Do not rechallenge. Consider filgrastim (G-CSF) or sargramostim (GM-CSF) during acute recovery phase.

BODY MASS INDEX (BMI)

Body Mass Index (BMI), kg/m^2
Height (feet, inches)

Weight (lb)	5'0"	5'3"	5'6"	5'9"	6'0"	6'3"
140	27	25	23	21	19	18
150	29	27	24	22	20	19
160	31	28	26	24	22	20
170	33	30	28	25	23	21
180	35	32	29	27	25	23
190	37	34	31	28	26	24
200	39	36	32	30	27	25
210	41	37	34	31	29	26
220	43	39	36	33	30	28
230	45	41	37	34	31	29
240	47	43	39	36	33	30
250	49	44	40	37	34	31

CYTOCHROME P450 ENZYMES AND DRUG METABOLISM

Background

There are five distinct groups of drug metabolizing which account for the majority of drug metabolism in humans. These enzymes "families", known as isoenzymes, are localized primarily in the liver. The nomenclature of this system has been standardized. Isoenzyme families are identified as a cytochrome (CYP prefix), followed by their numerical designation (eg, 1A2).

Enzymes may be inhibited (slowing metabolism through this pathway) or induced (increased in activity or number). Individual drugs metabolized by a specific enzyme are identified as substrates for the isoenzyme. Considerable effort has been expended in recent years to classify drugs metabolized by this system as either an inhibitor, inducer, or substrate of a specific isoenzyme. It should be noted that a drug may demonstrate complex activity within this scheme, acting as an inhibitor of one isoenzyme while serving as a substrate for another.

By recognizing that a substrate's metabolism may be dramatically altered by concurrent therapy with either an inducer or inhibitor, potential interactions may be identified and addressed. For example, a drug which inhibits CYP1A2 is likely to block metabolism of theophylline (a substrate for this isoenzyme). Because of this interaction, the dose of theophylline required to maintain a consistent level in the patient should be reduced when an inhibitor is added. Failure to make this adjustment may lead to supratherapeutic theophylline concentrations and potential toxicity.

This approach does have limitations. For example, the metabolism of specific drugs may have primary and secondary pathways. The contribution of secondary pathways to the overall metabolism may limit the impact of any given inhibitor. In addition, there may be up to a tenfold variation in the concentration of an isoenzyme across the broad population. In fact, a complete absence of an isoenzyme may occur in some genetic subgroups. Finally, the relative potency of inhibition, relative to the affinity of the enzyme for its substrate, demonstrates a high degree of variability. These issues make it difficult to anticipate whether a theoretical interaction will have a clinically relevant impact in a specific patient.

The details of this enzyme system continue to be investigated, and information is expanding daily. However, to be complete, it should be noted that other enzyme systems also influence a drug's pharmacokinetic profile. For example, a key enzyme system regulating the absorption of drugs is the p-glycoprotein system. Recent evidence suggests that some interaction originally attributed to the cytochrome system may, in fact, have been the result of inhibition of this enzyme.

The following tables represent an attempt to detail the available information with respect to isoenzyme activities. Within certain limits, they may be used to identify potential interactions. Of particular note, an effort has been made in each drug monograph to identify involvement of a particular isoenzyme in the drug's metabolism. These tables are intended to supplement the limited space available to list drug interactions in the monograph. Consequently, they may be used to define a greater range of both actual and potential drug interactions.

CYTOCHROME P450 ENZYMES AND RESPECTIVE METABOLIZED DRUGS

CYP1A2

Substrates

Acetaminophen
Acetanilid
Alosetron
Aminophylline
Amitriptyline (demethylation)
Antipyrine
Apomorphine
Betaxolol
Caffeine
Chlorpromazine
Clomipramine (demethylation)
Clozapine
Cyclobenzaprine (demethylation)
Desipramine (demethylation)
Estradiol
Estradiol and medroxyprogesterone
Fluvoxamine
Haloperidol (minor)
Imipramine (demethylation)
Levobupivacaine
Levomepromazine
Lidocaine
Maprotiline
Methadone
Metoclopramide
Mirtazapine (hydroxylation)
Nordiazepam
Nortriptyline
Olanzapine (demethylation, hydroxylation)
Ondansetron
Phenacetin
Phenothiazines
Pimozide (minor)
Propafenone
Propranolol
Riluzole
Ritonavir
Ropinirole
Ropivacaine
Tacrine
Theophylline
Thioridazine
Thiothixene
Trifluoperazine
Verapamil
Warfarin (R-warfarin, minor pathway)
Zileuton
Ziprasidone (minor)
Zopiclone

Inducers

Carbamazepine
Charbroiled foods
Cigarette smoke
Cruciferous vegetables (cabbage, brussels sprouts, broccoli, cauliflower)
Griseofulvin
Modafinil (weak)
Nicotine
Omeprazole
Phenobarbital
Phenytoin
Primidone
Rifampin
Ritonavir

Inhibitors

Albendazole (weak)
Anastrozole
Cimetidine
Ciprofloxacin
Citalopram (weak)
Clarithromycin
Diethyldithiocarbamate
Diltiazem
Enoxacin
Entacapone (high dose)
Erythromycin
Ethinyl estradiol
Estradiol
Fluvoxamine
Fluoxetine (high dose)
Grapefruit juice
Isoniazid
Ketoconazole
Lidocaine
Mexiletine
Mibefradil
Moricizine (possible)
Norfloxacin
Paroxetine (high dose)(weak)
Ritonavir
Sertraline (weak)
Tacrine
Tertiary TCAs
Ticlopidine (possible)
Zileuton

CYTOCHROME P450 ENZYMES AND DRUG METABOLISM
(Continued)

CYP2A6

Substrates

Dexmedetomidine	Nicotine
Letrozole	Ritonavir
Montelukast	Tolcapone

Inducers

Barbiturates

Inhibitors

Diethyldithiocarbamate	Methoxsalen
Entacapone (high dose)	Ritonavir
Letrozole	Tranylcypromine

CYP2B6

Substrates

Antipyrine	Ifosfamide
Bupropion (hydroxylation)	Lidocaine
Cyclophosphamide	Nicotine
Diazepam	Orphenadrine

Inducers

Modafinil (weak)	Phenytoin
Phenobarbital	Primidone

Inhibitors

Diethyldithiocarbamate	Orphenadrine

CYP2C
(Specific isozyme has not been identified)

Substrates

Antipyrine	Mestranol
Carvedilol	Mephobarbital
Clozapine (minor)	Ticrynafen

Inducers

Carbamazepine	Primidone
Haloperidol	Rifampin
Phenobarbital	Sulfinpyrazone
Phenytoin	

Inhibitors

Isoniazid	Ketoprofen
Ketoconazole	Miconazole

CYP2C8

Substrates

Carbamazepine
Cerivastatin
Diazepam
Diclofenac
Ibuprofen
Mephobarbital
Naproxen (5-hydroxylation)
Omeprazole

Paclitaxel
Pioglitazone
Retinoic acid
Rifampin
Rosiglitazone
Tolbutamide
Warfarin (S-warfarin)

Inducers

Carbamazepine
Phenobarbital
Phenytoin

Primidone
Rifampin
Rifapentine

Inhibitors

Anastrozole
Nicardipine
Omeprazole

Propoxyphene
Trimethoprim

CYP2C9

Substrates

Alosetron
Amitriptyline (demethylation)
Amoxapine
Carvedilol
Celecoxib
Dapsone
Diazepam
Diclofenac
Flurbiprofen
Fluvastatin
Glimepiride
Hexobarbital
Ibuprofen
Imipramine (demethylation)
Indomethacin
Irbesartan
Losartan
Mefenamic acid
Metronidazole
Mirtazapine

Montelukast
Naproxen (5-hydroxylation)
Nateglinide
Omeprazole
Phenytoin
Piroxicam
Quetiapine (minor pathway)
Rifampin
Ritonavir
Rosiglitazone (minor)
Sildenafil citrate (minor pathway)
Tamoxifen
Tenoxicam
Tetrahydrocannabinol
Tolbutamide
Torsemide
Warfarin (S-warfarin)
Zafirlukast (hydroxylation)
Zileuton

Inducers

Carbamazepine
Fluconazole
Fluoxetine
Phenobarbital

Phenytoin
Rifampin
Rifapentine

Inhibitors

Amiodarone
Anastrozole
Chloramphenicol
Cimetidine
Clopidogrel (high conc - *in vitro*)
Sulfamethoxazole and Trimethoprim
Diclofenac

Disulfiram
Drospirenone
Entacapone (high dose)
Flurbiprofen
Fluconazole
Fluoxetine
Fluvastatin

CYTOCHROME P450 ENZYMES AND DRUG METABOLISM
(Continued)

Fluvoxamine (potent)
Isoniazid
Ketoconazole (weak)
Ketoprofen
Leflunomide (*in vitro* only)
Metronidazole
Nateglinide
Nicardipine
Omeprazole
Phenylbutazone
Propoxyphene
Ritonavir

Sertraline
Sulfamethoxazole-trimethoprim
Sulfaphenazole
Sulfinpyrazone
Sulfonamides
Sulindac
Trimethoprim
Troglitazone
Valproic acid
Warfarin (R-warfarin)
Zafirlukast

CYP2C18

Substrates

Dronabinol
Naproxen
Omeprazole
Piroxicam
Proguanil

Propranolol
Retinoic acid
Tolbutamide
Warfarin

Inducers

Carbamazepine
Phenobarbital

Phenytoin
Rifampin

Inhibitors

Cimetidine
Fluconazole

Fluvastatin
Isoniazid

CYP2C19

Substrates

Amitriptyline (demethylation)
Amoxapine
Apomorphine
Barbiturates
Carisoprodol
Cilostazol (minor)
Citalopram
Clomipramine (demethylation)
Desmethyldiazepam
Diazepam (N-demethylation, minor pathway)
Divalproex sodium
Esomeprazole
Hexobarbital
Imipramine (demethylation)
Lansoprazole

Mephenytoin
Mephobarbital
Moclobemide
Olanzapine (minor)
Omeprazole
Pantoprazole
Pentamidine
Phenytoin
Proguanil
Propranolol
Ritonavir
Tolbutamide
Topiramate
Valproic acid
Warfarin (R-warfarin)

Inducers

Carbamazepine
Phenobarbital

Phenytoin
Rifampin

Inhibitors

Cimetidine
Citalopram (weak)
Diazepam

Disulfiram
Drospirenone
Entacapone (high conc)

Ethinyl estradiol
Felbamate
Fluconazole
Fluoxetine
Fluvastatin
Fluvoxamine
Isoniazid
Ketoconazole (weak)
Letrozole
Modafinil
Nicardipine
Omeprazole

Oxcarbazepine
Proguanil
Ritonavir
Sertraline
Telmisartan
Teniposide
Ticlopidine (potent)
Tolbutamide
Topiramate
Tranylcypromine
Troglitazone
Warfarin (R-warfarin)

CYP2D6

Substrates

Almotriptan
Amitriptyline (hydroxylation)
Amoxapine
Amphetamine
Betaxolol
Bisoprolol
Brofaromine
Bufuronol
Captopril
Carvedilol
Cevimeline
Chlorpheniramine
Chlorpromazine
Cinnarizine
Clomipramine (hydroxylation)
Clozapine (minor pathway)
Codeine (hydroxylation, o-demethylation)
Cyclobenzaprine (hydroxylation)
Cyclophosphamide
Debrisoquin
Delavirdine
Desipramine
Dexfenfluramine
Dextromethorphan (o-demethylation)
Dihydrocodeine
Diphenhydramine
Dolasetron
Donepezil
Doxepin
Encainide
Ethylmorphine
Fenfluramine
Flecainide
Fluoxetine (minor pathway)
Fluphenazine
Galantamine
Halofantrine
Haloperidol (minor pathway)
Hydrocodone
Hydrocortisone
Hydroxyamphetamine
Imipramine (hydroxylation)
Labetalol
Lidocaine
Loratadine
Maprotiline
m-Chlorophenylpiperazine (m-CPP)

Meperidine
Methadone
Methamphetamine
Metoclopramide
Metoprolol
Mexiletine
Mianserin
Mirtazapine (hydroxylation)
Molindone
Morphine
Nortriptyline (hydroxylation)
Olanzapine (minor, hydroxymethylation)
Ondansetron
Orphenadrine
Oxycodone
Papaverine
Paroxetine (minor pathway)
Penbutolol
Pentazocine
Perhexiline
Perphenazine
Phenformin
Pindolol
Promethazine
Propafenone
Propoxyphene
Propranolol
Quetiapine (minor pathway)
Remoxipride
Risperidone
Ritonavir (minor)
Ropivacaine
Selegiline
Sertindole
Sertraline (minor pathway)
Sparteine
Tamoxifen
Thioridazine**
Tiagabine
Timolol
Tolterodine
Tramadol
Trazodone
Trimipramine
Tropisetron
Venlafaxine (o-desmethylation)
Yohimbine

CYTOCHROME P450 ENZYMES AND DRUG METABOLISM
(Continued)

Inducers

Rifampin

Inhibitors

Amiodarone	Moclobemide
Celecoxib	Nicardipine
Chloroquine	Norfluoxetine
Chlorpromazine	Paroxetine
Cimetidine	Perphenazine
Citalopram	Primaquine
Clomipramine	Propafenone
Codeine	Propoxyphene
Delavirdine	Quinacrine
Desipramine	Quinidine (potent)
Dextropropoxyphene	Ranitidine
Diltiazem	Risperidone (weak)
Doxorubicin	Ritonavir
Entacapone (high dose)	Sertindole
Fluoxetine	Sertraline (weak)
Fluphenazine	Thioridazine
Fluvoxamine	Ticlopidine (weak)
Haloperidol	Valproic acid
Labetalol	Venlafaxine (weak)
Lobeline	Vinblastine
Lomustine	Vincristine
Methadone	Vinorelbine
Mibefradil	Yohimbine

CYP2E1

Substrates

Acetaminophen	Isoflurane
Acetone	Isoniazid
Aniline	Methoxyflurane
Benzene	Nitrosamine
Caffeine	Ondansetron
Chloral hydrate	Phenol
Chlorzoxazone	Ritonavir
Clozapine	Sevoflurane
Dapsone	Styrene
Dextromethorphan	Tamoxifen
Enflurane	Theophylline (minor pathway)
Ethanol	Venlafaxine
Halothane	

Inducers

Ethanol	Mitoxantrone (weak)
Isoniazid	

Inhibitors

Diethyldithiocarbamate (disulfiram metabolite)	Entacapone (high dose)
Dimethyl sulfoxide	Ritonavir
Disulfiram	

CYP3A3/4

Substrates

Acetaminophen
Alfentanil
Almotriptan
Alosetron
Alprazolam**
Amiodarone
Amitriptyline (minor)
Amlodipine
Amoxapine
Amprenavir
Anastrozole
Androsterone
Antipyrine
Apomorphine
Astemizole**
Atorvastatin
Benzphetamine
Bepridil
Bexarotene
Bromazepam
Bromocriptine
Budesonide
Bupropion (minor)
Buspirone
Busulfan
Caffeine
Cannabinoids
Carbamazepine
Cevimeline
Cerivastatin
Chlordiazepoxide
Chlorpromazine
Cilostazol (major)
Cimetidine
Cisapride**
Citalopram
Clarithromycin
Clindamycin
Clofibrate
Clomipramine
Clonazepam
Clorazepate
Clozapine
Cocaine
Codeine (demethylation)
Cortisol
Cortisone
Cyclobenzaprine (demethylation)
Cyclophosphamide
Cyclosporine
Dapsone
Dehydroepiandrostendione
Delavirdine
Desmethyldiazepam
Dexamethasone
Dextromethorphan (minor, N-demethylation)
Diazepam (minor; hydroxylation, N-demethylation)
Digitoxin
Diltiazem

Disopyramide
Docetaxel
Dofetilide (minor)
Dolasetron
Donepezil
Doxorubicin
Doxycycline
Dronabinol
Drospirenone
Enalapril
Erythromycin
Esomeprazole
Estradiol
Estradiol and medroxyprogesterone
Ethinyl estradiol
Ethosuximide
Etoposide
Exemestane
Felodipine
Fentanyl
Fexofenadine
Finasteride
Fluoxetine
Flutamide
Fluticasone
Galantamine
Gemfibrozil
Glyburide
Granisetron
Halofantrine
Haloperidol
Hydrocortisone
Hydroxyarginine
Ifosfamide
Imipramine
Indinavir
Isradipine
Itraconazole
Ketoconazole
Lansoprazole (minor)
Letrozole
Levobupivacaine
Levomethadyl acetate hydrochloride
Levonorgestrel
Lidocaine
Loratadine
Losartan
Lovastatin
Methadone
Mibefradil
Miconazole
Midazolam
Mifepristone
Mirtazapine (N-demethylation)
Modafinil
Montelukast
Nateglinide
Navelbine
Nefazodone
Nelfinavir**

CYTOCHROME P450 ENZYMES AND DRUG METABOLISM
(Continued)

Nevirapine
Nicardipine
Nifedipine
Niludipine
Nimodipine
Nisoldipine
Nitrendipine
Omeprazole (sulfonation)
Ondansetron
Oral contraceptives
Orphenadrine
Paclitaxel
Pantoprazole
Pimozide**
Pioglitazone
Pravastatin
Prednisone
Progesterone
Proguanil
Propafenone
Quercetin
Quetiapine
Quinidine
Quinine
Repaglinide
Retinoic acid
Rifampin (major)
Risperidone
Ritonavir**
Salmeterol
Saquinavir
Sertindole
Sertraline
Sibutramine##
Sildenafil citrate

Simvastatin
Sirolimus
Sufentanil
Tacrolimus
Tamoxifen
Temazepam
Teniposide
Terfenadine**
Testosterone
Tetrahydrocannabinol
Theophylline
Tiagabine
Ticlopidine
Tolcapone
Tolterodine
Toremifene
Trazodone
Tretinoin
Triazolam**
Troglitazone
Troleandomycin
Venlafaxine (N-demethylation)
Verapamil
Vinblastine
Vincristine
Warfarin (R-warfarin)
Yohimbine
Zaleplon (minor pathway)
Zatosetron
Zidovudine
Zileuton
Ziprasidone
Zolpidem**
Zonisamide

Inducers

Carbamazepine
Dexamethasone
Ethosuximide
Glucocorticoids
Nafcillin
Nelfinavir
Nevirapine
Oxcarbazepine
Phenobarbital
Phenylbutazone
Phenytoin

Primidone
Progesterone
Rifabutin
Rifapentine
Rifampin
Rofecoxib (mild)
St John's wort
Sulfadimidine
Sulfinpyrazone
Troglitazone

Inhibitors

Amiodarone
Amprenavir
Anastrozole (high conc)
Cannabinoids
Cimetidine
Clarithromycin**
Clotrimazole
Cyclosporine
Danazol
Delavirdine
Dexamethasone
Diethyldithiocarbamate

Diazepam
Diltiazem
Dirithromycin
Disulfiram (and metabolite diethyldithiocarbamate)
Drospirenone (weak)
Entacapone (high dose)
Erythromycin**
Ethinyl estradiol (weak)
Fluconazole (weak)
Fluoxetine
Fluvoxamine**

Gestodene
Grapefruit juice
Haloperidol
Indinavir
Isoniazid
Itraconazole**
Ketoconazole**
Lopinavir and Ritonavir
Metronidazole
Mibefradil**
Miconazole (moderate)
Mifepristone
Modafinil (minor)
Nefazodone**
Nelfinavir
Nevirapine
Nicardipine
Norfloxacin
Norfluoxetine

Omeprazole (weak)
Oxiconazole
Paroxetine (weak)
Propoxyphene
Quinidine (weak)
Quinine**
Quinupristin and dalfopristin
Ranitidine
Ritonavir**
Saquinavir
Sertindole
Sertraline
Troglitazone
Troleandomycin
Valproic acid (weak)
Verapamil
Vinorelbine
Zafirlukast
Zileuton

CYP3A4/5

Substrate

Argatroban (minor)

Inducer

Oxcarbazepine

CYP3A5-7

Substrates

Cortisol
Diazepam
Estradiol and medroxyprogesterone
Ethinyl estradiol
Nifedipine

Terfenadine
Testosterone
Triazolam
Vinblastine
Vincristine

Inducers

Phenobarbital
Phenytoin

Primidone
Rifampin

Inhibitors

Clotrimazole
Ketoconazole
Metronidazole

Miconazole
Propoxyphene
Troleandomycin

**Contraindications:
Terfenadine, astemizole, cisapride, and triazolam contraindicated with nefazodone
Pimozide contraindicated with CYP3A3/4 inhibitors
Alprazolam and triazolam contraindicated with ketoconazole and itraconazole
Terfenadine, astemizole, and cisapride contraindicated with fluvoxamine
Terfenadine contraindicated with mibefradil, ketoconazole, erythromycin, clarithromycin, troleandomycin
Thioridazine contraindicated with CYP2D6 inhibitors
Ritonavir contraindicated with triazolam, zolpidem, astemizole, rifabutin, quinine, clarithromycin, troleandomycin
Mibefradil contraindicated with astemizole
Nelfinavir contraindicated with rifabutin

##Do not use with SSRIs, sumatriptan, lithium, meperidine, fentanyl, dextromethorphan, or pentazocine within 2 weeks of an MAOI.

CYTOCHROME P450 ENZYMES AND DRUG METABOLISM
(Continued)

References

Baker GB, Urichuk CJ, and Coutts RT, "Drug Metabolism and Metabolic Drug-Drug Interactions in Psychiatry," *Child Adolescent Psychopharm News (Suppl).*

DeVane CL, "Pharmacogenetics and Drug Metabolism of Newer Antidepressant Agents," *J Clin Psychiatry,* 1994, 55(Suppl 12):38-45.

Drug Interactions Analysis and Management. Cytochrome (CYP) 450 Isozyme Drug Interactions, Vancouver, WA: Applied Therapeutics, Inc, 523-7.

Ereshefsky L, "Drug-Drug Interactions Involving Antidepressants: Focus on Venlafaxine," *J Clin Psychopharmacol,* 1996, 16(3 Suppl 2):375-535.

Ereshefsky L, *Psychiatr Annal,* 1996, 26:342-50.

Fleishaker JC and Hulst LK, "A Pharmacokinetic and Pharmacodynamic Evaluation of the Combined Administration of Alprazolam and Fluvoxamine," *Eur J Clin Pharmacol,* 1994, 46(1):35-9.

Flockhart DA, et al, *Clin Pharmacol Ther,* 1996, 59:189.

Ketter TA, Flockhart DA, Post RM, et al, "The Emerging Role of Cytochrome P450 3A in Psychopharmacology," *J Clin Psychopharmacol,* 1995, 15(6):387-98.

Michalets EL, "Update: Clinically Significant Cytochrome P450 Drug Interactions," *Pharmacotherapy,* 1998, 18(1):84-112.

Nemeroff CB, DeVane CL, and Pollock BG, "Newer Antidepressants and the Cytochrome P450 System," *Am J Psychiatry,* 1996, 153(3):311-20.

Pollock BG, "Recent Developments in Drug Metabolism of Relevance to Psychiatrists," *Harv Rev Psychiatry,* 1994, 2(4):204-13.

Richelson E, "Pharmacokinetic Drug Interactions of New Antidepressants: A Review of the Effects on the Metabolism of Other Drugs," *Mayo Clin Proc,* 1997, 72(9):835-47.

Riesenman C, "Antidepressant Drug Interactions and the Cytochrome P450 System: A Critical Appraisal," *Pharmacotherapy,* 1995, 15(6 Pt 2):84S-99S.

Schmider J, Greenblatt DJ, von Moltke LL, et al, "Relationship of *In Vitro* Data on Drug Metabolism to *In Vivo* Pharmacokinetics and Drug Interactions: Implications for Diazepam Disposition in Humans," *J Clin Psychopharmacol,* 1996, 16(4):267-72.

Slaughter RL, *Pharm Times,* 1996, 7:6-16.

Watkins PB, "Role of Cytochrome P450 in Drug Metabolism and Hepatotoxicity," *Semin Liver Dis,* 1990, 10(4):235-50.

DEPRESSION

Medications That May Precipitate Depression

Anticancer agents	Vinblastine, vincristine, interferon, procarbazine, asparaginase, tamoxifen, cyproterone
Anti-inflammatory & analgesic agents	Indomethacin, pentazocine, phenacetin, phenylbutazone
Antimicrobial agents	Cycloserine, ethambutol, sulfonamides, select gram-negative antibiotics
Cardiovascular/ antihypertensive agents	Clonidine, digitalis, diuretics, guanethidine, hydralazine, indapamide, methyldopa, prazocin, procainamide, propranolol, reserpine
CNS agents	Alcohol, amantadine, amphetamine & derivatives, barbiturates, benzodiazepines, chloral hydrate, carbamazepine, cocaine, haloperidol, L-dopa, phenothiazines, succinimide derivatives
Hormonal agents	ACTH, corticosteroids, estrogen, melatonin, oral contraceptives, progesterone
Miscellaneous	Cimetidine, disulfiram, organic pesticides, physostigmine

Medical Disorders & Psychiatric Disorders Associated With Depression

Endocrine diseases	Acromegaly, Addison's disease, Cushing's disease, diabetes mellitus, hyperparathyroidism, hypoparathyroidism, hyperthyroidism, hypothyroidism, insulinoma, pheochromocytoma, pituitary dysfunction
Deficiency states	Pernicious anemia, severe anemia, Wernicke's encephalopathy
Infections	Encephalitis, fungal infections, meningitis, neurosyphilis, influenza, mononucleosis, tuberculosis, AIDS
Collagen disorders	Rheumatoid arthritis
Systemic lupus erythematosus	
Metabolic disorders	Electrolyte imbalance, hypokalemia, hyponatremia, hepatic encephalopathy, Pick's disease, uremia, Wilson's disease
Cardiovascular disease	Cerebral arteriosclerosis, chronic bronchitis, congestive heart failure, emphysema, myocardial infarction, paroxysmal dysrhythmia, pneumonia
Neurologic disorders	Alzheimer's disease, amyotrophic lateral sclerosis, brain tumors, chronic pain syndrome, Creutzfeldt-Jakob disease, Huntington's disease, multiple sclerosis, myasthenia gravis, Parkinson's disease, poststroke, trauma (postconcussion)
Malignant disease	Breast, gastrointestinal, lung, pancreas, prostate
Psychiatric disorders	Alcoholism, anxiety disorders, eating disorders, schizophrenia

DISCONTINUATION OF PSYCHOTROPIC DRUGS

Withdrawal Symptoms and Recommendations

Drug	Withdrawal Symptoms	Recommendations
Amantadine	Neuroleptic malignant syndrome, drug-induced catatonia	In Parkinson's disease, dosage should be reduced gradually in order to prevent exacerbation of symptoms
Antipsychotics	Nausea, emesis, anorexia, diarrhea, rhinorrhea, diaphoresis, myalgia, paresthesia, anxiety, agitation, restlessness, insomnia	Reinitiate antipsychotic[1]
Benzodiazepines	Rebound symptoms, tachycardia, insomnia, tremor, seizures, psychosis	Taper dose slowly or switch to benzodiazepine with a long half-life at a high affinity (preferable) for the GABA benzodiazepine receptor site
Benztropine	Nervousness, craving, restlessness, depression, poor concentration, nausea, vomiting, headache, blurred vision, malaise	Dosage should be reduced gradually to prevent sudden increase in adverse symptoms; half-life of benztropine is 24 hours
Biperiden	Anxiety, depression, motor agitation, hallucinations, physical complaints	When discontinuing an antidyskinetic, taper gradually to avoid a rebound of adverse symptoms
Bromocriptine	Recurrence of symptoms, galactorrhea	No definitive information available on dosage reduction; however, when initiating therapy, begin with low dose and increase gradually (2.5 mg every 14-28 days for Parkinson's and 3-7 days for other indications) to prevent development of side effects
Diphenhydramine	Recurrence of insomnia, increased daytime restlessness, irritability, excessive blinking, increased defecation (rebound cholinergic reaction)	No specific recommendations reported
Levodopa	Confusion, fever, seizure activity, hyper-rigidity, profuse diaphoresis, tachycardia, tachypnea, muscle enzyme elevation	Gradually reduce dose to avoid the neuroleptic malignant-like syndrome (NLMLS); after discontinuation, dantrolene and/or bromocriptine have been used in patients with evident NLMLS to decrease fever and avoid a potentially lethal complication
Pergolide	Hallucinations, confusion, paranoid ideation, worsening parkinsonism symptoms	No recommendations reported
SSRIs	Dizziness, light-headedness, insomnia, fatigue, anxiety, agitation, nausea, headache, sensory disturbances	Restart SSRI or another antidepressant with a similar pharmacologic profile[2]
TCAs	Malaise, myalgia, anergy, diaphoresis, rhinitis, paresthesia, headache, nausea, vomiting, diarrhea, anorexia, insomnia, irritability, depressed mood	Administer antimuscarinic agents
Trihexyphenidyl	Anxiety, tachycardia, orthostatic hypotension, deterioration of sleep quality, extrapyramidal symptoms, deterioration of psychotic symptomatology, life-threatening respiratory difficulties	Reduce dose gradually to avoid withdrawal symptoms or an increase in psychotic symptoms

1. Dilsaver SC and Alessi NE, "Antipsychotic Withdrawal Symptoms: Phenomenology and Pathophysiology," *Acta Psychiatr Scand*, 1988, 77(3):241-6.

2. Zajecka J, Tracy KA, and Mitchell S, "Discontinuation Symptoms After Treatment with Serotonin Reuptake Inhibitors: A Literature Review," *J Clin Psychiatry*, 1997, 58(7):291-7.

FEDERAL OBRA REGULATIONS RECOMMENDED MAXIMUM DOSES

Antidepressants

Drug	Brand Name	Usual Max Daily Dose for Age ≥65	Usual Max Daily Dose
Amitriptyline	Elavil®	150 mg	300 mg
Amoxapine	Asendin®	200 mg	400 mg
Desipramine	Norpramin®	150 mg	300 mg
Doxepin	Adapin®, Sinequan®	150 mg	300 mg
Imipramine	Tofranil®	150 mg	300 mg
Maprotiline	Ludiomil®	150 mg	300 mg
Nortriptyline	Aventyl®, Pamelor®	75 mg	150 mg
Protriptyline	Vivactil®	30 mg	60 mg
Trazodone	Desyrel®	300 mg	600 mg
Trimipramine	Surmontil®	150 mg	300 mg

Antipsychotics

Drug	Brand Name	Usual Max Daily Dose for Age ≥65	Usual Max Daily Dose	Daily Oral Dose for Residents With Organic Mental Syndromes
Chlorpromazine	Thorazine®	800 mg	1600 mg	75 mg
Clozapine	Clozaril®	25 mg	450 mg	50 mg
Fluphenazine	Prolixin®	20 mg	40 mg	4 mg
Haloperidol	Haldol®	50 mg	100 mg	4 mg
Loxapine	Loxitane®	125 mg	250 mg	10 mg
Mesoridazine	Serentil®	250 mg	500 mg	25 mg
Molindone	Moban®	112 mg	225 mg	10 mg
Perphenazine	Trilafon®	32 mg	64 mg	8 mg
Promazine	Sparine®	50 mg	500 mg	150 mg
Risperidone	Risperdal®	1 mg	16 mg	4 mg
Thioridazine	Mellaril®	400 mg	800 mg	75 mg
Thiothixene	Navane®	30 mg	60 mg	7 mg
Trifluoperazine	Stelazine®	40 mg	80 mg	8 mg
Trifluopromazine	Vesprin®	100 mg	20 mg	–

FEDERAL OBRA REGULATIONS RECOMMENDED MAXIMUM DOSES (Continued)

Anxiolytics*

Drug	Brand Name	Usual Daily Dose for Age ≥65	Usual Daily Dose for Age ≤65
Alprazolam	Xanax®	2 mg	4 mg
Chlordiazepoxide	Librium®	40 mg	100 mg
Clorazepate	Tranxene®	30 mg	60 mg
Diazepam	Valium®	20 mg	60 mg
Halazepam	Paxipam®	80 mg	160 mg
Lorazepam	Ativan®	3 mg	6 mg
Meprobamate	Miltown®	600 mg	1600 mg
Oxazepam	Serax®	60 mg	90 mg
Prazepam	Centrax®	30 mg	60 mg

*Note: HCFA-OBRA guidelines strongly urge clinicians not to use barbiturates, glutethimide, and ethchlorvynol due to their side effects, pharmacokinetics, and addiction potential in the elderly. Also, HCFA discourages use of long-acting benzodiazepines in the elderly.

Hypnotics
(Should not be used for more than 10 continuous days*)

Drug	Brand Name	Usual Max Single Dose for Age ≥65	Usual Max Single Dose
Alprazolam	Xanax®	0.25 mg	1.5 mg
Amobarbital	Amytal®	105 mg	300 mg
Butabarbital	Butisol®	100 mg	200 mg
Chloral hydrate	Noctec®	750 mg	1500 mg
Chloral hydrate	Various	500 mg	1000 mg
Diphenhydramine	Benadryl®	25 mg	50 mg
Ethchlorvynol	Placidyl®	500 mg	1000 mg
Flurazepam	Dalmane®	15 mg	30 mg
Glutethimide	Doriden®	500 mg	1000 mg
Halazepam	Paxipam®	20 mg	40 mg
Hydroxyzine	Atarax®	50 mg	100 mg
Lorazepam	Ativan®	1 mg	2 mg
Oxazepam	Serax®	15 mg	30 mg
Pentobarbital	Nembutal®	100 mg	200 mg
Secobarbital	Seconal®	100 mg	200 mg
Temazepam	Restoril®	15 mg	30 mg
Triazolam	Halcion®	0.125 mg	0.5 mg

*Note: HCFA-OBRA guidelines strongly urge clinicians not to use barbiturates, glutethimide, and ethchlorvynol due to their side effects, pharmacokinetics, and addiction potential in the elderly. Also, HCFA discourages use of long-acting benzodiazepines in the elderly and also discourages the use of diphenhydramine and hydroxyzine.

HALLUCINOGENIC DRUGS

Principal Pharmacological Properties of Hallucinogenic Drugs

Drug; Chemical Structure	Duration of Acute Effect (h)	pKa	Route of Metabolism/ Excretion	Half-Life	Protein Binding (%)	V_d (L/kg)	Urine Screen Positive for	Duration of Psychotropic Effects	Doses of Abuse	Fatal Dose
Phencyclidine (PCP); arylcyclo-hexylamine	4-6	8.5	Hepatic/urine	1 h	65	6.2-0.3	2 wk	Up to 1 mo	1-9 mg	1 mg/kg
Cocaine; tropane alkaloid	0.5	5.6	Plasma hydrolysis*	48-75 min	9-90	1.2-1.9	4 days (benzoyl-ecgonine)	≤5-7 d	20-200 mg (intranasally)	1-1.2 g
Cannabis; monoterpenoid	0.5-3	10.6	Hepatic hydroxylation	25-57 h	97-99	10	Up to 4 d	≤6 h	5-15 mg THC	
LSD; indole alkylamine	0.7-8	7.8	Hepatic hydroxylation	2.5 h		0.27	5 d	May last for days	100-300 mcg	0.2 mg/kg
Psilocybin; tryptamine	0.5-6						Not detected	12 h	20-100 mushrooms	5-15 mg of psilocybin
Mescaline; phenylalkylamine	4.6	Not known	Hepatic/urine†	6 h	None	Not known		12 h	5 mg/kg	20 mg/kg
Morphine; alkaloid/ derivative of opium	4-5	8.05	Glucuronidation/ urine	1.9-3.1 h	35	3.2	48 h	≤6 h	2-20 mg	Variable – dependent on tolerance, nontolerant fatal dose is 120 mg orally or 30 mg parenterally

HALLUCINOGENIC DRUGS *(Continued)*

Principal Pharmacological Properties of Hallucinogenic Drugs *(continued)*

Drug; Chemical Structure	Duration of Acute Effect (h)	pKa	Route of Metabolism/ Excretion	Half-Life	Protein Binding (%)	V_d (L/kg)	Urine Screen Positive for	Duration of Psychotropic Effects	Doses of Abuse	Fatal Dose
Heroin; diacetylmorphine	3.4	7.6	Hepatic‡	3-20 min	40	25	~40 h	≤6 h	2.2 mg	Variable – dependent on tolerance
Amphetamine; β-(phenylisopropyl)-amine	Variable	9.93	Hepatic§	12 h¶	16-20	3-6	2-4 d	Delusions may remain for months	100-1000 mg/d	Variable – dependent on tolerance

*By serum cholinesterase.
†60% excreted unchanged.
‡Converted to morphine.
§Converted to phenylacetone.
¶Urine pH-dependent.

Reprinted with permission from Leikin JB, Krantz AJ, Zell-Kanter M, et al, "Clinical Features and Management of Intoxication Due to Hallucinogenic Drugs," *Med Toxicol Adverse Drug Exp*, 1989, 4(5):328.

LIQUID COMPATIBILITY

Liquid Compatibility with Antipsychotics and Mood Stabilizers

Vehicle	Carba-mazepine*	Lithium	Val-proate	Chlor-promazine*	Fluphen-azine	Halo-peridol	Loxa-pine	Mesori-dazine	Risperi-done	Thiori-dazine	Thio-thixene	Trifluo-perazine
Water	C	C	C	C	C	C		C	C	C	C	C
Saline	C	C	C	C	C	X			C	C		C
Milk		C		C	C	X			C	X	C	C
Coffee		C		U	C	X	C		C	X	X	U
Tea		C		U	X	X			X	X	X	C
Apple juice		X		X	X	C				X	X	X
Grape juice		C		X		X		C		X		X
Grapefruit juice		C		C	C	X	C	C		C		C
Orange juice		C		C	C	C	C	C	C	C	C	C
Prune juice		C		C	C					X	C	C
Cola		C	X	U	X	C	C		X	X	X	C
7-Up/Sprite		C	X	C	X		C			C		C

C = Compatible; X - Incompatible; U = Conflicting Data; Blank = No Data

* Carbamazepine is not compatible with chlorpromazine

MOOD STABILIZERS

Generic Name (Brand Name)	Dosage Forms	Half-Life (h)	Usual Dose	Therapeutic Range	Comments
Lithium (Eskalith®; Lithane®; Lithobid®; Lithonate®; Lithotabs®)	T, C, L	18-24	600-1800 mg/day	0.5-1.5 mEq/L*	Nausea, tremor, polydipsia, and polyuria common; may cause hypothyroidism with chronic use; FDA approved for bipolar disorder
Carbamazepine (Epitol®; Tegretol®; Tegretol-XR®)	T, L	15-50 initial 8-20 chronic	600-1800 mg/day	N/A	Nausea, headache, dizziness, and sedation common; blood levels >12 mcg/mL associated with toxicity; enzyme inducer
Valproate (Depakene®; Depakote®)	T, C, L	5-20	1-3 g/day	50-125 μg/mL*	Nausea, sedation, diarrhea, and tremor are common; also indicated for migraine prophylaxis; loading dose: 20 mg/kg PO; monitor LFTs if using combination anticonvulsants; FDA approved for mania
Gabapentin (Neurontin®)	C	5-6	500-3600 mg/day	N/A	Renally eliminated
Lamotrigine (Lamictal®)	T	24	100-500 mg/day	N/A	May have antidepressant and mood-stabilizing effects
Topiramate (Topamax®; Topamax® Sprinkle)	T, C	21	400-1600 mg/day	N/A	May be associated with weight loss

T = Tablet, C = Capsule, L = Liquid

N/A = Correlation between serum concentration and clinical response have not been established.

* = Obtain blood level 12 hours after the last dose in the evening

NONBENZODIAZEPINE ANXIOLYTICS & HYPNOTICS

Drug	Dosage Forms	Initial Dose	Usual Dosage Range	Onset	Half-Life	Comments
Buspirone	T	7.5 mg bid	30-60 mg/d	30 min to 1.5 h	2-3 h	Do not use for alcohol or benzodiazepine withdrawal; no sedation or dependence; do not use PRN; use 4 weeks for full therapeutic effect
Chloral hydrate	C, R, S	500 mg to 1 g qhs	500 mg to 2 g/d	30 min	8-11 h	GI irritating; tolerance to hypnotic effect develops rapidly
Diphenhydramine	Soln, C, T, Crm, Lot, S, E	25-50 mg qhs	25-200 mg/d	1-3 h	2-8 h	Anticholinergic; max hypnotic dose: 50 mg/d
Hydroxyzine	T, C, L, I, S	25-100 mg qid	100-600 mg/d	30 min	3-7 h	Anticholinergic
Propranolol	T, C, Soln, I	10 mg tid	80-160 mg/d	1-2 h	4-6 h	Useful for physical manifestations of anxiety (increased heart rate, tremor); second-line agent
Zaleplon	C	5-10 mg qhs	5-20 mg qhs	30 min	1 h	Do not use for alcohol or benzodiazepine withdrawal
Zolpidem	T	10 mg qhs	10 mg qhs	30 min	2.5 h	Do not use for alcohol or benzodiazepine withdrawal

R = rectal suppository; S = syrup; T = tablet; C = capsule; L = liquid; Crm = cream; Inj = injection; Lot = lotion; E = elixir; Soln = solution

PHARMACOKINETICS OF SELECTIVE SEROTONIN-REUPTAKE INHIBITORS (SSRIs)

SSRI	Half-life (h)	Metabolite Half-life	Peak Plasma Level (h)	% Protein Bound	Bioavailability (%)	Initial Dose
Citalopram	35	N/A	4	80	80	20 mg qAM
Fluoxetine	Initial: 24-72 Chronic: 96-144	Norfluoxetine: 4-16 days	6-8	95	72	10-20 mg qAM
Fluvoxamine	16	N/A	3	80	53	50 mg qhs
Paroxetine	21	N/A	5	95	>90	10-20 mg qAM
Sertraline	26	N-desmethyl-sertraline: 2-4 days	5-8	98	—	25-50 qAM

SEROTONIN SYNDROME

Diagnostic Criteria for Serotonin Syndrome

- Recent addition or dosage increase of any agent increasing serotonin activity or availability (usually within 1 day).

- Absence of abused substances, metabolic infectious etiology, or withdrawal.

- No recent addition or dosage increase of a neuroleptic agent prior to onset of signs and symptoms.

- Presence of three or more of the following:
  Altered mental status (seen in 40% of patients, primarily confusion or hypomania)
  Agitation
  Tremor (50% incidence)
  Shivering
  Diarrhea
  Hyper-reflexia (pronounced in lower extremities)
  Myoclonus (50% incidence)
  Ataxia or incoordination
  Fever (50% incidence; temperature >105°F associated with grave prognosis)
  Diaphoresis

Drugs (as Single Causative Agent) Which Can Induce Serotonin Syndrome

Specific serotonin reuptake inhibitors (SSRI)
MDMA (Ecstasy)
Clomipramine

Drug Combinations Which Can Induce Serotonin Syndrome*

Alprazolam – Clomipramine

Bromocriptine – Levodopa/carbidopa

Buspirone – Trazodone

Clomipramine – Clorgiline

Clomipramine – Lithium

Dihydroergotamine – Sertraline

Dihydroergotamine – Amitriptyline

Fentanyl – Sertraline

Fluoxetine – Carbamazepine

Fluoxetine – Lithium

Fluoxetine – Remoxipide

Fluoxetine – Tryptophan

Lithium – Fluvoxamine

Lithium – Paroxetine

Monoamine oxidase inhibitor – Fluoxetine

Monoamine oxidase inhibitor – Fluvoxamine

Monoamine oxidase inhibitor – Meperidine

Monoamine oxidase inhibitor – Sertraline

Monoamine oxidase inhibitor – Tricyclic antidepressants

Monoamine oxidase inhibitor – Tryptophan

Monoamine oxidase inhibitor – Venlafaxine

Nefazodone – Paroxetine

Nortriptyline – Trazodone

Paroxetine – Dextromethorphan

SEROTONIN SYNDROME *(Continued)*

Paroxetine – Dihydroergotamine

Paroxetine – Trazodone

Phenelzine, Trazodone – Dextropropoxyphene

S-adenosylmethionine – Clomipramine

Sertraline – Amitriptyline

Sumatriptan – Sertraline

Tranylcypromine – Clomipramine *

Tramadol – Sertraline

Trazodone– Lithium – Amitriptyline

Trazodone – Fluoxetine

Valproic acid – Nefazodone

Venlafaxine – Tranylcypromine

Venlafaxine – Selegiline

*When administered within 2 weeks of each other

Guidelines for Treatment of Serotonin Syndrome

Therapy is primarily supportive with intravenous crystalloid solutions utilized for hypotension and cooling blankets for mild hyperthermia. Norepinephrine is the preferred vasopressor. Chlorpromazine (25 mg I.M.) or dantrolene sodium (1 mg/kg I.V. – maximum dose 10 mg/kg) may have a role in controlling fevers, although there is no proven benefit. Benzodiazepines are the first-line treatment in controlling rigors and thus, limiting fever and rhabdomyolysis, while clonazepam may be specifically useful in treating myoclonus. Endotracheal intubation and paralysis may be required to treat refractory muscular contractions. Tachycardia or tremor can be treated with beta-blocking agents; although due to its blockade of 5-HTIA receptors, the syndrome may worsen. Serotonin blockers such as diphenhydramine (50 mg I.M.), cyproheptadine (adults: 4-8 mg every 2-4 hours up to 0.5 mg/kg/day; children: up to 0.25 mg/kg/day), or chlorpromazine (25 mg I.M.) have been used with variable efficacy. Methysergide (2-6 mg/day) and nitroglycerin (I.V. infusion of 2 mg/kg/ minute with lorazepam) also has been utilized with variable efficacy in case reports. It appears that cyproheptadine is most consistently beneficial.

Recovery seen within 1 day in 70% of cases; mortality rate is about 11%.

References

Gitlin MJ, "Venlafaxine, Monoamine Oxidase Inhibitors, and the Serotonin Syndrome," *J Clin Psychopharmacol*, 1997, 17(1):66-7.

Heisler MA, Guidery JR, and Arnecke B, "Serotonin Syndrome Induced by Administration of Venlafaxine and Phenelzine," *Ann Pharmacother*, 1996, 30(1):84.

Hodgman MJ, Martin TG, and Krenzelok EP, "Serotonin Syndrome Due to Venlafaxine and Maintenance Tranylcypromine Therapy," *Hum Exp Toxicol*, 1997, 16(1):14-7.

John L, Perreault MM, Tao T, et al, "Serotonin Syndrome Associated With Nefazodone and Paroxetine," *Ann Emerg Med*, 1997, 29(2):287-9.

LoCurto MJ, "The Serotonin Syndrome," *Emerg Clin North Am*, 1997, 15(3):665-75.

Martin TG, "Serotonin Syndrome," *Ann Emerg Med*, 1996, 28(5):520-6.

Mills K, "Serotonin Toxicity: A Comprehensive Review for Emergency Medicine," *Top Emerg Med*, 1993, 15:54-73.

Mills KC, "Serotonin Syndrome. A Clinical Update," *Crit Care Clin*, 1997, 13(4):763-83.

Nisijima K, Shimizu M, Abe T, et al, "A Case of Serotonin Syndrome Induced by Concomitant Treatment With Low-Dose Trazodone, and Amitriptyline and Lithium," *Int Clin Psychopharmacol*, 1996, 11(4):289-90.

Sobanski T, Bagli M, Laux G, et al, "Serotonin Syndrome After Lithium Add-On Medication to Paroxetine," *Pharmacopsychiatry*, 1997, 30(3):106-7.

Sporer KA, "The Serotonin Syndrome. Implicated Drugs, Pathophysiology and Management," *Drug Safety*, 1995, 13(2):94-104.

Sternbach H, "The Serotonin Syndrome," *Am J Psychiatry*, 1991, 148(6):705-13.

Van Berkum MM, Thiel J, Leikin JB, et al, "A Fatality Due to Serotonin Syndrome," *Medical Update for Psychiatrists*, 1997, 2:55-7.

STIMULANT AGENTS USED FOR ADHD

Generic Name (Brand Name)	Dosage	Formulations	Comments
Amphetamine (Various)	2.5-5 mg/d, increase by 2.5-5 mg/wk; maximum dose: 40 mg/d	Tablet: 5 mg, 10 mg	Also used for narcolepsy and exogenous obesity
Amphetamine and Dextroamphetamine (Adderall®)	2.5-5 mg qAM, increase by 2.5-5 mg/wk; maximum dose: 40 mg/d on bid schedule	Tablet: 5 mg, 10 mg, 20 mg, 30 mg	Also used for narcolepsy
Dextroamphetamine* (Dexedrine®)	2.5-5 mg qAM, increase by 2.5-5 mg/wk; maximum dose: 40 mg/d	Elixir: 5 mg/5 mL (16 oz bottle) Tablet: 5 mg, 10 mg Spansules, sustained release: 5 mg, 10 mg, 15 mg	Avoid evening doses; monitor growth; also used for narcolepsy and exogenous obesity
Dextromethamphetamine (Desoxyn®)	2.5-5 mg qd-bid, increase by 5 mg/wk until optimum response is achieved, usually 20-25 mg/d	Tablet: 5 mg Tablet, slow release: 5 mg, 10 mg, 15 mg	
Methylphenidate* (Ritalin®; Ritalin SR®)	2.5-5 mg before breakfast or lunch; increase by 5-10 mg/d at weekly intervals; maximum dose: 60 mg/d	Tablet: 5 mg, 10 mg, 20 mg Tablet, slow release: 20 mg	
Pemoline (Cylert®)	37.5 mg qAM, increase by 18.75 mg/d at weekly intervals; usual range: 56.25-75 mg/d; maximum dose: 112.5 mg/d	Tablet: 18.75 mg, 37.5 mg, 75 mg Tablet, chewable: 37.5 mg	See Warnings in Pemoline monograph

*Available in generic form

TERATOGENIC RISKS OF PSYCHOTROPIC MEDICATIONS

Drug	Risk Category	Possible Effects
ANXIOLYTICS		
Benzodiazepines	D	"Floppy baby," withdrawal, cleft lip
Buspirone	B	Unknown
Hypnotic benzodiazepines	X	Decreased intrauterine growth
ANTIDEPRESSANTS		
MAOIs	C	Rare fetal malformations; rarely used in pregnancy due to hypertension
SSRIs	C	Increased perinatal complications
TCAs	C/D	Fetal tachycardia, fetal withdrawal, fetal anticholinergic effects, urinary retention, bowel obstruction
ANTIPARKINSONIAN		
Amantadine	C	Increase in pregnancy complications
Benztropine	C	Increase in minor malformations
Diphenhydramine	B	Oral clefts
Procyclidine	C	Increase in minor malformations
Trihexyphenidyl	C	Increase in minor malformations
ANTIPSYCHOTICS		
Conventional	C	Rare anomalies, fetal jaundice, fetal anticholinergic effects at birth
Atypical, clozapine	B	Unknown
Atypical, risperidone, quetiapine, olanzapine, ziprasidone	C	Unknown
MOOD STABILIZERS		
Carbamazepine	D	Neural tube defects, minor anomalies
Lithium	D	Behavioral effects, Epstein's anomaly
Valproate	D	Neural tube defects

Pregnancy Categories: A = Controlled studies show no risk to humans; B = no evidence of risk in humans, but adequate human studies may not have been performed; C = risk cannot be ruled out; D = positive evidence of risk to humans, risk may be outweighed by potential benefit; X = contraindicated in pregnancy.

TCA = tricyclic antidepressant; MAOI = monoamine oxidase inhibitor; SSRI = selective serotonin reuptake inhibitor

TYRAMINE CONTENT OF FOODS

Food	Allowed	Minimize Intake	Not Allowed
Beverages	Milk, decaffeinated coffee, tea, soda	Chocolate beverage, caffeine-containing drinks, clear spirits	Acidophilus milk, beer, ale, wine, malted beverages
Breads/cereals	All except those containing cheese	None	Cheese bread and crackers
Dairy products	Cottage cheese, farmers or pot cheese, cream cheese, ricotta cheese, all milk, eggs, ice cream, pudding (except chocolate)	Yogurt (limit to 4 oz per day)	All other cheeses (aged cheese, American, Camembert, cheddar, Gouda, gruyere, mozzarella, parmesan, provolone, romano, Roquefort, stilton
Meat, fish, and poultry	All fresh or frozen	Aged meats, hot dogs, canned fish and meat	Chicken and beef liver, dried and pickled fish, summer or dry sausage, pepperoni, dried meats, meat extracts, bologna, liverwurst
Starches — potatoes/rice	All	None	Soybean (including paste)
Vegetables	All fresh, frozen, canned, or dried vegetable juices except those not allowed	Chili peppers, Chinese pea pods	Fava beans, sauerkraut, pickles, olives, Italian broad beans
Fruit	Fresh, frozen, or canned fruits and fruit juices	Avocado, banana, raspberries, figs	Banana peel extract
Soups	All soups not listed to limit or avoid	Commercially canned soups	Soups which contain broad beans, fava beans, cheese, beer, wine, any made with flavor cubes or meat extract, miso soup
Fats	All except fermented	Sour cream	Packaged gravy
Sweets	Sugar, hard candy, honey, molasses, syrups	Chocolate candies	None
Desserts	Cakes, cookies, gelatin, pastries, sherbets, sorbets	Chocolate desserts	Cheese-filled desserts
Miscellaneous	Salt, nuts, spices, herbs, flavorings, Worcestershire sauce	Soy sauce, peanuts	Brewer's yeast, yeast concentrates, all aged and fermented products, monosodium glutamate, vitamins with Brewer's yeast

TYRAMINE CONTENT OF FOODS

Food	Allowed	Minimize Intake	Not Allowed

PHARMACOLOGIC CATEGORY INDEX

ANTI-PARKINSON'S AGENT (DOPAMINE AGONIST) *(Continued)*

ANTI-PARKINSON'S AGENT (MONOAMINE OXIDASE INHIBITOR)

ANTIPSYCHOTIC AGENT, BENZISOXAZOLE

ANTIPSYCHOTIC AGENT, BENZOTHIAZOLYLPIPERAZINE

ANTIPSYCHOTIC AGENT, BUTYROPHENONE

ANTIPSYCHOTIC AGENT, DIBENZODIAZEPINE

ANTIPSYCHOTIC AGENT, DIBENZOTHIAZEPINE

ANTIPSYCHOTIC AGENT, DIBENZOXAZEPINE

ANTIPSYCHOTIC AGENT, DIHYDOINDOLINE

ANTIPSYCHOTIC AGENT, DIPHENYLBUTYLPERIDINE

ANTIPSYCHOTIC AGENT, PHENOTHIAZINE, PIPERAZINE

ANTIPSYCHOTIC AGENT, PHENOTHIAZINE, PIPERIDINE

ANTIPSYCHOTIC AGENT, PHENOTHIAZINE, ALIPHATIC

ANTIPSYCHOTIC AGENT, THIENOBENZODIAEPINE

ANTIPSYCHOTIC AGENT, THIOXANTHENE DERIVATIVE

ANTIVIRAL AGENT

BARBITURATE

BENZODIAZEPINE

BETA BLOCKER, NONSELECTIVE

BETA BLOCKER (WITH INTRINSIC SYMPATHOMIMETIC ACTIVITY)

CHOLINERGIC AGONIST

ERGOT DERIVATIVE

GENERAL ANESTHETIC

HERB

ALPHABETICAL INDEX

NOTES

NOTES

NOTES

NOTES

NOTES

NOTES

Other titles offered by Lexi-Comp, Inc.

DRUG INFORMATION HANDBOOK (International edition available)
by Charles Lacy, RPh, PharmD, FCSHP; Lora L. Armstrong, RPh, PharmD, BCPS; Morton P. Goldman, PharmD, BCPS; and Leonard L. Lance, RPh, BSPharm

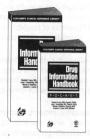

Specifically compiled and designed for the healthcare professional requiring quick access to concisely-stated comprehensive data concerning clinical use of medications.

The Drug Information Handbook is an ideal portable drug information resource, providing the reader with up to 29 key points of data concerning clinical use and dosing of the medication. Material provided in the Appendix section is recognized by many users to be, by itself, well worth the purchase of the handbook.

All medications found in the *Drug Information Handbook*, are included in the abridged *Pocket* edition (select fields were extracted to maintain portability).

PEDIATRIC DOSAGE HANDBOOK (International edition available)
by Carol K. Taketomo, PharmD; Jane Hurlburt Hodding, PharmD; and Donna M. Kraus, PharmD

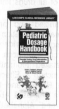

Special considerations must frequently be taken into account when dosing medications for the pediatric patient. This highly regarded quick reference handbook is a compilation of recommended pediatric doses based on current literature, as well as the practical experience of the authors and their many colleagues who work every day in the pediatric clinical setting.

Includes neonatal dosing, drug administration, and (in select monographs) extemporaneous preparations for medications used in pediatric medicine.

GERIATRIC DOSAGE HANDBOOK
by Todd P. Semla, PharmD, BCPS, FCCP; Judith L. Beizer, PharmD, FASCP; and Martin D. Higbee, PharmD, CGP

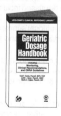

Many physiologic changes occur with aging, some of which affect the pharmacokinetics or pharmacodynamics of medications. Strong consideration should also be given to the effect of decreased renal or hepatic functions in the elderly, as well as the probability of the geriatric patient being on multiple drug regimens.

Healthcare professionals working with nursing homes and assisted living facilities will find the drug information contained in this handbook to be an invaluable source of helpful information.

An International Brand Name Index with names from 22 different countries is also included.

To order call toll free anywhere in the U.S.: 1-800-837-LEXI (5394)
Outside of the U.S. call: 330-650-6506 or online at www.lexi.com

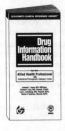
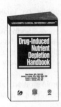
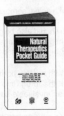

Other titles offered by Lexi-Comp, Inc.

DRUG INFORMATION HANDBOOK *for* ADVANCED PRACTICE
NURSING by Beatrice B. Turkoski, RN, PhD; Brenda R. Lance, RN, MSN; and Mark F.
Bonfiglio, PharmD   Foreword by: Margaret A. Fitzgerald, MS, RN, CS-FNP

1999 "Book of the Year" — *American Journal of Nursing*
Advanced Practice Nursing Category

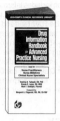

Designed specifically to meet the needs of nurse practitioners, clinical nurse specialists, nurse midwives, and graduate nursing students. The handbook is a unique resource for detailed, accurate information, which is vital to support the advanced practice nurse's role in patient drug therapy management. Over 4750 U.S., Canadian, and Mexican medications are covered in the 1000 monographs. Drug data is presented in an easy-to-use, alphabetically organized format covering up to 46 key points of information (including dosing for pediatrics, adults, and geriatrics). Cross-referenced to Appendix of over 230 pages of valuable comparison tables and additional information. Also included are two indexes, Pharmacologic Category and Controlled Substance, which facilitate comparison between agents.

DRUG INFORMATION HANDBOOK *for* NURSING
by Beatrice B. Turkoski, RN, PhD; Brenda R. Lance, RN, MSN; and Mark F. Bonfiglio, PharmD

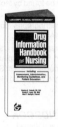

Registered Professional Nurses and upper-division nursing students involved with drug therapy will find this handbook provides quick access to drug data in a concise easy-to-use format.

Over 4000 U.S., Canadian, and Mexican medications are covered with up to 43 key points of information in each monograph. The handbook contains basic pharmacology concepts and nursing issues such as patient factors that influence drug therapy (ie, pregnancy, age, weight, etc) and general nursing issues (ie, assessment, administration, monitoring, and patient education). The Appendix contains over 230 pages of valuable information.

DRUG INFORMATION HANDBOOK *for* PHYSICIAN ASSISTANTS
by Michael J. Rudzinski, RPA-C, RPh and J. Fred Bennes, RPA, RPh

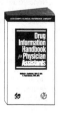

This comprehensive and easy-to-use handbook covers over 4100 drugs and also includes monographs on commonly used herbal products. There are up to 26 key fields of information per monograph, such as Pediatric and Adult Dosing With Adjustments for Renal/Hepatic Impairment, Labeled and Unlabeled Uses, Drug & Alcohol interactions, and Education & Monitoring Issues. Brand (U.S. and Canadian) and generic names are listed alphabetically for rapid access. It is fully cross-referenced by page number and includes alphabetical and pharmacologic indexes.

To order call toll free anywhere in the U.S.: 1-800-837-LEXI (5394)
Outside of the U.S. call: 330-650-6506 or online at www.lexi.com

Other titles offered by Lexi-Comp, Inc.

DRUG INFORMATION HANDBOOK *for* CARDIOLOGY

by Bradley G. Phillips, PharmD and Virend K. Somers, MD, Dphil

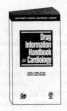

An ideal resource for physicians, pharmacists, nurses, residents, and students. This handbook was designed to provide the most current information on cardiovascular agents and other ancillary medications. Each monograph includes information on Special Cardiovascular Considerations and I.V. to Oral Equivalency. It is Alphabetically organized by brand and generic name. The Appendix contains information on Hypertension, Anticoagulation, Cytochrome P-450, Hyperlipidemia, Antiarrhythmia, and Comparative Drug Charts. The Special Topics/Issues include Emerging Risk Factors for Cardiovascular Disease, Treatment of Cardiovascular Disease in the Diabetic, Cardiovascular Stress Testing, and Experimental Cardiovascular Therapeutic Strategies in the New Millenium, *and much more . . .*

DRUG INFORMATION HANDBOOK *for* ONCOLOGY

by Dominic A. Solimando, Jr, MA; Linda R. Bressler, PharmD, BCOP; Polly E. Kintzel, PharmD, BCPS, BCOP; and Mark C. Geraci, PharmD, BCOP

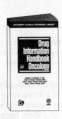

Presented in a concise and uniform format, this book contains the most comprehensive collection of oncology-related drug information available. Organized like a dictionary for ease of use, drugs can be found by looking up the *brand or generic name*!

This book contains individual monographs for both Antineoplastic Agents and Ancillary Medications.

The fields of information per monograph include: Use, U.S. Investigational, Bone Marrow/Blood Cell Transplantation, Vesicant, Emetic Potential. A Special Topics Section, Appendix, and Therapeutic Category & Key Word Index are valuable features to this book, as well.

ANESTHESIOLOGY & CRITICAL CARE DRUG HANDBOOK

by Andrew J. Donnelly, PharmD; Francesca E. Cunningham, PharmD; and Verna L. Baughman, MD

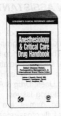

Contains the most commonly used drugs in the perioperative and critical care setting. This handbook also contains the following Special Issues and Topics: Allergic Reaction, Anesthesia for Cardiac Patients in Noncardiac Surgery, Anesthesia for Obstetric Patients in Nonobstetric Surgery, Anesthesia for Patients With Liver Disease, Chronic Pain Management, Chronic Renal Failure, Conscious Sedation, Perioperative Management of Patients on Antiseizure Medication, and Substance Abuse and Anesthesia.

The Appendix includes Abbreviations & Measurements, Anesthesiology Information, Assessment of Liver & Renal Function, Comparative Drug Charts, Infectious Disease-Prophylaxis & Treatment, Laboratory Values, Therapy Recommendations, Toxicology information, *and much more.*

International Brand Name Index with names from over 22 different countries is also included.

To order call toll free anywhere in the U.S.: 1-800-837-LEXI (5394)

Outside of the U.S. call: 330-650-6506 or online at www.lexi.com

Other titles offered by Lexi-Comp, Inc.

DRUG INFORMATION FOR MENTAL HEALTH
by Matthew A. Fuller, PharmD and Martha Sajatovic, MD

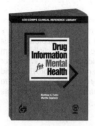

Formerly titled Drug Information Handbook for Psychiatry, this desk reference is a complete guide to psychotropic and nonpsychotropic drugs. The new 8 ½ x 11 size, presents information on all medications in a double column format. It is specifically designed as a tool for mental health professionals when assessing a client's medication profile with emphasis on a drug's Effect on Mental Status, as well as considerations for psychotropic medications. A special topics/issues section includes psychiatric assessment, major psychiatric disorders, major classes of psychotropic medications, psychiatric emergencies, special populations, patient education information, and DSM-IV classification. Also contains a valuable appendix section, Pharmacologic Index, Alphabetical Index, and International Brand Name Index.

RATING SCALES IN MENTAL HEALTH
by Martha Sajatovic, MD and Luis F. Ramirez, MD

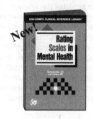

A basic guide to the rating scales in mental health, this is an ideal reference for psychiatrists, nurses, residents, psychologists, social workers, healthcare administrators, behavioral healthcare organizations, and outcome committees. It is designed to assist clinicians in determining the appropriate rating scale when assessing their client. A general concepts section provides text discussion on the use and history of rating scales, statistical evaluation, rating scale domains, and two clinical vignettes. Information on over 80 rating scales used in mental health organized in 6 categories. Appendix contains tables and charts in a quick reference format allowing clinicians to rapidly identify categories and characteristics of rating scales.

Coming Soon! **RATING SCALES TRAINING VIDEOS**
by Martha Sajatovic, MD and Luis F. Ramirez, MD

DRUG INFORMATION HANDBOOK FOR THE CRIMINAL
JUSTICE PROFESSIONAL by Marcelline Burns, PhD; Thomas E. Page, MA; and Jerrold B. Leikin, MD

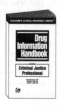

Compiled and designed for police officers, law enforcement officials, and legal professionals who are in need of a reference which relates to information on drugs, chemical substances, and other agents that have abuse and/or impairment potential. Contains over 450 medications, agents, and substances. Contains up to 33 fields of information including Scientific Name, Commonly Found In, Abuse Potential, Impairment Potential, Use, When to Admit to Hospital, Mechanism of Toxic Action, Signs & Symptoms of Acute Overdose, Drug Interactions, Reference Range, and Warnings/Precautions, *and much more.*

To order call toll free anywhere in the U.S.: 1-800-837-LEXI (5394)
Outside of the U.S. call: 330-650-6506 or online at www.lexi.com

Other titles offered by Lexi-Comp, Inc.

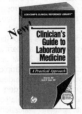
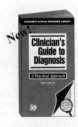
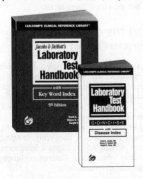

Other titles offered by Lexi-Comp, Inc.

DIAGNOSTIC PROCEDURE HANDBOOK by Frank Michota, MD

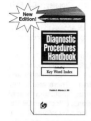

A comprehensive, yet concise, quick reference source for physicians, nurses, students, medical records personnel, or anyone needing quick access to diagnostic procedure information. This handbook is an excellent source of information in the following areas: allergy, rheumatology, and infectious disease; cardiology; computed tomography; diagnostic radiology; gastroenterology; invasive radiology; magnetic resonance imaging; nephrology, urology, and hematology; neurology; nuclear medicine; pulmonary function; pulmonary medicine and critical care; ultrasound; and women's health.

INFECTIOUS DISEASES HANDBOOK

by Carlos M. Isada, MD; Bernard L. Kasten Jr., MD; Morton P. Goldman, PharmD; Larry D. Gray, PhD; and Judith A. Aberg, MD

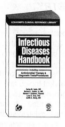

A four-in-one quick reference concerned with the identification and treatment of infectious diseases. Each of the four sections of the book contain related information and cross-referencing to one or more of the other three sections. The Disease Syndrome section provides the clinical presentation, differential diagnosis, diagnostic tests, and drug therapy recommended for treatment of more common infectious diseases. The Organism section presents the microbiology, epidemiology, diagnosis, and treatment of each organism. The Laboratory Diagnosis section describes performance of specific tests and procedures. The Antimicrobial Therapy section presents important facts and considerations regarding each drug recommended for specific diseases of organisms.

POISONING & TOXICOLOGY HANDBOOK

by Jerrold B. Leikin, MD and Frank P. Paloucek, PharmD

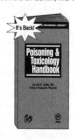

It's back by popular demand! The small size of our Poisoning & Toxicology Handbook is once again available. Better than ever, this comprehensive, portable reference contains 80 antidotes and drugs used in toxicology with 694 medicinal agents, 287 nonmedicinal agents, 291 biological agents, 57 herbal agents, and more than 200 laboratory tests. Monographs are extensively referenced and contain valuable information on overdose symptomatology and treatment considerations, as well as, admission criteria and impairment potential of select agents. Designed for quick reference with monographs arranged alphabetically, plus a cross-referencing index. The authors have expanded current information on drugs of abuse and use of antidotes, while providing concise tables, graphics, and other pertinent toxicology text.

To order call toll free anywhere in the U.S.: 1-800-837-LEXI (5394)
Outside of the U.S. call: 330-650-6506 or online at www.lexi.com

Other titles offered by Lexi-Comp, Inc.

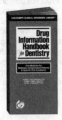
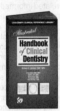
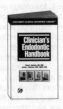

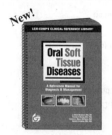
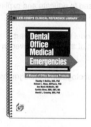
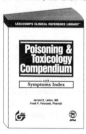

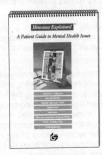
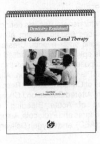
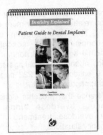

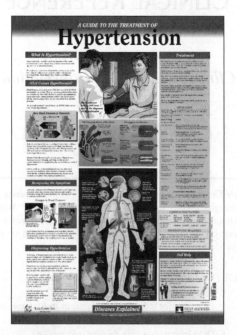